T0180396

Integrative Medicine for Breast Cancer

Mark A. Moyad, MD, MPH

Integrative Medicine for Breast Cancer

An Evidence-Based Assessment

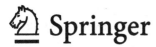 Springer

Mark A. Moyad, MD, MPH
Department of Urology
University of Michigan Medical Center
Ann Arbor, Michigan, USA

Jenkins/Pokempner Director of Complementary
& Alternative Medicine
University of Michigan Medical Center (Dept of Urology)
Ann Arbor, MI USA

ISBN 978-3-319-36389-9   ISBN 978-3-319-23422-9 (eBook)
DOI 10.1007/978-3-319-23422-9

Springer Cham Heidelberg New York Dordrecht London
© Springer International Publishing Switzerland 2016
Softcover re-print of the Hardcover 1st edition 2016

Printed on acid-free paper

Springer International Publishing AG Switzerland is part of Springer Science+Business Media (www.springer.com)

This book is dedicated to my cousin and one of my best friends that died of breast cancer at the age of 38. I miss you!

Acknowledgements

I want to thank Richard Hruska, Susan Westendorf, and Springer publishing for their guidance, assistance, and patience in helping to produce this unique first book on integrative medicine, breast cancer, and oncology. It is simply a book I wish I had when I was starting my career in integrative medicine almost 30 years ago, but at least now health care professionals and patients can utilize it as a regular reference guide to hopefully provide them with an objective and beneficial path for success in this often confusing and controversial area of medicine.

Contents

Chapter 1
Introduction

I lost my closest cousin to breast cancer. She was diagnosed in August of 1996 with metastatic breast cancer after feeling a lump a short time earlier and died 9 months later at the age of 38. I was so upset that I took a leave of absence from work and my medical education for several months to travel to all 50 states in an attempt to raise breast and overall cancer awareness and to try and increase government funding for cancer. I collected countless letters and took them with me to the Capitol and US Congress women and men and sent some of them to the White House including my letter (some excerpts from this letter are found at the end of this introduction).

A most unusual thing happened on my 50-state awareness, catharsis or self-medication tour (whatever you call it looking back over time). I would give a lecture and then I would receive countless questions on diet and lifestyle and alternative medicine and especially dietary supplements. I was constantly in awe and overwhelmed at the number and diversity of questions and there were many days I stayed after my lecture for 3, 4, and even more hours to answer them. I completely realized during this time there were few if any sources of objective (emphasis on objective) information on this topic especially in cancer. When I arrived home after all that time traveling I immediately dedicated myself to more than full-time to the field of complementary, alternative, holistic or the new and improved politically correct term "integrative medicine." Still, isn't evidence-based medicine just medicine, regardless if discussing a supplement or drug or acupuncture or dietary change or exercise? Sorry, I digressed-back to the story and this book.

I was going to be a full-time surgeon like my father and brother but quickly realized I had about as much talent for surgery as our family dog Chauncey. I also realized (as I should have at the age of 22 when I published my first medical journal article on cottonseed oil medicinal benefits and limitations) that my real passion and "calling" was for this field of integrative medicine that was then, and continues to be in dire need of full-time objective researchers, teachers, and clinicians. Not part-time but full time because this has become an overwhelming topic today with thousands of

© Springer International Publishing Switzerland 2016
M.A. Moyad, *Integrative Medicine for Breast Cancer*,
DOI 10.1007/978-3-319-23422-9_1

publications every year and countless new supplements. Yet it is tough to dedicate your life to this area because of the lack of even minimal financial resources or compensation especially for someone that does not proffer a serious or invasive procedure or even a royalty or sale of a dietary supplement out of their office. I recognized this very early in my career, which is why I am so grateful to the patients/friends (Epstein, Jenkins, Pokempner, Thompson, …) over the past 25 years that funded the dream so that we could help one starfish at a time (so to speak if you remember that story and its overall spiritual meaning). And the past and ongoing leadership of the surgical department I am a part of as a non-surgeon that took a chance on doing something different (from Dr. Montie and Dr. Pienta in the early days, to the "words cannot express my gratefulness now" to the current leadership of Dr. David Alan Bloom—mentor–friend–guidance counselor–voice-in-head—to always do the right thing). They taught me honor (along with my mom, Eva Moyad, and dad, Dr. Robert Moyad, best physician I have ever known), objectivity and most of all that to even slightly change the overall positive "system" you have to be a part of it, looking at it and dealing with its trials and tribulations/peaks and valleys from the inside and not from the outside looking in as many a Monday morning quarterback in integrative medicine have done almost as a profitable career unto itself.

Integrative medicine has arguably reached the point of being a specialty in its own right now because of the sheer amount of knowledge and information needed to fully evaluate a supplement or another intervention. Thus, this first of a kind book (I published one with Springer a few years ago in Prostate Cancer and Urology and I am so grateful to them and Richard A. Hruska, the indefatigable Senior Editor at Springer for again taking that massive leap of faith) is intended to be quick but pithy and cover enough items to establish a basic foundation of what I hear and observe in breast cancer and cancer overall. Breast and prostate cancer share a plethora of similarities for example (not just because they are both treated in many cases with some form of hormone manipulation or suppression) and research in one discipline has provided a mirror into the other, which is why you will notice some key references from both these fields throughout the book.

The first chapter covers my over 25+ years of experience in this field and what can be gleaned from all of the positive and negative issues I have observed in integrative medicine. Chapter 2 covers some of those positive and negatives of important lifestyle changes and supplements. Chapters 3–5 cover three naturally derived medications, which are arguably one of the most fascinating right now because of the heart and breast health nexus. These "naturally derived" pills (S.A.M.) have such a profound history in breast cancer (good and bad) and medicine that it was imperative to review them objectively despite being "drugs" (a good drug and supplement is virtually identical and interchangeable in the real world as you will notice multiple times in this book). Still, S.A.M. and the supplements that try to mimic them in Chaps. 3–5 are an excellent paradigm of how to approach and really learn from integrative medicine in breast cancer. Chapter 6 is a quick review of some lifestyle changes and supplements for breast cancer side effects and Chap. 7 is a free-for-all with many of the questions I receive on integrative therapies.

It must also be reiterated that this book is not about tinctures or homeopathy or exotic herbs and concoctions that are tough to find, or even when to meditate or do yoga or Pilates or …. Although my wonderful wife Mia and my fabulous kids (Nicholas and Holly) perform enough of these exercises regularly to satiate the entire family requirement—I am addicted to running. Rather, this book primarily covers the area that many oncologists and those working in or dealing with oncology (aka "patients"/ friends/family) do not feel comfortable discussing because of an ongoing lack of objective education especially in the field of dietary supplements [1]. Still, I would argue that wherever I traveled in the world over my career (virtually everywhere) patients want this information from you and if you cannot provide it then the risk of a patient going to a less credible source right down the street and succumbing to a misguided sales pitch increases exponentially.

Clinicians are an easy target for the "they are not educated on diet and supplements in medical school" almost cliché or jaded argument. However, good clinicians have so much positive intent and diverse knowledge about their patients that few harbors, so just because they do not hold one important piece of the health puzzle does not disqualify them, but rather should fully still qualify them, especially today when most are able and willing to access integrative medical information from some credible sources. This book should facilitate a better objective discussion with your patients because it is not "pro- or anti-supplements" and there is no "us versus them" agenda to stir up the masses, but rather real-world experience of someone that has worked a lifetime in this specialty mixed with best objective evidence to assist you in knowing what works and what is worthless.

Finally, I want to end this introduction with some of the final words I wrote to the President of the USA on August 15, 1997:

> My cousin was a beautiful woman with an equally beautiful personality. She was always like the sister I never had (I have 2 brothers in my family). Best of all she had this ability to make everyone laugh at any moment. I use to fly to Washington DC a few times a year just to be with her (and my older brother). I will never forget the time we walked together by the reflecting pool near the Vietnam Memorial and had a picnic and just appreciated the day for what it was, incredible. It was a great day to be alive and we laughed so much that we had tears streaming down our faces. I try to make that day part of my constant memories I have of her but unfortunately it is never that easy. Anyhow, the biggest tragedy was that of my cousin who never had the opportunity to live a full life. I hope that in some strange way her death will prevent many others from having to go through what she had to endure.

Sincerely yours,
Mark A. Moyad

Reference

1. Lee RT, Barbo A, Lopez G, Melhem-Bertrandt A, Lin H, Ol O, Curlin FA. National survey of US oncologists' knowledge, attitudes, and practice patterns regarding herb and supplement us by patients with cancer. J Clin Oncol. 2014;32:4095–101.

Chapter 2
25+ Observations Over 25+ Years for Surviving and Thriving in the Dietary Supplement Quality Control and/or Perception Versus Reality World

Introduction

"Vitamin E is dangerous!" "Herbal products have no evidence!" _____ does not treat or cure advanced cancer"? "Supplements don't do anything, so don't waste your money!" For almost 30 years I have watched not just patients, but especially some influential clinicians generalize, embellish, and misconstrue data on dietary supplements. This type of commentary just mirrors the lack of objective education in this area, does nothing to improve the clinician and patient relationship, and arguably sends countless individuals to less credible sources for information and misguided sales pitches (as it did through the years for many of my own family members). At the same time, I have watched many in the supplement industry embellish data and supplement efficacy and promote a "we vs. them" contentious milieu that only continues to confuse the public. Again, this acrimonious dichotomy or profound polarization does nothing for overall patient care [1].

A good example of the ongoing dual cacophony was a New York (NY) Times front-page article on quality control testing of dietary supplements. The New York State attorney general (NYAG) accused four national retailers (GNC, Target, Walgreens, and Walmart) of selling dietary supplements that were fraudulent and, in numerous cases, "contaminated with unlisted ingredients" [2]. A total of four out of every five products tested contained none of the herbs advertised on the label! And it seemed for critics of the supplement industry this added fuel to the ongoing fire while advocates for the industry fought back and stated that the NY state attorney general's office commissioned an independent testing group that actually performed the wrong test. And they have proof that exactly what is advertised in their products is what is in the products [3]. The NY investigation and accusation was based on testing of herbal products using "DNA barcoding." It is a very reliable method, but here is the key—it needs to be performed on the appropriate material. In other words, herbal extracts found in many supplements contain DNA but it is often of a low quality and broken down or degraded to a level that could make it

© Springer International Publishing Switzerland 2016
M.A. Moyad, *Integrative Medicine for Breast Cancer*,
DOI 10.1007/978-3-319-23422-9_2

really difficult to prove what is in the bottle based on this specific testing method. There is a chance that the supplement companies were primarily in compliance and the NY office was too quick in reaching a verdict. The problem at the time of this writing is that there has been no communication or release of the testing commissioned by the NYAG. In fact, NYAG has now shifted some of the focus on health claims made by these supplement companies and also quality control. This has all the makings of a reality TV show. Recently, research out of Canada showed similar findings of quality control issues but they also utilized DNA barcoding [4]. Regardless of who is right or who is wrong or semi-wrong there is little doubt that many supplements still have issues so perhaps the end will justify the mean with the NYAG situation. Even if the NYAG investigation was botched there appeared to be gluten for example found in "gluten free" advertised supplements.

Thus, I wanted to provide multiple rules or steps, questions I am asked, or really observations that have helped me when making a recommendation or finding the right product for patients that are as true today as they were almost 25+ years ago. This is critical because timeless advice is needed in this field rather than the need or desire to be attracted to the latest and greatest option only to be disappointed or taken to the cleaners so to speak. These will help you (health care professional, patient, …) in getting something desperately needed when reviewing the latest "groundbreaking" (how cliché are those words) supplement or dietary or lifestyle changes, and that is something called "objectivity." This what is desperately needed in the teaching of integrative medicine and especially dietary supplements, which is a business today, and I am glad it is a business because it initiating more and more research and interest, but the down side of that business is the nebulousness or demarcation of objectivity and subjectivity (of course conventional medicine is also as guilty at times of this problem). More and more health care professionals then ever before are selling or recommending supplements and get paid for doing so, and more and more consumers are selling them. This does not disqualify their expertise but makes it more difficult than ever before for a non-polarizing, non-royalty, or non-endorsing objective and experienced current up-to-date source of information, although I had my brief moments over my long career of having been often tempted or even succumbing temporarily to a disease called "JD" or "judgmental dysfunction," but at least I (or others) quickly reminded me of how to find the cure, which is actually appreciating the honor or privilege and trust you hold and earned over time with the public, patients, and health care professionals. Here in this chapter at least you will find that source of current information that I wish I had when I was starting my career as a complete greenhorn.

• **The difference between a clinically effective drug and supplement is perception and not reality. So, what are the rules or even politics of what becomes a supplement or a drug? What about FDA current Good Manufacturing Practices (cGMP) now required by supplement companies in the USA? Does that help to give a supplement drug like quality?**

In the words of the FDA: "A dietary supplement is a product intended for ingestion that contains a dietary ingredient intended to add further nutritional value to (supplement) the diet. A dietary ingredient may be one, or any combination, of the following substances: a vitamin, a mineral, an herb or other botanical, an amino acid, a dietary substance for use by people to supplement the diet by increasing the total dietary intake, a concentrate, metabolite, constituent, or extract ..." [5]. What?! And keep in mind that dietary supplements are not intended to diagnose, treat, cure or prevent and disease, but the FDA states that some supplements can be used to "help you reduce your risk of disease" [5]. What?!

Okay, now from those definitions above try and tell me the difference of what can become a supplement or a drug? It is pretty nebulous, which is why for example you can sell fish oil or omega-3 in the USA or you can also get it as a prescription drug (Epanova®, Lovaza®, Vascepa® ...) [1]. Thus, in my opinion the difference is usually researched based or the requirements of strict clinical trials for FDA approval (a drug) or no trials needed at all (a supplement) and political with an "us" versus "them" mentality which is why it is tough to regulate. In other words, in Congress you have staunch past and current advocates of legislation to maintain supplements as a standalone category (Senator Hatch from Utah, Senator Harkin from Iowa ... Republican and a Democrats joined together). And then you have others politically that are on the other side that are more quiet in general but try and monitor public concern, and since most Americans take supplements of some kind and most politicians I have met (hundreds over the years) consume supplements, then I think it is an unpopular position politically to suggest supplements should be tested or regulated like drugs.

The idea that there is no enforced safety net for pills that you consume is a little concerning. So, with some public pressure mounting on quality control the FDA came up with current good manufacturing practices (cGMP or GMP) rule many years ago, in 2007, that supplement companies are supposed to follow. However, if I told you the speed limit was 55 MPH but you knew there were few cops on the highways to enforce this law, then what speed would you drive? In other words, FDA does not have the person power to enforce cGMP so some companies say they are cGMP, but the public has no idea until they are actually inspected by the FDA or an outside third party (for example like NSF or USP). So, there are still a small number of companies operating with an "innocent until they catch me doing something wrong" mentality.

Still, I do not believe supplements should become prescriptions but at the same time anyone that wants to start a supplement company should have to abide by some credible third party independent quality control group like NSF. It makes no sense that tomorrow I could simply set up the "Dr Moyad supplement company" and there would be no one that could stop me or require me in some credible manner to prove that what I was proffering was at least safe (and do not get me started on the scientific part that also requires zero proof for some companies to start selling pills).

On the other side of the debate, you have the anti-drug movement folks and this is a reality. Some drugs today are so ridiculously and embarrassingly expense that this is why the name "big pharma" has become part of the US vernacular or lexicon and that term is obviously not complimentary. I had a colleague of mine at Harvard (notice how I threw in the word Harvard to impress the reader on my personal regular range of peers or colleagues) lean over to me at a lecture and tell me that sildenafil

(Viagra) was 40 dollars a single pill (at the time) for some men suffering from a medical condition (erectile dysfunction) after prostate surgery for example [1]. And by the way there is no justification for some of these prices such as Viagra's cost because research and development (R&D) was not that expensive for this once shelved drug to justify this ongoing cost. So, thanks to higher drug prices and I am sure numerous other reasons like shifting the profit to another source, there is also a strong movement that is anti-big pharma, which helps keep strong political advocacy in favor of NOT changing the supplement rules because what is the perceived antithesis of big pharma? In my opinion, the mom and pop supplement company or holistic practitioner just trying to sell their natural products to help people, and look at big pharma deliberately or personally getting in the way like some vendetta, or try to minimize the little alternative guy or gal (of course sarcasm because some of the biggest supplement companies are now pharmaceutical brands from Bayer to Pfizer and some of the biggest out of pocket profiting is from selling your own line of supplements/recommending them).

Supplements are a many billion-dollar industry (arguably 35–40 billion/year) [6, 7], and in some ways (ironically) it has taken on its own big pharma feel, and money doesn't talk but shouts! So, in reality there are massive money and political movements behind keeping things status quo. When I started 30 years ago in supplements and even in medical school, doctors would tell me all the time that a supplement might not help but "can't hurt" but we know that is not true anymore. *They can help, hurt or do nothing* (just like any other pill). The sheer amount of profit in the industry combined with the lack of good objective education to health care professionals and the public, and throw in the political forces, and you have somewhat of a blurred line between what can become or mimic a supplement and/or a drug. The bottom line again, is that the real difference to me is perception and reality, and also one is required to pass some threshold of evidence and the other does not have to pass a threshold of evidence (it is up to the individual company in the case of a supplement if they even want to risk their business model with something as silly as research—again sarcasm).

So, remember, there is no difference between an effective supplement and a drug. Some of the most widely used supplements in the USA are treated like regulated drugs in other countries. Ever heard of melatonin [1]? Alpha-Lipoic Acid [1]? S-adenosyl-methionine (SAM-e) or Zinc gluconate [1]?!

• **"This product is not intended to diagnose, treat, cure, or prevent any disease" is what most dietary supplements or commercials on supplements have to claim, because only a drug can make this claim. Excuse me? What? Yet this is precisely why physicians recommend them or not, and why many patients use them (or not)! The ongoing bane of the "structure/function" FDA allowed claims ("maintains," "promotes," or "supports" _____ Note: just fill in the organ system of interest and add the word "health" to it like breast, colon, immune, prostate health ...).**

Under the FDA Code of Federal Regulations, title 21, volume 2, the rules for dietary supplements are quite clear despite voluminous language. Under part 101, subpart F and section 101.93 (I am not kidding here) and stated under number 2 part C

"Text for disclaimer." It states that the rules are "This statement has not been evaluated by the Food and Drug Administration. This product is not intended to diagnose, treat, cure, or prevent any disease." The problem with this language is it also serves to provide a confusing chasm between reality and perception for families or individuals dealing with minor to devastating diseases. I often tell audiences that most of the effective supplements in the USA are actually prescription drugs or regulated like drugs in other countries such as S-adenosyl-methionine (SAM-e) for depression or osteoarthritis [8–10]. Thus, the line between an effective drug and supplement is only perception and not reality. Instead, what is permitted by the FDA for dietary supplements are what is known as "structure/function claims" (as long as some level of anemic general evidence is provided), which are non-disease claims and companies are allowed to suggest that something contributes or benefits "general well-being" or reduces "nutrient deficiency" or how a nutrient acts to "maintain such structure or function" [11].

In my experience, many companies have tried to follow structure/function claims by mentioning one of three words in advertising, so for example the suggestion that a supplement product may "maintain" or "promote" or "support" prostate health. For example, saw palmetto can advertise that it "supports prostate health," which is not only confusing vernacular to the consumer, but it is arguably now completely inaccurate (see below) [1, 12]. Thus, again these rules do not serve to provide clarity for clinicians and patients but rather perplexity. The current rules or system are scientifically confusing and health care professionals in everyday practice need to better educate the public and patients. Therefore, it is imperative to review a series of situations where supplements are utilized like a drug or not (clear demarcation), and why not allow over-the-counter exceptions or situation where some companies could advertise the benefits (especially when a part of clinical guidelines for a specialty) especially if they were part of the objective phase-3-like trial, while not allowing any suggestion of benefit for other products that have clearly failed phase-3-like trials. The solution does not have to be that difficult and it does not imply that supplements have to be strictly regulated by the government. *I am talking about rewarding the research (more on this later)!*

• **Please provide a review of some of the dietary supplements that are utilized as drugs (or not) by health care professionals and patients in the USA for specific diseases/medical conditions.**

Alzheimer Disease (AD) or completely different medical conditions known as "NAFLD" (non-alcoholic fatty liver disease) and "NASH" (non-alcoholic steatohepatitis) have somE-thing in common—vitamin E

Individuals with mild to moderate Alzheimer disease taking 2000 IU of vitamin E (DL-alpha-tocopheryl acetate or "synthetic" vitamin E from DSM Nutritional Products, Heerlen, Netherlands) per day in addition to standard medications—the acetylcholinesterase inhibitors (AChEI) drugs, experienced an over 6 month reduction in functional decline and reduced caregiver time by 2 h a day in one of the longest and best clinical trials conducted in the USA (known as the "TEAM-AD VA cooperative randomized trial" and published January 1, 2014 in the Journal of the American Medical Association) [13]. It is noteworthy that this is the second such phase-3-like trial to demonstrate this clinical benefit in Alzheimer patients with 2000 IU of vitamin E (again DL-alpha-tocopherol from Hoffman-LaRoche, Nutley, NJ) daily and the first trial was published on April 24, 1997 in the New England Journal of Medicine [14]!

AD patients need more options as exemplified by the recent Cleveland Clinic report that 99.6 % (244 out 245) of the Alzheimer's clinical trials have failed over the past decade [15], so why not? It is remarkable that no vitamin E supplement company is able to advertise these results (not even the company that provided the product for the clinical trial) so the only individuals that potentially suffer from this lack of objective information are the patients afflicted by Alzheimer disease and the other individuals that care about or for them.

It is also disconcerting that some practitioners have not been recommending vitamin E to Alzheimer patients because these supplements have been suggested to have shown some toxicity in other areas of medicine [16], so why utilize them in Alzheimer disease? This myopic thinking again somehow places an effective supplement for a devastating disease in a different category than how things would be treated for an effective drug with some standard limitations. If acetylcholinesterase inhibitors showed some toxicity in other disease scenarios, which they have significantly done already in mild cognitive impairment or Alzheimer patients (nausea, vomiting and diarrhea) [17, 18], then would practitioners quit using all these medications? This appears doubtful because the benefit exceeds the risk for many patients, which is similar to the situation with vitamin E. Additionally, in the TEAM-AD VA Cooperative Trial and in the first phase 3 trial published in 1997, the adverse effects of vitamin E were similar overall to placebo [13, 14]. Interestingly, vitamin E supplements have not shown an ability to prevent Alzheimer's or help those with mild cognitive impairment (MCI) at a dosage of 2000 IU per day (from DSM Nutritional Products, Heerlen, Netherlands) [19], but for those with mild to moderate or moderately severe impairment from Alzheimer's it should be discussed with a physician.

Interestingly, this situation and benefit is arguably similar to a different disease scenario occurring with NAFLD (non-alcoholic fatty liver disease) or NASH (non-alcoholic steatohepatitis) where 800 IU daily (400 IU twice a day) of vitamin E appears to have benefited children/young adults (age 8–17 years) and more clearly benefited adult patients from two major clinical trials (PIVENS trial used "natural" form vitamin E or D-alpha-tocopherol from Nature Made®, Pharmavite, LLC, Mission Hills or Northridge, CA and TONIC children/young adult trial also used Nature Made® vitamin E at the same dosage and form used in the PIVENS trial) [1].

Age-Related Macular Degeneration (AMD)

Individuals with intermediate to advanced stages of age-related macular degeneration (AMD) are now recommended to use a dietary supplement as one of the primary treatments for this disease, which can also prevent vision loss. The exact formulation recommended by the National Eye Institute (NEI) was derived from two phase-3 government funded trials known as AREDS1 (supplements provided by Bausch & Lomb, Bridgewater, NJ) conducted at 11 medical centers and AREDS2 [supplements from DSM Nutritional Products, Inc., Sisseln, Switzerland manufactured the constituents of the AREDS2 formulations and raw materials for active ingredients and placebos were produced into tablets (lutein + zeaxanthin) and gelatin capsules (EPA + DHA ethyl esters) by Tishcon Corp, Westbury, NY and Alcon Research Ltd, Fort Worth, TX provided raw materials for the four AREDS-type supplements and added into gelatin capsules Banner Pharmacaps Europe BV (Tilburg, the Netherlands)] conducted at 82 medical centers [20–22]. The following dosage is now a standard clinical recommendation for ophthalmologists dealing with AMD:

- 500 mg of vitamin C (ascorbic acid)
- 400 IU of vitamin E (DL-alpha-tocopheryl acetate)
- 25 or 80 mg of zinc (zinc oxide)
- 2 mg (cupric oxide—to prevent potential anemia with high-dose zinc)
- 10 mg Lutein
- 2 mg zeaxanthin

(Note: The lutein source was *Tagetes erecta*/Aztec marigold and zeaxanthin was synthesized at DSM via a patented process and omega-3's EPA + DHA failed to show a benefit in the AREDS2 clinical trail and all participants taking a multivitamin were required to switch to Centrum Silver®, now Pfizer, New York, NY, which was also provided to them, and in the AREDS1 trial the multivitamin allowed was Centrum®, Whitehall-Robins Healthcare, Madison, NJ and now Pfizer.)

Interestingly, this and a similar formula have not shown an ability to prevent this disease but appear to help those with the intermediate to advanced stages. Thus, it is critical that I reiterate the fact that this has become one of the primary or standard treatments for AMD (dry and wet form) along with conventional medicine to help preserve vision. Again, no direct advertisements or benefits are allowed by the companies that provided these products for the clinical trial despite the fact that they are a standard part of medical treatment. I am often frustrated by the fact that I am educating some patients with macular degeneration about these results and the specific formulation that they require, and immediately with the approval of their ophthalmologist they are utilizing these pills. There must be a better method of general education, right?

Antiaging?

Aging is not a medical condition per se, but some in the antiaging movement appear to be advertising that they are combating the aging process. High on this list is a dietary supplement known as "resveratrol." Resveratrol is a supplement that can cost 50–100 dollars a month and it is touted to have dramatic antiaging effects like increasing telomere length and other impressive vernacular, but the reality outside of the laboratory, is that many of the recent human studies have been a large disappointment. And even when preliminary clinical trials on the supplement were published [23], or a large pharmaceutical company (GlaxoSmithKline) invested heavily (arguably up to 750 million dollars for a resveratrol-like compound) it also turned out to be a preliminary disappointment [24]. I often tell patients to save their money until someone can actually prove it does something besides shrink your wallet, which ultimately can increase your stress and can accelerate the aging process [1, 25]. Why some practitioners are allowed to sell these expensive supplements and others out of their office, and profit from an overall lack of consistent beneficial evidence is concerning, especially based on the ongoing recent evidence [26]. Thus, when a supplement has drug-like efficacy it should be allowed to advertise to patients but at the same time if it fails to show overall efficacy then not even structure–function claims should be permitted.

BPH (Benign Prostatic Hyperplasia or non-cancerous prostate enlargement)— the story of saw palmetto and two phase-3-like and very well-done trials, or the story of chronic non-bacterial prostatitis: a tale of two urologic cities

One of the largest past reviews of clinical studies of saw palmetto for benign prostatic hyperplasia (BPH) found some interesting results in 1998 [27]. This analysis reviewed a total of 18 randomized trials ($n = 2939$ men) and found that most of the studies were limited by their short duration and study design. However, the existing evidence suggested that this herbal product improves urologic symptoms and flow measures. Compared with the FDA approved drug finasteride for this condition, saw palmetto produced similar improvement in urinary tract symptoms and urinary flow, with less side effects. However, saw palmetto had only been compared to current drug therapies for a maximum of approximately 12 months (still not a bad endorsement). More data was needed on this herbal product. Interestingly, the dosage of saw palmetto used in most randomized trials at this point in time was 320 mg/day and this dosage had no effect on PSA levels.

Four years after this notable 1998 review was published another one by similar authors added three new trials with 230 added male participants that translated into a meta-analysis of 21 randomized trials and the conclusions were similar stating that "The results of this update are in agreement with our initial review" [28]. In other words that saw palmetto could be an option that works as well as some pharmacologic agents but with less side effects.

The authors then updated their original meta-analysis again in 2009 and came to this conclusion "Serenoa repens was not more effective than placebo for treatment of urinary symptoms consistent with BPH" [29]. Next, in 2012 another follow-up review by similar authors concluded with the following comment on subjective and objective benefits of saw palmetto by noting: "Serenoa repens therapy does not improve LUTS or Q(max) compared with placebo in men with BPH, even at double and triple the usual dose" [30].

What happened that caused such a reversal in a long-standing recommendation or endorsement for saw palmetto? In the more recent meta-analysis for example there were nine new trials added to the analysis that included 2053 more men (about 65 % increase), and overall there were 5222 subjects from 30 randomized trials of a 4–60 week duration utilized for example [29, 30].

However, the answer to the question of what caused such a reversal in the saw palmetto enthusiasm lies in what is known as well-done non-biased or objective phase-3-like research. The first trial was a US government funded trial called "STEP" (The Saw palmetto for Treatment of Enlarged Prostates) [31], followed by the results of a more recent trial called "CAMUS" (Complementary and Alternative Medicine for Urological Symptoms) [32]—two outstanding phase-3 like trials that arguably should have settled the majority of the debate on saw palmetto itself.

The STEP trial was simply a very well done clinical trial [31], and the researchers and participants in this study should be commended for being a part of one of one the better herbal studies ever completed in medicine. Saw palmetto enjoys a tremendous amount of sales around the world. Some areas of Europe have made this herbal product a prescription, but in the USA there are literally hundreds of over-the-counter (OTC) brands. Florida and several coastal states are some of the largest exporters of this herbal product. This herbal product is so well known that it continues to be one of the more popular supplements taken by men to prevent prostate cancer despite having no relevant evidence that it prevents prostate cancer [33, 34]. Okay, another reason why a structure and function claim such as "supports prostate health" can confuse the public even more than it can clarify, and this is very concerning, because saw palmetto again never had any credible data that it reduces the risk of prostate cancer. So, then why are all these men taking it? Is it because they do not get enough saw palmetto in their diet, or could it be that when something supports prostate health it is very logical to assume that it may have some research against prostate disease prevention, including cancer? Regardless, all of the preliminary data was for the improvement of BPH symptoms. Some researchers suggest it has a finasteride (a drug approved for BPH) type effect, but unlike finasteride (also known as Proscar®) it has not been shown to have any impact on PSA levels. Regardless, there was an ample need to conduct a non-industry or non-biased supported clinical trial to determine if saw palmetto really does have some efficacy. And of course I was pulling for saw palmetto to work and work well given the lack of low cost options with reduced side effects at the time.

The STEP trial was funded by the National Institute of Diabetes and Digestive and Kidney Diseases (NIDDK) and by the National Center for Complementary and Alternative Medicine (NCCAM) [31]. In the STEP trial a total of 225 men with moderate-to-severe BPH symptoms were randomized to saw palmetto extract at a dosage of 160 mg twice a day (320 mg a day total) or placebo [31]. The primary outcomes were the change in score on the American Urological Association Symptom Index (AUASI, a subjective measurement completed by patients) and the maximal flow rate (an objective measure completed by the physician). There were also a number of secondary outcomes including: change in the prostate size, urine volume left in the bladder after urinating, quality of life, laboratory values and side effects. When the trial ended after 12-months of treatment there was no difference between saw palmetto and placebo in all the major areas of study including:

- AUASI score (only 0.04 point difference)
- Maximal urinary flow rate (only 0.43 ml difference)
- Prostate size or volume (only 1.22 ml difference)
- Residual volume after urinating (only a 4.51 ml difference)
- No difference in quality of life, PSA, or side effects

Interestingly, critics abound from these trials and it appears will do anything to shred a major well-done objective phase-3-like clinical trial. For example, some of the popular alternative medicine consumer books and websites had espoused for years the use of a saw palmetto with either 80–95 % combination of fatty acids and sterols or 85–95 % fatty acids and greater than 0.2 % sterols. The herbal extract used in this trial demonstrated consistent 90–92 % fatty acids and 0.33 % sterols and this was actually verified [31], which means it was right on target or even above the standards of what has been recommended in the past for effectiveness. Even the placebo had an odor similar to saw palmetto so that the participants could not tell the difference, which is always needed in a well-done clinical trial but had not been done in several past saw palmetto trials so I believe some of the participants could tell the difference. The placebo contained polyethylene glycol-400, which is a bitter-tasting liquid with an oil makeup. It contained no free fatty acids, and a brown coloring agent was used in order to ensure no difference in appearance between saw palmetto and placebo.

Some critics then argued that the study should have tested men with mild BPH symptoms or larger prostate glands. Perhaps including men with more mild BPH symptoms and not those with moderate-to-severe BPH would have been a better study, and perhaps men with larger prostates would have also been a better group. The reason for this is due to the suggestion that saw palmetto works similar to a drug (finasteride) that shrinks larger prostate glands. However, again in defense of the researchers in this trial, studying only mild BPH would have been filled with problems such as a large placebo effect, and the encouragement of medicating a condition that for many men needs no immediate intervention (aka overtreatment). Regardless, when the researchers looked at the small number of men with more or less symptoms than the average or with small or larger prostate glands there was still no difference between saw palmetto and placebo [31].

Additionally, what also did not receive attention from this trial was the fact that all of the potential participants in this trial were first placed in a 1-month, single-blind, placebo run-in phase and were not permitted in the trial unless they took 75 % or more of the placebo capsules [31]. In other words, in order to really determine who was committed to being compliant with the pills throughout this entire trial, the participants had to take placebo pills for 1-month prior to the start of the official study. It is interesting that there was actually a significant despite small improvement (or decrease) in symptom scores (AUASI) during this 1-month period! This demonstrates the impressiveness of the placebo effect, especially with BPH and it has to be accounted for, and the researchers made a good effort accounting for it.

Critics also complained of the short length of the trial. Yet this trial was one of the longest saw palmetto versus placebo trials in the history of medicine. The majority of the past trials were about 3 months or shorter [27, 28]. BPH trials of 6 months to 1 year or more are more than adequate to determine if a medication is effective. The researchers could have done this trial over 6 months, but in my opinion 1-year was the perfect duration to determine if saw palmetto was better than placebo. In fact, participants had eight clinic visits during the trial [31], which was also more than sufficient to determine the impact of saw palmetto.

If the STEP trial results were a surprise then the CAMUS results were arguably even more surprising in my opinion because of the higher doses of saw palmetto utilized [32]. Basically, the CAMUS researchers found that low (320 mg), moderate (640 mg), and high doses (960 mg) of saw palmetto given over 72 weeks did not work better than a placebo for BPH/LUTS. Saw palmetto was again as safe as a placebo, but not more effective than a placebo in the follow-up North American study to the STEP trial. CAMUS was a double-blind, multicenter, placebo-controlled randomized trial conducted at 11 North American clinics including Ontario, Canada [32]. A total of 369 men, approximate mean age, AUASI, peak urinary flow rate, and PVR (post-void residual) of 61 years, 14.5, and 14.9 ml/s and 41 ml were given escalating doses of saw palmetto or placebo over 72 weeks. Again, the intervention consisted of 1–3 chocolate covered gelcaps (320 mg each), and the starting dosage was 320 mg/day with a dose escalation at 24 (640 mg/day) and 48 weeks (960 mg/day) with the trial ending at 18-months of intervention compared to placebo. The saw palmetto used in CAMUS consisted of 85–95 % fatty acids, and it was a lipidic ethanolic extract of ripe, dried saw palmetto berries manufactured by Rottapharm/Madaus, Cologne, Germany, and sold as PROSTA-URGENIN UNO capsules. The placebo contained 375 mg of polyethylene glycol and a matched weight (475 mg), and participants were told to take all gel caps at same time.

Again, in the CAMUS trial the baseline and 72-week results found no significant differences between saw palmetto and placebo for any parameter [32]. For example, no differences were found for all of the following (impressive list):

- AUASI (primary outcome),
- BPH impact index,
- AUA SI QOL,
- Nocturia,
- Peak flow rate,
- Postvoid residual,
- PSA,
- IIEF (International Index of Erectile Function),
- Sleep dysfunction scale,
- Incontinence scale or
- NIH CPSI (Chronic Prostatitis Symptom Index).

Many items actually favored placebo except for the difference in AUASI for non-Caucasian participants, which favored saw palmetto (non-significantly). Some critics suggested the extraction process of saw palmetto was faulty resulting in an impure product. However, the STEP trial used a carbon dioxide extraction procedure for their saw palmetto preparation [31], compared to an ethanolic extraction procedure in the CAMUS trial [32]. In other words, some internet criticisms of the extraction procedure for saw palmetto after the STEP trial was addressed in the CAMUS trial and did not produce better results. This is again a beautiful testament to the researchers for these trials (many of them I know and respect, as is the case with many of the other clinical trials in this book that I thought I would mention to mildly impress the reader).

Interestingly, the most notable saw palmetto supplement/drug in the world (Permixon®) with the most positive clinical research (popular in Europe) apparently either did not or could not participate in this trial [35–38], despite being requested to participate by the North American researchers. Thus, the researchers were left with another agent from a different manufacturer in this trial, which again arguably demonstrated that North American saw palmetto rigorous studies do not demonstrate efficacy of this herbal product compared to placebo. However, should researchers discount the more positive European studies utilizing Permixon? Not necessarily, but since the most notable product outside the USA are not for sale in the USA, then both the STEP and CAMUS trial suggests that saw palmetto should not be allowed to make any prostate health claim without some future positive research. This would seem appropriate based on the fact that two of the most rigorous trials ever done in medical history showed no benefit over placebo. Regardless of the type of supplement and whatever the medical condition, if most of the rigorous trials result in failure then why is a structure/function claim still permitted?

Still, in order to maintain objectivity in this discourse, patients are left with unmet needs when it comes to prostate enlargement prescription FDA approved medications because numerous men are not able to tolerate them or they could be dangerous for some elderly men [39]. And recent costly drug combinations approved by the FDA did not even include a placebo arm and were still given FDA approval [40]? Also, in discussions with some of the researchers from the CAMUS trial there appeared to be no volunteers (despite being requested) from the pharmaceutical world to be placed up against saw palmetto or placebo when the original trial was being designed. Again, the patients get lost in this shuffle, so BPH is an area of medicine that would benefit from some dietary supplement that works modestly or moderately better than a sugar pill. And although there are some candidates like beta-sitosterol [25], it has been difficult to initiate more recent and rigorous clinical trials to determine if these agents are truly effective. Instead, high-priced combinations of ingredients are used in prostate health supplements that include beta-sitosterol and some of these companies use the old beta-sitosterol clinical data (normally a low cost single ingredient) as evidence as to why their product is effective? However, their product contains countless compounds and beta-sitosterol is just one of them and yet they are allowed to promote their product using the publications of beta-sitosterol as a stand-alone intervention? What?! This issue is not only symptomatic of some urologic supplements but symptomatic of the larger disease found with supplements in almost every medical specialty [1]. Some are bad and should never be allowed any claim, and others do not get the credit they deserve because research does not get rewarded enough in the world of dietary supplements so let's reward some more research before finishing this section.

On the other hand, it is fascinating and perplexing that in another area of urology, chronic non-bacterial prostatitis there are some dietary supplements (Cernilton pollen extract from a variety of sources such as Graminex LLC products, Deshler, OH; and quercetin generic and quercetin complexes from Farr Labs, Beverly Hills, CA such as Prosta-Q and Q-Urol) with adequate clinical evidence and no consistently effective FDA approved drugs [1, 25, 41, 42]. And countless clinicians from the Mayo Clinic to UCLA utilize and recommend these dietary supplements and yet no one is allowed to advertise their benefits?! And chronic non-bacterial prostatitis, by the way, consists of the vast the majority of the global cases of prostatitis, not infectious prostatitis [25].

Breast and Prostate Cancer Prevention/Treatment/Side Effects

Interestingly, there is no supplement that has shown evidence to reduce the risk or recurrence of these two common cancers. And, in fact, there is now plenty of evidence to suggest that getting too many supplements when completely healthy could increase the risk of these cancers, especially prostate cancer. For example, higher-dosages of selenium supplements (200 μg or more) when already ingesting ample selenium from dietary sources could increase the risk of aggressive prostate cancer [25, 43]. Additionally, the evidence of vitamin E supplements and an increased prostate cancer risk as well as potentially high-dose folic acid cannot be ignored [25]. Currently, there is no single supplement that could be considered to have ample evidence in the area of breast cancer prevention or recurrence. And the past 30 years are replete with supplements that claimed such a potential distinction or were deemed to potentially benefit by "experts" in the field. However, the evidence for dietary supplements to reduce the risk of side effects or treat side effects from breast and prostate cancer treatment are impressive (see Chap. 7).

Dry Eye and/or High Triglycerides

Fish oil has been touted for countless conditions but overall has failed most recent clinical trials from cardiovascular disease prevention to macular degeneration [22, 44, 45]. However, it continues to garner increasing research and recommendations in the area of dry eye syndrome [46–49], which is commendable because prescription drugs for this condition can be quite expensive. In the most recent meta-analysis of seven independent studies and almost 800 participants concluded with the following: "Consequently, our findings suggest that omega-3 fatty acids is an effective therapy for dry eye" [49].

These studies have attracted enough interest to initiate a large phase-3 like trial in collaboration with the National Eye Institute (NEI) at over 20 medical centers (2000 mg EPA and 1000 mg DHA) to determine if omega-3 can improve moderate to severe dry eye disease. This trial is known as "DREAM" (Dry Eye Assessment and Management Study) [50]. It will be interesting because the placebo contains olive oil, which also has some known anti-inflammatory properties (a controversial choice). Ophthalmologists are using this option in clinical practice but again how do patients in general discover this information [1]? And what of a cancer patient that experiences this specific problem as a side effect from conventional treatment. Why not try this low-cost option?

Interestingly, the American Heart Association (AHA) guidelines suggest 2–4 g of EPA + DHA (omega-3 from marine sources) per day provided as capsules under a physician's care for hypertriglyceridemia (500 mg/dl+) or simply "patients who need to lower triglycerides" [51]. Currently, three omega-3 prescription drugs have been approved by the FDA for the reduction of triglycerides and they include: Lovaza (approved in 2004), Vascepa (2012), and Epanova (2014) [52, 53]. However, the question remains whether low-cost over-the-counter omega-3 products (fish oil) are the same, better, or worse at lowering triglycerides compared to the more expensive prescription brands. In my experience, there is no difference except in price and the perception of quality control assurance, but most of the over-the-counter fish oil products have outstanding quality control based on serendipity [25]. This is due to the finding that fish oils are usually derived from short-lived nontoxic harboring fish such as anchovies, sardines, and mackerel. Most of the krill, shrimp, salmon, and even green-lipped mussel fish oils are also well-known for their high quality control, and ease of use/utilization compared to larger fish oils pills, but also high price in some cases, and lack of an impressive number of more rigorous trials with hard clinical endpoints found with low cost (aka cheap) fish oil supplements [1]. And if there is a reason to take fish oil but one needs to avoid large pills, then a children's flavored liquid easily suffices in terms of taste, quality control, concentration, and ease of use compared to any many fish oil pills or capsules.

Erectile Dysfunction (ED)

L-citrulline (an amino acid derived from watermelon rind) is arguably the most promising supplement for ED at 1500 mg/day because it can significantly raise nitric oxide (NO) levels better than the most commonly used products for this same purpose (L-arginine) [25, 54]. And preliminary clinical research demonstrates that it (L-citrulline free form) may be an adequate option for mild or moderate ED. Many other supplements touted for ED have little to no research. And in many parts of the USA some of ED prescription drugs are approximately 10–40 dollars a single pill. This will moderately change with sildenafil becoming generic but in the meantime other viable options to be utilized with and without prescription medications are being utilized by physicians. L-citrulline malate (or even free form) also has the potential to help with legal athletic enhancement (improve muscle blood flow/oxygenation and remove metabolic waste products to allow muscles to function longer) [55]. And since the only primary dietary source of citrulline is watermelon rind, supplementation is the only option for a medical condition [1, 25].

High LDL Cholesterol (aka "Statin intolerance")

Individuals with high cholesterol that cannot tolerate statin drugs have the option of using red yeast rice extract (RYR). However, in one of the more bizarre rulings by federal officials companies are NOT allowed to standardize the active ingredient known as "monacolin K" (basically identical to isolated lovastatin), which is responsible for the lowering of LDL cholesterol in RYR [25].

A meta-analysis of 9625 patients in 93 randomized trials involving three different commercial variants of RYR has summarized this alternative option for patients [56]. The mean reduction in total cholesterol, LDL, triglyceride, and increase in HDL was respectively the following: −35 mg/dl (−0.91 mmol/L), −28 mg/dl (−0.73 mmol/L), −36 mg/dl (−0.41 mmol/L), and +6 mg/dl (+0.15 mmol/L).

"Xuezhikang" is a commercial RYR product evaluated in a large, randomized, placebo-controlled clinical trial with robust endpoints [57]. The China Coronary Secondary Prevention Study (CCSPS) enrolled 4870 participants (3986 men, 884 women) with a previous myocardial infarction (MI), and a baseline mean total cholesterol, LDL, triglyceride, and HDL of approximately 208 mg/dl (5.38 mmol/L), 129 mg/dl (3.34 mmol/L), 165 mg/dl (1.85 mmol/L), and 46 mg/dl (1.19 mmol/L). Participants received RYR 600 mg twice daily (1200 mg total, monacolin K 2.5–3.2 mg/capsule) or matching placebo and followed for 4.5 years. The trial was conducted from May 1996 to December 2003 in 65 hospitals in China. The primary end point was nonfatal MI or death from coronary or cardiac causes. Secondary end points included total mortality from CV disease, total all-cause mortality, need for coronary revascularization procedure, and change in lipid levels. Fasting blood samples were drawn at baseline, 6–8 weeks after randomization, and at 6-month intervals. There were two interim analyses, and the second one demonstrated a significant difference for the primary endpoint. The study was stopped in June 2003. A total of 98 % of the participants completed the study. It is of interest that a plethora of clinical endpoints were significantly reduced with the exception of a nonsignificant reduction in fatal MI (see Chap. 4). Cancer mortality and all-cause mortality were reduced. Lipids were also modestly and significantly reduced. No serious adverse events were observed during this trial. Total adverse events and treatment cessation numbers were similar for RYR and placebo. The number needed to treat (NNT) to prevent a primary end-point over the 4.5 year duration of the trial is 21, which favorably compares to the NNT range (19–56) observed in previous secondary prevention trials [58]. Subsequent subgroup evaluations from the CCSPS trial have found equivalent benefits with RYR among diabetics [59], elderly (mean age 69 years) [60], and hypertensive participants [61]. Potential anticancer benefits found in the overall trial with RYR were also found among the elderly (significant reduction in cancer deaths) [57, 60], and included a 51 % reduction in cancer incidence [60]. Thus, the data has been consistent that RYR reduces lipid parameters, especially LDL [62–64], and appears to have a favorable impact on clinical endpoints [57]. Reviews of past studies in statin intolerant patients have demonstrated efficacy and safety [65], including a preliminary study in breast cancer patients where RYR was a primary ingredient in one supplement [66], so it could be an interesting current or future option in some cancer patients. The catch … searching for a supplement used in a positive clinical trial that one can rely on and some are mentioned in this text (for example, Sylvan Bioproducts at www.sylvaninc.com/bio/healthCare.html).

Low Testosterone (all perception and minimal to no reality)

There are currently no effective dietary supplements that can consistently increase low testosterone in men [12], and even when testosterone pills were utilized in drugs in many other countries there were health concerns, which is arguably why this form of testosterone was never FDA approved in the USA [1, 25]. In fact, many of the best selling supplements in this category contains fenugreek (*Trigonella foenum-grae-cum*), which has not only not worked consistently, but actually showed a significant reduction in free testosterone in one study [67]. Fenugreek was famous/infamous over a decade ago when female breast enhancement supplements used this as their primary ingredient (and it did not work in this situation either) [25]. Fenugreek the food has health benefits but the supplement being linked to testosterone or even estrogen consistent increase needs quality research and I am not optimistic despite the fact that having a supplement to increase testosterone would be well-received if safe because some forms of prescription testosterone replacement are expensive.

Insomnia

Melatonin is a well-known supplement that can help with jet lag but it can also help with occasional bouts of insomnia and has an excellent safety record [1]. Most melatonin supplements are immediate release, which means they do not remain in the body for long (short half-life), but they have still demonstrated efficacy. Currently there is another option known as PR (prolonged release) melatonin that has shown some benefit and is regulated like a drug in some European countries (known as "Circadin®") and it is approved in multiple counties for primary insomnia for individuals 55 years and older [68].

The preliminary benefit in utilizing melatonin for breast cancer patients with insomnia or even depressive symptoms with similar side effects to placebo also should be preliminarily impressive (for example one 3 mg melatonin supplement from Rugby Laboratories—a subsidiary of Watson Laboratories in Duluth, GA, USA—used in a Harvard study, or another 6 mg melatonin from Pharma Nord, Vejle, Denmark) [69, 70]. It is critical to continue to find short-term insomnia solutions especially since some of the prescription drugs have come under some scrutiny lately (for example eszopiclone and FDA concerns) because in rare situations higher dosages can lead to fugue states or "impairment," where the person performs activities, such as driving a vehicle, and does not recall them [71]. And it should be kept in mind that unintentional prescription drug abuse is a leading cause of mortality in the USA with opioids, antianxiety and then insomnia prescription drugs as the top three (in that order) medications that the CDC has identified as a source of this epidemic issue [1].

Migraine Prevention

Prescription drugs and painkillers work well for some migraine sufferers but what does a patient do when suffering from them regularly in terms of prevention? The American Academy of Neurology (AAN) guidelines recommend butterbur extract (Petadolex® brand licensed to multiple companies including Linpharma Inc., Oldsmar, FL—not identified by AAN, but utilized in the clinical trials) as having class A evidence (one of its highest recommendations) as a method to prevent migraine [72]. Additionally higher dosages of vitamin B2 (generic riboflavin) have excellent preliminary data (Level B recommendation) [72]. Yet how exactly does the patient figure all of this out without a reputable and highly specific source [1]?

Parkinson's Disease (PD): Another tale of two supplements—one promising and the other not so promising supplement

There are no effective treatments that slow the progression of this disease but few realize that one of the most interesting options being utilized now by some clinicians and tested in large clinical trials is inosine (from initial research funded by the Michael J. Fox Foundation, US Government/NIH and others and called "SURE-PD" Trial and inosine supplements were obtained from Kyowa Hakko USA Inc., New York, NY) to slow the progression of this disease by raising uric acid levels (making sure patients are monitored carefully by a health care professional because taking too much can increase the risk of kidney stones) [1, 73]. Inosine is also receiving research currently in Amyotrophic Lateral Sclerosis (ALS) and Multiple Sclerosis (MS) [1].

Creatine monohydrate is commonly associated with exercise enhancement but it was also being studied at 10 g a day in arguably one of the largest and well done trials in PD to potentially slow clinical decline and improve quality of life (45 clinical sites in the USA and Canada for a minimum of 5 years) [74]. After reviewing the data from an interim analysis of 955 patients enrolled at least 5 years in this trial there was no observation of efficacy, so the study was appropriately stopped [75].

Urinary Tract Infections (UTI)

Chronic antibiotic use for the prevention of recurrent UTIs may have efficacy but also have potential toxicity and the development of resistance. Cranberry dietary supplements have worked as well as cranberry juice in preventing UTI for individuals that suffer from recurrent UTIs but this is still preliminary data [76, 77]. Regardless, cranberry supplements only contain a few calories whereas cranberry juice contains about 125–150 calories per 8 ounces, which can increase your weight and waist, which in the long-term could theoretically increase the risk of UTIs [25]. Supplements with higher concentrations of the active ingredients, PAC-A (proanthocyanidin A), need more research [77, 78], but are arguably an option being utilized currently for antibiotic-intolerant patients based on benefit over risk ongoing research [25, 77–79]. Looking for reasonable priced supplement with a higher concentration of PAC or especially PAC-A is important since there is no stand out product from a major clinical trial (numerous products exist in Europe such as Anthocran, Cysticlean, Monoselect Macrocarpon-enteric-coated that are regulated).

Weight Loss

Green coffee bean extract, Garcinia cambogia, acai berry … there are a countless list of weight loss supplements that are controversial. However, protein powder isolates (no sugar or lactose) contain as much as 25 g of protein per 100 calories far exceeds what can be accomplished with almost any protein bar or dietary option [1]. It should be "first do no harm" when dealing with weight loss and dietary supplements. Research continues to accumulate that this or another protein powder is a potential option to encourage weight/waist loss and enhance lean muscle mass in association with resistance exercise/exercise and moderate calorie reduction from an analysis of 14 randomized trials [80]. Cancer patients experiencing sarcopenia from treatment should at least be informed of this data. Additionally, alpha-lipoic acid (ALA) has received some interesting rigorous trial results and it may just function as a less potent metformin mimic (see Chap. 6), but ALA is a regulated drug in many countries but it is a supplement in the USA (from multiple easy to access companies) [1].

• **Aspirin for up to 50 dollars a month?! Most dietary supplements are initially sold as generics and not patented compounds versus pharmaceuticals that start as patented compounds and then ultimately become generic. Watch for the old "bait and switch" when concerning dietary supplement prices based on this tactic. Adding a celebrity and more ingredients is not always tantamount to a better product but can dramatically increase the price, confusion and obscure the question of whether or not high-quality research was performed on the product itself.**

Excuse the distraction for a moment on the discussion of plant sterols (also see Chap. 4), but it is not only educational on some specific dietary supplements and nutrient added to foods and beverages (plant sterols and stanols) to lower cholesterol, but demonstrates what has become somewhat common when utilizing someone else's research to promote a new product that in and of itself has little to no research.

Phytosterols are found in a variety of plants and plant oils [81]. Phytosterols are similar in structure to cholesterol except for minor structural differences. They are not synthesized in humans and minimally absorbed, excreted more rapidly from the liver compared to cholesterol, and not found in high concentrations in human tissues. The main phytosterols found in diet are sitosterol, stigmasterol, and campesterol. Beta-sitosterol is arguably the phytosterol found in largest quantity in the diet (please keep this in mind). Phytosterols block the uptake of exogenous cholesterol from dietary and bile sources in the intestinal tract. LDL cholesterol is reduced by phytosterols, and HDL and triglycerides are not impacted. The blockage of cholesterol absorption may produce a relative cholesterol pool reduction that is followed by up regulation of cholesterol synthesis and LDL receptors, which can increase LDL removal. This is somewhat similar to how some healthy dietary fats found in many healthy foods such as almonds or pistachios may also reduce LDL and improve some health outcomes [82, 83].

An ample quantity (over 40) of clinical trials utilizing phytosterols themselves has been conducted that have ranged from 1 to 12 months in duration [81, 84, 85]. Plant sterols added to foods such as yogurt, margarine, orange juice, mayonnaise, olive oil, and milk have been shown to reduce LDL by approximately 10–15 % (mean of 10–11 %) when approximately 2000 mg or more per day is ingested. And 1600–3000 mg of plant sterol supplemental or tablet consumption can also reduce LDL approximately 4–15 %. Plant sterols may also reduce the absorption of some fat-soluble vitamins, so there has been some debate as to whether multivitamin consumption should occur with the use of these products, and I agree that one multivitamin per day should also be encouraged.

It is interesting that the primary mechanism of action of these sterols via cholesterol uptake reduction and a minor anti-inflammatory mechanism suggests, in my opinion, that they are weaker or less potent mimics of the drug ezetimibe (Zetia®), which can reduce LDL by approximately 20 % with 10 mg dose [86, 87]. Laboratory research suggests ezetimibe favorably impacts prostate tissue and reduces prostate enlargement [88]. Ezetimibe is also commonly added to statin therapy or other lipid lowering agents to achieve synergistic impacts and more favorably reduce LDL [86, 87]. Thus, it should not be surprising that beta-sitosterol by itself or with other lipid lowering medications could reduce non-cancerous prostate enlargement (BPH) symptoms. For example, despite some data to suggest no impact of statins on established BPH over a short period of time [89, 90], other epidemiologic and past laboratory studies suggest potentially favorable impacts on BPH prevention and progression with cholesterol lowering prescribed medications [91–94]. What does this have to do with supplements in general? No problem, we will arrive at this point very soon.

There were two critical and similar reviews that were published in 1999 that has allowed beta-sitosterol supplements to become a potential option for BPH [95, 96]. It is interesting that since this time period no other definitive clinical trials (positive or negative) have been published. The first systematic review was by Wilt et al. and appeared in BJU international that identified studies from 1966 to 1998 [95]. A total of four clinical trials that included 519 men met the inclusion criteria [97–100]. All four trials were randomized, double-blind, placebo-controlled that included men with mild to moderate symptomatic BPH, and the intervention was given from 4 to 26 weeks. Beta-sitosterol significantly improved symptom scores and flow measures compared to placebo. Beta-sitosterol had no impact on prostate size. Gastrointestinal side effects were the most common side effects and occurred in 1.6 % of men on beta-sitosterol compared to 0 % on placebo. Erectile dysfunction was reported in approximately 0.5 % of men on beta-sitosterol and none on placebo. The authors of this systematic review concluded that beta-sitosterol "improves urological symptoms and flow measures," but that more long-terms studies and standardization of beta-sitosterol preparations were needed. The beta-sitosterol utilized in these studies were known by the names "Harzol," "Azuprostat," or "WA184" (standardized like drugs in other countries), usually derived from South African star grass (*Hypoxis rooperi* or from species of Picea or Pinus). Studies used primarily purified extracts and three studies used "nonglucosidic B-sitosterol" again from 60 to 195 mg/day (two of these studies used Azuprostat, 65 mg TID or 195 mg/day with a 70 % beta-sitosterol content). The preparation generally contained 50 % or higher amounts of B-sitosterol.

The second review was published in 2000 and consisted of similar authors compared to the first review [96], except there may be the potential for beta-sitosterol to reduce getting up at night (nocturia) approximately one less time. The positive results observed in these trials compare with results from pharmaceutical agents. Although beta-sitosterol was considered the active ingredient in these clinical trials this has not been definitively proven but it is reasonable to conclude that it is the most likely or primary efficacious ingredient.

The clinical question is why not just utilize beta-sitosterol as a stand-alone cost-effective single ingredient pill as a patient or recommend it as a clinician? Beta-sitosterol is a heart healthy low-cost ingredient. However, the dosage recommended in cholesterol treatment guidelines is 2000–3000 mg a day to reduce LDL by 6–15 %, and in fact in these National Cholesterol Education Panel recommendations it states that the following: "Plant stanol/sterol esters (2 g/day) are a therapeutic option to enhance LDL cholesterol lowering" [101]. This should be kept in mind when consulting with patients about beta-sitosterol because it is important to be able to discuss the efficacious dosages from the older 1990 prostate studies (20–65 mg TID) compared to the evidence-based hearth healthy guidelines of just plant stanol/sterols to reduce LDL cholesterol (2000–3000 mg/day). Regardless, using just beta-sitosterols or plant sterols by themselves make clinical sense right, but perhaps does not make cents but dollars.

Currently there appears to be multiple costly prostate healthy products that patients are paying as much as 30–50 dollars or more per 1–2 months that appear to have diverse and numerous ingredients but promote their product utilizing the research mentioned earlier. This was not the research on their product but the research someone else conducted. This has ethical issues in some cases because it is my perception and reality that the patients believe the product being sold to them at a high price was the exact product utilized in the research! However, again this is not the case and more importantly they are a variety of other ingredients in these products that combined have never been tested in any clinical trial or any single rigorous clinical trial. For example, imagine if I sold you aspirin and then I sold you aspirin with ten other ingredients in the same pill and utilized the research on aspirin itself to sell the more expensive 10-item pill! Oh, and I also added a celebrity endorsement to promote the product with real verve. And this is exactly what has been done by some (small number but vociferous and profitable) companies in the supplement business, but one would hope that patients and clinicians would be wise enough to simply just recommend low-cost aspirin? Yet this is not the case in my opinion because they are not aware of what is happening in terms of the "bait and switch here." Thus, in this example I would simply just recommend beta-sitosterol from food or the lower priced single ingredient or primarily generic "plant sterol" supplement pill compared to any other product, and this would save the patient a large sum of money and would follow the research and it would appear to be the most ethical route. These tactics are not utilized only in prostate health products but throughout the supplement spectrum by a select number of companies so just being aware of this one teachable example, which can pave the way for future objectivity, success, and cost-savings for your patients. As I was writing this chapter coincidentally I observed multiple other celebrity endorsed weight loss and other products that are costly and utilize one ingredient or several from some other groups research and surround that ingredient with others that do not contain arguably any reliable clinical research (the beat goes on unless it is stopped at the grass roots or patients and health care professional level).

Plant sterols are an interesting option and they arguably will continue to garner positive data. For example, the early research in breast cancer suggests that this and other compounds in this class are heart healthy and breast healthy [102]. And lowering cholesterol by blocking the uptake of cholesterol from food is now again a legitimate pharmaceutical option (again ezetimibe or Zetia), especially after the recent conclusion of the IMPROVE-IT clinical trial of over 18,000 patients in a randomized, double-blind that included a placebo and statin arm versus statin and ezetimibe [103], and has preliminary anticancer effects via favorable lipid changes or a reduction in inflammation [104]. Please see Chap. 4 for more on this and other lipid lowering products (such as PCSK9 inhibitors) that will be utilized in clinical trials with cancer patients in the future.

  • **Remember, the primary goal with patients should be pill-free or the minimum number of pills needed (MNPN) and NOT to encourage a self-medication personality.**

The concept or belief that a pill is needed regardless of evidence or safety should be antiquated, but it is not. Patients should be instructed that based on an extensive evaluation of benefit-versus-risk a pill (supplement or prescription) should be considered. Ingesting countless pills, without evidence for this practice, I have found no different from an addict self-medicating for the pleasure derived from his or her drug of choice. The plethora of other negative outcomes with self-medication practices apart from dependence and abuse abound including: incorrect use, delay in care, adverse reactions, drug interactions, masking of another physical or mental health issue … [105]. When talking to patients about prescriptions or supplements I believe the initial mantra should be "less is more" and patients appear to appreciate that philosophy because it saves money and sets a philosophy from baseline that you are objective when it comes to pill ingestion (aka "not in the back pocket of the pharmaceutical or supplement industry").

• **There is nothing "natural" about taking pills if you are otherwise healthy unless the benefit exceeds risk (rare), and there is nothing healthy about the natural versus synthetic debate.**

Arsenic, tobacco, mercury, … are all natural but I do not recommend them. Pills contain all kinds of obscure compounds such as fillers and binders and compounds that are not natural at all and the body must metabolize and excrete them. And the longest-lived populations in the world from Andorra to Mediterranean to Singapore are not massive pill consumers (quite the contrary) [1]. There is also nothing natural about indoor pipes, heating and cooling systems, airplanes, highways …, but I am grateful they exist. The "natural" is better debate is one that I find is often used to create some kind of debate advantage that is usually tied into something financial or profitable in the industry. I often explain to the public and patients that I have no idea if something natural is better, worse or the same for you unless it is tested. For example, I have heard for years that natural vitamin E supplements are better compared to synthetic but in reality in major clinical trials the benefit and toxicity have been similar or with slight differences neither advantageous or disadvantageous. In fact, it could be argued that from eye disease to other medical conditions such as Alzheimer disease that synthetic vitamin E actually has slightly better efficacy data now [13, 14, 20–22], but in reality I treat them the same. It could also be argued that Centrum Silver is the most tested synthetic multivitamin in the history of medicine from the 11-year and over 14,000 individuals tested versus placebo in the Physicians Health Study II. Regardless of the modest reduction in cancer and cataracts the percentage of patients experiencing or reporting rash with the placebo or multivitamin was 27–29 %. In other words, ingesting any pill including a placebo has the potential to create some minor to major side effects. There is nothing "natural" about taking a pill unless one actually needs a pill.

• **"Tachyphylaxis" can occur with any pill including dietary supplements, as well as toxicity when higher dosages are utilized and/or saturation kinetics finally comes into play. The antiquated terms "water-soluble" and "fat-soluble" vitamins because they are all dangerous in excess.**

Many, if not most drugs have patients that experience "tachyphylaxis" (Greek, meaning "rapid" and "protection") or desensitization to a medication after it has been utilized for a short or long period of time. For example, histamine 2-receptor antagonists, antidepressants, statins, nitrates, and most classes of drugs have some patients that experience this phenomenon [106–109]. Yet there is little to no research on tachyphylaxis with dietary supplements. However, it is evident that in multiple past studies utilizing a well-known supplement a form of tachyphylaxis can easily occur, for example when larger doses of L-arginine are administered in patients with essential hypertension to increase nitric oxide levels [110]. It is also known that saturation kinetics does not allow some supplements to exceed a certain concentration without excessive displacement in the urine or other physiologic spaces or as another metabolic by-product. This is another form of tolerance, but whether or not tachyphylaxis is encouraged under these circumstances is not well known and does not matter simply because toxicity eventually surfaces because of this phenomenon. Ingesting too much of a compound eventually causes saturation of the blood or tissue and the rest of the compound is discarded or increases to unhealthy levels [25]. For example, overexposure to calcium and vitamin C supplements could increase the risk of kidney stones [111, 112]. Selenium can get deposited in soft tissues and increase the risk of nail or hair loss, and perhaps even diabetes, skin cancer recurrence, and other cancers in excessive amounts [1, 25]. Thus, the concept of tachyphylaxis and/or saturation kinetics needs to be explained to patients as another reason why a supplement should not be ingested without extensive analysis of the benefit-to-risk scenario. Folic acid has a metabolic by-product known as "UMFA" or unmetabolized serum folic acid that could be a future concern in those that ingest mega-quantities of this dietary supplement. Vitamin A can cause excessive damage to the liver in large amounts. Vitamin B6 can cause a sensory neuropathy at excessive intakes. And the list goes on and on .... The idea that "water-soluble" vitamins like the B-vitamins or vitamin C are harmless in excess if you take excess amounts that just get excreted in urine is obviously an antiquated thought process and designation, as is "fat-soluble" essentially (although fat in diet may increase their absorption). In other words, all of these compounds or supplements display toxicity in excess and this has already been known for some supplements and for the rest it is starting to reveal itself via good research.

• **Pill esophagitis? Ulcers? Kidney stones made of sand (silicon dioxide) oh my? The ongoing list of side effects from dietary supplements or pills. Another reason that pill ingestion is not "natural" unless needed.**

Pills come with unique side effects, and although life saving in many cases, another reason not to ingest a pill unless needed is due to "pill esophagitis." This is known in the pharmaceutical industry for example and often it is due to patients not drinking enough water or standing up when ingesting a pill [113]. The symptoms of pill esophagitis include difficulty swallowing, pain on swallowing, and retrosternal pain. Yet dietary supplements can also cause pill esophagitis and esophageal ulcers [114], so the concern or at least recognition over this side effect in the supplement industry should immediately match that of the pharmaceutical industry. Increasing awareness of dietary supplement side effects allows for the identification of pill side effects unique to the industry itself, especially when compounds such as "silicon dioxide" (aka "sand") are utilized in some products to a large extent (improve flow or anti-caking agent). Recently, recognition of an increased risk of 100 % silicate based kidney stones can occur in products that contain ample amounts of this compound [115]. And this is just one of many compounds uniquely utilized in pills, especially supplements that were believed to be inert in humans.

• **Reducing fluoride in water and why it is symbolic for the current status of diet and supplements and why nutritional education needs to shift from a primarily deficiency to sufficiency. Further proof that "less is more" in the twenty-first century compared to 1700s or 1800s, and medical education needs to reflect this shift, or the "over-antioxidation of the US (and other) population" and living in one of many "first world" countries.**

Grand Rapids, Michigan became the world's first city to add fluoride to its drinking water in 1945 and within 6 years of this landmark change a study showed dramatic reductions in tooth decay among children living in this area [116]. Next, the US surgeon general and others began to endorse it. Fast forward to now, and approximately 75 % of Americans receive fluoridated water. However, recently federal officials (aka Department of Health and Human Services) released a statement that they are lowering the recommended amount of fluoride in drinking water because some kids are getting too much, which could cause white splotches on their teeth (also known as "fluorosis"). This overexposure to fluoride appears to be permanent in many cases unless of course an individual receives some kind of tooth whitening procedure to correct it. In fact, in one study 40 % of adolescents had tooth spottiness or streaking. Thus, this recent announcement to lower fluoride is a smart move. Since 1962, the government has recommended a range of 0.7 mg/L for warmer areas where individuals consume more water to 1.2 mg in cooler areas. Now, the new government standard is simply 0.7 everywhere. Not dramatic, but a small significant step in the right direction. The CDC's advice for small children is to not use fluoride toothpaste for children under 2 unless recommended by a dentist and use only a pea-sized amount of toothpaste for children 2–6 and avoid fluoride mouthwash.

And regardless of what side of the fence you are when it comes to fluoridating water, the bigger implications of this latest government recommendation has even far broader implications when it comes to future nutrition and supplement recommendations! What? What is Dr. Moyad talking about? How is that related to the whole fluoride controversy—seems like an obvious non-sequitur Moyad, right? Nope!

Several years ago during my lectures I decided to review clinical studies with health care professionals that showed why getting more of something that is perceived to be healthy, if you are already healthy, has in general never been shown to be better. And the reason I added this to my teachings and regular lectures is due to the disturbing trend I began to see in countless situations, where a plethora of compounds were being added to the food or beverage supply in large amounts from so many directions including fluoride. You see, one of the biggest frustrations I was experiencing was antiquated nutritional lectures being given to health care professionals as if we were living in the year 1750 and mentioning for example that if you do not get enough vitamin C you can get scurvy. If you do not get enough vitamin B6, you can get nerve damage, not enough beta-carotene or vitamin A then night blindness, or if you do not get enough niacin you can get the disease "pellagra" [25]! Our clinics are not satiated by these medical conditions anymore.

Today the issue is not getting too little vitamin C, but some individuals are getting too much supplemental vitamin C, which is increasing their risk of kidney stones [25]. Too much supplemental B6 actually can increase the risk of nerve damage, too much supplemental beta-carotene in former and current smokers could increase the risk of lung cancer, too much supplemental vitamin A can increase the risk of liver toxicity, and consuming too much supplemental niacin is now linked to liver toxicity and potentially heart unhealthy changes. Physicians in the USA hardly ever see these nutritional deficiency diseases anymore unless they volunteer in third world countries. In fact, most of the nutritional deficiencies I see today are from the overuse of many medications, which is now "first world" country. For example, chronic use of acid reflux drugs can result in a deficiency of vitamin B12 and/or magnesium, which the FDA recognizes along with multiple other issues [117]. My point is that nutritional education needs to change to spend more time addressing what I call in medical publications the "over-antioxidation of our population" or "the over-antioxidation of the US population" [118].

We now live in a time where nutrition and supplements are a billion dollar industry where folks compete to add the latest and greatest nutrient to the food supply, which in some cases can result in an overexposure to many things. For example, selenium deficiency use to be a serious problem in some countries, and it is still can rarely cause a serious medical condition known as "Keshan disease" but today an overexposure of selenium is more common and could lead to problems [12, 25]. I remember only a few years ago attending multiple medical lectures where Keshan disease was mentioned as a reason for some individuals to supplement with selenium?!

In one of the largest dietary supplement studies ever completed in the world (SELECT Trial) in healthy individuals, researchers recently found the potential for an increased aggressive prostate cancer risk in men getting large amounts of selenium from food and then taking a higher dose of selenium as a supplement [43]. In other words, if you were already receiving sufficient selenium from the diet and then you added more in terms of a supplement (200 µg a day), then more was not better. However, it was not that long ago selenium was difficult to find in our food supply but in the 1990s when preliminary research showed a potential anticancer and overall health benefit of selenium it took only a few years before it started getting added to many nutritional products from protein powders to almost every basic multivitamin. So, by the time this landmark SELECT study started the minimal deficiency once seen in the USA with selenium was no longer an issue, and sufficiency or overexposure quickly became the problem [25]. There is also the concern that an overexposure to selenium can increase the risk of skin cancer returning after treatment. This is also somewhat similar to the story with calcium supplements in this country. Some US restaurants have now enriched their breads with calcium, and calcium is fortified in many foods and beverages from numerous almond milks that contain over 450 mg of calcium in just 8 ounces, to some multivitamins replete with calcium. Now, in most major clinical trials women are getting enough calcium from food and beverages to match or exceed the RDA so that by the time a clinical trial of calcium supplements and bone health is initiated, many of the participants are replete with calcium before the study even starts. This was observed not long ago in one of the largest clinical trials in the world to prevent bone loss and fractures known as "WHI" or the Women's Health Initiative [119]. The end result ... more kidney stones in the group taking calcium and recent concerns that more calcium is not better for women and men. Calcium and vitamin D deficiency used to be such a problem in the USA that the disease rickets (a bad bone disease) occurred, but now this has become rare, and it was only a few decades ago that not getting enough calcium caused an increase risk of kidney stones [25].

Now, think about the number 1 cause of acute liver failure in the USA. It is due to overexposure to the over-the-counter pain reliever acetaminophen, generally (not always) in combination with alcohol. However, acetaminophen has been around a long time and so has alcohol, so why only more recently did this become a problem? In my opinion it is due to the overexposure of a drug that use to be just sold as a pain reliever and during my lifetime it got added to almost everything you can imagine, from as many as 50 % of the cold and flu therapies, to many of other targets discomfort relievers [25]. We woke up one day and it was everywhere and it is now so easy to be overexposed to this drug. Acetaminophen is a good drug but the overexposure to it has led to devastating consequences.

And fluoride use to be fairly difficult to ingest in the USA and during my lifetime it got added to almost all the dental products such as toothpaste and mouthwashes and the drinking water supply [116]. Thus, the call for the reduction of fluoride by the US government (a first in over 50 years) in my opinion is a harbinger of things to come where sudden overexposure to certain compounds and ingredients and eventually the risk will exceed the benefit, and more government or simply personalized regulation will reduce the overexposure of what not to long ago was a "deficiency." It is not 1700 or 1850 and part of our challenge is accepting the benefits and limitations of past dietary and medical advice, and how it really pertains to the modern world. We need to be vigilant and be willing to admit when we have reached the point where more does not mean better, and at least with fluoride that moment has arrived. The question now is "What is next?"

Is there really anything the US population and other industrialized countries have an overt "deficiency" of today that might still exist 50 years from now in the population? There are a small number of subtle exceptions or true subtle "deficiencies" today and for objectivity and completeness of this discussion they are mentioned in the next section.

• **The only true long-term and extreme deficiencies that most patients are dealing with are dietary limitations for chronic disease prevention, for example fiber and/or especially potassium, which are basically part of the foundation of a heart healthy diet and lifestyle program. Otherwise, getting too much of a good thing is the norm.**

This will be reviewed in the next chapter, especially fiber but these two "deficiencies" I often lecture on are simply part of eating more heart healthy and primarily pertain to chronic disease prevention.

Low potassium is a problem for arguably 98–99 % of the population. Why? Few people realize that the suggested intake or arguably the recommended daily allowance (RDA) or recommended daily intake for adults is 4700 mg/day (only 1–2 % of the population) [1]. This is how much is needed to keep the body functioning normally in terms of disease prevention, for example stroke and hypertension, kidney stones … [120]. Say you eat a banana every day, but that only gives you 450 mg or less so where are you going to get another 4000+ mg during your day? Another 8+ or so bananas daily?

How about taking a simple potassium dietary supplement? However, you can only purchase tablets with 99 mg or less in them [1]; otherwise should everyone be on potassium prescription drugs? Plain yogurt, beans, fish, fruits, veggies, and even coconut water can contain almost as much potassium as a banana or more. So, the key to ingesting more potassium is simply eating a heart healthy diet! How about spinach? One cup has almost twice the amount of potassium compared to a banana and so does one cup of avocado.

In fact, there is new strong evidence to suggest that it is not excessive sodium alone increasing the risk of hypertension, but excessive sodium and sugar, with a reduced potassium intake [1]. It is the potassium that counteracts the effects of sodium and the reduced sugar reducing weight/waist and lowering blood pressure (foods high in sodium and sugar tend to be low in potassium and high potassium foods are low in sodium and sugar). In the most recent study from the CDC (Center for Disease Control in Atlanta, GA) of over 10,000 participants, researchers found the average American intake of sodium was 3659 mg/day and for potassium it was only 2745 mg/day [120]. So, the real message should be increase potassium intake from heart healthy foods and this will naturally cause you to lower your sodium (and sugar) intake.

The World Health Organization advocated for a sodium-to-potassium ratio of 1 or less [121], but in reality some of the best dietary studies to lower blood pressure (for example DASH = Dietary Approaches to Stop Hypertension) the target was 0.6 sodium-to-potassium ratio [122]! It is also interesting recent research is demonstrating not only blood pressure reductions with an increased consumption of potassium from food, but also a reduction in other medical conditions such as kidney stones, and perhaps in other situations from my personal experience in following some patients. For example, cancer medications being utilized in prostate cancer and being tested in breast cancer (such as abiraterone) that lower potassium in many patients could potentially ameliorate this side effect at greater rate if educated on how to get ample potassium in their diets. My favorite list of banana-competing sources of potassium, apart from just asking patients to generally eat more fruits and vegetables and beans and seeds, is the following [25]:

– Avocado
– Spinach
– Plain yogurt
– Coconut water (after an extensive workout)
– Lentils
– Carrot juice (6 ounces contains over 500 mg of potassium and only about 70 calories)
– Soybeans (half-cup contains almost 500 mg of potassium)
– Fish (Alaskan Salmon, Halibut, Tuna, …)
– Sweet potato
– Prunes or an orange

An ample discussion on fiber will occur in the next chapter, but the vast majority of the population cannot achieve 20–30 g/day. Arguably, this is due to the reliance of fiber from non-dietary sources such as pills and powders [1], and arguably the reason normal potassium ingestion is also difficult to achieve is the reliance on pills and powders or fortification to usually close this gap, but again this does not exist or is not permitted. Thus, once again dependence primarily on dietary sources.

• **"Inflammation," "Free Radicals," "Boost the Immune System," and other buzzwords help sales but not objective education of patients and health care professionals. Remember the hygiene-hypothesis?**

If a product claims to reduce inflammation it tends to appear to be a legitimate pathway and solution (I cannot help but use this term at times). However, upon further investigation like most things in life there are two sides to every story. Inflammation in healthy individuals is a necessary evolutionary process to signal the body to produce more protective compounds and items such as mitochondria [1, 25]. Thus, it appears that in some individuals suppressing inflammation does not allow the body to adapt to stress and actually could reduce the body's ability to handle extrinsic and intrinsic damaging compounds. It is for this reason recent research in athletes suggests a reduction in mega-doses of supplements in order to enhance exercise performance.

It is now appreciated that the generation of "free radicals" are critical signaling compounds that aid in promoting adaptive changes to exercise training such as intrinsic antioxidant defense system increases, insulin sensitivity, glucose uptake, mitochondrial mass or number increases, and growth factors involved in tissue repair (IL-6 ...) [123–128]. Recent research and discovery of "inflammasomes," which are multi-protein oligomers of the cell, that appear to function as a critical intracellular sensors and responders (maturation of inflammatory cytokines ...) to oxidative stress are now considered a part of the innate immune system [128]. Ongoing research in this area is needed to determine which supplements enhances or suppresses the role of this part of the immune system. Regardless, less appears to be more again.

I remember when it was critical to be clean (aka "hygienic") and ensure a lack of exposure to pathogens when growing up and currently the hygiene hypothesis is challenging this concept [129, 130]. Allowing the body to deal with germs or infectious agents to help the immune system demarcate self versus true extrinsic threats could be one pathway to reducing the ongoing increase in autoimmune disease and allergies (including some food-based sensitivities). I find this argument similar and as compelling to the potential reduction of athletic performance and fitness with mega-doses of antioxidants, and again just because a buzzword appears to make sense the clinician needs to explain to the patient while it is not always logical. Inflammation and the creation of free radicals are part of a necessary trigger for the body to adapt to stress and heighten defense and even endurance mechanisms. Patients should be told that it is more chronic or unmitigated stress or inflammation that is the real issue and not temporary or acute inflammation or stress.

Another example of this marketing phenomenon is products that promise to "boost your immune system." In reality patients should be told that better immune surveillance is what is really required because when boosting the immune system the result is also allergies and autoimmune disease. In cancer treatment, drugs that boost the immune system represent a breakthrough for melanoma and other disease, but it comes with the limitation of autoimmune (attacking of self) side effects, which can be quite serious [131]. Thus, these drugs of course are only reserved for those cancer patients where benefit can exceed risk. Therefore, if otherwise healthy or free from cancer why would I, or a patient want to ingest a supplement that claims to "boost the immune system." No thanks.

• **"When you have a hammer everything looks like a nail," but "when you have a mouth everything looks like a supplement." What is the difference between some conventional doctors that push a plethora of prescriptions versus a naturopathic doctor that pushes a plethora of dietary supplements? A good review with a patient with or at high-risk of a medical condition covers lifestyle changes and supplements (to take or not) and prescriptions (to take or not). The goal again is less pills, or lower dosages of the existing medications.**

I have reviewed this elsewhere in this book, but I believe this point needs reiteration because I find that it is becoming very relevant. I find it frustrating when a patient constantly seeks the attention of a medical doctor only to walk away with more and more prescription medications as the only solution to an isolated or related problem. Today, almost every issue in medicine has a lifestyle option (or not) or a supplement option (or not), or a prescription option (or not). In other words, it is just as critical to feel comfortable NOT recommending something as it is to recommending something. Exercise to reduce muscle/joint pain from aromatase inhibitors, weight loss for the reduction of acid reflux with the lowest dose of a proton pump inhibitor, acupuncture for hot flashes and not just progesterone [1, 25] .... The list is endless. However, when only a pill is presented it tends to set up a toxic, "one size certainly fits all," solution/dependence for patients. Occasionally I get frustrated with some conventional doctors that hand out scripts like candy to patients and suddenly 5–10 drugs later the patient becomes completely dependent on them, and polypharmacy and all its inherent issues abounds. However, I also become occasionally frustrated with naturopathic doctors that push supplements and sell them out of their office like candy. It is comical when I hear surgeons suffering from that old adage "when you have a hammer everything looks like a nail," but I find this no different than anyone else in medicine that wants to push a product out of their office or within their possession. So, I like to say "when you have a mouth everything looks like a supplement!" I meet breast and other cancer patients that visit with some naturopathic doctors and walk out purchasing or being recommended 5–10 different supplements when they have never even used one in the past. I find this so concerning because it simply reinforces the behavior of dependence on pills when in some cases many of these pills were never needed. *In reality, whether a good medical doctor or osteopathic or naturopathic or physician assistant or nurse practitioner or nutritionist or nurse or whatever ... I think we should share the common mantra that pill dependence, when not absolutely needed, is not good for patients, and not the reason we first entered into the medical profession.*

• **"Us" versus "Them"—Okay perhaps in politics but completely toxic in medicine!**

It is never my intention to have anyone perceive that I am personally endorsing or advertising a specific brand whether it is from a pharmaceutical or nutraceutical company. My only goal is to provide an audience with many things to consider when choosing any pill. One of the most critical factors has to be the human or clinical evidence that a product or procedure currently has compared to others. For example, the supplement that has the longest and most rigorous multivitamin clinical trial compared to a placebo is Centrum Silver [132]. There is simply no other multivitamin that has this amount of human evidence. Let me play devil's advocate here—if the Centrum trial would have failed, then their product and business would not have survived. This was an incredibly risky venture, as is the case with any supplement or drug that decides to actually test their product in a human research setting. This is also the reason some supplement companies never really want to test or invest in research.

My goal is to never engage in an "us" versus "them" scenario because in my opinion it is so toxic and unhealthy in so many areas from politics to television news to pharmaceutical versus nutraceutical companies. I am grateful for many pharmaceutical companies and the researchers behind them that have changed the course of AIDS or breast cancer or hepatitis C ... for many of my friends and family (not just patients). In fact, there are also some friends and family members that were not able to live a long life simply because a game changing drug for their disease (including breast cancer and Hepatitis C in the case of my family) was invented just a few years after they died. However, I have also been very vocal about other pharmaceutical companies that have provided no purpose to the overall health and well-being of individuals, and I will continue to be critical of them (spinning over and over different forms of a drug that was about to become generic).

Supplements are no different over my 25 years of experience—we have very good and very bad supplement companies. We have some that simply gauge the public and are dangerous and others that provide benefits. It is messy out there at times (especially now) and it takes a lot of information (evidence, cost, quality control, safety, ...) for someone to personally decide what they want or not to consume. I mention in my books, and in my articles and all my lectures, all the different factors someone should consider as if I am advising my own wife and kids. If you decide not to purchase Centrum or any other brand I think this is fabulous. Do what you are comfortable with after all the evidence is in. I will continue to push to extract the most information on these pills to help provide some guidance. Of course I would like to see all companies become more transparent with their consumers including Centrum or any other company. I also would like to see more supplement clinical trials that include women and minorities, which is a major past and current problem. I would like to see companies think twice before giving or offering kids supplements with no research, such as many gummi (primarily added sugar) variety brands. I would like to see more companies utilize less toxic ingredients but at the same time others need to quit hiding behind a "natural is better" label and really invest and test their specific product in a clinical research setting. Natural is better when proven to be better especially when it comes to taking a pill. Arsenic and tobacco again are natural but I do not recommend them. I cannot objectively educate future health care professionals on the positives of lifestyle and supplements without research. My list is endless for what I want to see change ASAP (more on that at a later time).

In the meantime, I can promise you that I will never take a side in a discussion simply because I have to pick a side and ignore the other important qualities offered in the argument. Health care professionals, patients and just consumers should try not to fall the "us" versus "them" debate from "big pharma versus supplements" to "medical doctors versus naturopaths" to "holistic/alternative versus conventional" … no one wins except the side that wants you to believe that you have to take their side in order to be right and profitable. Again, I will never take a side in a discussion simply because I have to pick a side and ignore the other important qualities offered in the argument.

This is a debate I clearly mention to my audience that I will promise to never engage in but will instead function like an old reliable news anchor that reports on the existing or past evidence or lack thereof. And I think this is exactly why many of us wanted to go into medicine—to be the trusted objective non-influenced advisor to the patients.

• **If I am not supposed to get overly excited if a supplement company claims (as mentioned in your rule number 1) they follow the FDA cGMP (current good manufacturing practices) how do I know I have a quality product? Look for a seal of approval on the company website, or even better on the product itself that is legitimate (NSF, USP, NPA, …). The top choice is arguably NSF (once every 6 months of auditing), but USP, NPA, and Informed Choice are also credible.**

In 2007, current Good Manufacturing Practices (cGMP) were established for dietary supplements sold in the USA, which means the FDA now has the authority to enforce and ensure that companies meet current requirements for the identity, strength, quality, and purity of their products [133]. And many companies like to claim that they follow the cGMP, but in reality again you have no idea if this is true unless someone actually tests this claim. Some companies claim to follow cGMP but we really do not know unless some outside party tests them or they get caught for doing something wrong by the FDA. So, do not rely on this self-advertisement to ensure that your herbal products are clean and contain what they report on the label. The FDA does not have the person power to enforce this ruling on a large scale, which is why following other steps will be helpful.

Imagine an independent and private third party testing group that most professional athletic organizations like the NFL, Major League Baseball (MLB), PGA, LPGA, NHL, and even Olympic athletes use to guarantee that the supplements (sport supplements in this case) they consume are clean and have exactly what they report on the label! Well, that company exists and it is known as NSF [25, 134]! It is in my opinion the best quality control insurance that exists right now for herbal supplements and supplements overall. In fact, it is also the only quality control company that actually does ON-SITE auditing or checking of a facility EVERY 6 MONTHS! That is simply outstanding quality control. So, whether the supplement provider is in China or India or Brazil or the USA they are there on-site every 6 months!

Why doesn't everyone just sign up with NSF? Good question. It costs money that many companies simply do not want to spend and every 6 months is really daunting for many companies. Yet in my opinion the cost is minimal because the risk in terms of potential insurance costs and litigation are large. Ideally, a perfect herbal or supplement has an NSF label (NSF or NSF Certified for Sport®) on the bottle itself, which means that individual product was tested versus an NSF label on the website, which is still of high quality and provides or identifies the facility that the supplement was produced follows the FDA rules on quality control. Again, ideally a supplement should have an NSF label on the bottle or container and the silver medal (almost as good) is an NSF label on the website (to help ensure cGMP). The company also tests for all sorts of bad things such as herbicides, pesticides, and heavy metals. And it also tests athletic or sports nutritional products for countless athletes and organizations around the world, and this program is known as "NSF certified for sport" (mentioned earlier).

Athletic or sports nutritional products have a history of contamination or quality control issues, so actually two quality control companies have stepped in to ensure compliance with the FDA and clean products. The first one was mentioned previously and this is NSF, but more specifically when the company or product states "certified for sport" by NSF this equates to outstanding quality control for that athletic enhancement product [134]. In addition, another group known as "informed choice" is another quality assurance program for sports nutrition products [135]. "Informed choice®" is a label with a check mark on it that identifies a product that has been tested especially for banded substances and helps to ensure good quality control in the sports nutritional area.

Another very good independent quality control group is USP and if the website or bottle contains the label then usually what is reported on the label is actually in the bottle [136]. When looking at the auditing or on-site monitoring accomplished by this group it appears to be longer than 6 months and seems to be on average every year or two which, is why I do not rank them number 1. Regardless, they are excellent. Again, the catch (similar to NSF) is that many companies or herbal products do not have a USP label. Additionally, The Natural Products Association or NPA label is another good group that appears to audit every year or more and when a company carries the NPA (Natural Products Association) label they are also appear to be following FDA quality control rules (yet audit every year or two) [137].

I am often asked the meaning of NSF or USP and things can be found in the history of these organizations, which were not originally designed to ensure quality control for dietary supplements, which is why the companies like to be known by their abbreviated name rather than their antiquated original name (NSF=National Sanitation Foundation and USP=United States Pharmacopeial Convention or United States Pharmacopeia).

• **Herbal supplements are a whole new and old wild animal, so make sure you treat them that way! Always look for some quality control seal/proof AND the standardized ingredient in the herbal that was found to be effective in the phase-3-like clinical trial for the medical condition it might reduce or resolve.**

I usually have little to worry about when it comes to basic vitamins and minerals in supplements like vitamin D or A or C or magnesium. The amount listed on the label is usually accurate so I am not obsessed with finding an NSF or USP label for example but that would a nice bonus. However, the real concern over quality control lately has been herbal products so if you think you might be purchasing one soon demand some level of quality control testing. In other words, look for a seal of approval as mentioned earlier and look on the website for some other types of quality control testing. I am often really surprised by large supplement companies that do not mention they are NSF certified until page 4 or 10 of their website. This should be on the first page!

Also, it is important to understand that almost every herbal product that has ever demonstrated a benefit from American ginseng to reduce cancer related fatigue (CRF) to ginger to reduce chemotherapy nausea have an active ingredient that was standardized in the more rigorous and definitive trial that demonstrated a benefit [1, 25]. So, look for the active ingredient on the website and label. For example, in many of the cancer-related fatigue (CRF) reducing studies of American ginseng the active ingredients were standardized to 3–5 % ginsenosides (the active ingredients, and the supplement was obtained from the Ginseng Board of Wisconsin) at a dosage of 1000–2000 mg/day for 8 weeks [138, 139], and it now appears this may be one of the only pill options for CRF and the only one that has similar side effects to a placebo [140]. Additionally, *Panax ginseng* (Asian ginseng) also has novel preliminary evidence (800 mg/day—7 % or greater ginsenosides) [141]. Ginger (Z. *officinale*) supplements at 500–1000 mg for chemotherapy-induced nausea (started 3 days before start of chemotherapy and for a total of 6 days) were also standardized (purified liquid extract of ginger root "with concentrated 8.5 mg of combined gingerols, zingerone, and shogoal content, equivalent to 250 mg of ginger root, in extra virgin olive oil …") [142]. Interestingly, the ginger was manufactured by Aphios Corporation in Woburn, MA, which is now testing their product (called Zindol®) in a phase III clinical trial and should be lauded for this wonderful dedication to research [143]! Again, the difference between a drug and supplement is perception and not reality, but the ginger product itself can be purchased right now as a dietary supplement (Zindol® DS) [144]. *In addition, it is critical to mention that the majority of the patients in all of these previously mentioned herbal studies were being treated for breast cancer* [138–142].

• **Several other outstanding quality control sites and/or publications on herbal/supplements reviewing quality and/or efficacy are the following:**

– **Center for Science in the Public Interest (CSPI or www.cspinet.org),**
– **Consumerlab.com,**
– **ConsumerReports.org,**
– **The "Natural Medicines Comprehensive Database" (www.naturaldatabase. com).**

CSPI is a very reputable group that reports on the evidence as well as periodic quality control testing of supplements. Overall, I find that they are objective and well-researched group and the staff that reports on dietary supplements is excellent. Since they follow quality control intermittently it is not the ideal place to get regular information but since they have regular evidence-based reviews of herbal products for medical conditions overall it is a good source. And their overall focus on nutritional information is really interesting. They have a newsletter that is low cost.

Consumerlab.com is a website that commissions independent testing on all types of dietary supplement brands so you know exactly what you are or are not getting in them. It was this site that informed me about many multivitamins and which ones passed their test. You probably have to pay a small fee to obtain the latest and greatest quality control information, but for those in need of the latest testing and who passed or not—it is usually there.

Consumer reports? Yes, the same independent and noncommercial group that tests everything from blood pressure monitors to cars and vacuum cleaners also regularly follows stories or issues with dietary supplements. Overall they are objective and interesting and tend to require a certain level of evidence to endorse any product. I do not always agree with their take on the clinical research (as with many other groups) but when it comes to protecting the safety of the public I agree with them. They may require a small fee for their newsletter or more extensive website access but it is worth it.

The Natural Medicines Comprehensive Database is essentially a group of health care professionals that claim they are a source of "unbiased, scientific clinical information on Complementary, Alternative, and Integrative Therapies" and in my opinion this is accurate. Thus, they really do not have a profound role in quality control testing but their regular information of clinical efficacy for supplements is very good. The cost of their information can be a little pricey but is worth it. There are few places on earth that one can find such good information on everything from drug and supplement interactions to clinical efficacy of supplements (apart from this and other Moyad texts …). Pharmacists are a large part of the writing and staff of this group, which again should provide some assurance that especially for drug and supplement interactions the information is up to date and excellent.

• **Pharmaceutical brand supplements have a lot to lose if they are wrong (Note: this does not mean I endorse any of these brands or want you to take one, but it is a simple tip for guidance).**

When a pharmaceutical company begins to market and sell supplements such as Pfizer (Centrum®) or Bayer (One-A-Day®) or Abbott Labs … they generally have very good quality control and overall their prices are competitive (aka low cost or cheap like me). Another reason I like some of them is personally I believe they have a lot to lose if they are wrong. In other words, bad products on the supplement side could be a disaster in terms of public relations and profit on the drug side. So, in general I find that these companies fly straight because they cannot afford to fly any other way.

Now here is the catch! I wrote this exact same tip on a popular website and about 10 % of those that read this tip were very upset. They thought I was endorsing "big pharma" and suggesting that the only products you should buy when it comes to supplements are pharmaceutical supplements?! This is never the intention, but instead I wanted readers to know that they could rely on these brands in terms of the accuracy of what is on their label is almost always in the bottle (for example this is exactly what consumerlab.com has found since 2007). In addition, I was upset that individuals somehow think that pharmaceutical supplements are all bad! Again, it is never my intention to have anyone perceive that I am personally endorsing or advertising a specific brand whether it is from a pharmaceutical or nutraceutical company.

My only goal is to provide the audience with many things to consider when choosing any pill. One of the most critical factors has to be the human or clinical evidence that a product or procedure currently has compared to others

Again, I would like to see more companies utilize less toxic ingredients but at the same time others need to quit hiding behind that "natural is better" label again, and really invest and test their specific product in a clinical research setting. Again, natural is better when proven to be better especially when it comes to taking a pill. Pharmaceutical brands have a history of containing exactly what they claim on the ingredient label and they should be complemented for this fact (see the next chapter—multivitamins section).

- **Multivitamin with herbal ingredients? No thanks!**

The largest and best objective multivitamin clinical trials like the Physicians Health Study II (PHSII) never used any herbal products in their multivitamin and they have the longest and best clinical study ever conducted in this area, and they still showed a benefit (slight reduction in risk of cancer and cataracts) [132]. The only other major phase-3-like multivitamin randomized trial that included healthy women and men (called "SU.VI.MAX" or The Supplementation en Vitamines et Mineraux Antioxydants) also did not use and herbals in their formulation [145]. In other words, I see no reason to purchase a multivitamin with any herbal ingredients on the label because you might as well mimic what worked best in the largest clinical trial of a multivitamin (Centrum Silver® or SU.VI.MAX but both were just one pill a day).

- **Only purchase a single ingredient supplement most of the time except in rare situations (like a multivitamin or when a clinical trial specifies/utilizes more than one ingredient, which rare). Dilution = Pollution? Don't be a clinical trial of 1! Proof and reward should be in the research and again in standardization of the active ingredient!**

Most well done clinical studies of supplements to help almost any condition usually used a single standardized ingredient. For example, melatonin use for jet lag, or insomnia (single ingredient) or even SAM-e supplements for mental health improvement or osteoarthritis (usually 1 ingredient) [1, 25]. Where consumers get in trouble is when they start to buy products with multiple ingredients in them that were never used in the largest and best studies. This process not only dilutes the active ingredient rendering it less effective, but also pollutes the product and can make it tougher on your liver to metabolize. Again, think about this for a second, you would never buy a bottle of aspirin that also contained multiple herbs and vitamins and compounds in the aspirin because it would not only make aspirin itself less effective, but increases the risk of further toxicity because now you are a clinical trial of one! Aspirin was only studied in most major clinical trials as a single ingredient and not combined with multiple other products.

There are exceptions such as macular degeneration (mentioned earlier) where several ingredients were used together (500 mg vitamin C, 400 IU vitamin E, 10 mg lutein, 2 mg zeaxanthin, 25–80 mg zinc, and 2 mg copper) but in those situations it is clear what was used in the clinical trial (called AREDS2 for macular degeneration) and you should only use those ingredients [20–22]. Another example is glucosamine sulfate (1500 mg daily) and chondroitin sulfate (800 mg daily) used together in notable clinical trials such as LEGS study [146]. So, do your research and again only buy or recommend what was used in the most impressive clinical trial and copycat that scenario (not different from a drug trial).

I am asked often asked what kind of saw palmetto I recommend for prostate issues and I tell audiences that since two very large clinical trials (called "STEP" and "CAMUS") both showed that saw palmetto works about as well as a placebo [31, 32], so I do not recommend it. However, butterbur extract for migraine prevention was given a "Level A" (one of the highest and means it is "effective") by a subcommittee of the American Academy of Neurology and the American Headache Society in 2012 in the medical journal "Neurology," which is highly reputable [72]. However, what they failed to emphasize was the product called "petadolex" (mentioned earlier) was the supplement (actually a drug in other countries) utilized in the best clinical studies. In other words, if I were going to recommend or use butterbur then petadolex (petadolex.com) would be my initial choice. For example, when the Mayo clinic and 40 other medical centers did a very large clinical trial of American ginseng to reduce fatigue from cancer treatment they found 2000 mg worked significantly better than placebo after 8 weeks (mentioned earlier) [138, 139]. However, what fails to be mentioned in other publications is that the Ginseng Board of ginseng (www.ginsengboard.com) provided the product and this is exactly what I recommended to patients with cancer inquiring about which ginseng to utilize for their fatigue. In other words, I reward and trust the products that have gone through the most human research on efficacy and safety. So, the next time you hear about a positive or negative herbal supplement study just look at the medical paper on line and check the materials and methods section to see exactly what commercial product was used.

• **Always reevaluate your situation and do not be afraid to be a part-time guinea pig (if benefit >>> risk). The A, B, C's of whether a pill is working and if you really need it (the impact on heart health and other parameters)! Look for non-pill pill-like options (the new calcium supplement)?!**

I often tell patients to only take the supplements that you and the doctor you trust (and a pharmacist …) think you need. Revisit your list every single 6-months to a year. Now, this sounds simplistic but I meet people daily that don't know why they are taking many of their supplements, and they have no idea if they are experiencing any benefit. In other words, I hear words like it has "antiaging" effects or "prevents free radicals" but this means nothing unless you feel or see some benefit. Would you follow this same approach with a drug? No. Most supplement pills have very low levels of heavy metals or other pollutants that are not a concern daily but when taken over years this amounts to a great deal of exposure and no one knows the implications.

Apart from a multivitamin, which helps a little (not much but a little) it is my opinion that this idea that supplements subtly change your life is primarily an advertising or marketing ploy. There are realities that I believe folks should contemplate. For example, many healthy individuals do not qualify for pills—not just supplements, but also drugs. I think we should embrace and celebrate a person when they are so healthy they need little to no pills. And I am convinced future generations will feel this way. Still, I apply A, B, and C rules (three of them) to determine if patients or individuals need a pill or supplement.

A. Subjective Test (aka guinea pig approach)

If you ever wonder whether or not a supplement is helping (which I am asked this question all the time) you need to embrace the Dr. Moyad guinea pig approach— stop the product for 1 month and tell me if you feel any better, or worse, or the same? For example how has anything you feel changed including your mood. This works very well. I often hear from folks that they actually feel better or no different and then they simply stop the pill and save a lot of time and money. There are also moments where someone says they feel worse or more fatigued and they get ill more often, especially after they stopped their supplement. Well, this is a good indication that you may need your pill.

B. Objective Test (aka laboratory or numbers approach)

Is the supplement you are taking changing any single parameter that suggests you are becoming more healthy? I like to first look at cardiovascular disease (CVD) parameters because CVD has been the number 1 cause of death in women and men for 114 of the last 115 years [25]. In fact, I do not like to take or recommend any pill unless I know what its impact is on heart health. "First do no harm" right?! So, is the pill you are taking dropping your cholesterol, blood pressure, blood sugar, or helping you lose weight? In other words, what is it objectively doing for you? If the answer is nothing then I would become a little skeptical. If it is increasing some number that is unhealthy such as your liver enzymes then this is another bad sign. What numbers are changing for the bad or good with this pill? Working with a good doctor is critical to getting number 2 answered. A doctor or pharmacist or another health care practitioner that applies broad strokes to supplements (all bad or all good for example) make me nervous. Patients should find one with an open and objective mind.

Ideally I want a pill to change both A and B above but if it can still change A or B then this increases the chances that what you are taking is actually helping you. People need to do this more often with their drugs or supplements. However, always remember rule number C.

C. Lifestyle Test (to reduce or determine pill count/dosage)

Is there a lifestyle change that can substitute for this pill or at least reduce the dosage?

I find that many people who are taking great care of their bodies and minds also take some of the largest number of supplements and this is what the research also shows [1, 25]. However, it is almost a form of self-medication and giving credit where the credit is not due. In other words, they claim all these benefits from taking these pills but they do not realize how much of what they are doing personally is simply making them feel and be healthier (not the pills).

Look at athletic supplements mentioned earlier and how research is now showing that mega-doses of supplements may actually be hindering the benefits of exercise by not allowing oxidative stress to help signal the body that it needs more mitochondria or cellular changes that in the long-term would build better fitness or endurance.

Additionally, we have too many individuals hooked on pills because many do not realize that moderate lifestyle changes could get them off these pills or reduce their dosage to a more safe range if they make these changes [1, 12, 25]. Higher or mega-dosages of drugs or supplements make no sense because ultimately there is some ugly price to pay. Look at cholesterol lowering drugs and the number of folks that rely on the maximum dosage to keep their cholesterol down. Now, you start to dramatically increase the risk of never imagined before side effects like type 2 diabetes, serious muscle discomfort .... Look at vitamin C-mega doses (1000 mg+) can dramatically increase oxalate levels in the urine and increase the risk of kidney stones [25]. Applying moderate lifestyle changes first and foremost allows you to determine how much of a drug or supplement you truly need or maybe you do not need it at all. Give yourself the chance to figure out what you can do on your own before turning toward pills as a solution. When you take better care of yourself this is the ultimate truth detector test of what your body really needs or not in terms of pills. And if you can replace a pill with a food or beverage of your liking then this is always an option (8 ounces of almond milk=455 mg of calcium or protein in food/powder instead of pills).

• **Do patients really need comprehensive testing via blood or genetics to determine their nutritional deficiencies if they are otherwise healthy? No. And get ready to buy a pill! Remember genes can also be changed or altered in some situations like "jeans."**

Comprehensive nutritional testing have not been comprehensively tested (ironic right?) to see if they change hard (not soft) clinical endpoints that matter, for example stroke or heart attack or cancer or whatever. In other words, just because a company says you need to increase your intake of X or Y does not mean you need to do this. Blood testing on nutrients is interesting but well within its infancy still so that we do not know what disease they do or do not predict. Look what has happened lately with the FDA and some home genetic testing companies. The FDA did a good job of exposing the fact that some of these tests would tell your chance of getting a disease but in reality did not have that kind of research to really predict this [147], so you end up creating a number of people that just live with a lot of unnecessary anxiety. Patients should be told that in some cases even when a genetic test demonstrates some risk, lifestyle changes can alter risk or even prevent that gene from being ultimately expressed (just because you have a gene does not mean you will express the clinical endpoint of that gene).

Another example of over testing the population for nutrient issues should be exemplified in the "homocysteine" blood test used by some companies and practitioners to generally screen asymptomatic healthy individuals. If the test was slightly abnormal many folks were placed on high doses of B-vitamins. However, no one had tested what happens when you bring that test level down on these high dosages. Now, decades later countless clinical trials later and arguably hundreds of millions of taxpayer dollars, and little to no benefit has been found in using this test to screen the general population [148]. It still has some merit in a minority of high-risk individuals but in the majority of folks they were found to be worthless.

Many nutritional blood tests also simply change dramatically in your favor with differing factors weight loss such as vitamin D [25]. And again many tests have not been validated in terms of the best assay and accuracy or correlation with end points (like vitamin D). And just because a blood test is low or high does not necessarily mirror the amount in your body tissues or vice versa. In other words, part of good testing is figuring out what type of test is really needed and what precise sample is needed for optimal testing—whole blood, red blood cells, plasma, tissue, lymphocytes … and this takes time and money and lots of research.

We live in an age of over testing but in supplements there is also huge profit tied to nutritional testing because what is the first thing I see patients receive when some blood test is low? A recommendation to buy a high priced supplement from the same office that provided the blood testing! That is a clear conflict of interest. Again, "when you have a hammer everything looks like a nail." However, when you sell supplements especially out of your office "everything looks like a mouth." Subconsciously or consciously it is easy to require a patient to take a supplement when behind the scenes you profit from recommending it. This is no better or worse than the old days of doctors being placed on advisory boards for pharmaceutical companies or having paid trips if they prescribed a drug more or willing to prescribe more of a drug from the company that is paying for their medical advisory trip in the Bahamas.

• **What is my best advice for determining what supplements an otherwise healthy person could need? Supplements are primarily for medical conditions and targeted dieting once again to the rescue.**

There are a few simple tips [25]:

– Get comfortable with your family disease tree. What were individuals in my family diagnosed with and suffer from and why? What did they die from and why? Thus, it allows you to determine what you may be at high-risk for and why you have what you have, or may be diagnosed with in the future. So, if you are starting to suffer from migraines and there is a family history of migraines you may want to be aggressive in taking something to prevent migraines. And this leads to the next point ….

– Try to put as much effort as is practical and realistic in becoming more heart and mentally healthy to determine if you need a pill for the major issues. This was mentioned many times before but also applies here. Diet, exercise …. Are you capable of achieving optimal cholesterol, blood pressure, blood sugar, and weight on your own. How about your mental health? If not you may need some pill support because these are the big preventive numbers that really make or break whether or not you are predicted to live a longer and better life. I find it interesting again that in the longest lived populations in the world such as Andorra [25], which is number 1 (I have been there also) in global population longevity, it is actually unusual to take any pills or supplements unless you have been diagnosed with a medical condition. Hmmm, interesting.

– Think of taking a supplement for a condition or to reduce the risk of recurrence of that condition and not for primary prevention (except perhaps for a multivitamin) unless you have already been diagnosed and treated for a condition. And think of taking a pill to reduce side effects of some conventional medical treatments (ginseng and cancer fatigue …). If you have been diagnosed with Celiac or bone loss or any other conditions then it makes sense to review what supplements have worked or is needed and which are worthless.

– If you are taking any prescription medications ask yourself and the doctor you trust if a supplement is needed to reduce any "quiet" side effects the drug is causing such as lowering vitamin B12 (with acid reflux drugs, metformin …) [1]. Many of the so-called "deficiencies" I see today again occur from other medications.

– If someone tells you that you have to take a pill or supplement, is there also a way you can just get it with targeted dieting. Look at calcium in food, mentioned earlier and almond milk (or cashew milk …) or look at protein pills and now protein powders have in many cases 25 g of protein in 100 or so calories with no sugar and excellent taste and these pills are not needed anymore.

The beauty of most supplements is not for preventing countless diseases but in treating diseases or side effects suffered from the treatment of a disease. Unfortunately the perception is the opposite of what I just mentioned.

• **What does the medical research suggest about the form of the supplement that should be ingested? Tablets? Capsules? Liquids? What should patients know about this and the best time of the day or situation to ingest a supplement for maximum efficacy? How about the half-life of supplements in the body? Following the path of compliance and flexibility and with aging metabolism, intestine, kidney, liver … changes (we also age on the inside). Never forget "20 %"? Children, adolescents, and supplements?**

The answer is similar to the drug world, where compliance is the biggest issue and everything else is a distant second. Research shows us that pill ingestion does not ever become routine and this has been my clinical experience. After a few years many begin to get bored or simply forget to take their drugs regularly, even if they are life saving in some cases [149]. This "non-adherence" as it is called is intentional in some cases, unintentional in others, neglectful in other cases by caregivers, and other possibilities abound. Yet it is a reality. In the famous Women's Health Initiative (WHI)—the largest clinical trial of calcium and vitamin D in the world to prevent bone loss and hip fractures published almost 10 years ago many people still believe the supplements did not work! And they used very cheap brands of calcium and vitamin D. However, a secondary look at the same trial actually showed for the women that took their supplements most days of the month (80 % of the time), they did work in slowing bone loss and preventing hip fractures by almost 30 % [119]!

Thus, the form (calcium carbonate) that was used in the phase-3 like study (one of my criteria) is important but compliance is just as important [1, 25]. Still, every year you have to ask yourself how much of this nutrient is now in foods and do I even need the pill anymore. Again, look at calcium supplements and a decade ago it made sense to take a supplement. However, 10 years later there are countless well fortified with calcium foods and beverages. Many almond, cashew, and hemp milks including the leading brands have 455–500 mg of calcium in just 8 ounces. So, you could just drink two cups a day and no longer need calcium supplements! ND, most multivitamins now carry larger amounts and numerous beverages (including milk substitutes) are now fortified so taking an individual vitamin D supplement is rarely necessary. The bottom line is that if you need a pill or supplement, you find the form or type used in the clinical study that was most definitive or the one that has the highest probability of working and then ingest it normally in the form (liquid, capsule, powder, …) that allows for the best individual compliance. It's all about the compliance!

Most of the time when asupplement says ingest "with a meal" it is to reduce gastrointestinal side effects and improve compliance and memory (remembering that you need to take a pill being tied or associated with meals) [1]. And in some other cases you get slightly better absorption with a meal but there are many exceptions. Iron supplements work better in terms of absorption without a meal, as do osteoporosis drugs. However, it seems that iron absorption is adequate enough if used right after a meal, and it can reduce many of the gastrointestinal side effects [150]. In fact, ingesting iron with some acidic foods and vitamin C (food and/or supplement) or using a non-enteric coated brand also increases absorption [151].

I find that most of this research in drugs and supplements was based on lowering side effects with a meal compared to make or break clinical changes or endpoints. I find that too many people get caught in the minutiae or specifics of how to take it and this just increases their anxiety and reduces the focus on what really matters—again regular compliance.

Absorption is often used as a way to sell a more expensive non-researched compound to a customer but I rarely am attracted by this approach. Again, just because you might absorb better does not mean you will be better until it is tested to prove this fact. It turns out that some low cost supplements (used in most supplement major clinical trials by the way) mentioned in this book absorb just fine when measuring blood levels.

There is an old saying about absorption I have been using for over 25 years, and that is "if you can hit a baseball 500 feet in Detroit Tiger Stadium then it is called a home run, but if you can hit a baseball 500 miles into Canada from Tiger stadium then this is so impressive that I am sure you will make more money in endorsement deals but it still counts as a home run!" In other words the body works by a threshold effect so that you do not need massive absorption for an impact, but just some absorption. It is kind of like asking me is it better to run 5 miles a day or 5.2 miles a day. Both are fine.

Still, I know there are some individuals that think the best time to take a certain pill is on a full moon in October after midnight, but again the research overall does not support this behavior. I tell patients that you should generally try and take your supplements right before or during or right after a meal (if you able) to lower side effects, and in some cases and it may or may not increase absorption. Groundbreaking drugs, such as metformin, were found to have reduced absorption with food, but this increased compliance (lowered gastrointestinal complications), which resulted in lowering the risk of type-2 diabetes and/or still providing adequate weight loss

[152]. So, taking a product with meals improves compliance and still gives clinical results even if food in some cases moderately reduces the absorption of the product. Patients appear to be often told to take their statin in the evening before bed because cholesterol production via the liver is highest at this time, but in the largest clinical trials this was not how they were generally utilized, and they still favorably changed clinical end points [153]. Still, the reality or bottom line is that a person should take a pill primarily at the time of day when they can best remember to take it.

The half-life of many supplements is not known, because research has not been adequate in this area. I mentioned earlier the WHI trial and we learned that you needed to take your calcium 6–7 days a week (80 % of the time) for the best results [119]. We know with red yeast rice for cholesterol lowering the half-life of the active ingredient is only a few hours, so you need to take it daily to keep your cholesterol lowering effects [25]. It should also be utilized with a meal if possible because the active ingredient is a lovastatin drug mimic, which does absorb better with food (this rarely or ever is mentioned in the medical literature).

It is a shame because in the drug world we can help people by knowing all the drug pharmacology, so I know if I recommend the cholesterol lowering drug rosuvastatin (Crestor®) that the drug half-life is long enough that ingesting the drug once a week still reduces cholesterol moderately well [154]. I know that taking alendronate (Fosamax) for osteoporosis or fracture prevention can be stopped after 5–10 years ("drug holiday"), which still allows for adequate bone protection in most individuals because the half-life of the drug itself is in years, and there are clinical studies that proved this [155, 156]! We just do not have this data with supplements, and all one can do is mimic the method from the clinical study that peaked your interest in utilizing or recommending it. As a broad rule of them, the majority of positive dietary supplement trials have used something you should take daily. Whenever the half-life of a supplement appears to increase that product ultimately turns into a drug (like melatonin in Europe) [68].

Finally, it needs to be remembered that aging is associated with gradual but tangible changes internally and not just externally [25]. Intestinal absorption decreases, liver metabolism is not as adequate and the kidney is not similar to the 16-year-old individual. Thus, pill consumption and analysis of needs or not should become even more critical with age. *In the most recent years of analysis, arguably due to greater awareness and monitoring, approximately 20 % of the serious hepatotoxic (liver failure, need for transplant, or death) events from pills occurred with dietary supplements (1 out 5) [157], which is the largest that I am aware of in US history. The average age of the person experiencing such an event was a 40-year-old healthy female ingesting a "fly by night" product (weight loss …). Every day countless men and women take a dietary supplement that has never been adequately tested for safety and efficacy and are essentially agreeing to be a clinical trial of 1!*

The earlier an adult or child is sent this message the better, which is why I often tell parents to try and not have your kids solve a perceived non-issue with a supplement or drug. In my experience, the teenager that embraces the 1–2 supplements today is the 30-year-old that ingests 5 of them and the 50-year-old that ingests 8 of them …. I find it interesting that one of the biggest predictors of childhood or adolescent pill consumption is if a parent(s) is an advocate of supplements/pills and/or the child or adolescent has a higher household income and more optimal health [158–160]. This is in many cases precisely the group that does not need them as a preventive option (adult data is not much different).

• **You cannot trust health TV shows? Maybe you cannot just trust what TV shows claim about dietary supplements?**

A recent study of the "Dr Oz" show and "The Doctors" television shows found that often their advice is not accurate and conflict of interest is revealed less than 1 % of the time [161]! The conclusion of this large research study was the following:

> Recommendations made on medical talk shows often lack adequate information on specific benefits or the magnitude of the effects of these benefits. Approximately half of the recommendations have either no evidence or are contradicted by the best available evidence. Potential conflicts of interest are rarely addressed. The public should be skeptical about recommendations made on medical talk shows.

I was a featured guest on Dr. Oz and it was a lifestyle piece and it was a wonderful moment. In general TV health shows have provided some valuable advice especially in regard to practical or lifestyle changes. However, apparently these shows have also had some negative moments. Researchers randomly selected 40 episodes and reviewed 80 recommendations total from both shows [161]. Less than half the time there was evidence to support a claim and over 50 % of the time there was no evidence or contradictory evidence, and this was for the Dr. Oz show and The Doctors demonstrated slightly better results. And again, less than 1 % of the recommendations from these shows included information on conflicts of interest.

When these shows begin to especially recommend dietary supplements they ran into some trouble. I think this can be cleaned up but will it keep their audience? In other words, I believe there are many people that want to believe in magic potions and miracle weight loss products and quick fix it situations. In fact, when any media source from a magazine to the nightly news appears to endorse a dietary supplement it tends to feed the self-medication or pill solution appetite and psyche. However, when a health show no longer promotes countless quick fix products or ideas then what happens to the ratings. And part of what is also driving this criticism or cacophony to end these shows is that I believe there are a plethora of jealous health care professionals that would like to have their own TV show.

Regardless, these TV shows need to do a better job of referring to well-done research especially in the area of dietary supplements, and if you think about it for a second, when it comes to surgery or taking pills how can you decide what is right for you in a several minute segment? I like Doctor Oz and The Doctors just like I like some reality TV shows but I am not about to imbibe specialized advice from them or refer consumers to them as their primary resource, but rather a piece of their potential large health puzzle that contains a variety of pieces. The glass is half-full here but patients should be told if deciding or thinking about taking a supplement because of a short endorsement like TV segment then this is precisely why you need to be careful, because supplements like drug, need a detailed benefit-to-risk assessment before utilizing them. Over 25+ years I cannot name a single supplements whose hype was matched by the eventual research (not acai berry, green tea, lycopene, magnesium, shark cartilage, vitamin C, D, E, K, zinc, …).

• **Any other advice? Doctors know more than they think about supplements. Family disease trees for better communication and supplements for medical conditions. Recommending one brand of supplements? Why the future looks great! Ground-to-Gut or Dirt-to-Duodenum!**

Circle of Trust

This might sound simplistic but I tell patients and health care professionals they need to assemble a team that can be trusted in regard to supplements. Doctors get criticized a lot for not knowing about supplements (almost cliché) but many of them know everything else about the patient (arguably more than anyone apart from the patient herself or himself) in terms of their health and they should defend that position. Just because they don't have specialized knowledge in this area does not make them invalid. Arguably, the health food store expert or another interesting source of information for some patients does not have the head-to-toe medical information that the health care professional harbors, so it is critical that they know supplement intake. The medical literature is now replete with good and bad supplement information in medical journals so the average supplement knowledge of many physicians has increased substantially. Objective pharmacists are arguably the best source for drug–herb interactions and objective nutritionists know about which foods might substitute for a pill and an objective naturopath could provide the latest information on a particular herbal and the beat goes on and on. Assemble a team you can trust.

Additionally, I often encourage clinicians to review a patient's family disease tree and this allows for an objective discussion of what, if any, supplements are needed for an otherwise moderately healthy individual. If the family disease tree suggests heart disease or cancer or Alzheimer disease or autoimmune disease is prevalent in a particular family then the heart health lifestyle approach in the next chapter has ample information for most patients. Otherwise, if there is macular degeneration or migraines then one can discuss those particular supplements if needed in the future. All of this provides a healthy and transparent bidirectional dialogue between the patient and the physician and in my experience reduces the risk of a patient becoming mesmerized by the latest and greatest pill advertised on the television. Also, it keeps the focus of pill use (supplement or drug) on medical conditions or high-risk medical situations and not for antiaging or esoteric and obscure prevention purposes.

Recommend A Brand or Line of Supplements? No thanks. Just Reward the Research

I favor no brands and this is my job. I have to go into any situation with objectivity and the "please prove it to me approach." So, my first job is to reward the research by explaining to patients and the public the product that was used in the most impressive clinical trial that shows a benefit or harm. Next, for each and every condition I need to know quality control and safety data for the product and study. And finally are there are products with the same or potentially cheaper and safer ingredients? I tend to find that companies that lead with their own research and boast about their quality control are the ones that grab my attention. I treat every situation separately as a new story and rather than subscribing to a brand, I subscribe to the supplement that shined or not for the individual condition [25]. Petadolex or generic riboflavin for migraine prevention [72, 162], red yeast rice for cholesterol lowering from Sylvan Bioproducts, Kittanning, Pennsylvania was used in several good trials and was tested and free of a contaminant called "citrinin" that could be found in some red yeast rice supplement [163, 164]. SAM-e from Pharmavite used in a fabulous preliminary clinical trial from Massachusetts General/Harvard in patients that were not responding to their conventional antidepressant drugs [165, 166], but keep in mind that SAM-e is considered a drug in many other countries [25]. How about the probiotic product "Align" (Bifidobacterium infantis 35624 from Procter & Gamble) used in moderately impressive several clinical trials of IBS and should be discussed with patients as an option [167, 168]. And the best goes on and on …. Health care professionals could never endorse one pharmaceutical company and only their drugs as the best option for countless medical conditions because the research has never supported this activity, and so why would it be any different in the dietary supplement world.

Dirt-to-Duodenum and Ground-to-Guts?

Currently an individual can get an herbal from the dirt/ground in China and then have it arrived to a center in Brazil, which then combines that herbal with other ingredients from three other countries so by the time it hits the duodenum/gut the patient is getting raw and processed materials from around the world with no certification or process to trace these components throughout all the steps or stops it takes in the process. Imagine if a contaminant is found, then what lots or boxes need to be stopped or not shipped? This scenario is not uncommon because personally I recently witnessed a recall of supplements potentially contaminated with the antibiotic "chloramphenicol" from India. There were at least 25 companies that would have received this supplement from this supplier/manufacturer if this error were not detected in the supplements (voluntary recall) [169, 170]. Chloramphenicol can rarely cause bone marrow suppression or aplastic anemia in otherwise healthy individuals. The mistake was caught and product or lots in question recalled (it was fortunate the problem was discovered early in the process).

The past may be partially prologue. In the early 1990s, an epidemic of rapidly progressive interstitial renal fibrosis and renal failure occurred in young female patients in Belgium taking a weight loss supplement with Chinese herbs [171, 172]. The cause of this problem was aristolochic acid (AA) and the condition it caused is now known as aristolochic acid nephropathy or AAN. Over 100 patients were impacted during this time. An investigation revealed that one component in the weight loss regimen (*Stephania tetrandra*) was replaced by *Aristolochia fangchi*. Other case series have occurred all over the world (Australia, China, Europe, Japan, Korea, Taiwan, …). And the only risk factor identified for this renal disease is cumulative AA exposure or dose. Currently, it is also known that AA is associated with an increased risk of urothelial cancer (upper urinary tract and bladder). This association is independent of even arsenic exposure (another bladder carcinogen).

The mechanism of action suggests extensive DNA damage when exposed to this compound. In the USA, the FDA issued an alert in 2001 on AA and the seizure of any product with AA is in place.

And when my career started as a student in the late 1980s/early 1990s while at the College of Public Health at the University of South Florida, the L-tryptophan dietary supplement outbreak or eosinophilia–myalgia syndrome (EMS) occurred among some users of this product. More than 1500 cases were documented and over 30 deaths (6-month period) [173], and the State of Florida had one of the top three (along with California and New York) occurrences of cases. My job while in school was to interview these patients and their current symptoms. Ultimately, one of the most famous cases of supplement contamination was traced back to a company in Japan, which was a supplier to American supplement manufacturers. The ban on L-tryptophan was removed in 2005 and there are still some concerns about this product but how can this kind of chaos be prevented?

How can all of these past issues be prevented with current technology? In the future, I believe most supplement companies will need to subscribe to an independent third party quality control group to survive and thrive, such as NSF and others mentioned in this chapter. Additionally, at the time of this writing and for transparency sake, I own stock in the Park City Group (PCYG) because food and supplement companies that use their service are forced to comply with standards and transparency from dirt-to-duodenum and ground-to-guts [174]. In other words, it forces all of the groups up and down the supply chain to follow the rules (via software monitoring batch by batch and company by company) and monitor each and every player in the game! In other words, this and other software companies will be arriving soon that will allow a consumer to feel more comfortable about the source of their pills from ground-to-guts or dirt-to-duodenum.

There are also companies that are looking at better bar coding so that in the future you can scan the product and see where all the parts of your supplement came from and what is in it. For example, a company called "DNA TREK" currently allows customers to "trace fresh produce, protein and processed foods back to their source in minutes," or from "fork to farm traceability" [175]. A product is sprayed directly onto food products and only one billionth of a gram is adequate to trace the product back through the entire food chain process. This type of similar technology is being developed in the dietary supplement world. So, the glass is half-full but it is a little dirty, and by following some of these rules in the future, which I am confident will occur, the glass will be very clean!

Conclusion

Table 2.1 is a brief summary of the observations and advice proffered in this chapter.

Dietary supplements are a full-time job today as opposed to 25 years ago or should be a full-time job. The reason I see a lot of doctors get into trouble trying to

Table 2.1 Recommendations and observations proffered over a 25+ dietary supplement career

Dr. Moyad and his 25+ observations over 25+ years in the dietary supplement world	Dr. Moyad commentary
1. The difference between an effective drug and supplement is perception and not reality	Some of the most effective supplements sold in the USA are drugs in other countries (SAM-e for depression and osteoarthritis, melatonin for insomnia, …)
2. Supplements are not allowed to "diagnose, treat, cure, or prevent any disease"? Instead they are usually allowed structure and function claims like "supports" or "maintains" or "promotes _____ health"? For example, "bone," "digestive," "immune" health	This is precisely how they are used by clinicians today—to prevent or actually treat numerous medical conditions from chronic non-bacterial prostatitis to migraine prevention to neural tube defect prevention, to statin intolerance …. Some supplements using structure and function claims are of course hinting at a drug-like benefit (wink-wink)
3. There are almost countless examples of dietary supplements that are utilized like drugs by health care professionals, and there are examples of supplements that should not be used by health care professionals	– Alzheimer Disease (2000 IU from TEAM-AD VA Cooperative Trial) – Age-Related Macular Degeneration (AMD) and AREDS1 and AREDS2 Trials – Antiaging and the failure of significantly consistent results with resveratrol – BPH and the failure of Saw palmetto in US Trials (STEP and CAMUS) and the need for more research with the European drug-like product Permixon® – Breast and Prostate Cancer and the failure of multiple supplements, especially the potential increased risk of prostate cancer (Vitamin E-400 IU) and aggressive prostate cancer with a supplement (200 μg selenium) in healthy individuals – Dry Eye and/or high triglycerides and the benefit of omega-3 supplements – Erectile Dysfunction and the benefit of L-citrulline supplements – High cholesterol or statin intolerance and the benefit with red yeast rice – Low testosterone and the lack of effective supplements – Insomnia and melatonin including prolonged release (PR) melatonin – Migraine prevention and butterbur extract (also used for seasonal allergies) or riboflavin – Parkinson Disease and the clinical research ongoing with inosine (also with MS or ALS research) – UTI and the potential benefit over cranberry supplements (with a high concentration of proanthocyanicins) over juice and to prevent antibiotic resistance

4. Most dietary supplements starts as generics and then some become proprietary or patented versus pharmaceuticals where most start out with a patent and then eventually become generic	– Beware of many supplements just throwing together a proprietary blend of compounds and using someone else's research along with a celebrity or "expert" to promote their product that they actually have not adequately tested. And look for drug copycats in some of these products like "salicin" used in pain relieving supplements at a high price, which is metabolically altered basically into the same compound or active metabolite of low-cost aspirin
5. The primary goal with patients should be no or a minimum number of pills (supplement or prescription) and never to encourage self-medication	– Lifestyle changes are powerful and provide key information in making the decision of whether or not a pill is needed and/or the lowest dose needed when otherwise taking care of you or being followed by a medical professional
6. There is nothing "natural" about taking pills and there is nothing healthy about the natural versus synthetic debate	– Pill use is minimal in the areas of the world with the longest life expectancy except when needed for a medical condition – And most of what surrounds humans and what we utilize is also "not natural" unless we need them—cars, highways, cooling, heating, plumbing, toilets, airplanes AED device, … – Natural is better than synthetic when proven to be better. For example, natural vitamin E supplements have data that is no better clinically versus synthetic in major clinical trials (a synthetic vitamin E increased the risk of prostate cancer SELECT trial) and a natural vitamin E may have increased the risk of cardiovascular complications (HOPE TOO) in diabetics and those with vascular disease. A natural vitamin E supplement appears to help kids and adults with NAFLD/NASH (PIVENS and TONIC Trials) and a synthetic vitamin E appears to have helped Alzheimer patients (TEAM-AD VA Cooperative trial)
7. All pills have the potential for "tachyphylaxis" and "saturation kinetics," which is also why we need to always review benefit-versus-risk	– Desensitization to medications is known to occur with a variety of drugs over time and in some cases even higher dosages are needed for an impact and this encourages pill addiction. Some supplements for example arginine and others may also cause this in some individuals – Ingesting too much of a compound eventually causes saturation of the blood or tissue and the rest of the compound is discarded or increases to unhealthy levels. For example, vitamin C in excess increases the risk of kidney stones and selenium can get deposited in soft tissues and increase the risk of nail or hair loss, and perhaps even diabetes, skin cancer recurrence and other cancers in excessive amounts

(continued)

Table 2.1 (continued)

Dr. Moyad and his 25+ observations over 25+ years in the dietary supplement world	Dr. Moyad commentary
8. Increased awareness has increased the risk of novel prescription pill like side effects in supplements such as pill esophagitis, esophageal ulcers, silicon-based kidney stones …	– Pill esophagitis and esophageal ulcers are known to rarely occur in the drug world but it also can occur now in the supplement world. In addition, novel side effects from the pill itself such as silicon-based kidney stones from the excess of silicon dioxide (aka "sand") used in some supplements is a concern. Another reason pill consumption is not "natural" and should only be used when benefit>>>risk
9. Fluoride levels in drinking water are symbolic for the need to realize that we are experiencing overexposure to a variety of ingredients with recent societal advancements including the "over-antioxidation of the population" in some cases Medical education needs to shift from discussing antiquated disease deficiencies from the lack of a nutrient (Keshan disease from selenium deficiency for example or vitamin C and scurvy …) to modern day overexposure to certain nutrients	– The recent Department of Health and Human Services request to lower fluoride levels in drinking water was smart because over the past decade fluorosis was increasing from overexposure to fluoride not just from water, but also in toothpastes and mouthwashes. The cumulative exposure over time was becoming concerning and this is symbolic for the nutrition world – The ongoing additions of nutrients to food are reducing the need for some pills, for example calcium exposure in some beverages (almond milk=455 mg per 8-ounce serving in some products). Increased exposure to pills and food sources of the same nutrient could be hazardous such as selenium (SELECT Trial) and an increased risk of cancer, calcium supplement excess and kidney stones or constipation … – Medical education needs to shift from not just emphasizing third world nutrient or antiquated needs (vitamin C to prevent scurvy), but to also reflect modern day or "first world" overexposure (excess vitamin C creates increased oxalate levels in urine and risk of kidney stones) – Acetaminophen became the number 1 cause of acute liver failure when this compound began to be found not just in pain pills but half of the cold and flu remedies …

10. The only consistent or true deficiencies are related to chronic disease prevention or cardiovascular disease (stroke, hypertension, …) and these are potassium (RDA basically 4700 mg/day—only 1–2 % of the population complies with this intake and the average intake is 2500–2700 mg) and fiber (average intake 10–15 g and intake should be at least 20–30 g)	– Fiber and potassium are difficult to achieve goal because heart healthy foods contain them (we do not consume enough) and because we have relied on pills and powder that can never meet the needs in the case of fiber and potassium (potassium supplement pills are only allowed to have 99 mg or less in them and some fiber pills are needed in mega-quantities for only a 3–5 g intake) – Many deficiencies are actually created by the use of pills and lifestyle today, such as increased zinc supplement intake and copper deficiency, or acid reflux and B12 and magnesium deficiencies. Increased weight/waist gain increases the risk of being diagnosed with a vitamin D deficiency
11. Buzzwords like "inflammation," "free radicals," "boosts the immune system" help sales of pills but not objective education of patients and health care professionals. Remember the hygiene-hypothesis?	– Temporary inflammation, or even the generation of free radicals, is a critical signaling in the human body, which is needed to improve exercise performance and overall bodily function. Suppressing of these signals with the use of pills comes at a price. This is also what is observed in the drug world and may be the reason for increased diabetes risk in some high-dose statin users – Allergies and autoimmune disease are caused by "boosted immune systems" but detrimental to health. Optimal immune surveillance is really what is needed and many can achieve this effect without pill unless critically needed for example in melanoma treatment – Hygiene-hypothesis states that the lack of allowing exposure to pathogens or a somewhat unclean environment raises the risk of allergies and autoimmune disease. Thus, trying to prevent every acute illness with pills when not really needed could be detrimental in teaching the body how to respond adequately to these insults
12. "When you have a hammer everything looks like a nail, but when you have a mouth everything looks like a supplement"	– Surgeons are subject to jaded commentary on desiring to do surgery to fix something. However, this can actually occur in any field of medicine including supplements – There is no difference between a conventional doctor that pushes a drug out of conflict of interest and a naturopath or conventional doctor that pushes a supplement, because of conflict of interest. The goal with patients again is minimal pill reliance and independence and not complete dependence on you and the products you (the health care professional) proffers

(continued)

Table 2.1 (continued)

Dr. Moyad and his 25+ observations over 25+ years in the dietary supplement world	Dr. Moyad commentary
13. "US" versus "Them" maybe okay in politics but it is completely toxic in medicine	– Medicine is evidence-based and whether it is a supplement or a drug it should be utilized or avoided as needed. However, the terms "big pharma" is used by some major advocates of alternative medicine, and "snake oil" by some in conventional medicine. This serves no purpose but to polarize consumers and patients in one direction that supports these radical agendas. The art and practice of medicine essentially follows evidence and when there is a lack of evidence making sure this is transparent to patients because in the end it is arguably their choice to be treated. I am grateful to some drug companies and not so much for others, and this is also true of supplement companies (grateful for some and can't stand others)
14. FDA cGMP sounds good but needs help. Look for NSF ideally, or USP, or Informed Choice, or NPA … contrary to popular belief there is a lot of support to help you decide supplements with quality and those without quality or efficacy. NSF is arguably my favorite because NFL, MLB, NHL, PGA/LPGA, Olympic athletes and most major athletic organizations use them to keep athletes clean and it has worked well	– In 2007, the FDA cGMP rules helped to moderately clean up the industry but this ruling is similar to requiring a 55 MPH speed limit on the highway with few highway patrol officers. The need for third party oversight or proof of cGMP is critical. Look for NSF labels (on website or on bottle and they audit companies anywhere in the world every 6 months), but also USP and NPA are adequate as well, and "Informed Choice" for sports supplements (and NSF Certified for Sport). Now some of these companies like NSF are also offering gluten free certification and other benefits
15. Herbal supplements are a whole new and old wild animal, so make sure you treat them that way! Always look for some quality control seal/proof AND the standardized ingredient in the herbal that was found to be effective in the phase-3-like clinical trial for the medical condition it might reduce or resolve	– I am not as concerned about labeling issues on simple ingredients like vitamins and minerals as I am on herbals, because of the potential for contamination and the need to demonstrate an active standardized ingredient among the other herbal compounds in the pill. For this reason, I only recommend the herbal used in the definitive clinical trial for example ginseng from the Ginseng Board of Wisconsin when used in the Mayo Clinic reduction in fatigue trial (cancer-related fatigue or CRF). And I look for some definitive quality control measure or seal

16. Several other quality control sites and/or publications on herbal/supplements follow quality and/or efficacy and include some the following:
  – Center for Science in the Public Interest (CSPI or www.cspinet.org)
  – Consumerlab.com
  – ConsumerReports.org
  – The "Natural Medicines Comprehensive Database" (www.naturaldatabase.com)
	Other sources of information on dietary and supplement efficacy and quality are good including Center for Science in the Public interest (CSPI), consumerlab.com, consumer reports, and the "Natural Medicines Comprehensive Database." All of them come with some small to moderate fee but are worth it if you are taking supplements or thinking about using them or even recommending them

17. Pharmaceutical brand supplements have a lot to lose if they are wrong (Note: this does not mean I endorse any of these brands or want you to take one but it is a simple tip for comparison guidance, for example how does your multivitamin compare to Centrum Silver in price, research, quality, ...). Quality control is rarely an issue—aka what it says on the label is in the bottle with pharma brands	– Pharmaceutical brand supplements known for their drugs (Bayer, Pfizer) have excellent quality control and also many are cost-competitive. The largest multivitamin trial in the world utilized a pharmaceutical brand (Centrum Silver® in the PHS2 trial). They need to continue to provide cleaner products but some of these options are at least partially evidence based (Centrum, or Align®-B. infantis 35624 by Procter & Gamble ...).
18. Multivitamin with herbal ingredients? No thanks!	The two largest multivitamin trials in the world were SU.VI.MAX (five ingredients) and PHS2 (or PHSII-30 ingredients) and both products used a limited or low number of ingredients and dosages (both were one pill a day) and did not include any herbal products. And the risk of adding an herbal to a multivitamin is not worth it and it is not even evidence based now or anytime soon
19. Only purchase a single ingredient supplement most of the time except in rare situations (like a multivitamin or when trial specifies/utilizes more than one ingredient, which is rare). Dilution = Pollution? Don't be a clinical trial of 1! Proof and reward should be in the research and again in standardization of the active ingredient!	– Most supplements for medical conditions consist of one ingredient or one standardized ingredient with a few exceptions (multivitamin, macular degeneration, ...). Multiple ingredients without evidence of efficacy and safety potentially dilute and pollutes the active ingredient and increases the risk of toxicity – For example, you would never buy an aspirin pill with ten ingredients in it for pain relief or heart protection or when given to someone having a heart attack. Melatonin and insomnia, and SAM-e and depression, or American ginseng standardized to 3–5 % ginsenoside ... all have that one compound that was the result of a benefit usually in a clinical trial

(continued)

Table 2.1 (continued)

Dr. Moyad and his 25+ observations over 25+ years in the dietary supplement world	Dr. Moyad commentary
20. Always reevaluate your situation and do not be afraid to be a part-time guinea pig (if benefit>risk). The A, B, C's of whether a pill is working and if you really need it! Look for non-pill pill-like options (the new calcium supplement)?!	We should embrace and celebrate a person when they are so healthy or getting healthier they need little to no pills or lower dosages. Still, I apply A, B and C rules (three of them) to determine if patients or individuals need a pill or supplement *A. Subjective Test (aka guinea pig approach)* Stop the product for 1 month at least and tell me if you feel any better, or worse, or the same? *B. Objective Test (aka laboratory or numbers approach)* Is the supplement you are taking changing any single important parameter that suggests you are becoming more healthy? Cholesterol, blood pressure, blood sugar, weight, … *C. Lifestyle Test (to reduce or determine pill count/dosage)* Is there a lifestyle change that can get me off this pill or at least reduce the dosage?
21. Do patients really need comprehensive testing via blood or genetics to determine their nutritional deficiencies if they are otherwise healthy? No. And get ready to buy a pill! Remember genes can also be changed in some situations like "jeans"	– The FDA did a good job of exposing the fact that some genetic tests would tell you your chance of getting a disease but in reality did not have that kind of research to really predict this, so you end up creating a number of people that just live with a lot of unnecessary anxiety. Patients should be told that in some cases even when a genetic test demonstrates some risk, lifestyle changes can alter risk or even prevent that gene from being ultimately expressed (just because you have a gene does not mean you will express the clinical endpoint of that gene) – Another example of over testing the population for nutrient issues should be exemplified in the "homocysteine" blood test used by many companies to generally screen asymptomatic healthy individuals and place some patients on high-dose B-vitamins – Some nutritional blood tests also simply change dramatically in your favor with lifestyle changes such as weight loss such as vitamin D. And many nutritional tests or specific assay have simply not been validated with any hard clinical endpoints (vitamin D …) – What is the first thing I see patients get when some blood comprehensive nutrient panel demonstrates that something is low? A recommendation to buy a high priced supplement from the same office that provided the blood testing or an office that recommends a supplement and gets paid on the back end without being transparent of that fact! That is a clear conflict of interest. When you sell supplements especially out of your office "everything looks like a mouth"

22. What then is my best advice for determining what supplements an otherwise healthy person could need? Supplements are primarily for medical conditions and targeted dieting once again to the rescue	Supplements mirror drugs in that they can be life altering or life wrecking in the wrong person. Supplements should be primarily used for high-risk medical conditions or medical conditions themselves – Currently in cancer supplements look like a good option to reduce some side effects of treatment and not for treatment itself (ginseng for cancer-related fatigue, ginger for chemotherapy-induced nausea, melatonin for insomnia, protein powder for weight loss or gain …) – Targeted dieting involves getting rid of a pill because of sufficient targeting of foods/beverages high in the nutrient of interest (calcium from foods and beverages and no longer in need of the supplement is easier than ever and so is vitamin D …)
23. When does the medical research suggest about the form of the supplement that should be ingested? Tablets? Capsules? Liquids? What should patients know about this and the best time of the day or situation to ingest a supplement for maximum efficacy? How about the half-life of supplements in the body? Following the path of compliance and flexibility and with ongoing aging metabolism, intestine, kidney, liver, … changes (we also age on the inside). Never forget "20 %"? Children, adolescents and supplements?	– The answer is similar to the drug world, where compliance is the biggest issue and everything else is a distant second – In the famous Women's Health Initiative (WHI)—the largest clinical trial of calcium and vitamin D in the world to prevent bone loss and hip fractures published a decade ago many people still believe the supplements did not work! However, a secondary look at the same trial actually showed for the women that took their supplements most days of the month (80 % of the time) they did work in slowing bone loss and preventing hip fractures by almost 30 % – Most of the time when a supplement says ingest "with a meal" it is to reduce gastrointestinal side effects and improve compliance and memory – My old saying about absorption I have been using for over 25 year, and that is "if you can hit a baseball 500 feet in Detroit Tiger Stadium then it is called a home run but if you can hit a baseball 500 miles into Canada from Tiger stadium then this is so impressive that I am sure you will make a lot of money in endorsement deals but it still counts as a home run!" Absorption is oversold – Groundbreaking drugs, such as metformin, were found to have reduced absorption with food, but this increased compliance (lowered gastrointestinal complications), which resulted in lowering the risk of type-2 diabetes or still providing adequate weight loss. Iron supplements appear to operate this way – 20 % of serious hepatotoxic events in the USA last year occurred with supplements and in generally healthy people. So, again take a supplement that has been tested if you qualify. Do not be a clinical trial of one! – The healthy kids of today that take pills are the adults of tomorrow that ingest more pills. And the parents that take pills usually are the kids that take pills

(continued)

Table 2.1 (continued)

Dr. Moyad and his 25+ observations over 25+ years in the dietary supplement world	Dr. Moyad commentary
24. You cannot trust health TV shows? Maybe you cannot just trust what TV shows claim about dietary supplements?	– A recent study of the Dr. Oz show and The Doctors television shows found that often their advice is not accurate and conflict of interest is revealed less than 1 % of the time – These shows do offer some very good advice especially on lifestyle and diet but appear to run into trouble when recommending supplements. Regardless, no pill should be suddenly ingested because of a short segment on a TV show. Instead use TV advice as part of the larger discussion of the health of the overall patient (one piece of the larger health puzzle)
25. Any other advice? Doctors know more than they think about supplements. Family disease trees for better communication and supplements for medical conditions. Recommending one brand of supplements? Why the future looks great! Ground-to-Gut or Dirt-to-Duodenum!	– Doctors know more than they think about supplements – Recommending a supplement line exclusively is like recommending one pharmaceutical line of drugs exclusively?! Let the evidence lead to the specific supplement brand recommendation (hey, like with drugs). I recommend Petadolex for migraine prevention, Pharmavite for SAM-e, Align for some IBS, Sylvan Bioproducts for red yeast rice … and the beat goes on! – Dirt-to-Duodenum and Ground-to-Guts is what new software and third party seals will allow in the future. Supplement companies should be required to sign up with one of these companies in order to sell their products. And it reduces their insurance costs and litigation – The future looks bright because transparency software and testing I believe will become a part of the supplement business (it is now in many cases—moving into food safety and next into supplements)

interpret the supplement research is they think they can dabble in this field and provide all the answers but the days of dabbling are over. It is time to respect that fact that over 5000 articles in diet and supplements are published yearly and this requires your full (not part-time) attention. Imagine if I dabbled in orthopedic surgery or dermatology … would one really then wonder why things could go very wrong and inaccuracies would abound?!

Still, the advice proffered in this chapter has provided a foundation for teaching and instructing and helping consumers and patients around the world. The field of dietary supplements appears bright because the sheer amount of clinical research has increased exponentially, and determining what is working and what is worthless gets easier year-to-year. On the other hand, it is a business and the good side of that business is more options for patients and the nefarious sides is also more trickery for some patients that I observe get financially abused and become no more salubrious or hurt. Yet it starts with the clinician because I have always argued that wherever I have traveled in the world patients want to hear these answers to their questions from you (the clinician), and if you are not able to objectively answer them, then going to less credible sources down the street will become the norm.

References

1. Moyad MA. The supplement handbook: a trusted expert's guide to what works & what's worthless for more than 100 conditions. New York: Rodale Publishing; 2014.
2. O'Connor A. New York Attorney General targets supplements at major retailers, 3 Feb 2015. wee.blogs.nytimes.com/2015/02/03/new-york-attorney-general-targets-supplements-at-major-retailers/?_r=0 Accessed 1 June 2015.
3. Esch M of Associated Press. Supplements industry derides NY attorney general's DNA tests, 8 Feb 2015. http://abcnews.go.com/Health/wireStory/supplements-industry-derides-ny-attorney-generals-dna-tests-28812984?page=2. Accessed 1 June 2015.
4. Newmaster SG, Grguric M, Shanmughanandhan D, Ramalingam S, Ragupathy S. DNA barcoding detects contamination and substitution in North American herbal products. BMC Med. 2013;11:222.
5. US Food and Drug Administration. What is a dietary supplement? www.fda.gov/AboutFDA/Transparency/Basics/ucm195635.htm. Accessed 1 June 2015.
6. Nahin RL, Barnes PM, Stussman BJ, Bloom B. Costs of complementary and alternative (CAM) and frequency of visits to CAM practitioners: United States, 2007. Natl Health Stat Report 2009;(18):1–14.
7. Bradley J. NBJ: the US supplement industry is 37 billion, not $12 billion. http://www.nutraingredients-usa.com/Markets/NBJ-The-US-supplement-industry-is-37-billion-not-12billion/?utm_source=newsletter_daily&utm_medium=email&utm_campaign=01-Jun-2015&c=Ql8IFB6tgmvkRJlzON1mnozAbR4uHGGV&p2=. Accessed 5 June 2015.
8. Papakostas GI. Evidence for S-adenosyl-L-methionine (SAM-e) for the treatment of major depressive disorder. J Clin Psychiatry. 2009;70 Suppl 5:18–22.
9. Soeken KL, Lee WL, Bausell RB, Agelli M, Berman BM. Safety and efficacy of S-adenosylmethionine (SAMe) for osteoarthritis. J Fam Pract. 2002;51:425–30.
10. Morelli V, Naquin C, Weaver V. Alternative therapies for traditional disease states: osteoarthritis. Am Fam Physician. 2003;67:339–44.
11. US FDA. Structure/function claims. http://www.fda.gov/Food/IngredientsPackagingLabeling/LabelingNutrition/ucm2006881.htm.

12. Moyad MA. Dr. Moyad's no BS diet health advice: a step-by-step guide to what works and what's worthless. Ann Arbor: Spry Publishing; 2008.

13. Dysken MW, Sano M, Asthana S, Vertees JE, Pallaki M, Llorente M, et al. Effect of vitamin E and memantine on functional decline in Alzheimer disease: the TEAM-AD VA Cooperative Randomized Trial. JAMA. 2014;311:33–44.

14. Sano M, Ernesto C, Thomas RG, Klauber MR, Schafer K, Grundman M, et al. A controlled trial of selegiline, alpha-tocopherol, or both as treatment for Alzheimer's disease. The Alzheimer's Disease Cooperative Study. N Engl J Med. 1997;336:1216–22.

15. Cummings JL, Morstorf T, Zhong K. Alzheimer's disease drug-development pipeline: few candidates, frequent failures. Alzheimers Res Ther. 2014;6:37. https://my.clevelandclinic.org/about-cleveland-clinic/newsroom/releases-videos-newsletters/cleveland-clinic-researchers-identify-urgent-need-for-alzheimers-disease-drug-development. Accessed 1 June 2015.

16. Dysken MW, Kirk LN, Kuskowski M. Changes in vitamin E prescribing for Alzheimer patients. Am J Geriatr Psychiatry. 2009;17:621–4.

17. Russ TC, Morling JR. Cholinesterase inhibitors for mild cognitive impairment. Cochrane Database Syst Rev. 2012;9:D009132.

18. Birks J. Cholinesterase inhibitors for Alzheimer's disease. Cochrane Database Syst Rev. 2006;1(1):CD005593.

19. Petersen RC, Thomas RG, Grundman M, Bennett D, Doody R, Ferris S, et al., for the Alzheimer Disease Cooperative Study Group. Vitamin E and donepezil for the treatment of mild cognitive impairment. N Engl J Med 2005;352:2379–88.

20. Age-Related Eye Disease Study Research Group. A randomized, placebo-controlled, clinical trial of high-dose supplementation with vitamins C and E, beta-carotene, and zinc for age-related macular degeneration and vision loss: AREDS report no. 8. Arch Ophthalmol. 2001;119:1417–36.

21. Chew EY, Clemons TE, Agron E, Sperduto RD, Sangiovanni JP, Kurinij N, et al., for the Age-Related Eye Disease Study Research Group. Long-term effects of vitamins C and E, β-carotene, and zinc on age-related macular degeneration: AREDS report no. 35. Ophthalmology 2013;120:1604–11.

22. Age-Related Eye Disease Study 2-AREDS2 Research Group. Lutein + zeaxanthin and omega-3 fatty acids for age-related macular degeneration: the Age-Related Eye Disease Study 2 (AREDS2) randomized clinical trial. JAMA. 2013;309:2005–15.

23. Yoshino J, et al. Resveratrol supplementation does not improve metabolic function in nonobese women with normal glucose tolerance. Cell Metab. 2012;16:658–64.

24. Popat R, Plesner T, Davies F, et al. A phase 2 study of SRT501 (resveratrol) with bortezomib for patients with relapsed and or refractory multiple myeloma. Br J Haematol. 2013;16:714–7.

25. Moyad MA. Complementary medicine for prostate & urologic disease. New York: Springer Publishing; 2014.

26. Poulsen MM, et al. High-dose resveratrol supplementation in obese men. Diabetes. 2013; 62:1186–95.

27. Wilt TJ, Ishani A, Stark G, MacDonald R, Lau J, Mulrow C. Saw palmetto extracts for treatment of benign prostatic hyperplasia: a systematic review. JAMA. 1998;280:1604–9.

28. Wilt T, Ishani A, Mac Donald R. Serenoa repens for benign prostatic hyperplasia. Cochrane Database Syst Rev. 2002;3:CD001423.

29. Tacklind J, MacDonald R, Rutks I, Wilt TJ. Serenoa repens for benign prostatic hyperplasia. Cochrane Database Syst Rev. 2009;2:CD001423.

30. MacDonald R, Tacklind JW, Rutks I, Wilt TJ. Serenoa repens monotherapy for benign prostatic hyperplasia (BPH): an updated Cochrane systematic review. BJU Int. 2012; 109:1756–61.

31. Bent S, Kane C, Shinohara K, Neuhaus J, Hudes ES, Goldberg H, et al. Saw palmetto for benign prostatic hyperplasia (BPH). N Engl J Med. 2006;354:557–66.

32. Barry MJ, Meleth S, Lee JY, Kreder KJ, Avins AL, Nickel JC, et al., for the Complementary and Alternative Medicine for Urological Symptoms (CAMUS) Study Group. Effect of

increasing doses of saw palmetto extract on lower urinary tract symptoms: a randomized trial. JAMA 2011;306:1344–51.

33. Bauer CM, Ishak MB, Johnson EK, Beebe-Dimmer JL, Cooney KA. Prevalence and correlates of vitamin and supplement usage among men with a family history of prostate cancer. Integr Cancer Ther. 2012;11:83–9.

34. Uzzo RG, Brown JG, Horwitz EM, Hanlon A, Mazzoni S, Konski A, et al. Prevalence and patterns of self-initiated nutritional supplementation in men at high risk of prostate cancer. BJU Int. 2004;93:955–60.

35. Debruyne F, Koch G, Boyle P, Da Silva FC, Gillenwater JG, Hamdy FC, et al. Comparison of a phytotherapeutic agent (Permixon) with an alpha-blocker (Tamsulosin) in the treatment of benign prostatic hyperplasia: a 1-year randomized international study. Eur Urol. 2002; 41:497–507.

36. Debruyne F, Boyle P, Calais Da Silva F, Gillenwater JG, Hamdy FC, Perrin P, et al. Evaluation of the clinical benefit of permixon and tamsulosin in severe BPH patients-PERMAL study subset analysis. Eur Urol. 2004;45:773–9.

37. Raynaud JP, Cousse H, Martin PM. Inhibition of type 1 and type-2 5alpha-reductase activity by free fatty acids, active ingredients of Permixon. J Steroid Biochem Mol Biol. 2002; 82:233–9.

38. Di Silverio F, Monti S, Sclarra A, Varasano PA, Martini C, Lanzara S, et al. Effects of long-term treatment with Serenoa repens (Permixon) on the concentration and regional distribution of androgens and epidermal growth factor in benign prostatic hyperplasia. Prostate. 1998;37:77–83.

39. Nickel JC, Sander S, Moon TD. A meta-analysis of the vascular-related safety profile and efficacy of alpha-adrenergic blockers for symptoms related to benign prostatic hyperplasia. Int J Clin Pract. 2008;62:1547–59.

40. Roehrborn CG, Siami P, Barkin J, Damiao R, Becher E, Minana B, et al., for the CombAT Study Group. The influence of baseline parameters on changes in international prostate symptom score with dutasteride, tamsulosin, and combination therapy among men with symptomatic benign prostatic hyperplasia and an enlarged prostate: 2-year data from the CombAT study. Eur Urol 2009;55:461–71.

41. Wagenlehner FM, Weidner W. Prostatitis: no benefit of alpha-blockers for chronic prostatitis. Nat Rev Urol. 2009;6:183–4.

42. Nickel JC, Krieger JN, McNaughton-Collins M, Anderson RU, Pontari M, Shoskes DA, et al. Alfuzosin and symptoms of chronic prostatitis-chronic pelvic pain syndrome. N Engl J Med. 2008;359:2663–73.

43. Kristal AR, Darke AK, Morris S, Tangen CM, Goodman PJ, Thompson IM, et al. Baseline selenium status and effects of selenium and vitamin E supplementation on prostate cancer risk. J Natl Cancer Inst. 2014;106(3):djt456.

44. Mozaffarian D, Marchiolli R, Macchia A, Silletta MG, Ferrazzi P, Gardner TJ, et al. Fish oil and postoperative atrial fibrillation: the Omega-3 Fatty Acids for Prevention of Post-operative Atrial Fibrillation (OPERA) randomized trial. JAMA. 2012;308:2001–11.

45. Risk and Prevention Study Collaborative Group. N-3 fatty acids in patients with multiple cardiovascular risk factors. N Engl J Med. 2013;368:1800–8.

46. Rand AL, Asbell PA. Nutritional supplements for dry eye syndrome. Curr Opin Ophthalmol. 2011;22:279–82.

47. Foulks GN, Forstot SL, Donshik PC, Goldstein MH, Lemp MA, Nelson JD, et al. Clinical guidelines for management of dry eye associated with Sjogren Disease. Ocul Surf. 2015; 13:118–32.

48. Bhargava R, Kumar P. Oral omega-3 fatty acid treatment for dry eye in contact lens wearers. Cornea. 2015;34:413–20.

49. Liu A, Ji J. Omega-3 essential fatty acids therapy for dry eye syndrome: a meta-analysis of randomized controlled studies. Med Sci Monit. 2014;20:1583–9.

50. DREAM (Dry Eye Assessment and Management) Clinical Trial. https://clinicaltrials.gov/ct2/show/NCT02128763?term=dream%26rank=5. Accessed 1 June 2015.

51. Fish   101.   http://www.heart.org/HEARTORG/GettingHealthy/NutritionCenter/Fish-101_UCM_305986_Article.jsp#aha_recommendation. Accessed 1 June 2015.
52. Blair HA, Dhillon S. Omega-3 carboxylic acids (Epanova): a review of its use in patients with severe hypertriglyceridemia. Am J Cardiovasc Drugs. 2014;14:393–400.
53. Zhao A, Lam S. Omega-3-carboxylic acid (epanova) for hypertriglyceridemia. Cardiol Rev. 2015;23:148–52.
54. Cormio L, De Siati M, Lorusso F, Selvaggio O, Mirabella L, Sanguedolce F, et al. Oral-L-citrulline supplementation improves erection hardness in men with mild erectile dysfunction. Urology. 2011;77:119–22.
55. Wax B, Kavazis AN, Weldon K. Sperlak. J Strength Cond Res. 2015;29:786–92.
56. Liu J, Zhang J, Shi Y, et al. Chinese red yeast rice (Monascus purpureus) for primary hyperlipidemia: a meta-analysis of randomized controlled trials. Chin Med. 2006;1:4.
57. China Coronary Secondary Prevention Study Group. China coronary secondary prevention study (CCSPS)-Lipid regulating therapy with xuezhikang for secondary prevention of coronary heart disease. Chin J Cardiol (Chin). 2005;33:109–15.
58. Ong HT. The statin studies: from targeting hypercholesterolemia to targeting the high risk patient. QJM. 2005;98:599–614.
59. Zhao SP, Lu ZL, Du BM, et al., Xuezhikang, an extract of cholestin, reduces cardiovascular events in type 2 diabetes patients with coronary heart disease: subgroup analysis of patients with type 2 diabetes from China Coronary Secondary Prevention Study (CCSPS). J Cardiovasc Pharmacol 2007;49:81–4.
60. Ye P, Lu ZL, Du BM, et al., for the CCSPS Investigators. Effects of xuezhikang on cardiovascular events and mortality in elderly patients with a history of myocardial infarction: a subgroup analysis of elderly subjects from China coronary secondary prevention study. J Am Geriatr Soc 2007;55:1015–22.
61. Li JJ, Lu ZL, Kou WR, et al., for the Chinese Coronary Secondary Prevention Study (CCSPS) Group. Long-term effects of Xuezhikang on blood pressure in hypertensive patients with previous myocardial infarction: data from the Chinese Coronary Secondary Prevention Study (CCSPS). Clin Exp Hypertens 2010;32(8):491–8.
62. Huang CF, Li TC, Lin CC, et al. Efficacy of Monascus purpureus Went rice on lowering lipid ratios in hypercholesterolemic patients. Eur J Cardiovasc Prev Rehabil. 2007;14:438–40.
63. Lin CC, Li TC, Lai MM. Efficacy and safety of Monascus purpureus Went rice in subjects with hyperlipidemia. Eur J Endocrinol. 2005;153:679–86.
64. Heber D, Yip I, Ashley JM, et al. Cholesterol-lowering effects of a proprietary Chinese red-yeast-rice dietary supplement. Am J Clin Nutr. 1999;69:231–6.
65. Moyad MA, Klotz LH. Statin clinical trial (REALITY) for prostate cancer: an over 15-year wait is finally over thanks to a dietary supplement. Urol Clin North Am. 2011;38:325–31.
66. Zanardi M, Quirico E, Benvenuti C, Pezzana A. Use of a lipid-lowering food supplement in patients on hormone therapy following breast cancer. Minerva Ginecol. 2012;64:431–5.
67. Poole C, Bushey B, Foster C, Campbell B, Willoughby D, Kreider R, et al. The effects of a commercially available botanical supplement on strength, body composition, power output, and hormonal profiles in resistance-trained males. J Int Soc Sports Nutr. 2010;7:34.
68. Lyseng-Williamson KA. Melatonin prolonged release: in the treatment of insomnia in patients aged ≥55 years. Drugs Aging. 2012;29:911–23.
69. Chen WY, Giobbie-Hurder A, Gantman K, Savoie J, Scheib R, Parker LM, et al. A randomized, placebo-controlled trial of melatonin on breast cancer survivors: impact on sleep, mood, and hot flashes. Breast Cancer Res Treat. 2014;145:381–8.
70. Hansen MV, Andersen LT, Madsen MT, Hagerman I, Rasmussen LS, Bokmand S, et al. Effect of melatonin on depressive symptoms and anxiety in patients undergoing breast cancer surgery: a randomized, double-blind, placebo-controlled trial. Breast Cancer Res Treat. 2014;145:683–95.
71. FDA Drug Safety Communication: FDA warns of next-day impairment with sleep aid Lunesta (eszopiclone) and lowers recommended dose. http://www.fda.gov/Drugs/DrugSafety/ucm397260.htm. Accessed 1 June 2015.

72. Holland S, et al., for the Quality Standards Subcommittee of the American Academy of Neurology and the American Headache Society. Evidence-based guideline update: NSAIDs and other complementary treatments for episodic migraine prevention in adults: report of the Quality Standards Subcommittee of the American Academy of Neurology and the American Headache Society. Neurology 2012;78:1346–53.

73. Parkinson Study Group SURE-PD Investigators. Inosine to increase serum and cerebrospinal fluid urate in Parkinson disease: a randomized clinical trial. JAMA Neurol. 2014;71: 141–50.

74. Elm JJ, NINDS NET-PD Investigators. Design innovations and baseline findings in a long-term Parkinson's Trial: the National Institute of Neurological Disorders and Stroke Exploratory Trials in Parkinson's Disease Long-Term Study-1. Mov Disord. 2012;27: 1513–21.

75. Writing Group for the NINDS Exploratory Trials in Parkinson Disease (NET-PD) Investigators. Effect of creatine monohydrate on clinical progression in patients with Parkinson disease: a randomized clinical trial. JAMA. 2015;313:584–93.

76. Jepson RG, Williams G, Craig JC. Cranberries for preventing urinary tract infections. Cochrane Database Syst Rev. 2012;10:CD001321.

77. Micali S, Isgro G, Bianchi G, Miceli N, Calapai G, Navarra M. Cranberry and recurrent cystitis: more than marketing? Crit Rev Food Sci Nutr. 2014;54:1063–75.

78. Ledda A, Bottari A, Luzzi R, Belcaro G, Hu S, Dugall M, et al. Cranberry supplementation in the prevention of non-severe lower urinary tract infections: a pilot study. Eur Rev Med Pharmacol Sci. 2015;19:77–80.

79. Caljouw MA, van den Hout WB, Putler H, Achterberg WP, Cools HJ, Gussekloo J. Effectiveness of cranberry capsules to prevent urinary tract infections in vulnerable older persons: a double-blind randomized placebo-controlled trial in long-term care facilities. J Am Geriatr Soc. 2014;62:103–10.

80. Miller PE, Alexander DD, Perez V. Effects of whey protein and resistance exercise on body composition: a meta-analysis of randomized controlled trials. J Am Coll Nutr. 2014;33: 163–75.

81. Jones PJ, AbuMweis SS. Phytosterols as functional food ingredients: linkages to cardiovascular disease and cancer. Curr Opin Clin Nutr Metab Care. 2009;12:147–51.

82. Berryman CE, Preston AG, Karmally W, Deckelbaum RJ, Kris-Etherton PM. Effects of almond consumption on the reduction of LDL-cholesterol: a discussion of potential mechanisms and future research directions. Nutr Rev. 2011;69:171–85.

83. Aldemir M, Okulu E, Neselioglu S, Erel O, Kayigil O. Pistachio diet improves erectile function parameters and serum lipid profiles in patients with erectile dysfunction. Int J Impot Res. 2011;23:32–8.

84. Guardamagna O, Abello F, Baracco V, et al. Primary hyperlipidemias in children: effect of plant sterol supplementation on plasma lipids and markers of cholesterol synthesis and absorption. Acta Diabetol. 2011;48(2):127–33. Epub 6 Nov 2010.

85. Malinkowski JM, Gehret MM. Phytosterols for dyslipidemia. Am J Health Syst Pharm. 2010;67:1165–73.

86. Hamilton P. Role of ezetimibe in the management of patients with atherosclerosis. Coron Artery Dis. 2009;20:169–74.

87. Dujovne CA, Suresh R, McCrary Sisk C, et al. Safety and efficacy of ezetimibe monotherapy in 1624 primary hypercholesterolaemic patients for up to 2 years. Int J Clin Pract. 2008; 62:1332–6.

88. Pelton K, Di Vizio D, Insabato L, et al. Ezetimibe reduces enlarged prostate in an animal model of benign prostatic hyperplasia. J Urol. 2010;184:1555–9.

89. Mills IW, Crossland A, Patel A, Ramonas H. Atorvastatin treatment for men with lower urinary tract symptoms and benign prostatic enlargement. Eur Urol. 2007;52:503–9.

90. Stamatiou KN, Zaglavira P, Skolarikos A, Sofras F. The effects of lovastatin on conventional medical treatment of lower urinary tract symptoms with finasteride. Int Braz J Urol. 2008;34:555–61.

91. Hall SA, Chiu GR, Link CL, et al. Are statin medications associated with lower urinary tract symptoms in men and women? Results from the Boston Area Community Health (BACH) Survey. Ann Epidemiol. 2011;21:149–55.
92. St Sauver JL, Jacobsen SJ, Jacobson DJ, et al. Statin use and decreased risk of benign prostatic enlargement and lower urinary tract symptoms. BJU Int. 2011;107:443–50.
93. Padayatty SJ, Marcelli M, Shao TC, Cunningham GR. Lovastatin-induced apoptosis in prostate stromal cells. J Clin Endocrinol Metab. 1997;82:1434–9.
94. Freeman MR, Solomon KR. Cholesterol and benign prostate disease. Differentiation. 2011;82:244–52.
95. Wilt TJ, Macdonald R, Ishani A. B-sitosterol for the treatment of benign prostatic hyperplasia: a systematic review. BJU Int. 1999;83:976–83.
96. Wilt TJ, Ishani A, MacDonald R, Stark G, Mulrow CD, Lau J. Beta-sitosterols for benign prostatic hyperplasia. Cochrane Database Syst Rev. 2000;2:CD001043.
97. Kadow C, Abrams PH. A double-blind trial of the effect of beta-sitosteryl glucoside (WA184) in the treatment of benign prostatic hyperplasia. Eur Urol. 1986;12:187–9.
98. Fischer A, Jurincic-Winkler CD, Klippel KF. Conservative treatment of benign prostatic hyperplasia with high-dosage b-sitosterol (65 mg): results of a placebo-controlled double-blind study. Uroscopy. 1993;1:12–20.
99. Berges RR, Windeler J, Trampisch HJ, Senge T. Randomised, placebo-controlled, double-blind clinical trial of beta-sitosterol in patients with benign prostatic hyperplasia. Beta-sitosterol Study Group. Lancet. 1995;345(8964):1529–32.
100. Kippel KF, Hiltl DM, Schipp B. A multicentric, placebo-controlled, double-blind clinical trial of b-sitosterol (phytosterol) for the treatment of benign prostatic hyperplasia. Br J Urol. 1997;80:427–32.
101. National Cholesterol Education Program (NCEP) Expert Panel on Detection, Evaluation, and Treatment of High Blood Cholesterol in Adults (Adult Treatment Panel III). Third report of the National Cholesterol Education Program (NCEP) Expert Panel on Detection, Evaluation, and Treatment of High Blood Cholesterol in Adults (Adult Treatment Panel III) final report. Circulation. 2002;106:3143–421.
102. Grattan Jr BJ. Plant sterols as anticancer nutrients: evidence for their role in breast cancer. Nutrients. 2013;5:359–87.
103. Cannon CP, Blazing MA, Giugilano RP, McCagg A, White JA, Theroux P, et al., for the IMPROVE-IT investigators. Ezetimibe added to statin therapy after acute coronary syndromes. N Engl J Med 2015;372(25):2387–97, Epub 3 June 2015.
104. Solomon KR, Pelton K, Boucher K, Joo J, Tully C, Zurakowski D, et al. Ezetimibe is an inhibitor of tumor angiogenesis. Am J Pathol. 2009;174:1017–26.
105. Ruiz ME. Risks of self-medication practices. Curr Drug Saf. 2010;5:315–23.
106. McRorie JW, Kirby JA, Miner PB. Histamine2-receptor antagonists: rapid development of tachyphylaxis with repeat dosing. World J Gastrointest Pharmacol Ther. 2014;5:57–62.
107. Targum SD. Identification and treatment of antidepressant tachyphylaxis. Innov Clin Neurosci. 2014;11(3–4):24–8.
108. Cromwell WC, Ziajka PE. Development of tachyphylaxis among patients taking HMG CoA reductase inhibitors. Am J Cardiol. 2000;86:1123–7.
109. Klemenska E, Beresewicz A. Bioactivation of organic nitrates and the mechanism of nitrate tolerance. Cardiol J. 2009;16:11–9.
110. Malczewska-Malec M, Goldsztajn P, Kawecka-Jaszcz K, Czamecka D, Siedlecki A, Siemienska T, et al. Effects of prolonged L-arginine administration on blood pressure in patients with essential hypertension (EH). Agents Actions Suppl. 1995;45:157–62.
111. Manson JE, Bassuk SS. Calcium supplements: do they help or harm? Menopause. 2014; 21:106–8.
112. Thomas LDK, Elinder C-G, Tiselius H-G, Wolk A, Akesson A. Ascorbic acid supplements and kidney stone incidence among men: a prospective study. JAMA Intern Med. 2013; 173:386–8.

113. Dag MS, Ozurk ZA, Akin I, Tutar E, Cikman O, Gulsen MT. Drug-induced esophageal ulcers: case series and the review of the literature. Drug-induced esophageal ulcers: case series and the review of the literature. Turk J Gastroenterol. 2014;25:180–4.

114. Gallego Perez B, Martinez Crespo JJ, Garcia Belmonte D, Marin Bernabe CM. L-Arginine pill induced esophageal ulcer: causes not reported previously esophagitis for pills. Farm Hosp. 2014;38:487–9.

115. Flythe JE, Rueda JF, Riscoe MK, Watnick S. Silicate nephrolithiasis after ingestion of supplements containing silica dioxide. Am J Kidney Dis. 2009;54:127–30.

116. National Public Radio (NPR) website. Feds say it's time to cut back on fluoride in drinking water. http://www.npr.org/sections/health-shots/2015/04/27/402579949/feds-say-its-time-to-cut-back-on-fluoride-in-drinking-water. Accessed 1 June 2015.

117. Proton Pump Inhibitors Information. US Food and Drug Administration. http://www.fda.gov/Drugs/DrugSafety/InformationbyDrugClass/ucm213259.htm. Accessed 1 June 2015.

118. Moyad MA. Heart healthy = prostate healthy: SELECT, the symbolic end of preventing prostate cancer via heart unhealthy and over anti-oxidation mechanisms? Asian J Androl. 2012;14:243–4.

119. Jackson RD, LaCroix AZ, Gass M, Wallace RB, Robbins J, Lewis CE, et al. Calcium and vitamin D supplementation and the risk of fractures. N Engl J Med. 2006;354:669–83.

120. Zhang Z, Cogswell ME, Gillespie C, Fang J, Loustalot F, Dai S, et al. Association between usual sodium and potassium intake and blood pressure and hypertension among U.S. adults: NHANES 2005–2010. PLoS One. 2013;8:e75289.

121. WHO website. http://whqlibdoc.who.int/trs/who_trs_916.pdf. Accessed 1 June 2015.

122. Svetkey LP, Simons-Morton D, Vollmer WM, Appel LJ, Conlin PR, Ryan DH, et al. Effects of dietary patterns on blood pressure: subgroup analysis of the Dietary Approaches to Stop Hypertension (DASH) randomized clinical trial. Arch Intern Med. 1999;159:285–93.

123. Mankowski RT, Anton SD, Buford TW, Leeuwenburgh C. Dietary antioxidants as modifiers of physiologic adaptations to exercise. Med Sci Sports Exerc 2015, Epub ahead of print.

124. Olesen J, Gilemann L, Bienso R, Schmidt J, Hellsten Y, Pilegaard H. Exercise training, but not resveratrol, improves metabolic and inflammatory status in skeletal muscle of aged men. J Physiol. 2014;592(Pt 8):1873–86.

125. Andersen MB, Pingel J, Kjaer M, Langberg H. Interleukin-6: a growth factor stimulating collagen synthesis in human tendon. J Appl Physiol. 2011;110:1549–54.

126. Valero T. Mitochondrial biogenesis: pharmacological approaches. Curr Pharm Des. 2014;20:5507–9.

127. Kruger K, Mooren FC. Exercise-induced leukocyte apoptosis. Exerc Immunol Rev. 2014;20:117–34.

128. Harijith A, Ebenezer DL, Natarajan V. Reactive oxygen species at the crossroads of inflammasome and inflammation. Front Physiol. 2014;5:352.

129. Taghipour N, Aghdael HA, Haghighi A, Mossafa N, Tabaei SJ, Rostami-Nejad M. Potential treatment of inflammatory bowel disease: a review of helminthes therapy. Gastroenterol Hepatol Bed Bench. 2014;7:9–16.

130. Rutkowski K, Sowa P, Rutkowska-Talipska J, Sulkowski S, Rutkowski R. Allergic diseases: the price of civilizational progress. Postepy Dermatol Alergol. 2014;31:77–83.

131. Venditti O, De Lisi D, Caricato M, Caputo D, Capolupo GT, Taffon C, et al. Ipilimumab and immune-mediated adverse events: a case report of anti-CTLA4 induced ileitis. BMC Cancer. 2015;15:87.

132. Gaziano JM, Sesso HD, Christen WG, Bubes V, Smith JP, MacFadyen J, et al. Multivitamins in the prevention of cancer in men: the Physicians' Health Study II randomized controlled trial. JAMA. 2012;308:1871–80.

133. US Food and Drug Administration. Facts about the current good manufacturing practices (cGMPs). http://www.fda.gov/Food/GuidanceRegulation/CGMP/ucm079496.htm. http://www.fda.gov/Drugs/DevelopmentApprovalProcess/Manufacturing/ucm169105.htm. Accessed 1 June 2015.

134. NSF International. www.nsf.org. Accessed 1 June 2015.
135. Informed Choice. http://www.informed-choice.org/registered-products. Accessed 1 June 2015.
136. USP-US Pharmacopeial Convention. www.usp.org. Accessed 1 June 2015.
137. Natural Products Association. www.npainfo.org. Accessed 1 June 2015.
138. Barton DL, Liu H, Dakhil SR, Linquist B, Sloan JA, Nichols CR, et al. Wisconsin ginseng (Panax quinquefolius) to improve cancer-related fatigue: a randomized, double-blind trial, N07C2. J Natl Cancer Inst. 2013;105(16):1230–8.
139. Barton DL, Soori GS, Bauer BA, Sloan JA, Johhnson PA, Figuera C, et al. Pilot study of Panax quinquefolius (American ginseng) to improve cancer-related fatigue: a randomized, double-blind, dose-finding evaluation: NCCTG trial N03CA. Support Cancer Care. 2010;18: 179–87.
140. Ruddy KJ, Barton D, Loprinzi CL. Laying to rest psychostimulants for cancer-related fatigue? J Clin Oncol. 2014;32:1865–7.
141. Yennurajalingham S, Reddy A, Tannir NM, Chisholm GB, Lee RT, Lopez G, et al. High-dose Asian ginseng (Panax Ginseng) for cancer-related fatigue: a preliminary report. Integr Cancer Ther 2015, Epub ahead of print.
142. Ryan JL, Heckler CE, Roscoe JA, Dakhil SR, Kirshner J, Flynn PJ, et al. Ginger (Zingiber officinale) reduces acute chemotherapy-induced nausea: a URCC CCOP study of 576 patients. Support Care Cancer. 2012;20:1479–89.
143. Zindol® for chemotherapy induced nausea and vomiting. http://www.aphios.com/products/therapeutic-product-pipeline/oncology/zindol.html. Accessed 1 June 2015.
144. Zindol® DS. http://www.aphioshwc.com/products/zindol-ds.html. Accessed 1 June 2015.
145. Hercberg S, Galen P, Preziosi P, Bertrais S, Mennen L, Malvy D, et al. The SU.VI.MAX Study: a randomized, placebo-controlled trial of the health effects of antioxidant vitamins and minerals. Arch Intern Med. 2004;164:2335–42.
146. Fransen M, Agallotis M, Nairn L, Votrubec M, Bridgett L, Su S, et al. Glucosamine and chondroitin for knee osteoarthritis: a double-blind randomized placebo-controlled clinical trial evaluating single and combination regimens. Ann Rheum Dis. 2015;74:851–8.
147. Yim SH, Chung YJ. Reflections on the US FDA's warning on direct-to-consumer genetic testing. Genomics Inform. 2014;12:151–5.
148. Wallace ML, Ricco JA, Barrett B. Screening strategies for cardiovascular disease in asymptomatic adults. Prim Care. 2014;41:371–97.
149. Gadkari AS, McHorney CA. Unintentional non-adherence to chronic prescription medications: how unintentional is it really? BMC Health Serv Res. 2012;12:98.
150. Harvey LJ, Dainty JR, Hollands WJ, Bull VJ, Hoogewerff JA, Foxall RJ, et al. Effect of high-dose iron supplements on fractional zinc absorption and status in pregnant women. Am J Clin Nutr. 2007;85:131–6.
151. Alleyne M, Horne MK, Miller JL. Individualized treatment for iron-deficiency anemia in adults. Am J Med. 2008;121:943–8.
152. Diabetes Prevention Program Research Group. 10-year follow-up of diabetes incidence and weight loss in the Diabetes Prevention Program Outcomes Study. Lancet. 2009;374: 1677–86.
153. Taylor F, Huffman MD, Macedo AF, Moore TH, Burke M, Davey Smith G, et al. Statins for the primary prevention of cardiovascular disease. Cochrane Database Syst Rev. 2013; 1:CD004816.
154. Kennedy SP, Barnas GP, Schmidt MJ, Glisczinski MS, Paniagua AC. Efficacy and tolerability of once-weekly rosuvastatin in patients with previous statin intolerance. J Clin Lipidol. 2011;5:308–15.
155. Watts NB, Diab DL. Long-term use of bisphosphonates in osteoporosis. J Clin Endocrinol Metab. 2010;95:1555–65.
156. Black DM, Schwartz AV, Ensrud KE, Cauley JA, Levis S, Quandt SA, for the FLEX Research Group. Effects of continuing or stopping alendronate after 5 years of treatment: the Fracture Intervention Trial Long-term Extension (FLEX): a randomized trial. JAMA. 2006;296: 2927–38.

157. Navarro VJ, Barnhart H, Bonkovsky HL, Davern T, Fontana RJ, Grant L, et al. Liver injury from herbals and dietary supplements in the US Drug-induced Liver Injury Network. Hepatology. 2014;60:1399–408.
158. Lee Y, Mitchell DC, Smiciklas-Wright H, Birch LL. Maternal influences on 5- to 7-year old girls' intake of multivitamin-mineral supplements. Pediatrics. 2002;109:E46.
159. Sien YP, Sahril N, Abdul Mutalip MH, Zaki NA, Abdul Ghaffar S. Determinants of dietary supplements use among adolescents in Malaysia. Asia Pac J Public Health. 2014;26(5 Suppl): 36S–43.
160. Wu CH, Wang CC, Kennedy J. The prevalence of herb and dietary use among children and adolescents in the United States: Results from the 2007 National Health Interview Survey. Complement Ther Med. 2013;21:358–63.
161. Korownyk C, Kolber MR, McCormack J, Lam V, Overbo K, Cotton C, et al. Televised medical talk shows-what they recommend and the evidence to support their recommendations: a prospective observational study. BMJ. 2014;349:g7346.
162. Petadolex. www.petadolex.com. Accessed 1 June 2015.
163. Sylvan Bio. www.sylvaninc.com/bio/healthCare.html. Accessed 1 June 2015.
164. Becker DJ, Gordon RY, Halbert SC, French B, Morris PB, Rader DJ. Red yeast rice for dyslipidemia in statin-intolerant patients: a randomized trial. Ann Intern Med. 2009;150:830–9.
165. Phamavite. www.pharmavite.com. Accessed 1 June 2015.
166. Papakostas GI, Mischoulon D, Shyu I, Alpert JE, Fava M. S-adenosyl methionine (SAMe) augmentation of serotonin reuptake inhibitors for antidepressant nonresponders with major depressive disorder: a double-blind, randomized, clinical trial. Am J Psychiatry. 2010;167: 942–8.
167. Align. www.aligngi.com. Accessed 1 June 2015.
168. Brenner DM, Chey WD. Bifidobacterium infantis 35624: a novel probiotic for the treatment of irritable bowel syndrome. Rev Gastroenterol Disord. 2009;9:7–15.
169. US Food and Drug Administration. http://www.accessdata.fda.gov/scripts/enforcement/enforce_rpt-Event-Detail.cfm?action=detail&id=66557&w=11202013&lang=eng. Accessed 1 June 2015.
170. US Food Safety. Dietary supplements recall for the potential of chloramphenicol. http://blog.usfoodsafety.com/2014/01/10/dietary-supplements-recall-for-the-potential-of-chloramphenicol/. Accessed 1 June 2015.
171. Gokmen MR, Cosyns J-P, Arit VM, Stiborova M, Phillips DH, Schmeiser HH, et al. The epidemiology, diagnosis, and management of aristolochic acid nephropathy. Ann Intern Med. 2013;158:469–77.
172. US Food and Drug Administration. Dietary supplements: aristolochic acid. Silver Spring, MD: US Food and Drug Administration; 2001. www.fda.gov/Food/DietarySupplements/Alerts/ucm095272.htm. Accessed 1 June 2015.
173. Allen JA, Peterson A, Sufit R, Hinchcliff ME, Mahoney JM, Wood TA, et al. Post-epidemic eosinophilia-myalgia syndrome associated with L-tryptophan. Arthritis Rheum. 2011;63: 3633–9.
174. Park City Group and Repositrak. www.repositrak.com or www.parkcitygroup.com. Accessed 1 June 2015.
175. DNA TREK. www.dnatrek.co. Accessed 1 June 2015.

Chapter 3
The Ideal 7-Step Breast Cancer Diet, Lifestyle, and Dietary Supplements Program for Prevention/Recurrence: Heart Healthy = Breast Healthy!

Introduction (Heart Health = Breast Health = All Healthy)

Before recommending the ideal breast cancer diet and lifestyle program, perhaps health concerns need to be triaged or probability based. Reviewing the most common causes of morbidity and mortality allow for an easier understanding of dietary changes that should be recommended for patients in general. These recommendations need to be simple, logical, and practical for the patient as well as the clinician. Thus, reviewing common causes of mortality are paramount to construing all other recommendations in this manuscript.

Cardiovascular disease (CVD) is the number 1 overall cause of mortality in the USA and in other industrialized countries [1, 2]. CVD is currently the number 1 cause of death worldwide, and is the number one cause of death in virtually every region of the world. Cancer is the second leading cause of death in the USA and in most developed countries, and it expected to potentially mirror the number of deaths from CVD in the next decade in various regions of the world. Regardless, CVD has been the number one cause of death in the USA every single year for the last 100 years, with the exception of 1918, which was the year of the influenza pandemic.

If cancer becomes the primary cause of mortality, the majority of what is known concerning lifestyle and dietary change for CVD prevention applies to cancer prevention [3]. Heart healthy changes are tantamount to overall health improvements regardless of the part of the human anatomy that is receiving attention, including the bladder, brain, breast, colon, kidney, liver, ovaries, pancreas, penis, or prostate. Heart healthy changes need to be advocated in cancer clinics because it places probability and the sum of the research into perspective. Triaging preventive medicine for breast health is providing probability based advice via evidence-based medicine.

The largest US and worldwide pharmaceutical-based breast cancer primary prevention trials exemplify the urgent need for a more proper and balanced perspective. For example, the P-1 trial for tamoxifen (breast cancer) chemoprevention was

© Springer International Publishing Switzerland 2016
M.A. Moyad, *Integrative Medicine for Breast Cancer*,
DOI 10.1007/978-3-319-23422-9_3

a landmark trial because it represented the first drug ever approved by the Food and Drug Administration (FDA) for the prevention of any major specific cancer [4]. Participants (premenopausal and postmenopausal) in this trial had a higher risk (Gail Score ≥1.66) of being diagnosed with breast cancer, but despite this drug reducing the risk of breast cancer by approximately 50 % few individuals and media outlets realized that four times as many heart disease deaths occurred in the drug and placebo arms of the trial versus breast cancer deaths (25 versus 6). This was arguably similar in multiple ways to the P-2 STAR (Study of Tamoxifen and Raloxifene) prevention trial [5], which allowed raloxifene to also receive FDA approval for breast cancer prevention. Approximately 20,000 postmenopausal women from nearly 200 clinical centers with 327 invasive breast cancer diagnosed found raloxifene to be as effective as tamoxifen. However, there were over 430 total cases of ischemic heart disease, stroke, and transient ischemic attack that occurred during the trial! However, there were 93 deaths from cancer, 30 from lung cancer, and six from breast cancer and there were 42 causes of death from cardiovascular disease (14 from ischemic heart disease). The updated analysis or 81-month median follow-up revealed a continuation of this trend [6]. In other words, the primary risk or concern for women at high-risk of breast cancer is lung cancer, cardiovascular disease, and then other cancers. In other words, reducing the risk of cardiovascular disease is of paramount importance to simply reduce all-cause morbidity and mortality whether this includes tobacco cessation or weight reduction.

Interestingly, research from both the P-1 and P-2 trial found a slight nonsignificant increased risk of invasive breast cancer with increased weight. In fact, compared with women with a BMI less than 25, the risk for premenopausal women was 59 % higher for BMI 25–29.9 and 70 % greater for BMI 30 or more [7]. Obviously, like tobacco, obesity is a risk factor for CVD and cancer. Heart health is again tantamount to breast and overall health.

Interestingly, when perceiving the landscape outside of breast cancer, especially the largest pharmaceutical clinical trials ever conducted, the results are no different. For example, the results of the Prostate Cancer Prevention Trial (PCPT) seem to have garnered attention plus controversy regarding the use of the drug finasteride daily versus placebo to reduce the risk of prostate cancer [8–10]. The discussion over the advantages and disadvantages of finasteride will continue, but one observation from this important trial has not received adequate exposure and debate in the medical literature. Over 18,000 men were included in this randomized trial, and five men died from prostate cancer in the finasteride and in the placebo arm, but 1123 men in total died during this primary prevention trial [8]. Thus, prostate cancer was responsible for approximately less than 1 % of the deaths, while the majority of the overall causes of mortality deaths were from CVD and other non-prostate cancer causes. Randomized trials tend to accurately provide a snap shot of day-to-day morbidity and mortality in this regard. This finding places the overall risk of morbidity and mortality in a more proper perspective. Men and women inquiring about the advantages and disadvantages of finasteride or dutasteride for prostate cancer or tamoxifen or raloxifene for prevention need to be reminded that the number 1 risk to them in general is CVD, and then the potential cancer risk-specific consult should occur after this first more relevant point is discussed, emphasized, reiterated, and in some cases even documented in the chart. Regardless, CVD prevention in terms of lifestyle changes mirrors cancer prevention.

Arguably, one of the largest dietary supplement studies conducted in women globally was the US Women's Health Initiative (WHI), a double-blind, placebo-controlled trial randomly assigned 36,282 postmenopausal women to 1000 mg calcium carbonate per day and 400 IU vitamin D per day (OsCal®, GSK Pharma US Consumer Division) or placebo with an average intervention of 7.0 years [11]. The study was designed to determine if these supplements would primarily reduce the risk of hip fractures and secondarily total fracture and colorectal cancer risk. When the overall results of the trial itself and post-interventional follow-up were completed the controversy over supplementation initiated, but the overall morbidity and mortality numbers, a reflection of what happens in real life, did not seem to garner attention. Invasive breast cancer occurred in 1667 women and myocardial infarction or stroke occurred in 2645 women and CVD death occurred in 1074 women and approximately one of three deaths were due to a CVD cause [12–14]. A total of 46 deaths occurred from breast cancer. Interestingly, the mean age at baseline was 62 years and the mean BMI was 29 (overweight), but there were more obese women compared to overweight and normal BMI women. Again, larger randomized clinical trials generally reflect the overall health status of that same population being studied.

The largest dietary supplement trial ever conducted in healthy men (essentially the mirror of the WHI) once again reiterates that risk needs to be placed in its proper perspective. The largest dietary supplement clinical trial to prevent prostate cancer was the selenium and vitamin E supplementation randomized trial (SELECT) [15]. It was terminated approximately 7 years early because of a lack of efficacy, and even a potential negative impact with these supplements at these specific dosages. CVD represented the primary cause of mortality overall in this study with over 500 deaths occurring from this cause compared to the one death from prostate cancer in just 5 years follow-up. Heart healthy programs simply need to receive more emphasis throughout medicine.

The lifestyle recommendations proffered in this chapter essentially serve to impact CVD and breast and overall health simultaneously. Patients can now be offered lifestyle changes that can potentially impact all-cause morbidity and mortality rather than just disease-specific morbidity and mortality.

General Heart Health = Breast Health Step #1 for your patients:
Know and always try to improve on the 4 low cost and proven heart healthy parameters:

- **Fasting cholesterol level (Total, LDL, HDL, and triglycerides)**
- **Blood pressure**
- **Blood glucose (and hemoglobin A1c)**
- **BMI and/or waist circumference (WC)**

The lack of general health knowledge exhibited by some patients and even future health care professionals can be concerning. For example, surveys of the general population indicate that a majority of individuals do not know their cholesterol values, or most risk factors for CVD and this finding is consistent regardless of age, race, and even gender [16–20].

In my experience when the dual concern of CVD and overall breast cancer prevention/recurrence risk is emphasized and promoted, patients tend to become familiar with all of their clinical values, numbers, and overall risks. It is of interest that at least in the USA the prevalence of cardiovascular disease is still high. For example, almost 15 % of men and 10 % of women have cardiovascular disease between the ages of 20–39, and that number increases to approximately 40 % from the ages of 40–59 years, and over 70 % from 60 to 79 years, and over 80 % from 80+ years of age [21]. These prevalence numbers are quite surprising for some patients, but again it places disease risk in perspective.

Approximately 150,000 individuals die annually of a cardiovascular event in the USA before the age of 65, and 15,000 women die yearly of CVD before the age of 55. One in two women die from heart disease or stroke compared to one in 25 women who will die of breast cancer [22], and since 1984, the number of CVD deaths for women has surpassed those for men [23]. I often remind women concerned about breast cancer that CVD was a "super epidemic" and now it is simply just an "epidemic." Thus, a woman or man attending a breast cancer awareness or screening would appear to be at risk of ending up with a myopic health and disease perspective unless other screenings, such as blood pressure, cholesterol, weight, and/or glucose were also proffered or at least emphasized equally.

Cholesterol

Patients should be educated regularly on the normal values of a cholesterol panel, which are updated by expert guideline groups such as the National Cholesterol Education Program (NCEP) [24, 25]. Patients need multiple resources, apart from the generally over burdened primary care practitioners, to emphasize and review basic optimal lipid and general health values. Table 3.1 is a modified quick review for patients and health care professionals of past cholesterol guidelines that are in flux but this at least gives some proper perspective [24, 25]. Despite the potentially ongoing changes in lipid and heart parameters the generally "less is more to a point" philosophy is still evidence-based and also plays a role in preventing all-cause morbidity and mortality (see Chap. 4). Additionally, the evolving recommendation on lipids and women's health is amply reviewed in Chap. 4 of this book, and Chap. 5 of this book also provides adequate review and perspective.

The NCEP suggests a first cholesterol screen at an age of 20 [24, 25], which is approximately at least 20–30 years before a suggested mammography screen or colonoscopy, but few if individuals in my experience have had a lipid test at this early age. Clinicians can assist patients in adhering to this early screening age. For example, women and men with a family history of breast or prostate cancer or an early diagnosis of most diseases often inquire about what their children or other family members should do, first and foremost, to prevent this condition from happening to the next generation. A common suggestion that I reiterate for children or adolescents is to just have an initial blood pressure, cholesterol, and glucose screening tests and to maintain a healthy weight and have their weight and waist

Table 3.1 A partial summary of the overall health goals for patients in regard to total cholesterol, LDL, HDL, and triglycerides with some modifications that can be utilized in a clinical setting [24, 25]

Blood test parameter	Measurement commentary
Total cholesterol (mg/dl or mmol/L)	*A lower number is better*
<160 or <4.1	Optimal
160–200 or 4.14–5.16	Desirable
200–239 or 5.16–6.19	Borderline high
≥240 or ≥6.22	High
LDL="bad cholesterol" (mg/dl or mmol/L)	*A lower number is better*
Less than 70 or <1.81	Optimal for some high-risk individuals[a]
Less than 100 or <2.59	Optimal
100–129 or 2.59–3.34	Near optimal
130–159 or 3.37–4.12	Borderline high
160–189 or 4.14–4.90	High
Equal to or greater than 190 or ≥4.92	Very high
HDL="good cholesterol" (mg/dl or mmol/L)	*A higher number is better*
Less than 40 or <1.04	Low
40–59 or 1.04–1.53	Normal
Equal to or greater 60 or ≥1.55	High (Optimal)
Triglyceride (mg/dl or mmol/L)	*A lower number is better*
Less than 150 or <1.70	Normal
150–199 or 1.70–2.25	Borderline high
200–499 or 2.26–5.64	High
Equal to or greater than 500 or ≥5.65	High

[a]*Note*: High-risk individuals (existing CVD disease or a previous CVD event) may be required to reduce their LDL below 70 mg/dl based on outcomes data provided to the Expert Panel

size monitored. In my experience, this tends to surprise and simplify patient concerns because this is an unexpected suggestion. The time is now more appropriate than ever for this approach because of the past and ongoing concern in abnormal lipid levels among adolescents screened in the USA, which is approximately 20–43 % based on a variety of factors, especially weight status (normal, overweight, or obese) [26]. Other novel cardiovascular markers such as high-sensitivity C-reactive protein (hs-CRP), or traditional ancillary markers such as hemoglobin A1c (arguably a better reflection of long-term glucose control even in non-diabetics), and evidence of subclinical atherosclerotic disease could also be discussed for example with the patient [3, 27]. All of these items tend to garner less attention than a novel genetic test for example in cancer, which is why lifestyle and these numerical parameters associated with them matter even more today.

Other tangible advantages may occur for the patient and clinician that continue to follow these overall cardiovascular markers. For example, cholesterol levels are an adequate indicator of how well a patient may be adopting lifestyle changes or even medication compliance following breast cancer screening or after some definitive therapy. If these numbers improve it appears more likely that the patient is following a breast health lifestyle program. High-density lipoprotein (HDL) provides a good indicator of the commitment to aerobic exercise and is, in a sense, the "truth serum" as to how much physical activity has recently occurred. HDL tends to rise, and at times substantially and acutely with a greater amount of aerobic physical activity [28]. Triglycerides are an indicator of changes in belly (visceral) fat because this compound is generally stored in this anatomic location with increasing blood levels. In addition, a large drop in triglycerides can reflect adequate dietary changes and/or weight loss. Although table one suggests a triglyceride level of below 150 mg/dl is ideal, personally when a patient carries a level less than 100 mg/dl, my experience suggests a serious commitment to dietary change or a reflection of profound changes during that period of time. One other point needs emphasis, which is the obsession some clinicians and patients have beyond basic lipids such as lipid particle sizes and a variety of other costly lipid parameters. In general, the vast majority of these esoteric parameters normalize when a patient reaches the ideal basic lipid values. Simplicity negates the need for complexity and anxiety.

Blood Pressure

Hypertension is becoming the leading cause of CVD mortality in women and it should receive more of an emphasis. Thus, blood pressure monitoring should also be emphasized as much as any other value. The Joint National Committee on Prevention, Detection, Evaluation, and Treatment of High Blood Pressure adequately and regularly defines a healthy blood pressure [29, 30]. Individuals and their partners should be informed that normal blood pressure is less than 120/80 mmHg and individuals with a systolic blood pressure of 120–139 mmHg or diastolic blood pressure of 80–89 mmHg are actually considered to be "prehypertensive," and lifestyle changes should be advocated in these individuals (see Table 3.2) [29, 30].

Blood pressure can be reduced with a healthier lifestyle [31], and again is a good indicator of lifestyle adherence or compliance. Interestingly, one of the more subtle but prevalent etiologies of high blood pressure may be excessive alcohol consumption [1], and this should be discussed with patients as much as sodium (or sugar) restriction, and moderate to excessive alcohol intake, regardless of the beverage source, is a risk factor for breast cancer [32].

Hypertension is also an earlier marker of a high-risk type II diabetes patient or "pre-diabetic." Regardless, patients that adopt healthy lifestyle and behavioral changes should always be given encouragement to continue these changes because

Table 3.2 A partial summary of the blood pressure guidelines for patients derived from the Joint National Committee on Prevention, Detection, Evaluation, and Treatment of High Blood Pressure [29, 30]

Blood pressure (systolic/diastolic)	What does this mean to patients?
Less than 120/80 mmHg	Normal = low-risk
120–139/80–89 mmHg	Prehypertensive (moderately high or pre-high blood pressure) = moderate-risk
140/90 mmHg or greater	Hypertensive (high blood pressure) = high-risk

Table 3.3 Temporary behavioral issues, apart from white coat hypertension, that could cause false elevations in blood pressure readings (at home or in the office) [36]

Patient behavior or situation	Blood pressure can increase as much as
A full or distended bladder	10–15 mmHg
Talking or engaged in a conversation or has not had at least 3 min of quiet time before the measurement	10–15 mmHg
Cuff over clothing or cuff size issues	10–40 mmHg (too tight = higher and too loose = lower)
Unsupported back and/or feet and/or arm	5–10 mmHg
Crossed legs	2–8 mmHg
Ingestion of caffeine or source of caffeine within the past 30 min	Variable increases
Exertion or brisk walking/running and/or lifting right before the measurement	Variable increases
Stress/anxiety right before the measurement	Variable increases

of the other potential profound impact these behaviors may have on overall and mental health [33, 34]. Due to the phenomenon of "white coat hypertension" it seems critical to encourage some patients to invest some money in a at home blood pressure measurement device [35]. These devices have become cost-effective and potentially more accurate of the patient's blood pressure status compared to 1 or 2 values derived annually for example from a medical office. And patients should also be given a review of the potential behaviors that can lead to minor and major temporary false elevations in blood pressure. A review of some of these behaviors that can elevate blood pressure dramatically, especially a distended or full bladder (up to 10–15 mmHg) for example, is provided in Table 3.3 [36].

Blood Glucose (and/or hemoglobin A1c)

Fasting blood glucose is as important as any other parameter for your patients. Abnormally high blood glucose and diabetes is considered such a high-risk cardiovascular situation that these patients are treated as if already having established cardiovascular disease in terms of lipid control. Diabetes also appears to be a risk factor for breast cancer from past meta-analyses [37], and even pre-diabetes may soon become an established risk factor [38]. The relationship between glucose intolerance and sexual dysfunction is already well established in women and men [39, 40]. Patients appear more motivated to continue healthy lifestyle changes when there is some tangible healthy outcome with the behavioral change, and this becomes more probable when all numbers are utilized in the consult including cholesterol, blood pressure and glucose for example as opposed to just other single or disease specific values or images. Please see Chap. 6 for more unique information of the glucose and breast cancer relationship.

Weight, BMI, Waist Circumference (WC)

The negative impact of being overweight or obese on overall morbidity and mortality is also well known. Body mass index (BMI) is a moderately reliable as an isolated anthropometric measurement, but at least it is a rapid method to determine who may be overweight or obese [41]. BMI is defined as the weight (in kilograms) divided by the square of the height in meters (kilograms per square meter). Another method to calculate the BMI is to take weight in pounds and divide it by the height in inches squared and to multiply this number by 704 (pounds/in. × 704). A BMI < 25 is considered normal by the Word Health Organization (WHO), whereas 25–29 is overweight, and ≥30 is defined as obese, and 35 or more is considered morbidly obese. BMI does not fully account for changes in lean muscle mass, which is why it is often criticized (for example a lean extremely muscular women or man could be easily considered overweight with a BMI measurement), but again this is just one ancillary measurement to be used with others to access adipose status.

Several of the largest and most recent preventive medicine randomized trials of women or men have demonstrated that most individuals in these studies are indeed overweight at baseline, and this includes trials to prevent specific health abnormalities with prescriptions, supplements, or just dietary change [15, 42]. Thus, it has become so common for participants of the major clinical trials to be overweight or obese that only a small percentage of individuals in these studies have a BMI in the healthy range (a mirror reflection of the prevalence of this condition in the USA and other populations).

Waist-to-hip ratio (WHR) may be another rapid measurement to determine obesity [41]. An individual must stand during the entire measurement of WHR. WHR more precisely measures abdominal adipose circumference or tissue and fat distribution. The waist is defined as the abdominal circumference midway between the costal margin and the iliac crest. The hip is defined as the largest circumference just below the iliac crest. However, it requires more time and detail, which is why waist circumference (WC) alone is perhaps the easiest and fastest method to currently access obesity, and is my preference together with pant size (waist size).

"Belly fat" (visceral adipose tissue) seems to have one of the best predictive values of CVD and potential all-cause mortality risk among all the other weight parameters from some of the largest prospective studies in the world [43–45]. However, the combination of WC with a BMI measurement may have added predictability. Still, WC is also one of the best predictors of heart unhealthy changes and/or future cardiovascular events, regardless of the age group and ethnic group studied [46, 47].

WC is also one of the five specific criteria of the metabolic syndrome. WC has a tangible advantage over BMI, which can be appreciated after an individual commits to resistance exercise. An increase in muscle mass from resistance activities such as weight lifting can actually again cause an increase in BMI, which could be frustrating to the patient and clinician [41]. However, this does not generally occur when additionally utilizing the WHR or especially the more simplistic WC measurement. Informing patients of their official WC and asking pant size allows these parameters

Table 3.4 Body mass index (BMI), and waist circumference (WC) values for women's and men's health discussions [41]

BMI number	Classification
Less than 18.5	Underweight
18.5–24.9	Normal weight
25–29.9	Overweight
30 or more	Obese
WC number	**Classification**
Less than 32.5 in. in WOMEN (less than 83 cm)	Normal
32.5–36 in. in WOMEN (or 93–92 cm)	Overweight
37 or more inches in WOMEN (or 94 or more centimeters)	Obese
Less than 35 in. (or less than 89 cm) in MEN	Normal
35 to 39 in. (or 89 to 101 cm) in MEN	Overweight
40 or more inches (over 102 cm) in MEN	Obese

to not only be documented in the chart, but allows for the patient to identify a goal of maintaining or reducing these numbers by the time of the subsequent clinical visit. Thus, reducing the emphasis on just the weight scale or trying to compete with a national standard. A patient with a BMI of 35 and a WC of 40 in. is not as concerning compared to an individual with similar measurements and a lack of aerobic fitness and some modicum of caloric control, or not being able to reduce their WC value slightly over time is more of an issue. A summary of the basic interpretation of the BMI and WC value are found in Table 3.4 [41].

The list of medical conditions increased or exacerbated by adipose tissue or weight gain is remarkable and could occupy a full-text. For example, kidney stones and renal cell carcinoma (RCC) may have a strong relationship with obesity [48–51]. A table of a more comprehensive list of conditions exacerbated by weight gain is remarkable and found later in this chapter.

Clinicians should begin to carry and utilize tape measures that can measure WC or some weight parameter, and I often argue that this is as critical as the stethoscope. Clinicians should also refer patients on a consistent basis to ancillary diverse weight management services such as: nutritionists, therapists, social workers, a variety of professional and even surgical weight-loss programs if needed, and recent weight loss consumer publications. Simply becoming familiar with local weight loss resources is an initial step in the appropriate direction for the patient and clinician. For example, inviting a medical director of a local weight loss program to give grand rounds on what kind of treatment plans they proffer to the community demonstrates commitment in my opinion to this cause.

Another method that may provide positive teaching experience is to discuss or at least remind patients about the importance of a healthy weight by mentioning the gastric bypass or surgical weight loss data. The intent is obviously not to advocate the use of gastric bypass or any type of surgery for every patient, but to demonstrate how weight loss clearly and at times quickly impacts health. For example, researchers in the USA and Sweden found in separate studies that obese individuals that had gastric bypass surgery had a 30–40 % lower risk of dying 7–10 years after having the surgery compared to those that did not have the surgery [52–54]. The Swedish study was one of the longest studies ever published at that time with long-term health outcomes [53]. Researchers at the Goteborg University compared 4047 individuals with a body mass index (BMI) of over 34, who received one of three types of surgery (banding, vertical-banded gastroplasty, or gastric bypass) or some dietary advice (control group). Some of the basic characteristics of these patients before the study started were the following:

- About 70 % of the patients were women, and about a third of the women were postmenopausal.
- The average age was 46–48 years.
- Average weight was 262 pounds
- Average BMI was 42.
- Average waist-to-hip ratio was about 1.
- Average waist circumference was about 49 in.
- Average cholesterol was 226 mg/dl and HDL ("good cholesterol") was in the lower 40s.
- Average triglyceride was 197 mg/dl.

After 10.9 years, those that received surgery lost 14–25 % of their original weight compared to 2 % in the other group. Out of the 2010 surgery patients, 101 died, and there were 129 deaths in the comparison group of 2037 patients. There was a 29 % significant reduction ($p=0.01$) in the risk of dying from any cause in the surgery group. There were also lower risk of dying from cardiac disease, and non-cardiovascular causes such as cancer. However, there was a higher rate of dying from infection (12 versus 3 patients) and sudden death (20 versus 14) in the surgery group. The most successful weight loss occurred in the gastric bypass group where the average reduction in weight was about 30 % loss of their original weight. Interestingly, the risk reduction in disease and death was much larger in the older patients (about 25 %) compared to younger subjects (6 %).

In the US study (funded by a US government grant, or branch of the National Institutes of Health), which was retrospective and not prospective like the first study mentioned above, researchers (University of Utah and other centers) looked at 7925 severely obese individuals who had gastric bypass [52]. These patients were matched to 7925 control individuals with identical weights and height. About 84 % of the patients were women and the average age was 39 years, and the average BMI was 45–47. After an average of follow-up of 7 years there were 213 deaths in the surgery group versus 321 deaths in the non-surgical group. A total of 136 lives were saved per 10,000 gastric bypass surgeries after an average of 7.1 years following the actual procedure. The following interesting and significant results were found:

- Deaths from all causes were reduced ($p<0.001$) by 40 %.
- Deaths from diabetes were reduced ($p=0.005$) by 92 %.
- Deaths from cancer were reduced ($p<0.001$) by 60 %.
- Deaths from cardiovascular disease were reduced ($p<0.001$) by 50 %.
- Deaths from heart disease were reduced ($p=0.006$) by 56 %.

However, the surgery group had a 58 % significantly ($p=0.04$) higher risk of dying from accidents, suicides and other causes not related to the diseases they were studying. None of the non-disease causes of death ("accident unrelated to death, poisoning of undetermined intent, suicide, and other nondisease causes") were significantly different but just higher, but as a combined group there was a significant difference. For example, 63 of the deaths out of 213 in the surgery group were from these causes (15 from suicide) compared to 17 of the 321 deaths in the control group. The researchers did mention that a large number of severely obese individuals have "unrecognized presurgical mood disorder or post-traumatic stress disorder or have been victims of childhood sexual abuse." Some bariatric surgery centers recommend that all patients have a psychological evaluation, and if necessary some kind of treatment before surgery and some type of surveillance after surgery, but arguably this should probably be the standard way patients are handled after reading this study. And this should be kept in mind when talking to any patient about surgery or another method for weight loss over time.

An examination of more recent surgical series should continue to impress the health care professional and patients. In the Swedish Obese Subjects (SOS) study, an ongoing review of outcomes from 25 public surgical departments and 480 primary health centers in Sweden, a total of 2010 obese patients matched to controls found a 53 % reduction in the number of cardiovascular deaths ($p=0.002$), and the total of first time cardiovascular events were reduced by 33 % ($p<0.001$) [55]. Gastric bypass and other surgical weight loss randomized controlled data for obese type 2 diabetics from the Cleveland Clinic also continued to demonstrate the profound and immediate changes with weight loss [56]. A significant reduction in the utilization of medications to lower glucose, lipid, and blood pressure occurred within 12 months of their study on 150 patients, which in some cases occurred before the patients were discharged from the hospital! In a similar study from Italy the complete remission rates of type 2 diabetics approached 75–95 % within 2 years [57].

Again, the profound health changes in individuals that lose weight from surgery is an adequate teaching tool for patients to understand the devastating consequences of abnormal weight gain of any type on the human body. Adipose tissue is not inert and secretes a variety of compounds (not just increased aromatase and estrogen) and other inflammatory signals to the rest of the body that essentially causes even innate immune responses to occur against self. In other words, I often tell patients that greater accumulation of adipose tissue is somewhat tantamount to an autoimmune condition.

General Heart Health=Breast Health Step #2 for your patients:

Avoid tobacco exposure (this includes second hand smoke). Quitting smoking can cause dramatic weight gain which should be addressed before smoking cessation.

Lung cancer is the number 1 cancer killer of women and men in the USA, killing more women each year than breast, ovarian, and uterine cancers combined [58]. Women with breast cancer who smoke appear to have a lower chance of both overall and breast cancer-specific survival [59]. A meta-analysis found a significant 33 % increased risk of death from breast cancer in women who were smokers at diagnosis compared to never smokers.

The challenge in smoking cessation is not just the issue of addiction but one of metabolism. Tobacco provides one with a metabolic advantage, which is why substantial weight gain (over 10 pounds in first year and 15 or more pounds overall) is common after cessation [60]. Thus, addressing this frustration before cessation and the need for caloric control and exercise … should also be emphasized in my opinion as much as the method suggested for smoking cessation.

Rarely discussed is the accumulating data to support second hand smoke (SHS) exposure with an increased risk of breast cancer [61]. A summary of three meta-analyses reported a 65 % increase in premenopausal breast cancer risk among never smokers that were impacted by SHS. An expert panel from Canada and breast cancer risk concluded that SHS is indeed a risk factor utilizing the most current data.

General Heart Health = Breast Health Step #3 for your patients:

Approximately 30–60 min of physical activity a day or more on average should be the goal or enough exercise to achieve optimal mental and physical personal health, which should include lifting weights/resistance exercises 2–3 times/week. Equal emphasis should be placed on aerobic and resistance exercise; one is not more important than the other. Numerous forms of exercise, including High Intensity Interval Training (HIIT) appear just as effective as moderate exercise of a greater duration. Exercise type should fit the personality of the patient.

Exercise is one of the only consistent findings in the literature, apart from maintaining a healthy weight, to lower breast cancer risk, recurrence and mortality [62, 63]. Yet it may be the ancillary benefits of aerobic and resistance exercise that can also motivate patients, such as a reduction in bone loss [64], or even an improvement in fitness without exacerbating lymphedema [65], which use to be a perpetuated theory without clinical evidence that might have and still deter many individuals from engaging in exercise.

More recently, a 1-year randomized trial ($n = 121$) of aerobic (150 min per week) and resistance exercise (supervised resistance activity twice a week) versus usual care in women on aromatase inhibitors (AI) demonstrated a reduction of 29 % in worst joint pain scores versus control group ($p < 0.001$), and pain and interference along with arthritic and disability scores also significantly ($p < 0.001$) and favorably changed versus controls [66]. This is a remarkable initial finding considering arthralgia can occur in 50 % of breast cancer patients on these medications and it is the primary cause of reduced compliance.

One of the best past reviews on physical activity and cardiovascular disease found ample evidence for exercise to favorably impact markers of heart disease including triglycerides, apolipoprotein B reduction, HDL, LDL particle size, and a reduction in coronary calcium [67]. Thus, aerobic and resistance activity need to be emphasized equally because of the documented synergism. Weight training can increase fat free mass, lean body weight, reduces sarcopenia, increases resting metabolic rate, and potentially reduce the risk of abdominal adipose deposition [68, 69]. Weight training or resistance training also appears to improve glucose parameters, including insulin sensitivity, and may slightly improve lipid levels, educe hypertension, and reduce bone loss [69, 70]. Muscle tissue like the rest of the body exists in a "use it or lose it" state and the only consistent method found to maintain or improve lean muscle mass is the actual regular stimulation or exercise of the tissue itself.

The mental health improvements with increased exercise appear to be just as notable as the physical health benefits [71, 72]. For example, one often referenced trial published over a decade ago included 156 adult volunteers with major depressive disorder (MDD) randomly assigned a 4-month course of aerobic exercise (30 min three times/week), sertraline therapy (one of the biggest selling antidepressants in US history), or a combination of exercise and sertraline [73, 74]. After 4 months patients in all three groups demonstrated significant mental health improvements; however, after 10 months, individuals in the exercise group had significantly lower recurrence rates compared to individuals in the medication group of the study. Exercising during the follow-up period was associated with a 51 % reduction in the risk of a diagnosis of depression at the end of the investigation.

Remarkably, the overall effects of exercise in clinical trials of depression for example are not generally interpreted in a manner suitable for impact in a clinician or patient patient's discussion. Recently, experts have come to an interpretive rescue so to speak by mentioning that most prescription antidepressants demonstrated a 2- to 3-point benefit over placebo on depression rating scales, but a majority of exercise studies (13 of 16) have found a 5-point improvement on the depression scale [75]!

Novel studies of MRI utilization have demonstrated the prevention of temporal lobe hippocampal atrophy with physical activity at a variety of ages because the hippocampus is a primary area of memory storage and retrieval [76], and many patients inquire about preventing memory loss. Even recent randomized studies of patients with significant comorbidities such as heart failure have significant improvements in physical and mental health with regular exercise [77]. It is important to explain to patients that if the overall results from exercise studies were viewed similar to a specific pharmacologic intervention than it probably would have already garnered attention worthy of a Nobel Prize in arguably multiple categories of medicine. And the ability of exercise to work synergistically with medication is also notable.

Still, despite the plethora of positive research, are health care professionals excited about recommending exercise to their patients? The National Health Interview Survey (NHIS) data are recorded throughout the year from the Centers for Disease Control and Prevention (CDC) National Center for Health Statistics (NCHS) by interviewers from the US Census Bureau [78]. It is a household-derived survey, and interviews are usually conducted in the respondent's homes. Questions were asked in 2000, 2005 and 2010 with over 20,000 in each of these years sampled that visited with a physician or other health care professional within the past 12 months. In most recent year of data gathering which was 2010, about 32 % of adults that had visited with a physician or other health care professional had been recommended to begin or continue exercise or some form of physical activity. Between the years of 2000 and 2010, the percentage of adults given exercise advice increased by approximately 10 %, and women were more likely that men to have been advised to exercise, and one-third of patients with cancer were also recommended exercise. Thus, only one in three adults who had seen a physician or health care professional in the past 12 months had been told to begin or continue exercise/physical activity. You have the ability to improve these numbers everyday in your practice and I would encourage you to take advantage of this situation.

One final motivational incentive should be provided to patients before they leave your office. When the diversity of the potential benefits of exercise is distributed to your patients on a handout I believe the potential for effectiveness is heightened. Exercise tends to be discussed in terms of singular benefits (reduces heart disease, breast cancer, colon cancer risk, …), and Table 3.5 provides just a partial list of the diverse overall benefits [79, 80]. In fact, a basic Medline search on the word "exercise" provides almost 30,000 citations! Again, it has to be emphasized that after

Table 3.5 The benefit of exercise/physical activity (aerobic and/or resistance) is now staggering with approximately 30,000 publications of evidence that it prevents or reduces the severity of countless medical conditions including those listed in this table [79, 80]

Atrial fibrillation	Hot flashes
Autoimmune diseases	IBS
Atrophy/aging	Incontinence
Breast cancer	Infections
Colon cancer	Infertility (men and women)
Blood clots	Kidney disease, kidney failure and need for dialysis
Blood pressure	Loss of coordination/balance/increased risk of falls and fractures
Bone loss	Low back pain
Chronic pelvic pain syndrome	Low testosterone
Dementia/Alzheimer disease/ memory loss	Lung disease
Depression	NAFLD/NASH (aka fatty liver)
Diabetes	Osteoarthritis
Erectile dysfunction	Parkinson disease
Eye disease	PCOS
Fatigue	Peripheral artery disease (PAD)
Female sexual dysfunction	Pregnancy complications
Gallbladder disease	Premature death
Heart disease	Prostate cancer/enlargement/inflammation
Heart failure	Sarcopenia (muscle loss)
High blood pressure	Stress/anxiety
High cholesterol (and low HDL)	Stroke
Hot flashes	Weight gain/obesity

countless decades of research, exercise is one of the only known lifestyle changes to potentially reduce the risk of breast cancer or recurrence.

General Heart Health = Breast Health Step #4 for your patients:
Reducing overall caloric intake to achieve or maintain a healthy weight, regardless of the method/fad diet utilized could provide similar positive heart and breast health outcomes. Fad diet should fit personality because the end justifies the means, and never forget The WINS versus WHEL weight loss lesson?!

The NCEP recommends that saturated fat be reduced to less than 7 % of total calories to reduce the risk of CVD [24]. In reality this is simply an indirect method to achieve partial caloric reduction in my opinion [79, 80]. Many foods that contain high levels of saturated fat also contained (in the past) the highest levels of trans fat ("partially hydrogenated fat"), cholesterol, and more importantly total calories. For example, there are almost twice as many calories in 8 ounces of whole milk (5 g of saturated fat) compared to skim, or soymilk (0 g of saturated fat each), and there are almost four times as many calories in whole milk compared to almond or cashew milks. Thus, identifying two similar products, such as milk, meats, dairy, chips, and choosing the item lower in saturated in general allows for a profound (at times) reduction in total caloric intake, which is critical to helping maintain or reach an appropriate weight or waist size and improving overall heart health.

Yet simply reducing all saturated fat in an individual's diet is not necessarily a practical and healthy dietary lifestyle change because some saturated fats in the diet may promote healthy parameters and encourage satiation [79, 80]. The cardiovascular goal of obtaining less than 7 % of calories from saturated fat seems ideal, but ingesting minimal to no calories from saturated fat is also excessive, and it actually appears to reduce levels of HDL ("good cholesterol") from past CVD and other health promoting clinical trials [81, 82]. Aggressively reducing saturated fat consumption also implies that this type of fat, in and of itself, is heart unhealthy, which is not accurate from the largest recent meta-analysis of prospective studies [83]. And in some countries around the world where overall caloric intake is very low compared to the USA, saturated fat may have some tangible cardiovascular benefits, but this also needs to be placed in perspective [79]. For example in some regions of the world, such as Japan, a closer look at healthy individuals with the largest intakes of saturated fat in this country would actually be suddenly placed in the lowest category of saturated fat intake in the USA if they were to immediately migrate to the USA [84]. Regardless, one potential positive impact of reducing saturated fat, in my opinion, is that it may reduce overall caloric intake and reduce weight and waist gains in some individuals (again in others it might encourage satiation). Another benefit of reducing saturated fat is that it allows for the opportunity to reduce dietary cholesterol intake and increase the consumption of other monounsaturated and polyunsaturated fats that have shown a greater reduction in CVD from past clinical trials and epidemiologic research [85, 86]. If the patient has normal weight, exercise and other heart healthy parameters then the concern over saturated fat intake should not be as acute because caloric restriction or caloric

Table 3.6 Types of dietary fat, some of their primary sources, and the impact on lipid levels and heart health [79]

Type of dietary fat	Commonly found?	Good or bad fat, and impact on lipids versus carbohydrates (sugars)
Monounsaturated fat (includes omega-9)	Healthy cooking oils (canola, olive, safflower, ...), nuts, ...	GOOD, Lowers LDL, Increases HDL
Polyunsaturated fat (includes omega-3 and 6 fatty acids)[a]	Healthy cooking oils (canola, soybean, ...), flaxseed, fish, nuts, soybeans, ...	GOOD, Lowers LDL, Increases HDL
Saturated fat (known also as hydrogenated fat)	Non-lean meat, high-fat dairy, some fast food	Controversial (because it is associated with high caloric intake in some and lower caloric intake in others), Increases LDL, Increases HDL
Trans fat (also known as partially hydrogenated fat)	Some margarine, fast food, snack foods, deep fried foods, ...	BAD, Increases LDL, Lowers HDL

[a]*Note*: Omega-3 (ALA, EPA, DHA) and some omega-6 (GLA for example) also have heart healthy and anti-inflammatory benefits

control in some form by these individuals is not as beneficial. A summary of the different types of dietary fat, food sources, and impacts on specific lipids are found in Table 3.6 [79].

The Women's Intervention Nutrition Study (WINS) was one of the most unique lifestyle clinical trials in breast cancer research history [87]. A total of 2437 women were involved in a randomized, prospective, multicenter clinical to determine the effect of dietary fat reduction in women with resected, early-stage breast cancer receiving conventional treatment. An interim analysis was conducted after a median follow-up of 5 years when funding for the trial ended. The reduction of relapse events in the low-fat group was 24 % lower compared to the control group and was significant ($p = 0.034$). In reality, despite all the discussion of a lower fat intake there was a clear significant reduction in overall daily calories at 5-years (−167 calories per day; $p < 0.0001$) and weight (−6 pounds; $p = 0.005$) versus the control group, which could be argued was the true reason for the benefit. Table 3.7 is a summary of the primary dietary parameters and changes that occurred at baseline, during and at the end of this trial [87].

However, another landmark randomized trial of over 3000 women of five vegetable servings plus 16 ounces of vegetable juice, three fruit servings, 30 g of fiber, and 15–20 % of energy from fat compared to a comparison group (print materials describing "5-A-Day" diet guidelines) was also conducted [88]. This trial was known as WHEL (Women's Healthy Eating and Living) trial and tried to determine if increasing vegetable, fruits and fiber and reducing fat intake can impact breast

Table 3.7 Key findings at baseline, during and at the conclusion of the WINS trial to reduce the risk of breast cancer relapse (low-fat diet versus control) [87]

Parameter	Baseline between groups (diet versus control difference)	After 1-year in the diet group (diet versus control difference)	After 3-years (diet versus the control group difference)	After 5-years (diet versus the control group difference)
Total fat intake (g)	No difference (57 versus 56)	−18 (33 versus 51)	−20	−19
Fat (g)	No difference (30 versus 30)	−9 (20 versus 29)	−9	−8
Saturated fat (g)	No difference (19 versus 19)	−6 (10 versus 16)	−7	−7
Polyunsaturated fat (g)	No difference (12 versus 12)	−3.5 (7.5 versus 11)	−4	−4
Monounsaturated fat (g)	No difference (21 versus 21)	−7 (12 versus 19)	−8	−8
Fiber (g/day)	No difference (18 versus 18)	−2.2 (19.5 versus 17.3)	−1.2	−2.4
Overall caloric intake (calories per day)	+27 (1687 versus 1660)	−71 (1460 versus 1531)	−142	−167
Weight (in pounds)	No difference (160 lbs versus 160 lbs)	−5 pounds	−4 pounds	−6

cancer recurrence or survival. And after 7.3 years of follow-up these modifications in diet did not reduce breast cancer events or mortality. Why? In my opinion, when looking closer at the more heart healthy changes between the groups in terms of endpoints there was minimal to no difference. In other words, as stated in the results section of the publication: "Study groups differed by less than 80 kcal/day in energy intake and by less than 1 kg in body weight at any study point." Interestingly, an ancillary study of the inflammatory marker CRP (C-Reactive Protein), a marker of acute inflammatory response, demonstrated a reduced survival in WHEL when CRP was 10 mg/L or higher [89].

It is of interest that heart healthy changes including exercise and weight reduction can reduce CRP. For example, recent evidence from the LEAN (Lifestyle, exercise, and nutrition) study demonstrated significant improvements in cardiovascular risk and some cancer markers in breast cancer patients in only 6 months [90]. This study included a total of 97 overweight or obese breast cancer survivors identified from the Yale Hospital Tumor registry and randomized to a usual care group ($n = 33$) or weight loss instruction ($n = 64$) from a registered dietician. On average, the group assigned to the dietician lost 6 % of body weight and the comparison group 2 %. However, the women in the intervention group experienced reductions in insulin, glucose, and even CRP was reduced by 30 % compared to 1 % in the usual care group, but they also had increases in IGF-1. It is also interesting that IGF-1 increased and this use to be thought of as a cancer marker, but I believe that exercise slightly increases growth hormone that allows this value to increase slightly. In other words, I think it is another indication that the human body responds very well and very quickly to caloric reduction, exercise and weight loss and slight increases in IGF-1 after achieving these benefits is an indication of a more optimal physiologic state that is attempting to increase lean muscle mass and repair muscle tissue after exercise.

After 30 years of working in the diet and lifestyle milieu I simply allow the fad diet to fit the patient's personality. It appears the end may justify the means, and whatever appears necessary to reduce caloric intake and improve activity and reduce weight seems appropriate. A recent non-industry funded review from Stanford and the University of Toronto may have provided further impetus for this novel approach [91]. Researchers utilized a total of six electronic databases and overweight or obese adults randomized to a named (aka "fad") diet for 3-months or longer were included (primarily analyzing weight loss and BMI changes at 6- and 12-months). Two reviewers independently procured this data and the analyses were adjusted for behavioral support and exercise. A total of 48 randomized trials including over 7200 individuals were included. The results of this analysis found that weight loss differences between fad diets were "small." And the conclusion was noteworthy: *"This supports the practice of recommending any diet that a patient will adhere to in order to lose weight."* This is a particularly relevant finding since a recent a comprehensive global report concluded that over the past 33 years not a single country has experienced success against the obesity epidemic [92]. This also relates to why the next patient recommendation/step number 5 also revolves around caloric restriction.

In conclusion as long as a patient can fulfill five Dr. Moyad criteria on any fad diet I am a personal advocate of it. These criteria include:

– Cholesterol or LDL improvements
   (*note*: as a bonus I might also recommend hs-CRP or another low-cost inflammatory marker which tends to be reduced with weight loss)
– Blood pressure improvements
– Blood Sugar improvement
– Weight and/or waist circumference reduction
– Stable mental health during the fad diet

The above parameters appear to be similar to the Step 1 recommendation in this chapter, which is also not a coincidence. Regardless, there is one final critical point that must be demonstrated to health care professionals and patients in terms of weight/waist gain and obesity. This medical condition (obesity) is now responsible for a striking number of diseases either in terms of increasing risk and/or exacerbating the risk of recurrence or severity or even death from almost countless medical conditions. This list of diseases, found in Table 3.8 [80], has increased so dramatically that I like to provide and overview during my lectures or discussions with individuals in the public, patients, and health care workers (everyone).

Table 3.8 Obesity is now the primary preventable cause of illness and premature death and arguably the strongest lifestyle factor (or second to exercise) in terms of breast cancer risk and increased risk of recurrence. Some of the medical conditions increased or worsened with obesity are found in this table [80]

Acid reflux (GERD)	Hot flashes
Atrial fibrillation	Immobility
Blood Clots	Incontinence
Breathlessness	Infertility (men and women)
Cancers (breast, cervix, colorectal, endometrial, esophageal, gallbladder, kidney, liver, multiple myeloma, non-Hodgkin's lymphoma, ovarian, pancreas, and prostate—may also increase risk of getting a more aggressive form of cancer)	Kidney disease, kidney failure and need for dialysis
Complications from surgical procedures	Low back pain (chronic)
Diabetes	Low testosterone
Eye disease that can lead to blindness	NAFLD/NASH (aka fatty liver)
Fetal defects from maternal obesity	Osteoarthritis
Gallbladder disease	PCOS
Gout	Pregnancy complications (preeclampsia …)
Heart disease	Sexual dysfunction (female sexual dysfunction and erectile dysfunction)
Heart failure	Sleep apnea
Hiatal hernia	Stroke
High blood pressure	Urinary tract infection
High cholesterol	Varicose veins …

General Heart Health = Breast Health Step #5 for your patients:

Consume a diversity of low-cost fruits and especially vegetables (veggies tend to be lower in calories and sugar compared to fruits) and do not consume high-calorie, high-cost, and high-antioxidant exotic or even traditional fruit juices (unless there is a low-calorie option). Many fruit juices now have as much or more sugar compared to a regular cola or can of sugary soda. The processed (juice) versus non-processed (whole fruit or vegetable) debate begins and ends here. Rainbow of fruits and vegetables (high in antioxidants) does not have more data/clinical endpoints compared to dull or plain appearing fruits and vegetables (lower in antioxidants). Why I could go into medical marketing and why the organic or inorganic debate will not matter one day soon?!

Media attention and research appears to focus on one fruit or vegetable with each passing year. Why? In my opinion it is because of good marketing and knee-jerk responses without the careful evaluation of the publication [80]. Clinicians need to be able to remain somewhat objective and explain to patients that these media reports do not necessarily represent any major research breakthrough, but rather supports the ongoing and past research that consuming a diversity of low-cost fruits and especially vegetables is just one practical and logical approach to improving heart health. Several examples of this controversy exist including the past attention garnered toward the compound lycopene and tomatoes in preventing cancer based on numerous epidemiologic studies and a notable meta-analysis [93]. However, this meta-analysis concluded by reminding readers that this is just further evidence that a diversity of fruits and vegetables were important for a healthy diet, but this appeared to be misconstrued. Tomatoes were never the only or necessarily the primary source of lycopene. A variety of other healthy products contain this compound such as: apricots, guava, and pink grapefruit [94–97]. Watermelon is also an outstanding source of lycopene, and is the largest source per gram compared to any other nutritional source, including tomato products. Regardless, lycopene has minimal overall beneficial data to solve various health issues, but at least the compound and products that contain this compound are generally safe or even heart healthy [98–100].

The ongoing pomegranate juice and supplement research has experienced a somewhat similar story, but with a slightly different message for clinicians. Although this is a story that is rooted in prostate cancer, it is a paradigm or lesson as to why other cancers including breast cancer should not succumb to preliminary data without more heart healthy studies to suggest it is a situation of "first do no harm." The first attention gathering study did not include a placebo group or another group of men that consumed another type of healthy juice product [101], and other studies have questionable methodology and results [102]. Yet this should not be construed as a lack of efficacy and some of these companies should be lauded for at least investing in research, but an objective overview of the preliminary research and the caloric contribution of these and other juices are necessary. Many brands of these novel juices contain at least 140 calories per 8 ounce serving, which is a similar caloric contribution than most commercial regular soft drinks and alcoholic drinks (approximately 100–150 calories) [79, 80]. A quick glance at the internet and commercialized products now demonstrates that many fruit juices have as much or more sugar per ounce than a can of cola! Thus, fad diets that also dramatically reduce sugar intake (ketogenic or high fat, high protein, …) also appear to provide favorable results for those that can comply with them over the short- or long-term.

Further, again in partial defense of some of these companies it is also laudable that some lower caloric exotic juice options from these same manufacturers are now becoming commercially available. Still, many of these juices are expensive in comparison to cheaper nutritious and lower calorie products. Additionally, drug and juice interactions are still being researched, which is important since grapefruit juice studies has provided a paradigm of medication interactions [103], but novel juices may also cause some potential concern with medications metabolized by CYP3A4 [104, 105]. In reality, if a patient believes in pomegranate juice or another product I often recommend lower calorie or a no calorie option and utilize weight and other heart healthy changes (Moyad 5 parameters above for an effective fad diet) as the primary driving force or whether or not to continue or advocate for or against this patient driven regimen. I am not optimistic that any "exotic" or fruit juice high in calories and sugar will be found to reduce cancer incidence, progression or survival. And I also find it interesting that there are no consistent examples of these juices in the literature assisting patients with cholesterol, blood pressure, blood sugar or weight/waist reduction. Although past preliminary laboratory data has now accrued for pomegranate juice and breast cancer [106], clinicians need to be cautious about making any claims in the area without some future heart healthy data. Again, I am not optimistic.

Patients should try and think of the "natural" or "processed" debate as particularly applying to fruits and vegetables. Fruits or vegetables in their natural state are generally associated with less cost, less calories, less sugar, and more fiber [79, 80]. An apple is better than apple juice or applesauce, and an orange is better than orange juice. It is interesting that it takes multiple oranges to produce one cup of orange juice and the extra sugar and minimal to no fiber also is carried into glass of what I call "liquid sugar." In terms of fullness and potentially helping to lower weight, fruit and especially vegetables can be of assistance and they also play a role in lowering blood pressure with their high potassium and low sodium content. Overall, the specific evidence for fruit and vegetable intake and heart health is moderately consistent but in the area of breast cancer prevention or to reduce recurrence the evidence is inconclusive or weak [107, 108].

Fruits and vegetables have unique and shared anticancer and anti-heart disease compounds that may contribute to improved overall health. Again, the overall data currently supports a slightly greater potential reduction in CVD risk and mortality [109], perhaps through assisting in weight loss or via another heart healthy compound(s) such as natural salicylates (aka aspirin derivatives) or other natural compounds in these products (please also refer to Chap. 5 in this book for more on the subject of food salicylates) [110]. Clinicians should recommend fruit and vegetable consumption for better overall and heart health, but not for cancer prevention where large-scale data appears to be less impressive [111]. There are also certain high risk factors for breast cancer (obesity, alcohol, genetics, lack of exercise, tobacco, ...) that cannot be simply fully eliminated or erased by improving one aspect of lifestyle such as increased fruit and vegetable consumption. In other words, triaging lifestyle changes or recommendations from most-to-least important is critical to a patient's success.

Another point is critical for your patients, because it appears that the public is inundated by "experts" espousing the regular consumption of the most colorful or diverse or a variety of fruits and vegetables with the most antioxidants for a greater potential benefit on health. However, this is not evidence-based and has a not proven when analyzing past research on heart health. It is difficult enough to consume regular quantities of fruits and vegetables and I do not advocate creating a lifestyle recommendation simply because it appears to make sense when it fact it is not supported by research. For example, in one of the largest epidemiologic studies to date to examine the issue of fruits and veggies and heart disease, a higher intake of fruits and veggies was associated with a lower risk of heart disease (only about 17 %—not dramatic but modest) [112]. However, there was no added advantage over consuming a diversity or variety of fruits and vegetables. Over 71,000 women from the

Nurses' Health Study and over 42,100 men from the Health Professionals Follow-Up-Study were followed for over 20 years and over 6000 cases of heart disease cases were diagnosed in this study (largest to date). It was also interesting that this study documented the effect of a threshold for fruits and veggies whereby up to five servings a day provided more protection and beyond five servings the impact was the same. Interestingly only 1 other study has looked at fruit and veggie variety and heart disease and again no difference was found for diversity or variety [113].

Again, it is difficult enough to consume several servings of fruits and veggies a day and this is reflected in the national average or just 2–3 servings! What happened to avocado, celery, cucumber, or kale? They might not be brightly colored but they have a lot to offer, so I simply tell patients to consume the ones they like to consume first and foremost. Pushing fruits or vegetables only because they are brightly color in my experience has also caused some patients to seek out exotic or novel juices from a variety of sources that are "high in antioxidants" such as mangosteen or acai or goji and they spend a lot of money and time doing this which reinforces quick-fix without hard clinical effects or endpoints behavior. In other words, these creates a great deal of disappointment and noncompliance versus boring or dull products or fruits and veggies which harbor more evidence, less cost, and greater overall benefit and mental health for patients. I think the latter increases compliance and reduces stress.

In order to further exhaust the point that marketing or what tends to feel good can drive dietary or fruit and vegetable recommendation, I will take a moment to impress the reader when it comes to this author's personal marketing skills. It could be argued that since 50,000 or more overall medical publications occur each month there are enough studies to espouse any position in medicine today if subjectively reviewing the data. I argue often that medicine is a courtroom with the preponderance of the evidence that provides the highest probability of the truth. However, if someone wanted to slant the truth when the subject of fruits and vegetables is discussed I have decided to provide a review in Table 3.9 of how any fruit or vegetable could be construed as life changing based on preliminary data of some the compounds in them and basic research [79, 80]. In this table (see Table 3.9) are only a small percentage of the compounds found in these products that tend to receive some form of health promotion (imagine if I decided to publish the comprehensive list).

Additionally, health care professionals and patients ask if fruits and vegetables in a capsule are healthy and similar to ingesting fruits and vegetables in terms of antioxidants. And although some research exists from these companies to support preliminary blood marker benefits, there are no clinical endpoints in general that are exciting for me (especially in terms of cardiovascular disease prevention). And the idea of promoting more pills rather than the real product has always been concerning and I discourage it. Healthy behaviors promote more healthy behaviors like a pendulum that continues to swing in just one direction. I want to see all the vitamins, minerals, and especially fiber that are derived from real fruits and vegetables that are not capable of being placed in a capsule. In my experience, when someone relies just on a capsule for their fruits and vegetables, apart from paying an enormous

Table 3.9 Fruit or vegetable brightly or dull colored and how it could prevent disease in the Dr. Moyad Marketing world [79, 80]

Fruit or vegetable	Healthy compounds from the medical literature	Disease it may prevent from the medical literature (generally laboratory studies but don't tell anyone)?
Acai (fruit or juice) (pronounced ah-sigh-EE)	– Twice the antioxidant capacity of blueberries – 20 vitamins and minerals (including iron and vitamin E) – Omega-3, 6, and 9 fatty acids	– Currently receiving research in a variety of areas – Anticancer – Anticancer – Anti-heart disease
Apples	– Quercetin—a flavonoid	– Anticancer – Improve lung function
Allium vegetables—onions, leaks, garlic, …	– Sulfur containing compounds – Quercetin—high in onions	– Anti-heart disease – Anticancer – Anti-gastrointestinal cancers and bladder cancer
Asparagus	– Folic acid – Phytoestrogens – Sulfur containing compound	– May reduce liver enzymes and toxicity – Asparagusic acid (1,2-dithiolane-4-carboxylic acid) creates odorous urine for added effect in some individuals
Avocado (Persea americana) (a fruit related to cinnamon and sassafras)	– Potassium (more than banana) – High in monounsaturated fat – Highest content of lutein among commonly eaten fruits (70 % of carotenoids) – No cholesterol – Haas avocados—most common are available year round – Do not ripen till picked—fresh ones will be as hard as a rock (ripe when skin is almost black and yields to soft pressure) – Vitamin E	– Anticancer – Anti-heart disease – Aztecs used it as a sexual stimulant (known as the "testicle tree")
Banana Note: When banana is picked—soluble pectin increases—gives off ethylene gas—changes its color and can make other items ripen as well—like a green tomato to red or avocado or other bananas ripen …	– Potassium (450 mg–only potatoes, some beans, avocados, and tomatoes may contain more) and 1 mg of sodium – Folic acid – 2.5 g of fiber (one of the highest in nature) – Small amount of pesticides and herbicides-thick outer covering	– Anti-stroke – Anti-colon cancer

(continued)

Table 3.9 (continued)

Fruit or vegetable	Healthy compounds from the medical literature	Disease it may prevent from the medical literature (generally laboratory studies but don't tell anyone)?
Beets	– One of highest sources of inorganic nitrate, which can be converted to nitric oxide in human (especially beet root juice)	– Anticancer – Athletic enhancement – Lowers blood pressure – Studied to improve female and male sexual function
Broccoli	– High in isothiocyanates	– A cruciferous vegetable with some of the most preliminary evidence of an anticancer effect
Celery	– Low calorie – High in fiber – Luteolin – Apigenin	– Anticancer – Anti-heart disease
Cherries	– Anthocyanins (class of plant pigments responsible for the color of many fruits)—antioxidants – Vitamin C and metabolite of vitamin C	– Antidiabetic – Anti-arthritic – Anti-gout
Cranberries	– Proanthocyanidins—antioxidants	– UTI prevention – Anticancer
Cruciferous vegetables—Broccoli, broccoli sprouts, cabbage, cauliflower, …	– Vitamin C – Sulforaphane – Beta-carotene – Calcium – Fiber – Folic acid – Indole-3-carbinol (I3C) – Lutein – Reddish fermented cabbage (sometimes radish)—vitamins A, B, C, and "healthy bacteria" = lactobacilli	– Anticancer (stomach, bladder cancer, skin cancer, and others) – Anti-heart disease – May change estrogen metabolism to make it less potent and safer – Anti-inflammatory or potentially analgesic properties
Grape	– Polyphenols	– Anti-heart disease – Reduces platelet stickiness – Increases nitric oxide (a vasodilator)

Grapefruit	– Vitamin C – Folic acid – Flavonoids such as naringin or naringenin (structurally related to genistein—a flavonoid from soybean that many reduce cholesterol)	– May reduce cholesterol or more specifically triglycerides (red perhaps more than blond grapefruit)
Mango	– Vitamin C – Fiber	– Anti-disease
Mangosteen	– Xanthones (a family of tricyclic isoprenylated polyphenols)	– Anti-disease
Mushrooms	– Beta-glucans – Vitamin D – Ergothioneine—antioxidant—cooking has no impact on concentrations – Exotic varieties like shiitake and oyster offer the most ergothioneine (than portobellos and cremini, and white button the least)	– Immune boost or improved immune health – Anticancer – Anti-heart disease
Noni juice	– Contains multiple vitamins/minerals/electrolytes	– Anti-disease
Orange	– Vitamin C – Folic acid – Flavonoids such as hesperidin are structurally related to genistein (flavonoid from soybean that may reduce cholesterol)	– Heart healthy – Colon health – Anticancer
Persimmons (orange looking fruit) (two varieties—Hachiya and Fuyu)	– Low in calories (about 100) – High in fiber – Vitamin A – Vitamin C	– Anti-disease

(continued)

Table 3.9 (continued)

Fruit or vegetable	Healthy compounds from the medical literature	Disease it may prevent from the medical literature (generally laboratory studies but don't tell anyone)?
Pomegranate	– Soluble polyphenols – Tannins – Anthocyanins	– Anti-heart disease – Anticancer
Prunes (also known as the "dried plum")	– High in fiber – Poly-phenolic compounds (powerful antioxidants) such as neochlorogenic acid and chlorogenic acid – Ranked as one of the highest oxygen radical absorbance capacities (ORAC) among the commonly consumed fruits and vegetables – Selenium and boron	– Anti-heart disease – Anticancer – Anti-osteoporosis
Pumpkin	– Carotenoids – Fiber – Plant sterols	– Seeds or oil from seeds promote prostate health
Red Guava (November to March and from June to August in stores—round or pear-shaped—about the size of a large plum and dark green on the outside with soft and reddish flesh)	– Higher concentration of antioxidants than apples, carrots, oranges, and tomatoes, but a little lower than blueberries …	– heart Healthy – Anticancer
Spinach	–Xanthophylls—lutein and zeaxanthin—block 50–60 % of oxidative damage from sunlight (UVB) – Folic acid	– Anti-cataracts and anti-macular degeneration – Anticancer – Anti-heart disease – Brain healthy – Popeye endorsed it so has to be healthy
Strawberries	– Folic acid – Ellagic acid	– Anticancer (famous for being associated with a reduced risk of some cancers in one of the largest studies of tomatoes and cancer risk)

Watercress (also known as *Nasturtium officinale* or "nose twister" which refers to plant's pungency. It was thought to prevent baldness by Greeks, and Francis Bacon told women to eat it to prevent signs of aging)	– Phenethyl isothiocyanate or PEITC released when chewed or cut – Vitamin A, C, minerals, …	– Inhibits numerous human cancer cell lines – Now extracts in clinical trials as a drug to prevent tobacco-causing cancers (lung …)
Watermelon	– Lycopene (one of the highest natural sources of lycopene-yes more than tomatoes in most cases) – l-citrulline (highest source of this amino acid—found primarily in the rind)	– Inhibits numerous human cancer cell lines – Anti-heart disease – Athletic enhancement – Increases nitric oxide and being studied for female and male sexual dysfunction

financial cost they pay an enormous health cost by promoting their own pill seeking behavior and then their pendulum can swing in the opposite direction.

I am also often asked about "organic" versus "non-organic" fruits and vegetables and this is one of many examples where I let the economic pressure of our time determine the outcome. Similar to the trans-fat debate many years over time it became economically problematic if food products continued to harbor them so many companies began to remove them. Similarly, it hurts the economic viability long-term of a company not to offer a more "organic" option, so in time I believe prices will continue to drop on organic fruits and vegetables, especially as all of the leading food chains have begun to offer them [80]. Currently, since compliance on fruits and vegetables is low and since organic for the most part is still costly I cannot ethically espouse their use in most patients especially ones that are economically disadvantaged, and there is no consistent evidence as of yet they personally provide a healthier clinical endpoint or outcome. I believe organic will be a better future choice for environmental and perhaps other health reasons, but there is only so much energy to expend in a day and I am allowing the passage of time and economic pressure to ultimately solve this issue. I am comfortable that soon an organic box of many fruits and vegetables will be the price of the non-organic option.

General Heart Health = Breast Health Step #6 for your patients:

Consume more (soluble and insoluble) dietary fiber (20–30 g/day, or 14 g per 1000 calories consumed), especially from food sources. "Fiber is nature's internal Botox for the human body" and both soluble and insoluble fiber have unique and synergistic benefits when found together (as in most healthy dietary sources [80].

General and numerous health benefits are derived from consuming dietary fiber that have been well documented and include reductions in the following [114–117]:

– Coronary heart disease (CHD) risk
– Stroke
– High blood pressure
– Diabetes
– Obesity
– All-cause mortality

For example, a pooled analysis of past cohort studies of dietary fiber for the reduction of CHD (coronary heart disease) included research from ten international studies and included the USA [118]. Over a period of 6–10 years of follow-up, and after multivariate adjustment it was revealed that each 10 g/day increase of calorie-adjusted total dietary fiber was correlated with a 14 % reduction in the risk of total coronary events and a 27 % reduction in risk of coronary death. These findings were similar for both genders, and the inverse associations occurred for both soluble ("viscous") and insoluble fiber.

Past studies have not observed a consistent benefit with one class of fiber over the other [119, 120]. Recent large US and other international studies have even found more striking overall potential benefits for consuming more dietary fiber. For example, the NIH-AARP US prospective cohort found not only a lower risk of dying from cardiovascular, respiratory and infectious disease with greater intakes but a significantly lower risk of dying younger ("total death") in men and women [121]. This study may represent a major shift into the research behind fiber intake because now the potential health impact may be so much larger than first realized since reductions in the death rates of some of the largest causes of mortality may occur with greater fiber intakes [121, 122].

Even minor additions of fiber can positively impact medication dosages. A total of 15 g of psyllium husk supplementation daily with a 10 mg statin (simvastatin) was demonstrated to be as effective as 20 mg of this statin by itself in reducing cholesterol in a preliminary placebo-controlled study of 68 patients over 12-weeks [123]. Although adding soluble fiber from commercial products appears to be safe and synergistic with cholesterol lowering medications [124], the first choice of increasing fiber intake should be food sources based on cost-effectiveness and simplicity.

A meta-analysis of 24 randomized placebo-controlled trials of fiber supplementation found a consistent impact on blood pressure reduction [125]. Supplementation with a mean dose of only 11.5 g/day of fiber reduced systolic blood pressure by −1.13 mmHg and diastolic pressure by −1.26 mmHg. The reductions were actually greater in older and more hypertensive individuals compared to younger and normotensive participants. Recent international studies continue to support the modest reduction or control in blood pressure with greater intakes of dietary fiber [126].

How much fiber should patients be consuming daily? Daily intakes of total fiber in the USA and many other Western countries is approximately 10–15 g/day, which is approximately only half or even less than half of the total amount consistently recommended by the American Heart Association (AHA) and American Dietetic Association (20–30 g/day) for adequate overall health [116, 117, 127]. Another perspective on recommended fiber intake for children and adults is that for every 1000 calories of food and beverage consumed there should be at least 14 g of fiber consumed.

Dietary fiber from food is easily achieved by low cost sources of soluble and insoluble fiber. For example, I often tell patients to just consume a third of a cup of a bran cereal such as All-Bran Buds® several times a week, which is approximately only the size of 1–2 liquor shot glasses, with flaxseed and some fruit, and before they leave the door in the morning approximately 20 g of fiber will have already been ingested toward the 25–30 g goal [79, 80]! Low-cost fiber sources such as flaxseed can provide potentially numerous heart healthy and overall healthy benefits and outcomes [128, 129]. Perhaps the low-cost and non-commercialization of this product on a large-scale has led to the lack of adequate education that I have observed on this product. Flaxseed is also one of the highest plant sources of heart healthy omega-3 fatty acids [129], and chia seed is arguably the largest plant source of fiber and omega-3 [130], and both of these additions to the overall diet would be ideal.

Interestingly, the preliminary clinical trial data on ground flaxseed (average of 30 g or three rounded tablespoons per day) in other hormone mediated cancers such as prostate disease and prostate cancer has been as or more impressive (reduced proliferation rates or Ki-67) versus a low-fat dietary intake [131–134]. Thus, it should not be a surprise that preliminary data of flaxseed in breast cancer is also impressive and similar to some of the prostate cancer observations. For example, human studies of 25 g/day of flaxseed for 4 weeks downregulated Ki-67 by 34 %, increased apoptosis by 30 %, and decreased HER2 neu by 71 % in breast cancer [135].

Flaxseed contains a high concentration of lignans, which are also considered phytoestrogens, which are structurally related to endogenous estrogens and tamoxifen [79, 136]. The primary circulating lignan is known as "enterolactone," a weak estrogen compared to estradiol. Flaxseed may favorably alter hormone pathways, growth factors, aromatase and inhibit cell growth in estrogen positive and negative cell lines. Flaxseed oil also has preliminary data against breast cancer [137], but this and other oils are a large source of calories (120–130 calories/tablespoon) and contain no fiber so rarely have I recommended them over low cost flaxseed powder (similar to the real whole non-processed fruit versus the fruit juice debate mentioned earlier).

Overall dietary fiber intake (again not pills or powders) continues to garner evidence as a method of breast cancer prevention. One of the largest meta-analyses reviewed 16 prospective studies found a lower risk primarily among studies with a large range of intakes or high levels of fiber consumption, which equated to 25 g or more per day [138]. Another meta-analysis of 10 prospective studies involving over 16,800 cases, and also found a significant reduction in risk with greater intake [139]. This correlation did not differ by geographic area, menopausal status, or follow-up length. And for every 10 g/day increase in dietary fiber consumption there was a significant 7 % reduction in breast cancer risk. Multiple mechanisms are potentially involved with this fiber benefit including:

- Reduction in estrogen via the suppression of bacterial beta-glucuronidase activity in the gastrointestinal tract which inhibits the reabsorption of estrogens in the colon and increases estrogen content of the feces,
- Increased sex-hormone binding globulin (SHBG),
- Reduction in insulin and growth factors/mitogens related to this compound,
- Reduction in inflammatory compounds potentially via production of short-chain fatty acids when fibers are fermented in the colon by flora and products of fermentation such as butyrate and propionate enter the circulation,
- A plethora of heart healthy changes altering breast cancer risk/recurrence (lower weight/waist, reduced cholesterol and blood sugar)

Still, fiber itself appears to have become overtly commercialized, and in my experience some patients are turning primarily toward powders and pills to solve their fiber deficit, and this is not only costly, but it also provides primarily small amounts of soluble fiber that make it difficult to reach their total fiber goal utilizing only these sources. For example, I often ask audiences and students how many fiber capsules/pills are needed to be consumed daily to obtain just 20–30 g of fiber, and the answer always seems to provide adequate shockvalue (the answer is 30–50 pills a day or more depending on the commercial source) [80]! A bolus of only soluble fiber without insoluble fiber can also create excessive bloating and other gastrointestinal issues because soluble fiber is utilized by gut bacteria and then subsequently converted to gaseous compounds.

Processed soluble fibers abound today in protein bars and cookies and these items need to be avoided not only for a lack of evidence but again gastrointestinal discomfort with moderate to high intakes [80]. Research continues to support the overall and heart healthy health benefits of fiber, especially when it is primarily derived from food sources [116], because these sources also provide a unique and optimal balance of soluble and insoluble fiber. Another comprehensive list of dietary fiber benefits are found in Table 3.10 and this is why I often tell patients that "nature's greatest internal Botox" has to be dietary fiber! The plethora of internal antiaging effects it provides is noteworthy, from preventing cholesterol and glucose changes to preventing hemorrhoids, and it is easy to forget that humans do not just age externally but internally with time. Botox for cosmetic antiaging is attention grabbing but why isn't fiber just as notable for preventing internal aging? Table 3.10 can help level this playing field so to speak [79, 80].

Table 3.10 Fiber should be considered nature's great internal Botox for preventing and treating a diversity of aging effects on the human body [79, 80]

Antiaging and other benefits of fiber	
(1)	Helps with weight control because it delays the emptying of gastric contents, delays the absorption of fats, and promotes a feeling of fullness
(2)	Improves glucose or sugar balance by delaying the movement and absorption of carbohydrates into the small intestine—burn fuel more efficiently and evenly
(3)	Reduces cholesterol levels by binding with bile (cholesterol carrying products) in the intestine and causing it to be excreted or eliminated.
(4)	Increases the weight of the stool and softens the stool—so it promotes regular and smooth bowel movements
(5)	Reduces the colon transit time so that the stool goes through intestines faster
(6)	Reduces pressure within the colon
(7)	Reduces the risk of multiple cancers?
(8)	Reduces the risk of diverticulosis and diverticulitis
(9)	Reduces symptoms of Irritable Bowel Syndrome (IBS)
(10)	Reduces inflammation and inflammatory markers (CRP …)
(11)	Reduces the risk of acid reflux or gastroesophageal reflux disease (GERD)
(12)	Reduces the risk of and may even treat hemorrhoids or constipation
(13)	Reduces blood pressure
(14)	May reduce the risk of preeclampsia
(15)	Is an ideal prebiotic, thus reducing the dependence or need for probiotic pills
(16)	Reduces cardiovascular disease, stroke, and appears to favorably impact all-cause mortality (increase life span)

Table 3.11 Soluble and insoluble fiber have unique benefits to each and also share health benefits, which is why both are ideally needed in the same product and most health dietary sources harbor both types [79, 80]

Specific benefits of soluble and insoluble fiber		
Benefit	Soluble fiber	Insoluble fiber
Lowers total cholesterol and "bad" (LDL) cholesterol	YES	NO
Reduces sugar or glucose blood levels after a meal	YES	NO
Reduces the absorption of sugar or glucose from the small intestine	YES	NO
Delays gastric emptying or increases the amount of time it takes for food to leave the stomach—thus giving a sense of fullness and discouraging higher caloric intakes	YES	NO
Increases the production of intestinal gas	YES	NO
Increases the speed at which the stool moves the intestines—reduces the impact time that carcinogens have on the intestine	YES	YES
Increases the size of the stool and the frequency of bowel movements	YES	YES
Reduces the amount of essential nutrients absorbed by the body	NO (not in moderation)	NO (not in moderation)

Additionally, an appreciation of the two broad categories of fiber-soluble and insoluble fibers, are needed in order to understand why consuming both is critical for overall health. I find it interesting that most fruits, veggies, beans, bran, oatmeal, and other dietary sources of fiber are primarily an equal mix of soluble and insoluble fiber or insoluble fiber actually predominates over soluble in these products, while again most commercial products are basically almost all soluble fiber. They are both needed to improve compliance and health effects and a generalization or broad summary (there are exceptions) of what that they can do for patients are found in Table 3.11 [79, 80].

The reason one can consume two medium apples (about 10 g of fiber total) without experience significant bloating or gas or discomfort is the majority of the fiber is insoluble (about 30 % soluble). However, the reason one cannot consume a large bolus of processed or commercialized fiber supplements or powders is that the vast majority is soluble fiber. In other words, nature's fiber ratio provides all the health benefits and minimizes the side effects and cost [79, 80].

General Heart Health = Breast Health Step #7 for your patients:

Consume moderate (approximately two servings or more) weekly intakes of a variety of healthy fatty fish, but fried and high mercury concentrated fish should be generally discouraged. Other healthy plant-based sources of omega-3 fatty acids (for example nuts and healthy plant cooking oils) should also be equally emphasized (especially so for non-fish eaters). Pills have not replaced these dietary sources.

Numerous types of oily fatty fish contain high concentrations of marine-based omega-3 fatty acids (compounds known as "EPA and DHA"). Fish are also the best natural food source of vitamin D3 (cholecalciferol), and they contain high concentrations of high-quality protein and a diversity of minerals [79, 80]. Omega-3 fatty acids from food sources have exhibited numerous benefits in terms of reducing the risk of a variety of prevalent chronic diseases [140, 141], especially some aspects of cardiovascular disease [142–148]. There is also growing evidence for an ability of omega-3 from fish to reduce the risk of a diversity of unique health conditions including kidney stones [149, 150].

A variety of health fatty/oily fish contain high levels of omega-3 fatty acids, vitamin D, and protein including salmon, tuna, sardines, anchovies, Great Lakes whitefish and a variety of other baked, broiled, raw, but not fried fish are potentially beneficial [79]. Diversity should be encouraged to increase compliance and exposure to a range of nutrients.

The true clinical impact of mercury from fish on adult individuals remains controversial [151, 152], and it is possible that mercury may reduce some of the benefits of fish consumption [153]. Four types of larger predatory fish have been most concerning (king mackerel, shark, swordfish, and tilefish) because they have the ability to concentrate larger amounts of methyl-mercury over their longer life spans. However, moderate and recommended consumption (2–3 times/week) of most fish should have minimal impact on human mercury serum levels. A large investigation of moderate mercury serum levels in older individuals found little to no negative long-term impacts on neurobehavioral parameters [154]. A randomized trial of mercury exposure from dental amalgam in children also found no significant health issues [155]. The positive impact of consuming fish appears to outweigh the negative impact in the majority of individuals with the exception of women considering pregnancy or who are pregnant (although this is also controversial—see ongoing ALSPAC or Avon Longitudinal Study of Parents and Children in the medical literature).

One of the largest US cohorts to evaluate this issue found lower cardiovascular disease risk in adult men and women consuming higher amounts of fish regardless of mercury exposure (Benefit > risk) [156]. Interestingly, low-cost and low-mercury fish such as anchovies and sardines have some of the highest concentrations of omega-3 oils that are used in omega-3 fatty acid clinical trials utilizing dietary supplements for heart disease and cancer [79]. It should also be kept in mind that the American Heart Association (AHA) recommends approximately two servings of fish per week and plant (not just fish) omega-3 consumption [157], which I try to reiterate often to patients. Thus, the healthiest sources of omega-3 compounds in food are coincidentally very low in mercury.

Fish oil supplements for completely healthy individuals or for chronic disease prevention does not have data, and the use of fish oil to prevent heart disease in a primary or secondary prevention setting has mixed results because of potential subgroup benefit or harm [158–161]. For example, three recent phase-3 like trials from atrial fibrillation [162], to overall cardiovascular disease prevention in high-risk women and men [163], and even moderate to severe macular degeneration [164] have shown no benefit for omega-3 or fish oil supplementation. Thus, it would be prudent to wait to let the research on fish oil supplements in otherwise healthy individuals mature before providing a verdict.

The data for omega-3 and fish oil tends to mirror the cardiovascular prevention research, and suggests if there is any impact on breast cancer it is derived primarily from dietary or food sources [165, 166]. For example one of the largest reviews of 21 independent prospective cohort studies and approximately 21,000 cases of breast cancer were conducted [166]. Regardless of whether marine intake of omega-3 was derived from dietary recall or tissue biomarkers there was a 14 % modest reduction when higher versus lower intakes were compared.

The role of fish oil supplementation is garnering more research and attention in reducing side effects from conventional breast cancer treatment rather than for treatment itself. For example, improving cognitive function, prevention of sarcopenia or peripheral neuropathy has indirect human clinical data that simply needs more research in breast cancer patients [167–170]. Furthermore, one of the major omega-3 compounds in fish oil, docosahexaenoic acid (DHA), is being tested in combination with the chemotherapy drug paclitaxel to provide a potential for better tumor site delivery of chemotherapy itself [171].

Patients that are not consumers of fish could also utilize algae based sources of omega-3 supplementation or consume foods high in plant omega-3 (flaxseed, chia, nuts, ...) or alpha-linolenic acid (ALA) that is converted to a marine form of omega-3 (EPA) in the human body at variable amounts [79, 80].

Tree nuts share some similar clinical positive impacts of marine omega-3 oils. A consistent reduction in the risk of CHD and/or sudden cardiac death has been associated with an increased consumption of a diversity of nuts in prospective studies, and they can also reduce inflammatory markers that impact a variety of organ systems [172–177]. Nuts contain a variety of potential beneficial compounds such as: ALA (the primary plant-based omega-3 fatty acid), other polyunsaturated fats, monounsaturated fats, vitamin E, magnesium, potassium, fiber, and flavonoids [79]. Nut consumption via an improvement in heart health may also improve other aspects of health impacted by breast cancer such as diabetes [178]. However, the primary limitation of tree nuts is their high caloric content when going beyond several servings a day. Healthy plant oils utilized for cooking such as soybean, canola, olive oil, and safflower also contain a high concentration of omega-3 fatty acids, monounsaturated fat, and numerous other vitamins and minerals such as natural vitamin E [79]. Most cooking oils contain 120 calories/tablespoon; therefore, moderation again is the cornerstone to good health and nutrition.

Overall, minimal research into nut consumption and breast cancer status has been conducted, but again the overall findings on heart health and reduction in insulin resistance is sufficient to recommend them to patients dealing with various aspects of breast cancer. In my clinical experience many patients are now utilizing more macadamia nuts (high in fat and lower in carbohydrates) as part of their weight loss or ketogenic or semi-ketogenic protocol or for more other fad diets they appear to provide some positive role in moderation. Still, all form of nuts and even seeds contain some health characteristics that could be learned and utilized from the high content of fiber in almonds to the high plant omega-3 level in walnuts [79].

General Heart Health = Breast Health Steps and Recommendation Summary and Synergism for your patients:

Educate patients on the first seven heart healthy lifestyle changes because only 1–2 % of individuals are able to follow these on a regular basis. It is the sum of what is accomplished in moderation that has the highest probability of impacting heart and breast health compared to just one or several lifestyle changes in extreme (similar to cardiovascular disease prevention). Add other parameters as personally needed and triaged (sodium reduction, potassium increase, alcohol in moderation, coffee/caffeine in moderation, protein supplementation, pill reduction or addition, adult vaccines, …).

If multiple lifestyle changes, or if achieving numerous healthy parameters over time appears to be associated with the largest improvements in overall health then this theory should be tested. And it has been tested over the years and the results are profound. For example, data from the National Health and Nutrition Examination Survey (NHANES) was utilized that included 44,959 US adults 20 years of age or older [179]. Mean age was 46–47 years and approximately half of the participants were women. Median follow-up was 14.5 years. A total of only 1–2 % of the participants met all seven of the health parameters. Amazingly, there were a 51 % reduction in all-cause mortality, 76 % reduction in cardiovascular mortality, and 70 % reduction in ischemic heart disease (IHD) mortality for participants meeting 6 or more metrics compared to 1 or fewer. Achieving a higher number of cardiovascular health parameters also appeared to be correlated with a lower risk for all-cancer mortality. The following seven goals/parameters were utilized in this study (do they look familiar?!):

– Total cholesterol equal to or less than 200 mg/dl
– Blood pressure equal to or less than 120/80
– Fasting blood glucose less than 100 mg/dl
– Avoiding all tobacco products
– Being physically active almost every day of the week
– BMI 25 or less
– Overall diet that is moderately heart healthy (fruits/veggies/fiber/fish, …)

Another classic example of the benefit of just following one or two of the above healthy lifestyle parameters is derived from the Nurses' Health Study which reviewed 24-years of follow-up data in 116,564 women who were 30–55 years old in the 1970s and were healthy and not diagnosed with cancer or cardiovascular disease [180]. During the 24 years of study, a total of 10,282 deaths occurred mostly from cancer (5223 deaths) and cardiac disease (2370), but 2689 deaths occurred from other causes. Regardless of whether the researchers looked at dying from any cause there was interesting trend that occurred when multivariate relative risks were utilized. Women that were of normal weight and that exercised about 30 min a day had the lowest risk of dying of any cause compared to any other type of woman in this cohort. However, the researchers also found that thin women that hardly exercised had a greater chance of dying of any cause compared to thin women that exercised regularly. Obese women that rarely exercised had the highest chance of dying early, but the researchers also found that obese women (of the same general weight) that exercised about 30 min a day had a lower risk of dying from any cause compared to the obese women that rarely exercised! Thus, the greatest probability of living longer can be found in normal weight individuals that exercise 30 min daily or more and follow other healthy lifestyle parameters, but even if an individual is overweight or obese and exercises it still counts as an investment in long-term health. Interestingly, this same data and results can easily be derived from notable male cohort studies [181, 182].

Other past general health comprehensive lifestyle studies have demonstrated that few (less than 5 %—usually 1–2 %) individuals have reported adhering to numerous moderate healthy behaviors at one time [183]. Again, the collective sum of what is accomplished, rather than 1 or 2 specific behavioral changes have the largest impact on cardiovascular markers, CVD, cancer, and all-cause mortality [184]. Thus, I often use checklists derived and modified from the Mediterranean diet US study [185], and the INTERHEART study and other lifestyle studies to ensure verve and compliance in patients [79, 80, 186–190]. These studies essentially found that regardless of race, age, genetics and geographic location around the world, the ability to essentially maintain numerous consistent features of lifestyle and/or diet was associated with a 85–95 % reduced risk of a cardiovascular event (regardless of age or gender or race), and similar behaviors and changes in other recent studies demonstrated an improved ability to live far beyond average life expectancy with minimal mental or physical morbidity. The critical characteristics in these individuals included behavioral changes with no commentary or benefit or detriment in taking a dietary supplement or another pill.

Table 3.12 is a modified often utilized handout or checklist that I created and provide to individuals seeking to increase their odds or probability of living longer and better-through dietary changes adapted from a Mediterranean diet (moderation in everything diet) [79]. How many patients or even colleagues have all of these features or need to work on these changes? How many health conditions could be prevented or improved with these heart healthy changes? Keep in mind, I am not a primary advocate for a Mediterranean diet in breast cancer (remember diet fits personality and numerous diverse programs can help), but instead I use it as a paradigm of a "moderation in everything" approach that also can be beneficial.

Many health professionals find themselves at critical moments in a patient's care that could determine the future adherence to life changing lifestyle changes. The impact of mentioning just one study in consultation with a patient could be profound. For example, sodium intake also appears to follow a U-shaped curve. However, arguably one of the best clinical trials that could have an educational role for overall health and sodium consumption was from the DASH diet study [191–193]. Basically, the Dietary Approaches to Stop Hypertension (DASH) study was organized and financed by the National Heart, Lung, and Blood Institute (NHLBI) to look at the effects of overall dietary changes on blood pressure and then sodium

Table 3.12 US Mediterranean diet study (paradigm for an everything-in-moderation diet)—individuals with scores of 6 or more on the checklist had a lower risk of early mortality compared to those with scores of 4 or less. Just review the checklist, and add up the points [79, 185]

Beverage or food	Answer Yes or No (1 point for each question answered "yes" and zero points for a "no")
Alcohol—two drinks a day or less for men and one drink or less for women	
Fat intake focused on healthy fats, mostly monounsaturated and polyunsaturated (canola, olive, safflower oil, etc.)	
Fish—at least two or more servings per week	
Fruit—four or more servings a day	
Legumes/beans—two or more servings a week	
Meat—one or less servings a day	
Nuts and seeds—two or more servings a week	
Vegetables (other than potatoes)—four or more servings a day	
Whole grains (for example whole/multigrain and whole wheat foods with high amount of fiber and protein)—two or more servings a day	
Total score	

Note: Traditional Mediterranean diets also allow moderate intakes of dairy, such as cheese, milk, and yogurt

restriction in addition to these dietary changes. The DASH study involved 459 adults age 22 years or older with a systolic blood pressure lower than 160 mmHg and a diastolic blood pressure 80–95 mmHg, which is considered prehypertension or stage 1 hypertension. None of these individuals were taking blood pressure medications. *Approximately 50 % of the individuals were women, and 60 % were African Americans, which is a landmark clinical trial simply because women and minorities have been completely underrepresented in past trials especially of lifestyle changes.* The participants of DASH were assigned to one of three groups over an 8-week period:

1. A control or moderate diet similar to a normal American diet, but lower in calcium, magnesium and potassium intake.
2. Similar to the control diet but more fruits and vegetables.
3. A DASH diet which included fruits and vegetables, low-fat dairy, whole grains, chicken, fish, nuts, and low in fats, low in red meat, low in sweets, and low in beverages that are high in sugar.

Thus, the DASH diet is high in calcium, magnesium, potassium, and fiber, but low in saturated fat, low in trans fat, and low in cholesterol. All three diets contained the same amount of sodium or salt at 3000 mg/day, but participants were allowed 500 mg of extra sodium daily if they wanted. Alcohol consumption was limited to two drinks or fewer per day, and weight was not supposed to be decreased or increased during the study. It is interesting that the 3000 mg of salt per day is actually still about 20 % below the US average, but it is still above the recommended average consumption of 2400 mg of day.

After the original DASH study was concluded researchers conducted a similar study of a control diet compared to the DASH diet. In each diet group (control or DASH) participants ingested three different rotating levels of sodium intake in random order for 30 days each including: 3000 mg of salt per day, 2400 mg of salt per day or 1500 mg of salt per day. Therefore, each individual ingested all three sodium daily amounts on his or her assigned diet, which was either DASH or control diet. Researchers found that reducing salt intake lowered systolic and diastolic blood pressure significantly in both the control and DASH dietary group. The impressive findings in this part of the study were:

- The DASH diet itself lowered blood pressure at all the levels of sodium ingestion.
- Reducing salt intake to 1500 mg/day reduced the blood pressure by two times as much as the higher sodium intakes.
- The impact of lowering salt intake AND following the DASH diet on blood pressure was much greater when it was combined; so overall dietary changes and salt reduction is a far more powerful combination then either change by itself.
- Overall, the combined impact of the DASH diet and reducing sodium to 1500 mg a day was a decrease of −8.9 mmHg systolic and −4.5 mmHg diastolic.
- Overall, the combined impact of the DASH diet and reducing sodium to 1500 mg a day in normal blood pressure patients was a decrease of −7.1 mmHg systolic and −3.7 mmHg diastolic.
- Overall, the combined impact of the DASH diet and reducing sodium to 1500 mg a day in high blood pressure patients was a decrease of −11.5 mmHg systolic and −5.7 mmHg diastolic.

These findings are ground breaking in terms of lifestyle changes to reduce blood pressure! Patients should be first given the choice of eating an overall healthy diet and lowering salt intake (increasing potassium) before necessarily being offered medication, or regardless of medication status they should be offered this diet and salt reduction to reduce blood pressure. Also, another ground breaking conclusion; even patients with normal blood pressure can significantly reduce their blood pressure with dietary change and a lowering intake of salt. Whether a person has high blood pressure or not, and whether or not they are on a blood pressure medication or not the message is very clear. Moderately changing diet to reduce blood pressure includes the following changes derived from the DASH diet:

- more grains (7–8 daily servings)
- more vegetables (4–5 servings a day)
- more fruits (4–5 servings a day)
- low-fat or no fat dairy products (2–3 servings a day)
- low to moderate meat, poultry, or fish (two or less servings a day)
- more nuts, seeds, and dry beans (4–5 servings a week)
- low fats and oils (2–3 servings a day, the DASH diet had 27 % of total calories as fat, which is moderate)

- low in sweets (five servings a week, also low in fat)
- 1500 mg or less of sodium per day or 2400 mg a day, depending on the individual situation, and keep in mind that most sodium reduction comes from eating healthier and reducing intake of processed foods—not from the salt shaker.

Again, the findings from the government funded DASH study are profound, and should be reviewed by health care professionals and patients. The impact of the DASH protocol is now beginning to show potentially dramatic results in other areas of medicine. For example, in the Health Care Professionals Follow-up Study of 45,821 men with 18-years of follow-up and the Nurses' Health Study I and II of approximately 195,000 women with 14–18 years of follow-up, researchers constructed a DASH diet score and evaluated kidney stone risk [194]. A total of 5645 kidney stones were documented during this time period. The group with higher DASH scores (greater intakes of potassium, magnesium, oxalate, calcium, and vitamin C and lower sodium intake) experienced a 40–45 % reduction in the risk of a kidney stone. Again, this suggests that the sum of personal lifestyle behaviors and parameters are far more powerful on heart and overall health compared to one or just a few changes. I find it compelling that a comprehensive heart healthy lifestyle program appears to have the greatest risk reduction on the majority of diseases that cause morbidity and mortality in women and men.

One more critical note needs to be reviewed with patients and the DASH diet. One could also argue that the large increases in potassium and fiber intake and reduction in sugar and sodium and mild weight/waist reduction accounted for the dramatic drops in blood pressure (similar to what is observed with pharmaceutical drugs) [79, 80]. And this is my point of view—that it was the synergism that resulted in the clinical outcome or change. It is difficult to simply reduce sodium intake without dramatically increasing potassium intake in foods and also lowering sugar intake when consuming a DASH diet.

Bonus/Extra Credit After Reviewing the 7-Steps:
Less is more when it comes to the consumption of pills for preventive health.
Unless a patient qualifies for a pill there is no convincing evidence that high doses of concentrated antioxidants prevent breast cancer or recurrence in otherwise healthy individuals. Heart healthy dietary supplements that also mimic prescription medications when needed will arguably demonstrate the largest impact in overall disease prevention or adjuvant off-label breast cancer treatment. Dietary supplements will primarily and arguably have more of a role in mitigating side effects of some cancer treatments (American ginseng for cancer-related fatigue, melatonin for insomnia, protein powder for sarcopenia and weight loss or gain, ...) versus treating cancer itself.

What is missing from the first seven ideal health recommendations for your patients? The utilization of pills (supplements or prescriptions) to prevent cardiovascular or breast cancer, especially in otherwise healthy individuals because the benefit has not been found or the studies above and their participants were not regularly consumers of pills and medications. Is this a surprise? There is also minimal data to suggest a dietary supplement can prevent breast cancer recurrence.

For example, despite minimal scientific evidence, multivitamins are the largest selling supplements in the USA by men and women with over 40 % of the population utilizing them [195, 196]. They are also the primary supplement utilized by participants in notable prostate cancer screening studies [197], male health prevention trials [198], male physicians [199], and notable women's studies [200]. Why such overall and diverse endorsement without data especially in women? Perhaps it is the perception of the evidence compared to the reality, but in reality the vast majority of the observational data has been unimpressive thus far [201]. Thus, until higher quality evidence finds some realistic benefit with these supplements the potential even for some harm when taking them in excess seems concerning, especially in terms of other medical conditions or hormone mediated cancers [202, 203]. For example, an increased risk of advanced and fatal prostate was found in one of the largest prospective epidemiologic studies of multivitamins for those taking more than one per day, and the greater use of other supplements were also associated with an even greater risk [203]. Men with a family history of prostate cancer experienced the largest and most significant elevated risks of this condition. Other large male observational studies have found somewhat similar results [204, 205].

It is interesting that some recent studies in breast cancer has somewhat mirrored these negative findings [206, 207]. Overall, the data is not impressive thus far in a positive or negative direction and it is plausible that a good deal of confounding occurs.

Multivitamins are replete in my experience with higher doses of B-vitamins, which have also recently been found to potentially have no impact on health or increase the risk of some cancers from one of the largest and most recent meta-analysis of clinical trials [208, 209]. Since there is no consistent suggestion of benefit with a larger intakes (2 or more per day) of multivitamins, and since there is a suggestion of either no impact or serious harm it would be prudent to wait for more clarity [210, 211], or in my opinion begin to tell most men and patients to reduce their dosage of adult multivitamins to one pill a day maximum based on recent data that will be discussed next in this chapter.

A partial level of insight may have been provided in the Supplementation en Vitamines et Mineraux Antioxydants (SUVIMAX) randomized, placebo-controlled trial that included several vitamins and minerals at very moderate or low dosages not usually utilized in clinical trials [212], and commonly found in current children's or older adult formulations from my experience. SUVIMAX was a randomized, double-blind, placebo-controlled primary prevention trial (participants were healthy at the start of the trial) of healthy individuals. A total of 13,017 French adults (7876 women aged 35–60 years and 5141 men aged 45–60 years) were included in this study. All of the individuals took either a placebo or a daily capsule that consisted of:

- 120 mg of vitamin C
- 30 mg of vitamin E
- 6 mg of beta-carotene
- 100 μg of selenium
- 20 mg of zinc

These individuals were than followed for 7.5 years. Nothing notable occurred in the group as a whole, but men experienced a nonsignificant ($p = 0.54$) 18 % reduction in ischemic cardiovascular risk, a significant ($p = 0.008$) 31 % reduction in risk of being diagnosed with cancer, and a significant ($p = 0.02$) 37 % reduction in the risk of dying from any cause. It appeared that taking a low-dose multivitamin minimally based formula could provide a potential benefit for some men, but no benefit was found for women. The researchers from this study suggested that men benefited only because they had lower levels of these vitamins and minerals in their blood from less than optimal dietary patterns at the beginning of the study compared to the women that consumed a more healthy diet on average. For example, approximately 50 % of the men were former smokers compared to 29 % of the women and BMI in women was 23 versus 25 in men and cholesterol and glucose were lower in women. This clinical trial is arguably one of the best pieces of evidence to date for men's and women's health and the consumption of a mixed dietary supplement product. Thus, I will repeat an often cited mantra of mine that it would be wise not to take anything larger than a children's or older version of an adult 1 pill a day multivitamin (see PHS2 next) until someone can demonstrate that "more is better," which as mentioned earlier is currently not the case.

PHS2-The only major multivitamin randomized trial of healthy individuals-Less is More.

The largest multivitamin randomized clinical trial ever conducted in healthy individuals was the Physicians' Health Study II (PHS2), which included 14,641 physicians age 50–70 years old consuming a Centrum Silver® or placebo for approximately 11 years [213, 214]. Unfortunately, no women were included in this trial but it still should be reviewed with women concerned about breast cancer to help apply an objective discourse on the subject.

The primary endpoints were cancer and cardiovascular events and the results have provided more clarity on the multivitamin issue. PHS2 found a significant ($p = 0.04$) 8 % cancer reduction in total cancer incidence compared to placebo. Cancer incidence was reduced in men with and without a personal history of cancer. However, a larger nonsignificant 18 % reduction was found for men age 70 and over at baseline and those with a personal (not familial) history of cancer (−27 %), but no benefit was found for those with a parental history of cancer. Current smokers (less than 4 % of the participants) appeared to receive a large benefit (−28 %) compared to former and never smokers. The side effects were similar to a placebo, although in the placebo and supplement arms approximately 27 % and 29 % of the men in their respective groups complained of a rash at one time or another (even a placebo carries some side effects). Further subgroup analysis found that men consuming seven or more fruits and vegetables per day benefitted as much as those that consumed less than four servings a day, and those with a normal BMI benefited as much as overweight or obese men.

There was no increased or decreased risk of this multivitamin on cardiovascular events in PHS2, which is reassuring [214]. Yet fatal myocardial infarction (a secondary endpoint) was reduced by 39 % ($p = 0.05$; 27 versus 43 deaths) in the multivitamin group, but especially in those men without a baseline history of CVD (−44 %, $p = 0.03$; 22 versus 39 deaths). Men with a history of cardiovascular disease did not have an increase or a decrease in the risk of dying from a myocardial infarction with the multivitamin compared to placebo (5 deaths versus 4). Since so few fatal myocardial infarctions occurred in this trial it appears the researchers are suggesting that this finding was due to chance. There were sufficient numbers of cardiovascular events (stroke, death from heart disease, ...) overall to demonstrate that the multivitamin did not increase or decrease the risk of cardiovascular disease overall.

More recently, a slight reduction in cataract risk was found in the PHS2 (−9 %, $p = 0.04$) [215] and this is a consistent finding in previous randomized clinical trials [216, 217], and meta-analysis for women and men [218].

It is interesting that the original Centrum Silver utilized during this trial from 1997 to 2011 is not the over the counter product offered to consumers currently because over time these nutritional formulations appear to change based on some science and marketing demand. Therefore, if one is impressed by this data, a single children's multivitamin could be recommended for an adult because this dosage appears to be similar to an older Centrum Silver or the patient should just consume the newest Centrum Silver or something close to the formula in another product, which is detailed in the clinical trial publication and found in Table 3.13. Women interested in consuming one multivitamin a day can compare and contrast their product of interest with this product.

Thus, for pennies a day it is possible to modestly or mildly reduce the risk of being diagnosed with cancer and perhaps cataracts with similar side effects to a placebo. Additionally, the modest amounts of other vitamins and minerals suggest this is all that is needed if a multivitamin is even needed at all. I was surprised at how critical some alternative and conventional medical "experts" acted when this study was released. Some conventional folks argued the results were not impressive enough and some alternative experts suggested a different multivitamin would have had a better result? Centrum Silver should be applauded and rewarded for volunteering to be in this study because they risked their business by being a part of this research. *The biggest flaw of this study was the lack of women participants in*

Table 3.13 The 30-ingredient Centrum Silver® multivitamin utilized versus placebo during the Physicians' Health Study II randomized trial of over 14,000 male physicians for approximately 11.2 years [213]

Vitamin A = 5000 IU (50 % as beta-carotene)	Vitamin B12 = 25 µg	Copper = 2 mg
Vitamin C = 60 mg	Biotin = 30 µg	Manganese = 3.5 mg
Vitamin D = 400 IU	Pantothenic acid = 10 mg	Chromium = 130 µg
Vitamin E = 45 IU	Calcium = 200 mg	Molybdenum = 160 µg
Vitamin K = 10 µg	Iron = 4 mg	Chloride = 72.6 mg
Vitamin B1 = 1.5 mg	Phosphorus = 48 mg	Potassium = 80 mg
Vitamin B2 = 1.7 mg	Iodine = 150 µg	Boron = 150 µg
Niacin = 20 mg	Magnesium = 100 mg	Nickel = 5 µg
Vitamin B6 = 3 mg	Zinc = 15 mg	Vanadium = 10 µg
Folic acid = 400 µg	Selenium = 20 µg	Silicon = 2 mg

Note: IU = international units, mg = milligrams, µg = micrograms *the original design and trial* [219] *and this is a major flaw, but overall it should still be perceived as arguably the most rigorous and informative trial ever conducted on multivitamins. And the message is the same in healthy women and men-less is more!*

I am often cornered after a lecture by an advocate of another multivitamin product that is far more expensive, and claim more research than Centrum Silver. Yet these individuals are never able to produce a randomized trial of their product versus placebo with over 14,000 individuals for more than 14 years (not even close). Others argue that I am promoting Centrum Silver when in reality I am just fulfilling my moral and ethical duty to clearly mention the product used in this trial because no two multivitamin formulations are identical and I would conduct myself in the same fashion if this were the result of a drug trial. Transparency is critical here because no two multivitamins are identical. Finally, others complain that Centrum Silver is not a "clean" product and other more expensive multivitamins with less additives or fillers or dyes should be recommended and my response is that the list of ingredients in terms of vitamins and minerals are provided in Table 3.12, and if someone desires to take something cleaner then this then it is their prerogative and of course I also support their position on this matters (if this truly matters to them). The results of the PHS2 are impressive but modest or slight at best and it appears as the population continues to quit smoking and nutrients continued to get added to the food supply in record amounts the need for multivitamins in otherwise healthy individuals will probably diminish. And this is another reason I believe the results appeared to be greater in the PHS2 for the current smokers (only 3–4 % of the participants) versus the nonsmokers.

Regardless, how much more evidence do health care professionals and patients need throughout medicine, especially when the recent results of the SELECT trial (an all male trial), the largest chemoprevention trial of dietary supplements in medical history in healthy individuals that demonstrated a significant increased risk of prostate cancer when utilizing 400 IU daily of vitamin E [220]. And there was a nonsignificant increased risk of aggressive prostate cancer in all the dietary supplement groups compared to placebo [220], and an increased risk of hemorrhagic stoke in another similar randomized trial [221]. Recently, there was also a report from the SELECT trial that men assigned to selenium supplements already replete with selenium from diet and other sources at baseline experienced a significant increased risk of being diagnosed with aggressive prostate cancer [222]. And two more clinical (not basic science) reports of a higher risk of accelerating the growth of potential cancer precursors or increasing the risk of death from prostate cancer with higher selenium supplemental intake and other nutrients [223, 224]. It should "first do no harm" so why would higher doses of supplements be encouraged for otherwise healthy individuals concerned about breast cancer-another primary hormone mediated tumor type. *The only current consistent rationale utilization currently for supplements in breast cancer is for the prevention or treatment of side effects from treatment* [80], *which arguably a wonderful example of the benefits that can be derived for supplements (aka drugs) in the right evidence-based situation.*

Calcium and/or Vitamin D (negative acute phase reactant?)

Other dietary supplements do not have adequate chemoprevention or treatment data in healthy individuals for breast health, for example calcium supplementation

Table 3.14 Sources of calcium (and vitamin D) from food/beverages/multivitamin that allow for many individuals to cease utilizing calcium supplements [79, 80]

Beverage or food	Milligrams per serving
Almond milk/cashew/hemp and other newer fortified dairy milk alternatives	450–500 (8 ounces = 1 cup)
Multivitamin (Women's-new)	200–500 (per single multivitamin pill)
Yogurt (plain, low-fat)	400–425
Sardines (in oil with bones)	300–325
Cheddar cheese (and other cheeses)	275–300
Milk (skim and other types)	275–300 (8 ounces = 1 cup)
Orange juice (calcium fortified)	200–250
Salmon (with bones)	200–225
Cottage cheese	125–150
Spinach	100–125
Kale	75–100
Breakfast cereal (ready to eat)	75–100 (some brands contain more)
Soy milk	75–100 (some brands contain more)

Important bottom line:
– Try to work with a nutritionist. Keep in mind that dietary sources of calcium count toward your total recommended daily allowance of calcium (1000–1200 mg/day), so if you are having trouble calculating your current daily intake of calcium from beverages and foods talk to a hospital, private or doctor recommended nutritionist. For example, if you get on average 800 mg of calcium daily from beverages and foods than all you need to do now is get 400 mg a day from a dietary supplement (total = 800 + 400 = 1200 mg—you have met your goal)
– *Note*: RDA for calcium is 1000 mg in 19–50 year old males and females, 1000 mg in 51–70 year old males, 1200 mg in females 51 years and older and males 71+ years

(unless needed for bone health in breast cancer patients). And since calcium is so replete in multivitamins, food and fortified beverages today it has become easier than ever before to attain the recommended 1000–1200 mg/day (1000 mg in 19–50 year old males and females, 1000 mg in 51–70 year old males, 1200 mg in females 51 years and older and males 71+ years). Table 3.14 is a representation of how much easier it is to reach the RDA goal of calcium without having to take separate calcium supplements (see Table 3.14) [79, 80]. In fact, in the largest dietary supplement trial ever conducted on calcium supplements (WHI) the baseline intake of calcium from foods, beverages, and supplements was already approximately 1150 mg/day of calcium before randomization to the calcium or placebo groups!

Vitamin D dietary or supplements have studies that suggest harm from obtaining excessive intakes, which is also what has been preliminarily found in prostate cancer [225, 226]. The latest Institute of Medicine (IOM) report should also be a reminder that despite the perception, the recommended intakes of vitamin D have only increased by 200 IU (5 μg) in most groups and vitamin D supplements have the potential to increase the risk of hypercalcemia and nephrolithiasis [227]. Vitamin D is important for bone health, but the amount needed has been embellished and exaggerated in my opinion. Vitamin D tends to function more like a hormone, which is why caution should be followed because the potential for a U or even J-shaped risk curve does exist. One of the largest and longest randomized trials in elderly women found that excessively high blood levels of vitamin D from high-dose supplementation compared to placebo was actually associated with an increased risk of falls and fractures [228].

The vitamin D blood tests have a history of uncertainty based on the assay utilized [229, 230], and it is costly. Clinicians need to also remind patients that vitamin D blood levels may simply be a marker of healthy behavior. A lean woman or man, with a low cholesterol that consumes fish and exercises regularly is more likely to have a higher blood level of vitamin D compared to a physically inactive overweight or obese woman or man with a high cholesterol level and other heart unhealthy parameters [231, 232]. So, is it really the vitamin D supplement providing the majority of the benefit for health, or the finding that normal or just higher vitamin D levels could be found on average in more healthy women and men? It is for this reason that there is mounting evidence that vitamin D or *rather 25-OH vitamin D also functions as a negative acute phase reactant* [233]. Medical conditions with higher inflammatory disease status appear to greatly reduce the blood marker of vitamin D status. Regardless, patients should be reminded that improvement in heart healthy parameters could increase vitamin D levels without or with additional smaller increments in supplementation. *In other words, this moment represents a wonderful opportunity to emphasize heart healthy lifestyle changes first before relying on increasing the pill count of the average patient.*

S.A.M. (Statins–Aspirin–Metformin.)—"Natural Options"

Interestingly, the additional issue is that until a supplement or drug is found to be safe and heart healthy (benefit >>> risk), I am not an advocate for recommending it to patients, especially as a preventive or ancillary treatment. And dietary supplements again should be advocated for specific oncologic situations. It is interesting that in the field of breast or prostate cancer prevention perhaps the most intriguing medications for prevention or for ancillary treatment in my opinion may be heart healthy prescriptions or over-the-counter medicines that have been tested for long periods of time. In other words, these pills now all have generic options, and are heart healthy in the appropriate patients and all are derived from "natural" sources (statins from a fungus, aspirin from willow bark, and metformin from the French Lilac) [80]. Statins, aspirin, and metformin (S.A.M.-acronym that helps to remember to discuss with patients and SAM is a unisex name) [234] are garnering some impressive indirect data [235–242], and one (metformin) has a phase-3 breast cancer trial to prevent recurrence and mortality, and already has impressive metabolic or heart healthy changes from this intervention in the actual phase-3 trial itself [243]. Yet these medications all have the ability to cause more harm than good in the wrong patient [244–246]. I believe effective dietary supplements currently will be ones that are heart healthy or heart neutral and mitigate side effects from breast cancer treatment and this is actually occurring now in breast and other cancers (again direct data for ginseng for cancer fatigue, ginger for nausea, melatonin for insomnia, and indirect data for protein powder for weight gain or loss) [247–251]. And these evidence-based dietary supplement changes need to be embraced. And I believe effective chemoprevention or prevention of recurrence of breast or prostate or another cancer with a supplement will be accomplished when a particular product is able to mimic some of the mechanisms of heart healthy effects observed with S.A.M. [234]. For example, please see Chaps. 4, 5, and 6 on S.A.M., which include statins and the commentary on red yeast rice supplements [252] or salicin and aspirin, or perhaps berberine or alpha-lipoic acid and metformin [80]. And in the worst case scenario if a heart healthy pill does not work but reduces the risk of the number 1 cause of death in women and men (cardiovascular disease) then I believe it is a step forward in medicine, and not a lateral or backwards move, which appears to be the norm lately.

Conclusion

Countless simplistic lifestyle changes could have been proffered in this manuscript but why belabor the minutiae over the profound? Let me remind the reader of the heart healthy goals/parameters that could have such a profound impact on overall heath and longevity and mirror the data of what is potentially beneficial against breast cancer and these are:

- Total cholesterol equal to or less than 200 mg/dl
- Blood pressure equal to or less than 120/80
- Fasting blood glucose less than 100 mg/dl
- Healthy BMI (less than 25) and waist circumference (WC)
- Avoiding all tobacco products
- Being physically active almost every day of the week
- Overall diet that is heart healthy (fruits/veggies/fiber/fish, ...)

Again, only 1–2 % of patients can achieve these parameters? Is it possible that as hundreds of millions of tax payer dollars have been utilized attempting to identify the ideal dietary supplement or pharmacologic agent for cancer prevention and health, but in reality the ideal lifestyle program had already been tapping us on the shoulder all along?! Clinicians now have access to a wealth of data that suggests that an ideal breast cancer program for prevention and ancillary utilization along with conventional treatment diet and lifestyle program does exist to reduce the primary causes of morbidity and mortality in women and men and a plethora of these recommendations were outlined in this chapter. A quick review of the 7-step heart and overall health program from this chapter can be found in Table 3.15.

Health care professionals should embrace lifestyle and dietary changes for everything from cancer to kidney stones, and several ways to demonstrate your commitment to lifestyle changes in your medical practice from my experience are outlined in Table 3.16. One of the most common questions I am asked by health care practitioners around the world is how to encourage healthy lifestyle changes in such a short time that is allotted with each patient? Some of the most successful tips that have worked in my opinion are briefly reviewed for the health care professional in Table 3.16.

A cumulative review of the potential impacts of lifestyle changes and supplements on a variety of aspects of breast health and breast cancer are reviewed in Table 3.17 for those that need a quick A to Z guide as a refresher or even a brief list that can be given to patients from this chapter and other sources [79, 80, 253].

Table 3.15 A review of the Ideal Heart Health = Breast Health Lifestyle Program and Checklist (*note*: only 1–2 % of the population are able to achieve all seven steps consistently)

7 Step IDEAL LIFESTYLE PROGRAM Review (reviewed and discussed by patient and health care professional)	Your score (1 point if ideal or "normal" and 0 points if "abnormal" or needs more work)
1. Cholesterol? Blood pressure? Blood Glucose? BMI and/or Waist Circumference?	4-point maximum
2. Avoid tobacco and second hand smoke	1-point maximum
3. Approximately 30–60 min of physical activity a day or more on average should be the goal or enough exercise to achieve optimal mental and physical personal health, which should include lifting weights/resistance exercises 2–3 times/week	1-point for aerobic and 1-point for resistance activity (*note*: resistance and aerobic can be combined for example with certain types of yoga, Pilates, and essentially pick the exercises that give you the most enjoyment and compliance)
4. Reduce overall caloric intakes to achieve or maintain a healthy weight, regardless of the method/fad diet utilized as long as changes in step one improve, and mental health status is healthy or improves. Fad diet should fit personality	1-point wherever the reduction (alcohol, sugar, …)
5. Consume a diversity of low-cost fruits and especially vegetables (veggies tend to be lower in calories and sugar compared to fruits) and do not consume high-calorie, high-cost, and high-antioxidant exotic or even traditional fruit juices (unless there is a low or zero-calorie non-weight gaining option)	1-point maximum for avoiding fruit juices or caloric beverages with sugar and 1-point for beating the national average on fruit and veggie daily consumption (3 per day total)
6. Consume more (soluble and insoluble) dietary fiber (20–30 g/day, or 14 g per 1000 calories consumed), especially from food sources. "Fiber is nature's internal Botox" and both soluble and insoluble fiber have unique and synergistic benefits when found together (as in most healthy dietary sources)	1-point for ingesting 20–30 g/day of total fiber and 1-point for achieving your fiber goals without pills or powder or gimmick foods with processed fiber
7. Consume moderate (approximately two servings or more) weekly intakes of a variety of healthy fatty fish, but fried and high mercury concentrated fish should be generally discouraged. Other healthy plant-based sources of omega-3 fatty acids (for example nuts, flaxseed, and other healthy plant-based products/oils) should also be equally emphasized	1-point for two servings or more of plant and/or marine omega-3 sources
Bonus: What pills do I really need, and which ones can be reduced or eliminated as I adhere to more healthy lifestyle changes?	1-point every time a pill is reduced completely or a dosage is reduced for a pill due to better self-education on the need or because of a lifestyle change!

Additional Personalized Recommendations for your patients:

Table 3.16 Dr. Moyad's ten suggestions on how to immediately improve patient adherence/compliance in your medical practice with heart healthy = breast healthy lifestyle changes [79, 80, 253]

Improving adherence/compliance to the ideal lifestyle and diet program	Example and/or commentary
1. Simplify practical but pithy recommendations for patients (less than one sentence is enough in many cases) and redirect medical minutiae toward the life changing seven steps	1. Heart health = Breast Health or Heart Healthy = Prostate Healthy, Heart Healthy = Bladder/Brain/Colon/Kidney/Sexual Health … The seven steps in this chapter should help maintain a forest over tree approach, so if someone is obsessed by the trivial such as cell phones and brain tumor risk then redirect the conversation to the seven steps and explain the reason for doing this (Heart Healthy = All Healthy)
2. Practice and also appear to be exactly what you preach (perception should match the reality)	2. Clinicians should not only appear to be fit but follow the specific lifestyle recommendations they advocate
3. Motivate patients to practice what you preach by teaming up at least once a year	3. Pick a charity event annually such as a fun run, biking event, walk … that you and your patients can participate in yearly
4. Get to know ancillary behavioral assistance in your community and provide specific examples to your patients, which will provide credibility	4. Familiarize yourself with local nutritionists, trainers, health clubs, weight loss programs, health classes, etc. and precisely what these services have to offer the patient
5. Do not solve the world's problems in one visit … pick a single goal for your patients, or triage their preventive health and then write a quick personalized (from the desk of Dr._____ for example) lifestyle prescription to the patient or letter for the patient's employer	5. Better to know and recommend a variety of smoking cessation programs when talking to tobacco utilizing patients compared to spending additional time on environmental toxins or specific dietary changes. Also, better to be able to discuss the specifics of weight loss programs compared to specific dietary supplements for obese patients. Write an exercise prescription on a pad just like a drug prescription and occasionally write employer of your patient asking for some exercise time to help reduce employer and employee insurance costs

Improving adherence/compliance to the ideal lifestyle and diet program	Example and/or commentary
6. Office pictures are worth a thousand words. Show patients the moment they walk into and through your office that lifestyle changes are paramount to your practice setting	6. Handouts in the waiting room, BMI or waist circumference posters in the exam rooms, advertisements for exercise and cooking classes, a variety of health magazines, …
7. Office staff are just as important as you in sending the message	7. All members of the office staff should be as excited about lifestyle changes including providing information to patients on goals, local classes, fitness events, health coupons, …
8. Encourage the patient's spouse or another family member to attend the office visit	8. Ask the scheduling staff to remind the patient that you like to have at least one other family member in the room to improve quality of the patient visit
9. Encourage patients to give back to the community in your practice ("spiritual health screening"), which will develop cohesiveness and charity within and outside the practice setting	9. Ask patients to volunteer, donate blood, exercise for charity or another identified community need for a bidirectional health benefit
10. Personalize your practice to the patients whenever the opportunity arises	10. Dr_____ top ten lifestyle tips after breast cancer treatment. Feel free to give one-page handouts on your specific lifestyle recommendations before or after a particular procedure, recipes, …. Provide personal health book or DVD recommendations, …

Table 3.17 Heart healthy, heart unhealthy, and other cardiovascular disease (CVD) parameters and interventions and their potential correlation with the risk of breast cancer and breast cancer recurrence [79, 80, 253]

CVD parameter/interventions	Correlation with prostate cancer risk
Alcohol (*Note:* Moderation is still one drink a day in women and two drinks a day in men. A drink is defined as one 12-ounce beer, 4–6 ounces of wine, and 1.5 ounce liquor shot) (One drink in moderation usually contains 10–15 g of alcohol)	– A fairly consistent risk factor for breast cancer (all types of alcohol at a variety of regular intakes from moderate to excessive). Alcohol may mimic a "weak estrogen," reduce levels of key dietary nutrients (for example folic acid), promote immune suppression, create direct cellular damage, increase weight/waist size, increases insulin, increase triglycerides, … – Alcohol also tends to change bone markers in a favorable way in moderation but increases the risk of osteoporosis in excess (toxic to osteoblasts …). Other notable effects of excessive alcohol consumption include: increased histamine-like effects (can exacerbate allergies), increases in blood pressure (vasoconstrictor in excess), increase in multiple GI cancers (a definite carcinogen), disruption in deep phases of sleep, memory issues, and addiction issues
Aspirin (low dose) (low cost, generic, and "natural"-derived from the Willow Bark and Meadowsweet) (three forms of aspirin primarily exist-immediate release with the majority of the research, buffered, and enteric-coated)	– Determine if an individual concerned about breast cancer qualifies for aspirin based on CVD risk working with their health care professionals and utilizing risk scores such as Reynolds Risk Score (determine if benefit > risk overall-in general benefit more likely in women 65 and older) – Aspirin may be associated with a lower risk of breast cancer and recurrence. Currently, aspirin does appear to lower colorectal cancer risk in women and men, especially from recent research from the Women's Health Study (after 10-years of low-dose aspirin use even every other day) – Beware of expensive pain relief copycat dietary supplements that contain "salicin," which is arguably just similar to cheap aspirin in disguise because salicin like cheap aspirin is metabolized to "salicylic acid" which then exerts analgesic, anti-inflammatory and anti-fever effects (but salicin appears not to provide blood thinning effects like with low-cost aspirin/acetyl-salicylic acid)
B-vitamins (folic acid, B12, B6, ….)	B-vitamins especially folic acid from dietary sources could reduce the risk of some cancers (colorectal …) and lower concentrations of folic acid due to alcohol intake could increase the risk of breast cancer – However, B-vitamin dietary supplements have no evidence to reduce the risk of cancer, and have been actually implicated in some clinical trials (such as B-PROOF clinical trials) as potential stimulators of already established tumors especially gastrointestinal tumors and also some hormone driven cancers such as prostate cancer. B-vitamin supplements have not shown any potential to reduce breast risk or recurrence-only no impact or slight increased risk – B12 (and magnesium) blood levels needs to be monitored on acid reflux or metformin because these drugs are known to reduce these nutrients

Calcium and calcium supplements (Adult RDA for calcium is 1000–1200 mg/day) (RDA for calcium is 1000 mg in 19–50 year old males and females, 1000 mg in 51–70 year old males, 1200 in females 51 years and older and males 71+ years)	– No impact on breast cancer overall but may reduce the risk of bone loss and hip fracture in women who get regular adequate intakes (from WHI trial—80 % compliance per year with daily intakes). However, many foods now fortified with calcium may make calcium supplements antiquated. For example, one 8 ounces cup of some almond milk contain 455 mg of calcium! Only need two cups a day to support almost all of your calcium needs – Three forms of supplements over the counter A. Calcium carbonate-most studied and most concentrated so less pills need, but needs to be used with a meal to increase absorption and can increase the risk of kidney stones and constipation B. Calcium citrate-next most studied and you need to take more pills cause less concentrated so more expensive but can be used with or without meals and does not appear to increase stone risk but increases risk of constipation – Calcium phosphate-least studied and concentrated so less pills and need to assume similar issues as with calcium carbonate until proven otherwise *Note*: Magnesium (50–100 mg or more) is often used in or with a calcium supplement to soften the stool *Note*: The concern over calcium supplements increasing the rate of a cardiovascular event is controversial, but in excess harm ≫ benefit anyway and going above the RDA is not needed
Caloric control or reduction/diet (*Note*: The WINS trial demonstrated a significant reduced risk of breast cancer relapse after treatment with a low fat or really a reduction in calories and average of 6 pounds of weight loss when the trial concluded versus the WHEL trial that showed no difference in breast cancer outcomes with comprehensive dietary changes, but there were not significant weight or caloric reductions at any point during the WHEL trial. This may explain the difference in the observations from these trials)	– Reducing caloric intake to assist in preventing weight gain may reduce breast cancer risk and recurrence. Regardless of the method to reduce calories (high fat, low fat, high protein, low carb, moderate carb, …) as long as Dr. Moyad's five parameters are maintained or improved there should be support for the heart healthy diet program. The five parameters of a successful Dr. Moyad diet include: – Reduce cholesterol (LDL and/or triglycerides and maintain or increase HDL), – Reduce blood pressure, – Reduce blood glucose, – Reduce weight/waist, and – Improve or stable mood/mental health As an added bonus following a inflammatory marker on a diet such as hs-CRP is a good additional option to monitor diet success

(continued)

Table 3.17 (continued)

CVD parameter/interventions	Correlation with prostate cancer risk
Coenzyme Q10 supplements (also known as "ubiquinone")	– CoQ10 is produced in human cells from a mixture of compounds including one of the backbones of cholesterol synthesis, which is why statins can reduce blood levels of this compound significantly – Recommended for statin-induced myalgia (SIM) but mixed and controversial results. Perhaps more intriguing is the preliminary research to determine if these supplements reduce the risk of statin-induced diabetes. Currently, a high-priced supplement in general, so the buyer needs to careful and look for lower cost products if this supplement is actually needed
Coffee/caffeine and other "healthy" non-caloric caffeinated beverages (green, white, oolong, black tea, … all come from green that is oxidized)	– No to minimal calories can be part of a reduced calorie program that can help to achieve a healthy weight/waist – Preliminary evidence that caffeinated coffee could reduce the risk of breast cancer or have some anticancer effects, which is also observed in breast cancer – More definitive evidence that caffeine/coffee has a role against liver injury (reduce liver enzymes in some cases) and in type 2 diabetes prevention. Also receiving research in terms of improving cognitive function, reducing depression, and improve athletic workouts and recovery – Different tea forms have no or low calories and are healthy but data to support an anticancer effect is also preliminary – Green tea is oxidized slightly to "white tea" and then more oxidized to" oolong tea" and then fully oxidized to produce "black tea." Caffeine content varies among tea types so check the individual one of interest
Diabetes/glucose intolerance	Associated with a higher risk of breast cancer and breast cancer recurrence. Insulin and molecules impacted by insulin appears to serve as mitogens or growth factors for breast cancer
Dyslipidemia (high cholesterol)	Associated with a neutral or increased risk of breast cancer but more so could be associated with an increased risk of breast cancer recurrence
Exercise (aerobic and resistance) and HIIT (high intensity interval training)	– Associated with a lower risk of breast cancer and breast cancer recurrence and arguably has the strongest data of any lifestyle change except for maintaining a healthy weight or weight/waist loss – Exercise has countless benefits in all aspects of medicine from reducing side effects of aromatase inhibitors, increasing energy levels, reducing depression, reducing stress and anxiety, improving cognitive function, improving heart health … all of these diverse benefits should be presented to patients – Resistance exercise also reduces diabetes risk, bone loss and sarcopenia risk, reduces fatigue and does not exacerbate lymphedema so can be used in most breast cancer patients (except for those with metastatic bone disease–need to be careful here). Remember that resistance exercise includes any force on muscle and bone tissue so not just weight lifting but resistance against the body such as yoga or Pilates or push up type exercises – HIIT involves aggressive aerobic training in half the time or less of regular aerobic exercise (to the point of quick exhaustion intervals) and preliminary evidence demonstrates similar benefits to regular and longer endurance exercise

Fiber (*Note*: There are two beneficial types of fiber-soluble and insoluble. Most healthy foods contain as much insoluble as soluble fiber and in most cases actually contain more insoluble fiber than soluble)	– 20–30 g/day from non-supplemental sources such as fruits, veggies, beans and breakfast cereals/oatmeal is ideal. They contain both soluble and insoluble fiber for maximum benefits and lower cost – Preliminary evidence suggests dietary fiber may reduce the risk of breast cancer or potentially recurrence because of weight loss, glucose, blood pressure, cholesterol, and other heart healthy changes – Regardless, fiber should be encouraged as nature's greatest internal Botox because of the plethora of internal anatomical "antiaging" human benefits with consumption (reduces hemorrhoids, constipation, diverticulitis, heart unhealthy changes, …) – Regular fiber consumption also allows for a decreased need to purchase a probiotic supplement because fiber is an ideal prebiotic that establishes healthy flora in the gut with greater consumption – Fiber pills or supplements and processed fibers (cookies, bars, in liquid products, …) should be discouraged as well as liquid sugars without fiber such as fruit juice. The research with these products is minimal and they do not appear to promote overall health behaviors – Some fiber powders allow for 5–10 g of primarily soluble fiber a day and are an option but should be only a small part of daily intake
Fish and fish oil supplements (contain one or both primary omega-3 fatty acids EPA and DHA)	– Overall no strong association with breast cancer but dietary fish consumption is heart healthy – Supplements should only be used in those with abnormally high triglyceride levels (FDA approved for example 500 mg/dl+) but no clarity on CVD clinical endpoints in these individuals as of yet. Fish oil supplements are being studied to reduce side effects of breast cancer treatment (cognitive dysfunction, sarcopenia, …) but keep in mind that they have recently failed three major phase-3 trials outside of breast cancer (atrial fibrillation, high risk for CVD events, and macular degeneration) – *Note*: Arsenic, Cadmium, Lead, Mercury are always a concern. Just like mercury can concentrate in fish at the top of the marine food chain because they are larger and older animals, we are probably no different. Methyl mercury is water-soluble so when lead, cadmium, and others generally do NOT end up in the pills when oil is extracted to create them, which is arguably why most fish oils have good quality control (also they come from short-lived smaller fish–anchovies, sardines, mackerel, …) – Organic pollutants are oil-soluble so these are more concerning and should be addressed by companies – Most of the krill, shrimp, salmon, and even green-lipped mussel fish oils are also known for their high quality control but also high priced in some cases and lack of impressive number of more rigorous trials with clinical endpoints found with low cost (aka cheap) fish oil supplements. However, if one cannot consume fish or fish oil then these and other marine sources (algae) become an option as well as plant omega-3 fatty acids – Prescription omega-3 medications have excellent quality control but can be costly. And many over the counter fish oil supplement also have good quality control because of the fish utilized to extract most oils – If there is a reason to take fish oil but one needs to avoid large pills then a children's flavored liquid easily suffices in terms of taste, quality control, concentration, and ease of use compared to any many fish oil pills or capsules

(continued)

Table 3.17 (continued)

CVD parameter/interventions	Correlation with prostate cancer risk
Flaxseed, chia and other good sources of plant omega-3 (ALA or alpha-linolenic acid)	Flaxseed powder has preliminary data that it may provide anti-breast cancer effects via anti-estrogen, heart healthy, and antiproliferative effects. Regardless, flaxseed and chia powder are cost effective low-caloric products that also contain a good source of soluble and insoluble fiber – Omega-3 plant oils from supplements or flaxseed oil have minimal to no data and contain no fiber and can be a high source of calories
Fruits and vegetables (non-processed)	– Fruits and vegetables appear to reduce the risk of cardiovascular disease (CVD) up to five servings a day but beyond these levels the extra benefit may be minimal. Current research suggests minimal to no impact on cancer including breast cancer (unless part of a low-calorie or weight loss program). Fruits and veggies also appear to contain minimal amounts of "salicylic acid," which is similar one of the active ingredients in aspirin after it is partially metabolized – Dull or plain colored fruits and veggies have as much evidence as the more brightly colored products with more antioxidants – Fruits juices (processed) contain none of the fiber of the whole food product and can be a high source of calories, and sugar without fiber and could encourage weight gain. It takes numerous oranges and apples along with all that sugar and minimal fiber … to create a minimal amount of juice – Fruits and especially veggies are low in calories, contain numerous nutrients, and fiber. Fruit and vegetable dietary supplements do not enjoy all the medical research benefits currently found with whole low-cost fruits and vegetables
Hypertension (Note: Apart from white-coat hypertension as a cause of a temporary increase in blood pressure, a distended or full bladder can increase blood pressure 10–15 points so anytime a blood pressure reading is needed the patient should first urinate/ empty their bladder)	Part of the spectrum of metabolic syndrome that overall could increase the risk of breast cancer. Regardless, hypertension is becoming the number one cause of cardiovascular death
Intermittent fasting	Preliminary research suggests it may be as good as caloric reduction in improving overall CVD parameters

Iron dietary supplements	Not associated with an increased or decreased risk of breast cancer, but recent research suggests weight gain could lower iron levels and reduce duodenal iron absorption in body because it creates an inflammatory reaction that increases hepcidin levels (protein that when reduced allows for more absorption and when increased such as inflammatory states discourage iron absorption). Also, although iron supplements are absorbed better on an empty stomach, when used with a meal and some vitamin C the absorption is adequate and side effects are reduced and compliance increases
Metformin (low cost, generic, and "natural" – derived from the French Lilac)	– Reduces IGF-1, leptin, diabetes risk, weight, gluconeogenesis (glucose and insulin), which could reduce the risk of breast cancer and recurrence. Regardless it could be argued that since it does reduce the risk of diabetes from the Diabetes Prevention Program trial (first published in the New England Journal of Medicine in 2002) that it can be considered in some breast cancer patients currently to reduce weight, improve CVD risk, and provide anti-breast cancer effects – B12 deficiency can occur on metformin and magnesium deficiency – There are currently numerous clinical trials of metformin and breast cancer prevention and treatment being conducted with early success in at least lowering weight and improving heart health – Some dietary supplements including "berberine" currently and potentially "alpha-lipoic acid" could partially mimic metformin and are being investigated as options
Multivitamin (The number one supplement utilized by health care professionals and patients)	-One pill a day of a low-dose and low-cost multivitamin or children's multivitamin in adults such as Centrum Silver that was used in the only major multivitamin trial (PHS2) with or without a personal history of cancer appears safe and may lower overall cancer risk (but more than one multivitamin a day may increase risk of some cancers). However, data with women are lacking from the PHS2 trial but a potential lower risk of cataract could also be a potential benefit along with reducing minimal nutrient deficiencies caused by diet, exercise, alcohol, or even medications (acid reflux drugs, metformin, …) – Regardless, multivitamins have modest evidence and Centrum and other popular brands need to reduce many dyes and others compounds in their product to create a healthier pill. Gummi multivitamins and supplements are problematic because they contain numerous dyes, sugar and ample excess calories when consumed over long-periods of time
Obesity/overweight (from BMI and or waist circumference measurements)	– Associated with an increased risk of breast cancer and recurrence. Arguably the most important lifestyle factor (except for perhaps exercise) that can impact breast cancer risk or recurrence. In one of the most impressive trials to date (WINS) a weight loss of only 6 pounds over time may have been sufficient enough to reduce the risk of relapse after definitive treatment! – Obesity also appears currently to increase the severity of hot flashes and poor bone quality. Weight gain is now associated with so many negative health outcomes that the diversity and range of them should be discussed with patients

(continued)

Table 3.17 (continued)

CVD parameter/interventions	Correlation with prostate cancer risk
Protein powder supplementation (Animal based-whey, egg white, casein or plant based-brown rice, hemp, pea, soy, …)	– Excellent source of protein and minimal to no sugar and lactose in the best products. For example, ideal whey protein isolates have good taste with water, 25 g of protein and no sugar or lactose. Plant proteins are garnering more research and appear to be "catching up" with animal-based protein powders in terms of health benefits. Regardless, taste needs to be improved with many protein powders. They also may function as an appetite suppressant in moderate amounts (25–50 g/day)
Note: Chocolate milk is also an option but more so for extreme athletes because these milks still contain a lot of sugar and calories for the average exerciser	– Synergistic with exercise to increase muscle protein synthesis and lean muscle mass and reduce fat tissue
Note: Protein powder should not replace the emphasis on food sources of concentrated protein for example legumes, chicken, fish, turkey, and other lean or even game meats	– Protein powders can also help with weight gain in some patients (cachexia) because high amount help increase muscle and stimulate some insulin secretion
Note: It should be remembered that the maximum protein intake per day is usually weight in pounds divided by 2, so that a 150 pound person should consume up to a maximum of 75 g a day of total protein. And in the future this maximum could increase with increasing age and adequate kidney function	

S.A.M. (statins, aspirin, metformin)	The acronym for teaching students and patients to remember the potential for aggressive breast cancer prevention appears to now be immersed in CVD prevention, not just for lifestyle changes but also especially in regard to pill interventions. Statins, aspirin, and metformin are all derived originally from "natural" sources, primarily generic, low-cost, and have a long history of providing CVD protection in individuals that qualify for these medications. Additionally, they continue to garner data in breast cancer that is arguably more impressive than any dietary supplement
	– Three dietary supplements appear to mimic S.A.M. to some moderate degree. Red yeast rice (RYR), which has a lovastatin (statin) equivalent in it, salicin which is also derived form willow bark and is metabolized to salicylic acid similar to aspirin, and berberine or alpha–lipoic acid that appear to impact AMPK somewhat similar to metformin. None of these supplements works as well as the lower cost S.A.M. drugs but are interesting in their own right
Selenium dietary supplements (adult RDA for selenium is 55 μg/day)	High-dose (200 μg) selenium supplements may increase the risk of diabetes and increase the risk of aggressive prostate cancer in men already replete with selenium from dietary sources. It may also increase the risk of skin cancer recurrence (basal and squamous). Therefore, in other hormone mediated cancers such as breast cancer these individual supplements should be avoided (the amount of selenium in one multivitamin pill is more than adequate)
Smoking/tobacco/second hand smoke	Lung cancer is the number 1 cancer killer of women (breast cancer is second) and COPD is now one of the top five overall killers of women in the USA. Tobacco increases the risk of countless cancers (for example half the bladder cancer cases are smoking related) and potentially breast cancer recurrence and triple negative breast cancer, and reduces the blood level of numerous antioxidants. Former and current smokers appear to have a greater risk for lung cancer when consuming individual beta-carotene supplements. Second hand smoke may increase the risk of several cancers including lung and breast cancer
Sodium versus potassium (sodium is targeted for blood pressure reduction but arguably potassium consumption increases have more consistent evidence as part of a heart healthy diet)	Consuming heart healthy foods high in potassium will naturally lower your sodium intake. Potassium is arguably the greatest deficiency in the USA today since the RDA is 4700 mg/day and the average intake is 2500 and only 1–2 % of Americans consume 4700 mg/day. Healthy foods such as fruits, veggies, fish, nuts, seeds, plain yogurt contain potassium and only small amounts of sodium and sugar

(continued)

Table 3.17 (continued)

CVD parameter/interventions	Correlation with prostate cancer risk
Soy controversy? (aka the suggestion by some "experts" that soy contains a high concentration of plant isoflavones or "plant estrogens" and could increase the risk of breast cancer or recurrence or stimulate tumor growth)	– In 1999 the FDA approved a health claim for soy protein that states: "25 g of soy protein a day, as part of a diet low in saturated fat and cholesterol, may reduce the risk of heart disease. A serving of (name of food) provides _____ grams of soy protein."
	– Soy protein has been recognized from meta-analysis and major health organization (AHA) to potentially reduce LDL cholesterol by 2–7 % on average
	– Soy protein is one of the most concentrated protein sources among plants. And of the most developed commercial protein powders with acceptable taste
	– Soy protein arguably enjoys more research now compared to any other time as a potential part of a breast healthy program (as part of other heart health and weight loss measures) especially in Asian countries and no overall consensus in the USA or Western countries; HOWEVER, this is the reality and unfortunately the perception by some "experts" is that soy may increase the risk of breast cancer/recurrence
	– Traditional soy protein products (soybeans/edamame, soy protein, soy milk, tofu, tempeh, …) and the beneficial heart health research should be supported, but NOT soy pills or processed products
	– One of the largest cohort studies to address the soy and breast cancer recurrence was the "The Shanghai Breast Cancer Survival Study" (cohort study of 5042 female breast cancer survivors in China) and soy protein was associated with a reduced risk of death and recurrence
	However, 94 % of the women in this study were of normal or overweight BMI and only 6 % were obese, and approximately 66 % were of normal weight. Thus, it is difficult to compare this group with the USA and other countries where 70 % or more are overweight and 33 % are obese. This may be the reason soy may be more beneficial in Asian countries versus Western countries
	– Regardless, there are enough small studies of excessive soy supplementation to suggest the potential for an unfavorable effect on breast cancer tissue in a subset of patients. Thus, again when traditional soy food sources are a part of a lower caloric weight loss or overall heart healthy diet it appears that benefit>risk. Otherwise, avoiding soy supplements is a good idea. And there is minimal to no consistent evidence that soy dietary supplements reduce hot flashes or significantly reducing bone loss and fractures
	– There is also no solid evidence to suggest soy foods interfere with traditional breast cancers treatments (AIs, SERM, …)
	– And it should be kept in mind that traditional soy foods are low in calories, and high in healthy nutrients and protein and fiber, and associated with an overall healthy diet and this should be kept in mind

Sugar (sucrose-combination of fructose and glucose)	Hidden sugar in foods especially items such as fruit juice, which in some cases has more sugar than cola drinks are arguably one of the biggest contributors to caloric excess
Statins (low cost, generic, and "natural"-derived from Fungi)	– Associated with a lower risk of breast cancer recurrence from preliminary studies. .Higher dosages/duration of statins appear to be associated with a higher risk of type 2 diabetes – CoQ10 supplementation is being studies to reduce the risk of diabetes from statins and already has modest and controversial evidence to reduce the risk of statin-induced myalgia (SIM) – Red yeast rice (RYR) dietary supplements have good evidence as an option for those that are statin intolerant and this supplement contains "monacolin k," which is identical to the drug "lovastatin." Additionally based on new evidence (IMPROVE-IT trial) the intestinal cholesterol absorption inhibitor "ezetimibe" (Zetia) is also a good option to lower LDL for statin intolerant patients or could be added to a lower dose of a statin drug for maximum LDL lowering effects
Vitamin D supplements (adult RDA for vitamin D is 600 IU/ day for those up to the age of 70 and 800 IU/day for those 71 years and older)	– Potentially a U- or J-shaped curve with higher blood levels showing an increased risk breast caner and normalization of deficient or insufficient levels showing a reduction in breast cancer risk. However, the vitamin D blood test may just be a marker (negative acute phase reactant) of overall health since obesity, lack of exercise, poor vitamin D based diet, high cholesterol, inflammatory disease … all of these items can reduce blood levels of vitamin D (25-OH vitamin D) – Recommendation of vitamin D up to 1000 IU/day in those at increased risk of bone loss from breast cancer treatment is an option unless blood testing in an otherwise health person suggests to add more vitamin D – Otherwise the amount of vitamin D in most multivitamins and fortified foods is adequate
Vitamin E supplements (adult RDA for vitamin E is 15 mg or 22.4 IU/day)	High-dose vitamin E supplements (400 IU) significantly increases the risk of non-aggressive prostate cancer, and has shown no impact in breast cancer but since prostate cancer is hormone mediated then using them in breast cancer should be discouraged. The amount of vitamin E in one multivitamin pill is more than adequate
Zinc supplements (adult RDA for zinc is 8 mg in women and 11 mg in men per day)	High-dose individual zinc supplements have not been shown to reduce risk and may actually increase risk of aggressive prostate cancer, which again is another reason not to use them in breast cancer. One exception is an effective macular degeneration supplement from the AREDS1 and AREDS2 clinical trials (for those with intermediate to advanced stages of the disease usually contains 25 or 80 mg zinc oxide) and if it is a matter of preventing vision loss the benefit> risk here Otherwise, the amount of zinc in one multivitamin pill is more than adequate

A commitment to these lifestyle changes in all aspects of our behavior is not an easy task. It is difficult today when attending global cancer meetings to find an ample amount of time dedicated to diet and lifestyle. When the field of oncology begins to place as much of an emphasis on lifestyle as we do on pills and procedures I believe a dramatic shift in patient behavior will also begin to occur and this is how smoking cessation began to dramatically increase [80]. I believe oncology has done as well as any other field of medicine in trying to emphasize lifestyle research and teaching, but what does that tell you about the status of this information in other areas of medicine. Currently, there is a global obesity epidemic that has already had profound negative impacts of all aspects of medicine and perhaps if the glass of life is really half-full in your practice this may be the best opportunity in the history of oncology to impact the overall quality and quantity of the lives of the individuals that put their trust in your care. If the enthusiasm displayed by practitioners of all ages that I come in contact with lately and globally are an indication of the verve for these lifestyle changes to be implemented in clinical practice then I am more optimistic than ever that the field of oncology will provide the leadership needed to assist in reversing numerous unhealthy parameters.

References

1. Go AS, Mozaffarian D, Roger VL, Benjamin EJ, Berry JD, Borden WB, et al., for the American Heart Association Statistics Committee and Stroke Statistics Subcommittee. Heart disease and stroke statistics—2013 update: a report from the American Heart Association. Circulation 2013;127:e6–245.
2. World Heart Federation website. http://www.world-heart-federation.org. Accessed 20 Mar 2014.
3. Eyre H, Kahn R, Robertson RM, Clark NG, Doyle C, Hong Y, et al., for the American Cancer Society; American Diabetes Association, and the American Heart Association. Preventing cancer, cardiovascular disease, and diabetes: a common agenda for the American Cancer Society, the American Diabetes Association, and the American Heart Association. Circulation 2004;109:3244–55.
4. Fisher B, Costantino JP, Wickerham DL, Redmond CK, Kavanah M, Cronin WM, et al. Tamoxifen for prevention of breast cancer: report of the National Surgical Adjuvant Breast and Bowel Project P-1 Study. J Natl Cancer Inst. 1998;90:1371–88.
5. Vogel VG, Costatino JP, Wickerham DL, Cronin WM, Cecchini RS, Atkins JN, et al. Effects of tamoxifen vs raloxifene on the risk of developing invasive breast cancer and other disease outcomes. JAMA. 2006;295:2727–41.
6. Vogel VG, Costantino JP, Wickerham DL, Cronin WM, Cecchini RS, Atkins JN, et al. Update of the National Surgical Adjuvant Breast and Bowel Project Study of Tamoxifen and Raloxifene (STAR) P-2 Trial: preventing breast cancer. Cancer Prev Res. 2010;3:696–706.
7. Cecchini RS, Costantino JP, Cauley JA, Cronin WM, Wickerham DL, Land SR, et al. Body mass index and risk of developing invasive breast cancer among high-risk women in NSABP P-1 and START breast cancer prevention trials. Cancer Prev Res (Phila). 2012;5:583–92.
8. Thompson IM, Goodman PJ, Tangen CM, Lucia MS, Miller GS, Ford LG, et al. The influence of finasteride on the development of prostate cancer. N Engl J Med. 2003;349:215–24.
9. Scardino PT. The prevention of prostate cancer–the dilemma continues. N Engl J Med. 2003;349:297–9.

10. Kaplan SA, Roehrborn CG, Meehan AG, Liu KS, Carides AD, Binkowitz BS, et al. PCPT: Evidence that finasteride reduces risk of most frequently detected intermediate- and high-grade (Gleason score 6 and 7) cancer. Urology. 2009;73:935–9.
11. Jackson RD, LaCroix AZ, Gass M, Wallace RB, Robbins J, Lewis CE, et al. Calcium and vitamin D supplementation and the risk of fractures. N Engl J Med. 2006;354:669–83.
12. Cauley JA, Chlebowski RT, Wactawski-Wende J, Robbins JA, Rodabough RJ, Chen Z, et al. Calcium plus vitamin D supplementation and health outcomes five years after active intervention ended: the Women's Health Initiative. J Womens Health (Larchmt). 2013;22(11):915–29.
13. Hsia J, Heiss G, Ren H, Allison M, Dolan NC, Greenland P, et al. Calcium/vitamin D supplementation and cardiovascular events. Circulation. 2007;115:846–54.
14. Chlebowski RT, Johnson KC, Kooperberg C, Pettinger M, Wactawski-Wende J, Rohan T, et al. Calcium plus vitamin D supplementation and the risk of breast cancer. J Natl Cancer Inst. 2008;100:1581–91.
15. Lippman SM, Klein EA, Goodman PJ, Lucia MA, Thompson IM, Ford LG, et al. Effect of selenium and vitamin E on risk of prostate cancer and other cancers: the Selenium and Vitamin E Cancer Prevention Trial (SELECT). JAMA. 2009;301:39–51.
16. Nash IS, Mosca L, Blumenthal RS, Davidson MH, Smith SC, Paternak RC. Contemporary awareness and understanding of cholesterol as a risk factor: results of an American Heart Association National Survey. Arch Intern Med. 2003;163:1597–600.
17. Choi EJ, Jekal Y, Kim S, Yoo JS, Kim HS, Oh EG, et al. Middle-aged women's awareness of cholesterol as a risk factor: results from a national survey of Korean Middle-aged Women's Health Awareness (KomWHA) study. Int J Nurs Stud. 2010;47:452–60.
18. Hickey A, O'Hanlon A, McGee H, Donnellan C, Shelley E, Horgan F, et al. Stroke awareness in the general population: knowledge of stroke risk factors and warning signs in older adults. BMC Geriatr. 2009;9:35.
19. Jones SP, Jenkinson AJ, Leathley MJ, Watkins CL. Stroke knowledge and awareness: an integrative review of the evidence. Age Ageing. 2010;39:11–22.
20. Reiner Z, Sonicki Z, Tedeschi-Reiner E. The perception and knowledge of cardiovascular risk factors among medical students. Croat Med J. 2012;53:278–84.
21. Rogers VL, Go AS, Lloyd-Jones DM, Benjamin EJ, Berry JD, Borden WB, et al. Heart disease and stroke statistics—2012 update: a report from the American Heart Association. Circulation. 2012;125:e2–220.
22. Agency for Healthcare Research and Quality (2009). Cardiovascular disease and other chronic conditions in women: recent findings. www.ahrq.gov/research/womheart.htm. Accessed 1 June 2015.
23. American Heart Association (2012). AHA 2020 Goal—2012 statistical fact sheet. www.heart.org/dc/groups/heart-public/@wcm/@sop/@smd/documents/downloadable/ucm_319831.pdf. Accessed 1 June 2015.
24. The Expert Panel. Executive summary of the third report of the National Cholesterol Education Program (NCEP). Expert Panel on Detection, Evaluation, and Treatment of High Blood Cholesterol in Adults (Adult Treatment Panel III). JAMA. 2001;285:2486–98.
25. Grundy SM, Cleeman JI, Merz CN, Brewer Jr HB, Clark LT, Hunninghake DB, et al. Implications of recent clinical trials for the National Cholesterol Education Program Adult Treatment Panel III Guidelines. Circulation. 2004;110:227–39.
26. Centers for Disease Control and Prevention (CDC). Prevalence of abnormal lipid levels among youths—United States, 1999–2006. MMWR Morb Mortal Wkly Rep. 2010;59:29–33.
27. Ridker PM. Clinical application of C-reactive protein for cardiovascular disease detection and prevention. Circulation. 2003;107:363–9.
28. Kraus WE, Houmard JA, Duscha BD, Knetzger KJ, Wharton MB, McCartney JS, et al. Effects of the amount and intensity of exercise on plasma lipoproteins. N Engl J Med. 2002;347:1483–92.
29. Chobanian AV, Bakris GL, Black HR, Cushman WC, Green LA, Izzo Jr JL, et al., for the Joint National Committee on Prevention, Detection, Evaluation, and Treatment of High

Blood Pressure. National Heart, Lung, and Blood Institute; National High Blood Pressure Education Program Coordinating Committee. Hypertension 2003;42:1206–52.

30. James PA, Oparil S, Carter BL, Cushman WC, Dennison-Himmelfarb C, Handler J, et al. 2014 evidence-based guideline for the management of high blood pressure in adults: report from the panel members appointed to the Eighth Joint National Committee (JNC 8). JAMA. 2014;311:507–20.

31. Whelton SP, Chin A, Xin X, He J. Effect of aerobic exercise on blood pressure: a meta-analysis of randomized, controlled trials. Ann Intern Med. 2002;136:493–503.

32. Scoccianti C, Lauby-Secretan B, Bello PY, Chajes V, Romieu I. Female breast cancer and alcohol consumption: a review of the literature. Am J Prev Med. 2014;46(3 Suppl 1):S16–25.

33. Strijk JE, Proper KI, Klaver L, van der Beek AJ, van Mechelen W. Associations between VO2max and vitality in older workers: a cross-sectional study. BMC Public Health. 2010;10:684.

34. Blair SN, Morris JN. Healthy hearts—and the universal benefits of being physically active: physical activity and health. Ann Epidemiol. 2009;19:253–6.

35. Baguet JP. Out-of-office blood pressure: from measurement to control. Integr Blood Press Control. 2012;5:27–34.

36. AMA Wire. How a doctor quickly improved patients' blood pressure readings. http://www.ama-assn.org/ama/ama-wire/post/doctor-quickly-improved-patients-blood-pressure-readings. Accessed 1 June 2015.

37. Liao S, Li J, Wei W, Wang W, Zhang Y, Li J, et al. Association between diabetes mellitus and breast cancer risk: a meta-analysis of the literature. Asian Pac J Cancer Prev. 2011;12:1061–5.

38. Salinas-Martinez AM, Flores-Cortes LI, Cardona-Chavarria JM, Hernandez-Guiterrez B, Abundis A, Vazquez-Lara J, et al. Prediabetes, diabetes, and risk of breast cancer: a case-control study. Arch Med Res. 2014;45:432–8.

39. Isidro ML. Sexual dysfunction in men with type 2 diabetes. Postgrad Med J. 2012;88:152–9.

40. Copeland KL, Brown JS, Creasman JM, Van Den Eeden SK, Subak LL, Thom DH, et al. Diabetes mellitus and sexual function in middle-aged and older women. Obstet Gynecol. 2012;120(2 Pt 1):331–40.

41. Moyad MA. Current methods used for defining, measuring, and treating obesity. Semin Urol Oncol. 2001;19:247–56.

42. Writing Group for the Women's Health Initiative Investigators. Risks and benefits of estrogen plus progestin in healthy postmenopausal women: principal results from the Women's Health Initiative randomized controlled trial. JAMA. 2002;288:321–33.

43. Pischon T, Boeing H, Hoffmann K, Bergmann M, Schulze MB, Overvad K, et al. General and abdominal adiposity and risk of death in Europe. N Engl J Med. 2008;359:2105–20.

44. Jacobs EJ, Newton CC, Wang Y, Patel AV, McCullough ML, Campbell PT, et al. Waist circumference and all-cause mortality in a large US cohort. Arch Intern Med. 2010;170:1293–301.

45. Seidell JC. Waist circumference and waist/hip ratio in relation to all-cause mortality, cancer and sleep apnea. Eur J Clin Nutr. 2010;64:35–41.

46. Zhu S, Heymsfield SB, Toyoshima H, Wang Z, Pietrobelli A, Heshka S. Race-ethnicity-specific waist circumference cutoffs for identifying cardiovascular disease risk factors. Am J Clin Nutr. 2005;81:409–15.

47. Chandramohan G, Kalantar-Zadeh K, Kermah D, Marie Go SC, Vaziri ND, Norris KC. Relationship between obesity and pulse pressure in children: results of the National Health and Nutrition Survey (NHANES) 1988–1994. J Am Soc Hypertens. 2012;6:277–83.

48. Taylor EN, Stampfer MJ, Curhan GC. Obesity, weight gain, and the risk of kidney stones. JAMA. 2005;293:455–62.

49. Scales Jr CD, Smith AC, Hanley JM, Saigal CS, Urologic Diseases in America Project. Prevalence of kidney stones in the United States. Eur Urol. 2012;62:160–5.

50. Moyad MA. Obesity, interrelated mechanisms, and exposures and kidney cancer. Semin Urol Oncol. 2001;19:270–9.
51. Mathew A, George PS, Ildaphonse G. Obesity and kidney cancer risk in women: a meta-analysis (1992–2008). Asian Pac J Cancer Prev. 2009;10:471–8.
52. Adams TD, Gress RE, Smith SC, Halverson RC, Simper SC, Rosamond WD, et al. Long-term mortality after gastric bypass surgery. N Engl J Med. 2007;357:753–61.
53. Sjostrom L, Narbro K, Sjostrom CD, Karason K, Larsson B, Wedel H, et al., for the Swedish Obese Subjects Study. Effects of bariatric surgery on mortality in Swedish obese subjects. N Engl J Med 2007;357:741–752.
54. Bray GA. The missing link-lose weight, live longer. N Engl J Med. 2007;357(8):818–9.
55. Sjostrom L, Peltonen M, Jacobson P, et al. Bariatric surgery and long-term cardiovascular events. JAMA. 2012;307:56–65.
56. Schauer PR, Kashyap SR, Wolski K, Brethauer SA, Kirwan JP, Pothier CE, et al. Bariatric surgery versus intensive medical therapy in obese patients with diabetes. N Engl J Med. 2012;366:1567–76.
57. Mingrone G, Panunzi S, De Gaetano A, Guidone C, Iaconelli A, Leccesi L, et al. Bariatric surgery versus conventional medical therapy for type 2 diabetes. N Engl J Med. 2012;366:1577–85.
58. Siegel R, Naishadham D, Jemal A. Cancer statistics, 2013. CA Cancer J Clin. 2013;63:11–30.
59. Berube S, Lemiux J, Moore L, Maunsell E, Brisson J. Smoking at time of diagnosis and breast cancer-specific survival: new findings and systematic review with meta-analysis. Breast Cancer Res. 2014;16:R42.
60. Aveyard P, Lycett D, Farley A. Managing smoking cessation-related weight gain. Pol Arch Med Wewn. 2012;122:494–8.
61. Johnson KC, Miller AB, Collishaw NE, Palmer JR, Hammond SK, Salmon AG, et al. Active smoking and secondhand smoke increase breast cancer risk: the report of the Canadian Expert Panel on Tobacco Smoke and Breast Cancer Risk (2009). Tob Control. 2011;20(1):e2.
62. Lorinzi PD, Cardinal BJ, Winters-Stone K, Smit E, Loprinzi CL. Physical activity and the risk of breast cancer recurrence: a literature review. Oncol Nurs Forum. 2012;39:269–74.
63. Chen X, Lu W, Zheng W, Gu K, Matthews CE, Chen Z, et al. Exercise after diagnosis of breast cancer in association with survival. Cancer Prev Res (Phila). 2011;4:1409–18.
64. Pant S, Shapiro CL. Aromatase inhibitor-associated bone loss: clinical considerations. Drugs. 2008;68:2591–600.
65. Cormie P, Galvao DA, Spry N, Newton RU. Neither heavy nor light load resistance acutely exacerbates lymphedema in breast cancer survivor. Integr Cancer Ther. 2013;12:423–32.
66. Irwin ML, Cartmel B, Gross CP, Ercolano E, Li F, Yao X, et al. Randomized exercise trial of aromatase inhibitor-induced arthralgia in breast cancer survivors. J Clin Oncol. 2015;33:1104–11.
67. Ahmed HM, Blaha MJ, Nasir K, Rivera JJ, Blumenthal RS. Effects of physical activity on cardiovascular disease. Am J Cardiol. 2012;109:288–95.
68. Poehlman ET, Melby C. Resistance training and energy balance. Int J Sport Nutr. 1998;8:143–59.
69. Braith RW, Stewart KJ. Resistance exercise training: its role in the prevention of cardiovascular disease. Circulation. 2006;113:2642–50.
70. Hurley BF, Roth SM. Strength training in the elderly. Sports Med. 2000;30:249–68.
71. Blake H, Mo P, Malik S, Thomas S. How effective are physical activity interventions for alleviating depressive symptoms in older people? A systematic review. Clin Rehabil. 2009;23:873–87.
72. Deslandes A, Moraes H, Ferreira C, Veiga H, Silveira H, Mouta R, et al. Exercise and mental health: many reasons to move. Neuropsychobiology. 2009;59:191–8.
73. Blumenthal JA, Babyak MA, Moore KA, Craighead WE, Herman S, Khatri P, et al. Effects of exercise training on older patients with major depression. Arch Intern Med. 1999;159:2349–56.

74. Babyak M, Blumenthal JA, Herman S, Khatri P, Doraiswamy M, Moore K, et al. Exercise treatment for major depression: maintenance of therapeutic benefit at 10 months. Psychosom Med. 2000;62:633–8.
75. Blumenthal JA, Doralswamy PM. Exercise to combat depression. JAMA. 2014;312: 2166–7.
76. Biedermann SV, Fuss J, Steinle J, Auer MK, Dormann C, Falfan-Melgoza C, et al. The hippocampus and exercise: histological correlates of MR-detected volume changes. Brain Struct Funct 2014, Epub ahead of print.
77. Blumenthal JA, Babyak MA, O'Connor C, Keteyian S, Landzberg J, Howlett J, et al. Effects of exercise training on depressive symptoms in patients with chronic heart failure: the HF-ACTION randomized trial. JAMA. 2012;308:465–74.
78. Barnes PM, Schoenborn CA. Trends in adults receiving a recommendation for exercise or other physical activity from a physician or other health professional. NCHS Data Brief. 2012;86:1–8.
79. Moyad MA. Dr Moyad's no bogus science health advice. Ann Arbor, MI: Ann Arbor Media Group; 2009.
80. Moyad MA. The supplement handbook. New York, NY: Rodale Publishing; 2014.
81. Yu JN, Cunningham JA, Rosenberg Thouin S, Gurvich T, Liu D. Hyperlipidemia. Prim Care. 2000;27:541–87.
82. Ornish D, Weidner G, Fair WR, Marlin R, Pettengill EB, Raisin CJ, et al. Intensive lifestyle changes may affect the progression of prostate cancer. J Urol. 2005;174:1065–9.
83. Siri-Tarino PW, Sun Q, Hu FB, Krauss RM. Meta-analysis of prospective cohort studies evaluating the association of saturated fat with cardiovascular disease. Am J Clin Nutr. 2010;91:535–46.
84. Yamagishi K, Iso H, Yatsuya H, Tanabe N, Date C, Kikuchi S, et al., for the JACC Study Group. Dietary intake of saturated fatty acids and mortality from cardiovascular disease in Japanese: the Japan Collaborative Cohort Study for Evaluation of Cancer Risk (JACC) Study. Am J Clin Nutr 2010;92:759–65.
85. Mozaffarian D, Micha R, Wallace S. Effects of coronary heart disease of increasing polyunsaturated fat in place of saturated fat: a systematic review and meta-analysis of randomized controlled trials. PLoS Med. 2010;7:e1000252.
86. Chiuve SE, Rimm EB, Sandhu RK, Bernstein AM, Rexrode KM, Manson JE, et al. Dietary fat quality and risk of sudden cardiac death in women. Am J Clin Nutr. 2012;96(3):498–507. Epub 1 Aug 2012.
87. Chlebowski RT, Blackburn GL, Thomson CA, Nixon DW, Shapiro A, Hoy MK, et al. Dietary fat reduction and breast cancer outcome: interim efficacy results from the Women's Intervention Nutrition Study. J Natl Cancer Inst. 2006;98:1767–76.
88. Pierce JP, Natarajan L, Caan BJ, Parker BA, Greenberg ER, Flatt SW, et al. Influence of a diet very high in vegetables, fruit, and fiber and low in fat on prognosis following treatment for breast cancer: the Women's Healthy Eating and Living (WHEL) randomized trial. JAMA. 2007;298:289–98.
89. Villasenor A, Flatt SW, Marinac C, Natarajan L, Pierce JP, Patterson RE. Postdiagnosis C-reactive protein and breast cancer survivorship: findings from the WHEL study. Cancer Epidemiol Biomarkers Prev. 2014;23:189–99.
90. Loftfield E, Harrigan M, Li F, Cartmel B, Zhou Y, Playdon M, et al. Lifestyle, exercise and nutrition study (LEAN). J Clin Oncol. 2014;32:5s. abstract number 1505 ASCO 2014 Annual Meeting.
91. Johnstone BC, Kanters S, Bandayrel K. Comparison of weight loss among named diet programs in overweight and obese adults: a meta-analysis. JAMA. 2014;312:923.
92. Ng M, Fleming T, Robinson M, Thomson B, Graetz N, Margono C, et al. Global, regional, and national prevalence of overweight and obesity in children and adults during 1980–2013: a systematic analysis for the Global Burden of Disease Study 2013. Lancet. 2014;384: 766–81.

93. Giovannucci E. Tomatoes, tomato-based products, lycopene, and cancer: review of the epidemiologic literature. J Natl Cancer Inst. 1999;91:317–31.
94. Moyad MA. The ABCs of nutrition and supplements for prostate cancer. Ann Arbor, MI: JW Edwards Publishing; 2000.
95. www.usda.gov. Accessed 25 Oct 2010.
96. Clinton SK. Lycopene: chemistry, biology, and implications for human health and disease. Nutr Rev. 1998;56:35–51.
97. Mourvaki E, Gizzi S, Rossi R, Rufini S. Passionflower fruit—a "new" source of lycopene? J Med Food. 2005;8:104–6.
98. Ilic D, Forbes KM, Hassed C. Lycopene for the prevention of prostate cancer. Cochrane Database Syst Rev. 2011;11:CD008007.
99. Ilic D, Misso M. Lycopene for the prevention and treatment of benign prostatic hyperplasia and prostate cancer: a systematic review. Maturitas. 2012;72:269–76.
100. Ried K, Fakler P. Protective effect of lycopene on serum cholesterol and blood pressure: meta-analyses of intervention trials. Maturitas. 2011;68:299–310.
101. Pantuck AJ, Leppert JT, Zomorodian N, Aronson W, Hong J, Barnard RJ, et al. Phase II study of pomegranate juice for men with rising prostate-specific antigen following surgery or radiation for prostate cancer. Clin Cancer Res. 2006;12(13):4018–26.
102. Forest CP, Padma-Nathan H, Liker HR. Efficacy and safety of pomegranate juice on improvement of erectile dysfunction in male patients with mild to moderate erectile dysfunction: a randomized, placebo-controlled, double-blind, cross-over study. Int J Impot Res. 2007;19:564–7.
103. Uno T, Yasui-Furukori N. Effect of grapefruit juice in relation to human pharmacokinetic study. Curr Clin Pharmacol. 2006;1:157–61.
104. Komperda KE. Potential interaction between pomegranate juice and warfarin. Pharmacotherapy. 2009;29:1002–6.
105. Jarvis S, Li C, Bogle RG. Possible interaction between pomegranate juice and warfarin. Emerg Med J. 2010;27:74–5.
106. Rocha A, Wang L, Penichet M, Martins-Green M. Pomegranate juice and specific components inhibit cell and molecular processes critical for metastasis of breast cancer. Breast Cancer Res Treat. 2012;136:647–58.
107. Aune D, Chan DS, Vieira AR, Rosenblatt DA, Vieira R, Greenwood DC, et al. Fruits, vegetables and breast cancer risk: a systematic review and meta-analysis of prospective studies. Breast Cancer Res Treat. 2012;134:479–93.
108. van Gils CH, Peeters PH, Bueno-de-Mesquita HB, Boshulzen HC, Lahmann PH, Clavel-Chapelon F, et al. Consumption of vegetables and fruits and risk of breast cancer. JAMA. 2005;293:183–93.
109. Walker C, Reamy BV. Diets for cardiovascular disease prevention: what is the evidence? Am Fam Physician. 2009;79:571–8.
110. Duthie GG, Wood AD. Natural salicylates: foods, functions and disease prevention. Food Funct. 2011;2:515–20.
111. Boffetta P, Couto E, Wichmann J, Ferrari P, Trichopoulos D, Bueno-de-Mesquita HB, et al. Fruit and vegetable intake and overall cancer risk in the European Prospective Investigation into Cancer and Nutrition (EPIC). J Natl Cancer Inst. 2010;102:529–37.
112. Bhupathiraju SN, Wedick NM, Pan A, Manson JE, Rexrode KM, Willet WC, et al. Quantity and variety in fruit and vegetable intake and risk of coronary heart disease. Am J Clin Nutr. 2013;98:1514–23.
113. Oude Griep LM, Verschuren WM, Kromhout D, Ocke MC, Geleijnse JM. Variety of fruits and vegetable consumption and 10-year incidence of stroke. Public Health Nutr. 2012;15:2280–6.
114. Van Horn L. Fiber, lipids, and coronary heart disease. A statement for healthcare professionals from the Nutrition Committee, American Heart Association. Circulation. 1997;95:2701–4.
115. Brown L, Rosner B, Willett WW, Sacks FM. Cholesterol-lowering effects of dietary fiber: a meta-analysis. Am J Clin Nutr. 1999;69:30–42.

116. Anderson JW, Baird P, Davis Jr RH, Ferreri S, Knudtson M, Koraym A, et al. Health benefits of dietary fiber. Nutr Rev. 2009;67:188–205.
117. Slavin JL. Position of the American Dietetic Association: health implications of dietary fiber. J Am Diet Assoc. 2008;108:1716–31.
118. Pereira MA, O'Reilly E, Augustsson K, Fraser GE, Goldbourt U, Heitmann BL, et al. Dietary fiber and risk of coronary heart disease: a pooled analysis of cohort studies. Arch Intern Med. 2004;164:370–6.
119. Pietinen P, Rimm EB, Korhonen P, Hartman AM, Willett WC, Albanes D, et al. Intake of dietary fiber and risk of coronary heart disease in a cohort of Finnish men: the Alpha-Tocopherol, Beta-Carotene Cancer Prevention Study. Circulation. 1996;94:2720–7.
120. Rimm EB, Ascherio A, Giovannucci E, Spiegelman D, Stampfer MJ, Willett WC. Vegetable, fruit, and cereal fiber intake and risk of coronary heart disease among men. JAMA. 1996;275:447–51.
121. Park Y, Subar AF, Hollenbeck A, Schatzkin A. Dietary fiber intake and mortality in the NIH-AARP diet and health study. Arch Intern Med. 2011;171:1061–8.
122. Eshak ES, Iso H, Date C, Kikuchi S, Watanabe Y, Wada Y, et al. Dietary fiber intake is associated with reduced risk of mortality from cardiovascular disease among Japanese men and women. J Nutr. 2010;140:1445–53.
123. Moreyra AE, Wilson AC, Koraym A. Effect of combining psyllium fiber with simvastatin in lowering cholesterol. Arch Intern Med. 2005;165:1161–6.
124. Agrawal AR, Tandon M, Sharma PL. Effect of combining viscous fibre with lovastatin on serum lipids in normal human subjects. Int J Clin Pract. 2007;61:1812–8.
125. Streppel MT, Arends LR, van't Veer P, Grobbee DE, Geleijnse JM. Dietary fiber and blood pressure: a meta-analysis of randomized placebo-controlled trials. Arch Intern Med. 2005;165:150–6.
126. Vernay M, Aidara M, Salanave B, Deschamps V, Malon A, Oleko A, et al. Diet and blood pressure in 18–74 year old adults: the French Nutrition and Health Survey (ENNS, 2006–2007). J Hypertens. 2012;30(10):1920–7. Epub 12 July 2012.
127. Marlett JA, McBurney MI, Slavin JL, for the American Dietetic Association. Position of the American Dietetic Association: health implications of dietary fiber. J Am Diet Assoc 2002;102:993–1000.
128. Pan A, Yu D, Demark-Wahnefried W, Franco OH, Lin X. Meta-analysis of the effects of flaxseed interventions on blood lipids. Am J Clin Nutr. 2009;90:288–97.
129. Rodriguez-Leyva D, Dupasquier CM, McCullough R, Pierce GN. The cardiovascular effects of flaxseed and its omega-3 fatty acid, alpha-linolenic acid. Can J Cardiol. 2010;26:489–96.
130. Jin F, Nieman DC, Sha W, Xie G, Qiu Y, Jia W. Supplementation of milled chia seeds increases plasma ALA and EPA in postmenopausal women. Plant Foods Hum Nutr. 2012;67:105–10.
131. Demark-Wahnefried W, Price DT, Polascik TJ, Robertson CN, Anderson EE, Paulson DF, et al. Pilot study of dietary fat restriction and flaxseed supplementation in men with prostate cancer before surgery: exploring the effects on hormonal levels, prostate-specific antigen, and histopathologic features. Urology. 2001;58:47–52.
132. Demark-Wahnefried W, Robertson CN, Walther PJ, Polascik TJ, Paulson DF, Vollmer RT. Pilot study to explore effects of low-fat, flaxseed-supplemented diet on proliferation of benign prostatic epithelium and prostate-specific antigen. Urology. 2004;63:900–4.
133. Demark-Wahnefried W, Polascik TJ, George SL, Switzer BR, Madden JF, Ruffin 4th MT, et al. Flaxseed supplementation (not dietary fat restriction) reduces prostate cancer proliferation rates in men presurgery. Cancer Epidemiol Biomarkers Prev. 2008;17:3577–87.
134. Zhang W, Wang X, Liu Y, Tian H, Flickinger B, Empie MW, et al. Effects of dietary flaxseed meric extract on symptoms of benign prostatic hyperplasia. J Med Food. 2008;11:207–14.
135. Thompson LU, Chen JM, Tong L, Strasser-Weippt K, Goss PE. Dietary flaxseed alters tumor biological markers in postmenopausal breast cancer. Clin Cancer Res. 2005;11:3828–35.

136. McCann SE, Edge SB, Hicks DG, Thompson LU, Morrison CD, Fetterly G, et al. A pilot study comparing the effect of flaxseed, aromatase inhibitor, and the combination on breast tumor biomarkers. Nutr Cancer 2014;66:566–75.

137. Mason JK, Fu M, Chen J, Thompson LU. Flaxseed oil enhances the effectiveness of trastuzumab in reducing the growth of HER2-overexpressing human breast tumors (BT-474). J Nutr Biochem. 2015;26:16–23.

138. Aune D, Chan DS, Greenwood DC, Vieira AR, Rosenblatt DA, Vieira R, et al. Dietary fiber and breast cancer risk: a systematic review and meta-analysis of prospective studies. Ann Oncol. 2012;23:1394–402.

139. Dong JY, He K, Wang P, Qin LQ. Dietary fiber intake and risk of breast cancer: a meta-analysis of prospective cohort studies. Am J Clin Nutr. 2011;94:900–5.

140. Morris MC, Evans DA, Bienias JL, Tangney CC, Bennett DA, Wilson RS, et al. Consumption of fish and n-3 fatty acids and risk of incident Alzheimer disease. Arch Neurol. 2003;60:940–6.

141. Morris MC. The role of nutrition in Alzheimer's disease: epidemiological evidence. Eur J Neurol. 2009;16 Suppl 1:1–7.

142. Moyad MA. An introduction to dietary/supplemental omega-3 fatty acids for general health and prevention: part I. Urol Oncol. 2005;23:28–35.

143. Moyad MA. An introduction to dietary/supplemental omega-3 fatty acids for general health and prevention: part II. Urol Oncol. 2005;23:36–48.

144. Bucher HC, Hengstler P, Schindler C, Meier G. N-3 polyunsaturated fatty acids in coronary heart disease: a meta-analysis of randomized controlled trials. Am J Med. 2002;112:298–304.

145. Kris-Etherton PM, Harris WS, Appel LJ, for the Nutrition Committee. Fish consumption, fish oil, omega-3 fatty acids, and cardiovascular disease. Circulation 2002;106:2747–57.

146. Harris WS. N-3 fatty acids and serum lipoproteins: human studies. Am J Clin Nutr. 1997;65(5 Suppl):1645S–54.

147. Cabo J, Alonso R, Mata P. Omega-3 fatty acids and blood pressure. Br J Nutr. 2012;107 Suppl 2:S195–200.

148. Albert CM, Campos H, Stampfer MJ, Ridker PM, Manson JE, Willett WC, et al. Blood levels of long-chain n-3 fatty acids and the risk of sudden death. N Engl J Med. 2002;346:1113–8.

149. Siener R, Jansen B, Watzer B, Hesse A. Effect of n-3 fatty acid supplementation on urinary risk factors for calcium oxalate stone formation. J Urol. 2011;185:719–24.

150. Yasui T, Suzuki S, Itoh Y, Tozawa K, Tokudome S, Kohri K. Eicosapentaenoic acid has a preventive effect on the recurrence of nephrolithiasis. Urol Int. 2008;81:135–8.

151. Guallar E, Sanz-Gallardo MI, van't Veer P, Bode P, Aro A, Gomez-Aracena J, et al. Mercury, fish oils, and the risk of myocardial infarction. N Engl J Med. 2002;347:1747–54.

152. Yoshizawa K, Rimm EB, Morris JS, Spate VL, Hsieh CC, Spiegelman D, et al. Mercury and the risk of coronary heart disease in men. N Engl J Med. 2002;347:1755–60.

153. Virtanen JK, Laukkanen JA, Mursu J, Voutilainen S, Tuomainen TP. Serum long-chain n-3 polyunsaturated fatty acids, mercury, and risk of sudden cardiac death in men: a prospective population-based study. PLoS One. 2012;7:e41046.

154. Weil M, Bressler J, Parsons P, Bolla K, Glass T, Schwartz B. Blood mercury levels and neurobehavioral function. JAMA. 2005;293:1875–82.

155. DeRouen TA, Martin MD, Leroux BG, Townes BD, Woods JS, Leitao J, et al. Neurobehavioral effects of dental amalgam in children: a randomized clinical trial. JAMA. 2006;295:1784–92.

156. Mozaffarian D, Shi P, Morris JS, Spiegelman D, Grandjean P, Siscovick DS, et al. Mercury exposure and risk of cardiovascular disease in two U.S. cohorts. N Engl J Med. 2011;364:1116–25.

157. Kris-Etherton PM, Harris WS, Appel LJ, AHA Nutrition Committee. American Heart Association. Omega-3 fatty acids and cardiovascular disease: new recommendations from the American Heart Association. Arterioscler Thromb Vasc Biol. 2003;23:151–2.

158. GISSI-Prevenzione Investigators. Dietary supplementation with n-3 polyunsaturated fatty acids and vitamin E after myocardial infarction: results from the GISSI-Prevenzione trial. Lancet. 1999;354:447–55.
159. Marchioli R, Barzi F, Bomba E, Chieffo C, Di Gregorio D, Di Mascio R, et al. Early protection against sudden cardiac death by n-3 polyunsaturated fatty acids after myocardial infarction: time-course analysis of the results of the Gruppo Italiano per lo Studio della Sopravvivenza nell'Infarto Miocardico (GISSI)-Prevenzione. Circulation. 2002;105:1897–903.
160. Yokoyama M, Origasa H, Matsuzaki M, Matsuzawa Y, Saito Y, Ishikawa Y, et al. Effects of eicosapentaenoic acid on major coronary events in hypercholesterolaemic patients (JELIS): a randomized open-label, blinded endpoint analysis. Lancet. 2007;369:1090–8.
161. Kwak SM, Myung SK, Lee YJ, Seo HG, et al., for the Korean Meta-Analysis Study Group. Efficacy of omega-3 fatty acid supplements (eicosapentaenoic acid and docosahexaenoic acid) in the secondary prevention of cardiovascular disease: a meta-analysis of randomized, double-blind, placebo-controlled trials. Arch Intern Med 2012;172:686–94.
162. Mozaffarian D, Marchiolli R, Macchia A, Silletta MG, Ferrazzi P, Gardner TJ, et al. Fish oil and postoperative atrial fibrillation: the Omega-3 Fatty Acids for Prevention of Post-operative Atrial Fibrillation (OPERA) randomized trial. JAMA. 2012;308:2001–11.
163. Risk and Prevention Study Collaborative Group. N-3 fatty acids in patients with multiple cardiovascular risk factors. N Engl J Med. 2013;368:1800–8.
164. Age-Related Eye Disease Study 2 Research Group. Lutein + zeaxanthin and omega-3 fatty acids for age-related macular degeneration: the Age-Related Eye Disease Study 2 (AREDS2) randomized clinical trial. JAMA. 2013;309:2005–15.
165. Li D. Omega-3 polyunsaturated fatty acids and non-communicable diseases: meta-analysis based systematic review. Asia Pac J Clin Nutr. 2015;24:10–5.
166. Zheng JS, Hu XJ, Zhao YM, Yang J, Li D. Intake of fish and marine n-3 polyunsaturated fatty acids and risk of breast cancer: meta-analysis of data from 21 independent prospective cohort studies. BMJ. 2013;346:f3706. Epub ahead of print.
167. Fabian CJ, Kimler BF, Hursting SD. Omega-3 fatty acids for breast cancer prevention and survivorship. Breast Cancer Res. 2015;17:62.
168. Ghoreishi Z, Esfahani A, Djazayeri A, Djalali M, Golestan B, Ayromlou H, et al. Omega-3 fatty acids are protective against paclitaxel-induced peripheral neuropathy: a randomized double-blind placebo controlled trial. BMC Cancer. 2012;12:355.
169. Smith GI, Atherton P, Reeds DN, Mohammed BS, Rankin D, Rennie MJ, et al. Dietary omega-3 fatty acid supplementation increases the rate of muscle protein synthesis in older adults: a randomized controlled trial. Am J Clin Nutr. 2011;93:402–12.
170. Smith GI, Julliand S, Reeds DN, Sinacore DR, Klein S, Mittendorfer B. Fish oil-derived n-3 PUFA therapy increases muscle mass and function in healthy older adults. Am J Clin Nutr. 2015;102(1):115–22. Epub 20 May 2015.
171. Fracasso PM, Picus J, Wildi JD, Goodner SA, Creekmore AN, Gao F, et al. Phase 1 and pharmacokinetic study of weekly docosahexaenoic acid-paclitaxel, Taxoprexin, in resistant solid tumor malignancies. Cancer Chemother Pharmacol. 2009;63:451–8.
172. O'Neil CE, Keast DR, Nicklas TA, Fulgoni 3rd VL. Nut consumption is associated with decreased health risk factors for cardiovascular disease and metabolic syndrome in U.S. adults: NHANES 1999–2004. J Am Coll Nutr. 2011;30:502–10.
173. Albert CM, Gaziano JM, Willett WC, Manson JE. Nut consumption and decreased risk of sudden cardiac death in the physicians' health study. Arch Intern Med. 2002;162:1382–7.
174. Ellsworth JL, Kushi LH, Folsom AR. Frequent nut intake and risk of death from coronary heart disease and all causes in postmenopausal women: the Iowa Women's Health Study. Nutr Metab Cardiovasc Dis. 2001;11:372–7.
175. Fraser GE, Shavlik DJ. Risk factors for all-cause and coronary heart disease mortality in the oldest-old: the Adventist Health Study. Arch Intern Med. 1997;157:2249–58.
176. Sabate J, Wien M. Nuts, blood lipids and cardiovascular disease. Asia Pac J Clin Nutr. 2010;19:131–6.

177. Casas-Agustench P, Bullo M, Salas-Salvado J. Nuts, inflammation and insulin resistance. Asia Pac J Clin Nutr. 2010;19:124–30.
178. Afshin A, Micha R, Khatibzadeh S, Mozaffarian D. Consumption of nuts and legumes and risk of incident heart disease, stroke, and diabetes: a systematic review and meta-analysis. Am J Clin Nutr. 2014;100:278–88.
179. Yang Q, Cogswell ME, Flanders WD, Hong Y, Zhang Z, Loustalot F, et al. Trends in cardiovascular health metrics and associations with all-cause and CVD mortality among US adults. JAMA. 2012;307:1273–83.
180. Hu FB, Willett WC, Tricia L, Stampfer MJ, Colditz GA, Manson JE. Adiposity as compared with physical activity in predicting mortality among women. N Engl J Med. 2004;351(26):2694–703.
181. Ajani UA, Lotufo PA, Gaziano JM, Lee IM, Spelsberg A, Buring JE, et al. Body mass index and mortality among US male physicians. Ann Epidemiol. 2004;14:731–9.
182. Baik I, Ascherio A, Rimm EB, Giovannucci E, Spiegelman D, Stampfer MJ, et al. Adiposity and mortality in men. Am J Epidemiol. 2000;152:264–71.
183. Platz EA, Willet WC, Colditz GA, Rimm EB, Spiegelman D, Giovannucci E. Proportion of colon cancer risk that might be preventable in a cohort of middle-aged US men. Cancer Causes Control. 2000;11:579–88.
184. Trichopoulou A, Costacou T, Bamia C, Trichopoulos D. Adherence to a Mediterranean diet and survival in a Greek population. N Engl J Med. 2003;348:2599–608.
185. Mitrou PN, Kipnis V, Thiebaut AC, Reedy J, Subar AF, Wirfalt E, et al. Mediterranean dietary pattern and prediction of all-cause mortality in a U.S. population: results from the NIH-AARP Diet and Health Study. Arch Intern Med. 2007;167:2461–8.
186. Yusuf S, Hawken S, Ounpuu S, Dans T, Avezum A, Lanas F, et al. on behalf of the INTERHEART Study Investigators. Effect of potentially modifiable risk factors associated with myocardial infarction in 52 countries (the INTERHEART study): case-control study. Lancet 2004;364:937–52.
187. Joshi P, Islam S, Pais P, Reddy S, Dorairaj P, Kazmi K, et al. Risk factors for early myocardial infarction in South Asians compared with individuals in other countries. JAMA. 2007;297:286–94.
188. Wilcox BJ, He Q, Chen R, Yano K, Masaki KH, Grove JS, et al. Midlife risk factors and healthy survival in men. JAMA. 2006;296:2343–50.
189. Yates LB, Djousse L, Kurth T, Buring JE, Gaziano JM. Exceptional longevity in men: modifiable factors associated with survival and function to age 90 years. Arch Intern Med. 2008;168:284–90.
190. Terry DF, Pencina MJ, Vasan RS, Murabito JM, Wolf PA, Hayes MK, et al. Cardiovascular risk factors predictive for survival and morbidity-free survival in the oldest-old Framingham Heart Study participants. J Am Geriatr Soc. 2005;53:1944–50.
191. Appel LJ, Moore TJ, Obarzanek E, Vollmer WM, Svetkey LP, Sacks FM, et al. A clinical trial of the effects of dietary patterns on blood pressure. DASH Collaborative Research Group. N Engl J Med. 1997;336:1117–24.
192. Sacks FM, Svetkey LP, Vollmer WM, Appel LJ, Bray GA, Harsha D, et al. Effects on blood pressure of reduced dietary sodium and the Dietary Approaches to Stop Hypertension (DASH) diet. DASH-Sodium Collaborative Research Group. N Engl J Med. 2001;344:3–10.
193. Karanja N, Erlinger TP, Pao-Hwa L, Miller ER, Bray GA. The DASH diet for high blood pressure: from clinical trial to dinner table. Cleve Clin J Med. 2004;71(9):745–53.
194. Taylor EN, Fung TT, Curhan GC. DASH-Style diet associates with reduced risk for kidney stones. J Am Soc Nephrol. 2009;20:2253–9.
195. Rock CL. Multivitamin-multimineral supplements: who uses them? Am J Clin Nutr. 2007;85(Suppl):277S–9.
196. Gahche J, Bailey R, Burt V, Hughes J, Yetley E, Dwyer J, et al. Dietary supplement use among U.S. adults has increased since NHANES III (1988–1994). NCHS Data Brief 2011;(61):1–8.

197. Barqawi A, Gamito E, O'Donnell C, Crawford ED. Herbal and vitamin supplement use in a prostate cancer screening population. Urology. 2004;63:288–92.
198. Kristal AR, Arnold KB, Schenk JM, Neuhouser ML, Goodman P, Penson DF, et al. Dietary patterns, supplement use, and the risk of symptomatic benign prostatic hyperplasia: results from the prostate cancer prevention trial. Am J Epidemiol. 2008;167:925–34.
199. Muntwyler J, Hennekens CH, Manson JE, Buring JE, Gaziano M. Vitamin supplement use in a low-risk population of US male physicians and subsequent cardiovascular mortality. Arch Intern Med. 2002;162:1472–6.
200. Shikany JM, Patterson RE, Agurs-Collins T, Anderson G. Antioxidant supplement use in Women's Health Initiative participants. Prev Med. 2003;36:379–87.
201. Neuhouser ML, Wassertheil-Smoller S, Thomson C, Aragaki A, Anderson GL, Manson JE, et al. Multivitamin use and risk of cancer and cardiovascular disease in the Women's Health Initiative cohorts. Arch Intern Med. 2009;169:294–304.
202. Giovannucci E, Chan AT. Role of vitamin and mineral supplementation and aspirin use in cancer survivors. J Clin Oncol. 2010;28:4081–5.
203. Lawson KA, Wright ME, Subar A, Mouw T, Hollenbeck A, Schatzkin A, et al. Multivitamin use and risk of prostate cancer in the National Institutes of Health-AARP Diet and Health Study. J Natl Cancer Inst. 2007;99:754–64.
204. Stevens VL, McCullough ML, Diver WR, Rodriguez C, Jacobs EJ, Thun MJ, et al. Use of multivitamins and prostate cancer mortality in a large cohort of US men. Cancer Causes Control. 2005;16:643–50.
205. Neuhouser ML, Barnett MJ, Kristal AR, Ambrosone CB, King IB, Thornquist M, et al. Dietary supplement use and prostate cancer risk in the Carotene and Retinol Efficacy Trial. Cancer Epidemiol Biomarkers Prev. 2009;18:2202–6.
206. Larsson SC, Akesson A, Bergkvist L, Wolk A. Multivitamin use and breast cancer incidence in a prospective cohort of Swedish women. Am J Clin Nutr. 2010;91:1268–72.
207. Berube S, Diorio C, Brisson J. Multivitamin-multimineral supplement use and mammographic breast density. Am J Clin Nutr. 2008;87:1400–4.
208. Clarke R, Halsey J, Lewington S, Lonn E, Armitage J, Manson JE, et al. Effects of lowering homocysteine levels with B vitamins on cardiovascular disease, cancer, and cause-specific mortality. Arch Intern Med. 2010;170:1622–31.
209. Collin SM, Metcalfe C, Refsum H, Lewis SJ, Zuccolo L, Smith GD, et al. Circulating folate, vitamin B12, homocysteine, vitamin B12 transport proteins, and risk of prostate cancer: a case-control study, systematic review, and meta-analysis. Cancer Epidemiol Biomarkers Prev. 2010;19:1632–42.
210. Ng K, Meyerhardt JA, Chan JA, Niedzwiecki D, Hollis DR, Saltz LB, et al. Multivitamin use is not associated with cancer recurrence or survival in patients with stage III colon cancer: findings from CALGB 89803. J Clin Oncol. 2010;28:4354–63.
211. Li Q, Chuang SC, Eluf-Neto J, Menezes A, Matos E, Koifman S, et al. Vitamin or mineral supplement intake and the risk of head and neck cancer: pooled analysis in the INHANCE consortium. Int J Cancer. 2012;131:1686–99.
212. Hercberg S, Galan P, Preziosi P, Bertrais S, Mennen L, Malvy D, et al. The SU.VI.MAX study: a randomized, placebo-controlled trial of the health effects of antioxidant vitamins and minerals. Arch Intern Med. 2004;164:2335–42.
213. Gaziano JM, Sesso HD, Christen WG, Bubes V, Smith JP, MacFadyen J, et al. Multivitamins in the prevention of cancer in men: the Physicians' Health Study II randomized controlled trial. JAMA. 2012;308:1871–80.
214. Sesso HD, Christen WG, Bubes V, Smith JP, MacFadyen J, Schvartz M, et al. Multivitamins in the prevention of cardiovascular disease in men: the Physicians' Health Study II randomized controlled trial. JAMA. 2012;308:1751–60.
215. Christen WG, Glynn RJ, Manson JE, MacFadyen J, Bubes V, Schvartz M, et al. Effects of multivitamin supplement on cataract and age-related macular degeneration in a randomized trial of male physicians. Ophthalmology. 2014;121:525–34.

216. Milton RC, Sperduto RD, Clemons TE, Ferris 3rd FL, for the Age-Related Eye Disease Study Research Group. Centrum use and progression of age-related cataract in the Age-Related Eye Disease Study: a propensity score approach. AREDS report no. 21. Ophthalmology 2006;113:1264–70.

217. Clinical Trial of Nutritional Supplements and Age-Related Cataract Study Group. A randomized, double-masked, placebo-controlled clinical trial of multivitamin supplementation of age-related lens opacities. Clinical trial of nutritional supplements and age-related cataract report no. 3. Ophthalmology. 2008;115:599–607.

218. Zhao LQ, Li M, Zhu H, for the epidemiological evidence-based eye disease study research group. The effect of multivitamin/mineral supplements on age-related cataracts: a systematic review and meta-analysis. Nutrients 2014;6:931–49.

219. Christen WG, Gaziano JM, Hennekens CH. Design of Physicians' Health Study II—a randomized trial of beta-carotene, vitamins E and C, and multivitamins, in prevention of cancer, cardiovascular disease, and eye disease, and review of results of completed trials. Ann Epidemiol. 2000;10:125–34.

220. Klein EA, Thompson Jr IM, Tangen CM, Crowley JJ, Lucia MS, Goodman PJ, et al. Vitamin E and the risk of prostate cancer: the Selenium and Vitamin E cancer prevention trial (SELECT). JAMA. 2011;306:1549–56.

221. Sesso HD, Buring JE, Christen WG, Kurth T, Belanger C, MacFadyen J, et al. Vitamins E and C in the prevention of cardiovascular disease in men: the Physicians' Health Study II randomized controlled trial. JAMA. 2008;300:2123–33.

222. Kristal AR, Darke AK, Morris JS, Tangen CM, Goodman PJ, Thompson IM, et al. Baseline selenium status and effects of selenium and vitamin e supplementation on prostate cancer risk. J Natl Cancer Inst. 2014;106(3):djt456. Epub 22 Feb 2014.

223. Kenfield SA, Van Blarigan EL, DuPre N, Stampfer MJ, Giovannucci L, Chan JM. Selenium supplementation and prostate cancer mortality. J Natl Cancer Inst. 2014;107:360.

224. Gontero P, Marra G, Soria F, Oderda M, Zitella A, Baratta F, et al. A randomized double-blind placebo controlled phase I–II study on clinical and molecular effects of dietary supplements in men with precancerous prostatic lesions. Chemoprevention or "chemopromotion"? Prostate. 2015;75(11):1177–86. Epub 20 Apr 2015.

225. Ordonez-Mena JM, Schottker B, Fedriko V, Jenab M, Olsen A, Halkjaer J, et al. Pre-diagnostic vitamin D concentrations and cancer risks in older individuals: an analysis of cohorts participating in the CHANCES consortium. Eur J Epidemiol 2015, Epub ahead of print.

226. Barnett CM, Beer TM. Prostate cancer and vitamin D: what does the evidence really suggest? Urol Clin North Am. 2011;38:333–42.

227. Ross AC, Taylor CL, Yaktine AL, Del Valle HB, editors. Institute of Medicine of the National Academies. Dietary reference intakes for calcium and vitamin D. Washington, DC: National Academies Press; 2011.

228. Sanders KM, Stuart AL, Williamson EJ, Simpson JA, Kotowicz MA, Young D, et al. Annual high-dose oral vitamin D and falls and fractures in older women. JAMA. 2010;303: 1815–22.

229. Zerwekh JE. Blood biomarkers of vitamin D status. Am J Clin Nutr. 2008;87(Suppl):1087S–91.

230. Isenor JE, Ensom MH. Is there a role for therapeutic drug monitoring of vitamin D level as a surrogate marker for fracture risk. Pharmacotherapy. 2010;30:254–64.

231. Ardawi MS, Siblany AM, Bakhsh TM, Qari MH, Maimani AA. High prevalence of vitamin D deficiency among healthy Saudi Arabian men: relationship to bone mineral density, parathyroid hormone, bone turnover markers, and lifestyle factors. Osteoporos Int. 2012;23:675–86.

232. Jaaskelainen T, Knekt P, Marniemi J, Sares-Jaske L, Mannisto S, Heliovaara M, et al. Vitamin D status is associated with sociodemographic factors, lifestyle and metabolic health. Eur J Nutr. 2013;52:513–25.

233. Waldron JL, Ashby HL, Comes MP, Bechervaise J, Razavi C, Thomas OL, et al. Vitamin D: a negative acute phase reactant. J Clin Pathol. 2013;66:620–2.

234. Moyad MA, Vogelzang NJ. Heart healthy equals prostate healthy and statins, aspirin, and/or metformin (S.A.M.) are the ideal recommendations for prostate cancer prevention. Asian J Androl 2015, Epub ahead of print.
235. Rothwell PM, Fowkes FG, Belch JK, Ogawa H, Warlow CP, Meade TW. Effect of daily aspirin on long-term risk of death due to cancer: analysis of individual patient data from randomized trials. Lancet. 2011;377:31–41.
236. Jalving M, Gietema JA, Lefrandt JD, de Jong S, Reyners AK, Gans RO, et al. Metformin: taking away the candy for cancer? Eur J Cancer. 2010;46:2369–80.
237. Diabetes Prevention Program Research Group. 10-year follow-up of diabetes incidence and weight loss in the Diabetes Prevention Program Outcomes Study. Lancet. 2009;374:1677–86.
238. Platz EA, Till C, Goodman PJ, Parnes HL, Figg WD, Albanes D, et al. Men with low serum cholesterol have a lower risk of high-grade prostate cancer in the placebo arm of the Prostate Cancer Prevention Trial. Cancer Epidemiol Biomarkers Prev. 2009;18:2807–13.
239. Moyad MA. Why a statin and/or another proven heart healthy agent should be utilized in the next major cancer chemoprevention trial: part I. Urol Oncol. 2004;22:466–71.
240. Moyad MA. Why a statin and/or another proven heart healthy agent should be utilized in the next major cancer chemoprevention trial: part II. Urol Oncol. 2004;22:472–7.
241. Moyad MA. Heart healthy equals prostate healthy equals statins: the next cancer chemoprevention trial: part I. Curr Opin Urol. 2005;15:1–6.
242. Moyad MA. Heart healthy equals prostate healthy equals statins: the next cancer chemoprevention trial: part II. Curr Opin Urol. 2005;15:7–12.
243. Goodwin PJ, Parulekar WR, Gelmon KA, Shepherd LE, Ligibel JA, Hershman DL, et al. Effect of metformin vs placebo on weight and metabolic factors in NCIC CTG MA.32. J Natl Cancer Inst 2015;107, Epub ahead of print.
244. De Berardis G, Lucisano G, D'Ettorre A, Pellegrini F, Lepore V, Tognoni G, et al. Association of aspirin use with major bleeding in patients with and without diabetes. JAMA. 2012; 307:2286–94.
245. Dell'Aglio DM, Perino LJ, Kazzi Z, Abramson J, Schwartz MD, Morgan BW. Acute metformin overdose: examining pH, lactate level, and metformin concentrations in survivors versus nonsurvivors: a systematic review of the literature. Ann Emerg Med. 2009;54:818–23.
246. Zaharan NL, Williams D, Bennett K. Statins and risk of treated incident diabetes in a primary care population. Br J Clin Pharmacol. 2013;75:1118–24.
247. Barton DL, Liu H, Dakhil SR, Linquist B, Sloan JA, Nichols CR, et al. Wisconsin ginseng (Panax quinquefolius) to improve cancer-related fatigue: a randomized, double-blind trial, N07C2. J Natl Cancer Inst. 2013;105(16):1230–8.
248. Ryan JL, Heckler CE, Roscoe JA, Dakhil SR, Kirshner J, Flynn PJ, et al. Ginger (Zingiber officinale) reduces acute chemotherapy-induced nausea: a URCC CCOP study of 576 patients. Support Care Cancer. 2012;20:1479–89.
249. Hansen MV, Andersen LT, Madsen MT, Hagerman I, Rasmussen LS, Bokmand S, et al. Effect of melatonin on depressive symptoms and anxiety in patients undergoing breast cancer surgery: a randomized, double-blind, placebo-controlled trial. Breast Cancer Res Treat. 2014;145:683–95.
250. Chen WY, Giobbie-Hurder A, Gantman K, Savoie J, Scheib R, Parker LM, et al. A randomized, placebo-controlled trial of melatonin on breast cancer survivors: impact on sleep, mood, and hot flashes. Breast Cancer Res Treat. 2014;145:381–8.
251. Miller PE, Alexander DD, Perez V. Effects of whey protein and resistance exercise on body composition: a meta-analysis of randomized controlled trials. J Am Coll Nutr. 2014;33:163–75.
252. Moyad MA, Klotz LH. Statin clinical trial (REALITY) for prostate cancer: an over 15-year wait is finally over thanks to a dietary supplement. Urol Clin North Am. 2011;38:325–31.
253. Moyad MA. Complementary & alternative medicine for prostate and urologic health. New York: Springer Books; 2014.

Chapter 4
S.A.M. and Breast Cancer—Focus on Statins, Red Yeast Rice, Sterols, and Other Integrative Cholesterol Medicines: The Real "Natural" Options

Introduction

The leading cause of death in the USA for women and men is cardiovascular disease (CVD), and this has been the case for 116 of the last 117 years [1]. CVD causes more deaths than cancer and chronic lower respiratory diseases (CLRD) combined. CVD causes one death per minute among females in the USA or over 400,000 deaths, which is approximately the same number of female lives lost by cancer, CLRD, and Alzheimer disease combined. The most recent US statistics have recorded the following: approximately 41,000 deaths from breast cancer, 70,500 female deaths from lung cancer, one in 30 deaths are from breast cancer whereas 1 in 7 was from coronary heart disease (CHD), and 1 in 4.5 females died of cancer and 1 in 3.1 died of CVD. CVD is also still a disease of the young and old. Approximately 150,000 Americans died of CVD last year who were less than 65 years of age and over one third of CVD deaths occurred before the age of 75 years (life expectancy is 78.7 years). The number 1 cause of death in women and men from age 65 and older is CVD (number 2 is cancer). Thus, it could be argued that the overall impact of lipid lowering with statins or lifestyle changes should be of paramount importance in women treated for breast cancer, concerned about prevention and a reduction in all-cause mortality.

Statins and primary prevention

"When used for primary prevention, statins are associated with lower rates of all-cause mortality, major vascular events, and revascularizations compared with placebo. Statin therapy is not associated with increased rates of life-threatening adverse effects such as cancer [2, 3]." This was the conclusion of one of the largest and most current and extensive meta-analyses of statins and primary prevention. Is there another pill in medical history ever invented that in otherwise healthy individuals can make this claim? I am not aware of one, which is reason enough to discuss this finding with the appropriate patients. This extensive meta-analysis included the following [2, 3]:

© Springer International Publishing Switzerland 2016
M.A. Moyad, *Integrative Medicine for Breast Cancer*,
DOI 10.1007/978-3-319-23422-9_4

- Number of randomized trials: 18
- Number of participants: 56,934
- Men = 60 % of the participants and Women: 40 %
- Mean age: 57 (range of 28–97 years)
- Countries: 17 trials from the USA, Japan, and Europe; one trial from South America, Israel, South Africa, and Russia
- Average LDL reduction versus placebo: 39 mg/dl (multiply by 0.0259 to convert to millimoles per liter)
- All-cause mortality: 14 % Reduction (Number Need to Treat or NNT for 5-years of 138)
- Fatal and Nonfatal CVD (combined): 25 % Reduction (NNT for 5-years of 49)
- Fatal and Nonfatal Coronary Heart Disease (CHD) Events: 27 % Reduction (NNT 88)
- Fatal and Nonfatal Stroke: 22 % Reduction (NNT 155)
- Coronary Revascularization (Stents, Coronary Artery Bypass Grafting or CABG, …): 38 % Reduction (NNT 96)
- Incidence of cancers, myalgia, rhabdomyolysis, liver enzyme increases, arthritis, or renal dysfunction: No difference between statin and placebo groups.
- Increase diabetes was found in one of two trials (18 % increase, 95 % CI, 1.01–1.39, NNT 198)

The overall quality of the studies was high, and they were funded by pharmaceutical companies. A total of three trials, which comprised almost 50 % of the recruited group, were stopped early because of a significant reduction in the primary endpoint. The median control group CVD rate was 15 % over 10 years and NNT would be 25–75 over 5 years to reduce CVD rates to 10 % over 10 years. Hemorrhagic stroke could be increased by statins but none of the individual studies provided clarity on this issue. Overall, the result of this unique analysis suggests the benefits of statins outweigh the risk of life-threatening events. Another method of analyzing the full results for statins and the Primary Prevention of CVD are found in Table 4.1 [2, 3].

Still, there are other issues that need to be resolved. For example, one recent 6-month primary prevention trial found reduced energy and fatigue with exertion [4], but more quality of life data is needed from long-term trials to address this and other issues such as changes in memory. Overall, in these trials individuals treated with statins were just as likely to discontinue treatment compared to placebo (12 %) [2, 3].

Interestingly, the most recent American College of Cardiology/American Heart Association (ACC/AHA) guidelines on the treatment of cholesterol to reduce cardiovascular risk in adults recommends moderate- to high-intensity statin treatment for primary prevention (class I recommendations) for the following [5]:

- LDL cholesterol of 190 mg/dl or higher
- Aged 40–75 years with type 1 or 2 diabetes
- Aged 40–75 years with LDL between 70 and 189 mg/dl and 7.5 % or higher estimated 10-year risk of CVD

The group also suggests it could be reasonable to offer statin therapy in those with a 10-year risk of 5 % to less than 7.5 % (class IIa recommendation).

Table 4.1 Cumulative research for the primary prevention of CVD [2, 3]

Outcome (# of trials)	Events Statins	Total in statin group	Events Placebo/control	Total in control group	Relative risk (95 % CI)	NNT—5 years (95 % CI)
All-cause mortality (13)	1077	24,408	1223	23,652	0.86 (0.79–0.094)	138
Total CVD (9)	1103	11,892	1444	11,913	0.75 (0.70–0.081)	49
Total CHD (14)	820	24,217	1114	23,832	0.73 (0.67–0.080)	88
Total stroke events (10)	345	20,302	442	19,993	0.78 (0.68–0.89)	155
Revascularization (7)	286	21,166	461	21,237	0.62 (0.54–0.72)	96
Any adverse event (12)	5748	20,718	5090	19,998	1.00 (0.97–1.03)	NA
Type 2 diabetes (2)	342	12,205	290	12,202	1.18 (1.01–1.39)	99

The cholesterol guideline cutoffs were derived from the placebo group of 3 notable primary prevention only trials:

- Air Force/Texas Coronary Atherosclerosis Prevention Study (AFCAPS/TexCAPS) [6],
- Management of Elevated Cholesterol in the Primary Prevention Group of Adult Japanese (MEGA) study [7], and
- Justification for the Use of Statins in Primary Prevention: an Intervention Trial Evaluating Rosuvastatin (JUPITER) [8].

Statins, safety, and Type 2 diabetes

The sum of the recent data and meta-analyses provides a large source of evidence that should quench some of the overall controversy of utilizing statins in so-called "healthy individuals" (primary prevention) [2, 3, 9]. In the appropriate individuals statins reduce all-cause mortality, CVD events, especially costly cardiovascular procedures, and are of low cost (5 are now generic) and well-tolerated overall. Regardless, the primary issue that still needs to be resolved is whether or not statins significantly increase the risk of diabetes, and if so is that risk negligible or relevant? For example, it may be dose-related, or primarily in those with diabetes risk factors. In the notable JUPITER trial there were 2.5 CVD events or deaths avoided for each potential case of diabetes with rosuvastatin [10]. Thus, for most qualifying individuals the benefit appears to outweigh the risk, but more answers and clarity on this topic are desperately needed. The association of statins and type-2 diabetes is indeed a real finding from meta-analyses but causality has not been proven, but it appears women, the elderly, and those on higher dosages may be at higher risk [11, 12].

Recent laboratory evidence suggests a potential mechanism of action whereby statins increase the risk of diabetes [13]. Investigators from McMaster University in Ontario, Canada have found that these drugs may activate an immune response pathway that hinders insulin signaling. Multiple statins activate NLRP3/caspase-1 inflammasome, a multiprotein complex, which is known to encourage inflammation and insulin resistance. Interestingly, combining a statin with the drug glyburide (an inhibitor of NLRP3/caspase-1) suppressed these harmful effects in fat tissue of obese mice. These negative effects of statins were also not found in mice genetically engineered to lack expression of NLRP3/caspase-1 inflammasome. Thus, especially in high-risk patients there may be value in monitoring insulin sensitivity during statin use and using antidiabetes medications may further reduce risk. Ultimately, if the overall risk of type 2 diabetes becomes consistently clinically significant researchers may find a way to improve this drug class, for example CoQ10 supplementation is also being investigated for this purpose.

Still, one mantra of this drug class (and others) that now seems more relevant than ever is the need to encourage patients to be on the lowest dosage of a statin, along with moderate to aggressive lifestyle change to maintain small dosage needs (or no drug). In fact, there is also recent data to suggest that consistent lifestyle changes such as exercise may provide similar benefits to these and other preventive medications at least in a secondary prevention setting. For example, a total of four exercise and 12 drug meta-analyses and the addition of three recent exercise trials were utilized in a recent investigation for a total of 305 randomized control trials with over 339,000 participants [14]. A total of over 14,700 participants were randomized to exercise in 57 trials. Four conditions with evidence on the impact of exercise on mortality outcomes were the focus: secondary prevention of coronary heart disease, rehabilitation of stroke, treatment of heart failure, and the prevention of diabetes. No statistical differences were found between exercise and drug interventions in the secondary prevention of heart disease and pre-diabetes. Exercise was more effective compared to drug treatment among patients with stroke, and diuretics were more effective than exercise in heart failure. More studies are needed but current randomized data suggest the mortality benefits of exercise and prescription medications are similar in the secondary prevention of heart disease, rehabilitation after stroke, prevention of diabetes, and even provide unique benefits in heart failure. It will be of enormous interest in the future to determine the impact of exercise on a variety of other diverse and similar medical conditions. It is also interesting that after countless dollars and studies have been conducted in breast cancer, one of the only lifestyle modifications that may prevent or reduce the recurrence of this disease is exercise.

Statins and women

Interestingly, in the AFCAPS/TexCAPS study, the effect of lovastatin on the risk of first major coronary event was greater in woman versus men (−46 % versus −37 %), but the number of women having such an event was small (20 out of 997), so there was no treatment difference between genders [6, 15]. In the MEGA study, which used pravastatin, there was a 37 % reduction in men versus 29 % for women [7, 15]. Almost 70 % of the participants in MEGA were women, but interestingly the average BMI was 23–24, which is far below what is observed in US trials (BMI of 27–28) for men and women. In the JUPITER trial, which was stopped in 1.9 years because of its significant impact on reducing CVD events the average LDL reduc-

Table 4.2 Statin primary prevention trials only and impact on women [15]

Trial name	Statin treatment	Women (%)	Primary endpoint	Relative risk in women (95 % CI)
AFCAPS/TexCAPS	Lovastatin 20–40 mg/day versus placebo	997 (15)	Sudden cardiac death, MI, unstable angina	0.54 (0.22–1.35)
JUPITER	Rosuvastatin (Crestor)—20 mg/day versus placebo	6801 (38)	MI, stroke, unstable angina, CHD death, revascularization	0.54 (0.37–0.80)
MEGA	Pravastatin 5–20 mg + diet versus diet alone	5356 (69)	CHD, MI, sudden cardiac death, angina, revascularization	0.71 (0.44–1.14)

tions were 50 % and high-sensitivity C-reactive protein (hs-CRP) was reduced by 37 % [8, 15]. Positive impacts were observed in all subgroups evaluated and risk reduction in the rosuvastatin group was −46 % for women and −42 % for men. Women in JUPITER experienced a significant reduction in revascularization/unstable angina (−76 %, 95 % CI 0.11–0.51), and there was a nonsignificant reduction in nonfatal myocardial infarction (−44 %) or CHD death (−27 %). However, it needs to be reiterated that this trial was stopped in 1.9 years for already meeting its primary endpoint and other primary prevention trials also had short follow-up and smaller numbers of events. Thus, I find it striking in primary prevention that some "experts" make claims that the impact of statins in women is not known or of no benefit. Simply the potential dramatic reduction in the need of a revascularization procedure should be further explored and discussed with women at higher risk of a cardiovascular event (also see Chaps. 5, 6 and Reynolds Risk Score).

Table 4.2 is a summary of the statin data and primary prevention trial results for women.

Statins and breast cancer (incidence versus recurrence)

Overall, there has been no lucid association between statins and breast cancer incidence [16]. Yet there is accumulating data that statins may impact cancer progression more than cancer incidence, including breast cancer [17–19]. Numerous prospective studies suggest a reduction in recurrence including:

– A 2008 Kaiser Permanente US study of 1945 early stage breast cancer survivors and 210 recurrences were reported and primarily lovastatin or simvastatin (lipophilic statins) were utilized. An overall RR = 0.67 (0.39–1.14) [20] was observed. Mean duration of statin use was only 1.96 years and there was reduced risk of recurrence with increasing duration of statin use (p trend = 0.02). This study suggested post-diagnostic statin use was beneficial.
– In the 2011 Danish Breast Cancer Cooperative Group registry (n = 18,769), simvastatin (highly lipophilic statin) was associated with a reduced risk of breast cancer recurrence with an RR = 0.70 (0.57–0.86) [21].

- In an MD Anderson Cancer Center (Houston, TX) US study statins were associated with a significant ($p < 0.001$) reduction with an HR-0.40 (0.26–0.67) with the use of atorvastatin or simvastatin [22].
- A 2013 study from Germany of 3024 patients at risk of recurrence (stage I–III) found nonsignificant reduction in recurrence and HR=0.83 (0.54–1.24) and reduced breast cancer-specific mortality (HR=0.89, 0.52–1.49) with the use of any statin [23].
- A Seattle, WA USA 2014 study of 4216 women found a nonsignificant reduction in recurrence with lipophilic statins with an HR=0.76 (0.55–1.06) [24].
- A 2014 Finnish Cancer Registry cohort (31,236 cases) found the potential for a significant lower risk of breast cancer death especially with pre-diagnostic statin use with an HR=0.54 (0.44–0.67) [25].

Pre-surgery and statins

Pre-surgical clinical trials have demonstrated reduced proliferation activity and enhanced apoptosis in high-grade breast cancer tissue only in patients randomized to high (80 mg/day) or low-dose (20 mg/day) fluvastatin for 3–6 weeks before mastectomy [26]. Antiproliferative effects were also demonstrated in another presurgical clinical study of atorvastatin (80 mg/day) on invasive breast cancer utilized for 2 weeks before mastectomy, primarily in tumors expressing the rate limiting enzyme for cholesterol in breast cancer tissue [27].

Mechanisms of action (not just cholesterol but pleiotropic effects)

It is well-known that statins block the rate-limiting enzyme in the cholesterol synthesis pathway, 3-hydroxy-methylglutaryl (HMG) CoA reductase. However, there are multiple diverse mechanisms (including lipid lowering) whereby statins my disrupt cancer growth and include the following [28–31]:

- Decreased localized and systemic inflammation
- Helps normalize cell signaling (intracellular lipid-rafts)
- Inhibit thrombotic process (anticoagulant properties, enhance fibrinolysis, ...)
- Inhibit tumor cell proliferation
- Induction of cell cycle arrest
- Induction of apoptosis
- Reversion of multidrug resistance
- Inhibit cell-signaling pathways involved in invasion and metastasis
- Induction of tumor differentiation
- Modulate immune responses
- Reduces cholesterol intermediates and by-products that assist in cell growth and tumor promoting effects of oncogenes
- Reduces levels of estrone sulfate and estrogen mimic compounds
- Improve vascular endothelium function
- Reduce oxidative stress
- Modulate smooth muscle cell proliferation
- Stabilize plaques
- Stimulate bone growth/repair
- Upregulation of nitric oxide synthase

Table 4.3 FDA approved statins and the minimum dosage needed for a 30–40 % LDL reduction [32, 33]

Drug	Dosage (mg/day)	LDL reduction (%)
Atorvastatin (generic)	10	39
Fluvastatin (generic)	40–80	25–35
Lovastatin (generic)	40	31
Pitavastatin (Livalo®)	2 mg	35–40
Pravastatin (generic)	40	34
Rosuvastatin (Crestor®)	5	39–45
Simvastatin (generic)	20–40	35–41

Differences and similarities in statins

Currently available statins (in alphabetical order), and the minimum doses needed to reduce LDL cholesterol by at least 30–40 % are found in Table 4.3 [32, 33].

Other notable differences between FDA approved statins include the following [32, 33]:

- Statin drugs that are NOT negatively impacted by grapefruit juice includes: fluvastatin, pitavastatin, pravastatin, and rosuvastatin.
- Lovastatin, pravastatin and simvastatin are derived from fungal metabolites and have half-lives of 1–3 h, so daily compliance is critical for LDL reduction.
- Atorvastatin, fluvastatin, pitavastatin, and rosuvastatin are synthetic compounds with half-lives that range from 1 h (fluvastatin) to 19 h (rosuvastatin).
- Lipophilic statins include: Atorvastatin, fluvastatin, lovastatin, pitavastatin, and simvastatin (most lipophilic), which are more susceptible to undergo cytochrome P450 enzyme metabolism (except for pitavastatin). And passive diffusion through the hepatocyte membrane allows for their hepatic effects.
- Relatively hydrophilic statins, which are not metabolized by P450 enzymes include pravastatin and rosuvastatin. An active-carrier mediated process allows hydrophilic statins to impact hepatic cells.

Bias of industry funded statin trials?

A systematic review and network meta-analysis included 183 randomized trials of statins. A total of 146 industry-sponsored trials were found and 64 were placebo controlled and no differences were found in outcomes (especially LDL changes) from non-industry funded studies [34, 35].

Statins—Discovered from a natural source

Patients and health care professionals should be reminded that statins are naturally derived drugs. The story of their discovery is fascinating and will allow a greater appreciation of this drug class and the dietary supplement "red yeast rice" (RYR), which is arguably one of the better options today for statin intolerant patients.

It took approximately 2 years and thousands of moldy broth samples for a researcher named "Akira Endo" to identify something that actually lowered cholesterol [36, 37]. His discovery, taken from a mold like the one that grows on fruit turned out to be the very first in a class of drugs that in the past and also currently grosses billions a year for pharmaceutical companies. Dr. Endo is credited with discovering the first statin in 1973 from a natural source or one normally produced in nature. It was a fungal byproduct that shares the same basic chemical structure to three of the biggest selling statin drugs of all time: lovastatin (Mevacor®), pravastatin (Pravachol®), and simvastatin (Zocor®). All three drugs have now lost their patents by mid-2006 and are now also sold as generics. Some researchers hypothesize that it is three billion years of natural selection that helped Dr. Endo find this original product. This may be part of the recent ongoing trend in some small scientific circles to reexamine the possibility of finding compounds from nature.

Dr. Endo, now 81 years old was born on a farm in the snowy north of Japan [36, 37]. He remembers being taught by his grandfather about the fungi that grew in his geographic area. Dr. Endo was interested in one poisonous mushroom that killed flies but not people. He was fascinated by the fact that a natural compound could have such an impact. His original research came at a time when there was a general enthusiasm from natural products to treat infections. For example, penicillin is a compound produced by a mold to kill bacteria, and was accidentally discovered in 1928 by Alexander Fleming. Fleming had allowed his untidy lab with bacteria to sit during a vacation. He came back to find that mold had grown in one plate and the mold had a bacteria-free zone around it. Amazingly, penicillin was later mass produced during World War II and saved millions of lives. After the war a new discovery for tuberculosis occurred. The drug known as "streptomycin" was developed by researchers at Rutgers University, who investigated microorganisms from the soil, and it eventually became the first antibiotic that could be utilized to cure tuberculosis.

Dr. Endo became employed after college by a Tokyo-based pharmaceutical company, Sankyo and his job was to research food ingredients [36, 37]. He investigated some 250 kinds of fungi to find just one that produced an enzyme to make fruit juice less pulpy. This product was a success, and in 1966 the company allowed Dr. Endo to travel to Albert Einstein College of Medicine in New York to pursue his real strong interest in cholesterol research. During this time, cholesterol was a popular topic in research circles because of some evidence that it might play a major role in heart disease. Dr. Endo was surprised to find such strong interest by Americans in diet and dieting. "I thought it was really strange that people would cut off the fat before eating their steak. This was a culture shock, something inconceivable in Japan." Dr. Endo has stated.

Clofibrate was an anticholesterol drug already being used, but it came with notable side effects. Several companies recognized that inhibiting a vital enzyme in the body's production of cholesterol known as "HMG-CoA reductase" might be a better drug [36, 37]. However, researchers could not find a substance with this mechanism that actually worked in living animals. Dr. Endo, with his unique background had a different idea: find something in fungi that might block the enzyme. He already was well aware of the penicillin and streptomycin stories of discovery and in college he actually read a Japanese translation of a Fleming biography. Dr. Endo had realized that bacteria, like humans, needed cholesterol to maintain the integrity of their cell walls. He figured that some fungus most likely had evolved a compound that would block this HMG-CoA reductase enzyme as a way of keeping enemy bacteria from using cholesterol and eventually killing them. So, it was a matter of locating the right fungus. Dr. Endo convinced the Sankyo company to give him assistance. A chemist who had just joined the company named "Masao Kuroda" and two lab assistants joined his team. In April 1971 they began brewing fungal broths and tested each of them for their ability to block the cholesterol enzyme, which they got from ground up rat livers. "It was a bet, just like the lottery," said Dr. Endo. For more than 2 years, he and his team worked countless hours at their lab next to a train depot in southern Tokyo. "We were doing grunt work every day until we got sick of it," he said. Some chemicals were successful at inhibiting the enzyme but were not accepted because they were too toxic.

After testing some 6000 fungal broths, they found the perfect one in August 1973 [36, 37]. A compound made by a mold called "*Penicillium citrinum*," which was similar to a mold that grows on outdated oranges, and it produced a strong inhibitor of the enzyme that helps the body produce cholesterol. This was the first statin. However, Dr. Endo ran into a problem because the compound soon to be named "compactin" hardly worked in rats. More research would later find that rats actually differ in how they make cholesterol. Dr. Endo was puzzled until he happened to meet a colleague at a local watering hole near the laboratories one evening. The colleague suggested he use some hens for research, because they were about to be destroyed, and later the substance worked in these animals.

However, there was disagreement with Dr. Endo and the company on whether or not this research should be further pursued because companies working with other compounds that also held some promise. Therefore, Dr. Endo embarked on a surreptitious experiment at Osaka University. Akira Yamamoto was treating patients at this university hospital that had very high levels of cholesterol because of a genetic defect. Dr. Endo remembers calling Dr. Yamamoto from home at night so colleagues would not learn of the experiment. Dr. Endo personally prepared the samples of the potential drug and brought them to Osaka. Today, this would not be allowed because a review board would have to approve the experiment but following this procedure was not needed at that time.

The first patient (patient zero) in the entire world to receive a statin was an 18-year old woman. She was also the first to experience a side effect that even today can occur with these drugs: muscle pain (myalgia). Dr. Yamamoto gave her such a high dose she was weak and unable to walk. Dr. Yamamoto was advised apparently by his boss to stop the testing, but insisted he should continue the research. He stopped the drug on the first patient and she recovered. He also tried compactin on other patients but in lower dosages. This procedure lowered cholesterol in nine patients by an average of 27 %, according to a paper he later published. The first patient apparently has since been treated with other drugs and lives today in Southern Japan and she even had a daughter.

The Sankyo company agreed to place Dr. Endo's drug in clinical trials, and he felt he had done enough at this point and took a job as a professor at Tokyo Noko University. He apparently did not leave the job on friendly terms with the company.

Dr. Endo still mentions that the company told the researchers in his lab not to even assist him with placing his boxes of papers on the moving truck. Sankyo apparently in a one-page agreement in 1976 with Merck allowed access to its data and procedures associated with Dr. Endo's statin. Companies often do release such information when interested in partnering with another business group. However, Merck had also been working on its own cholesterol compound and did not have any official affiliation with Sankyo. In 1978, Merck found a different fungus with a compound that was essentially identical to Dr. Endo's and called it "lovastatin." Dr. Endo claims he also discovered this compound independently, during his first several months at Tokyo Noko University. Merck held the patent rights in the USA, and in 1987 began marketing this compound in the USA as "Mevacor®"—the very first FDA-approved statin drug.

Eventually, Sankyo no longer pursued compactin, but instead focused on another statin with a similar structure [36, 37]. It licensed this compound outside of Japan to Bristol-Myers Squibb Company, which began selling it in the USA in 1991 as "Pravachol®." In the early to mid-1990s, with strong research behind them, statins became to gain enormous popularity and Merck even released another statin known as "Zocor®" in 1992. Pfizer's "Lipitor®" is a statin with a structure different from Dr. Endo's original discovery, and it became the world's number 1 selling drug with approximately $12 billion in sales per year.

As the popularity of statins continued to grow Dr. Endo received little to no attention. For example, on the Sankyo website the discovery of compactin is mentioned but not Dr. Endo [36, 37]. However, some Sankyo spokesperson mentions Dr. Endo as a key figure in the discovery. Michael S. Brown and Joseph Goldstein won a Nobel Prize for their research in cholesterol and wrote in 2004: "The millions of people whose lives will be extended through statin therapy owe it all to Akira Endo." Dr. Endo apparently never earned a penny from his statin discovery. He left Sankyo in December 1978 and was making less than $2000 a month. Later in his time at the University doing more research on fungal byproducts he found applications for some compounds for use in cosmetics, chewing gum, and other products. He is now retired from the University, and he maintains an office in a two-room apartment in western Tokyo, with closets full of files he has maintained for years. Interestingly, several years ago Dr. Endo had a daylong health exam and was found to have a slightly abnormal cholesterol level. He claims the doctor did not know him and told him, "We have good drugs for that." Dr. Endo also claims he took Mevacor® for a while but discontinued the drug. At his physical in 2004, his LDL or "bad cholesterol" was 155 mg/dl, but instead of going on a statin he decided to first exercise more and brought his number down to 130 mg/dl. Dr. Endo used a Japanese proverb "The indigo dyer wears white trousers" to explain why he has not yet taken a drug that was partly from his own research and invention.

Thus, numerous statins and multiple other drugs have been derived from natural sources (approximately one third of current medications on the market), but Akira Endo's is arguably one of the most notable. Again, the statins derived from natural sources as well as several other naturally derived drug examples are listed in Table 4.4 [36].

Table 4.4 Several popular drugs derived from natural sources [36]

Drug name	Where it is used	Launch date	Where it comes from
Aspirin	Painkiller	1899	Willow bark
Penicillin	Antibiotic	1940s	Fungus
Mevacor	Cholesterol-statin	1987	Fungus
Pravachol	Cholesterol-statin	1991	Fungus
Zocor	Cholesterol-statin	1992	Fungus
Taxol	Cancer	1993	Pacific yew tree
Byetta	Diabetes	2005	Gila monster saliva

Red Yeast Rice (RYR)

Lost in the overall story of Akira Endo was that he found another fungus that was able to block cholesterol synthesis that was also utilized as part of the statin discovery. Dr. Akira Endo also found that a Monascus yeast strain naturally produced a substance that inhibits cholesterol synthesis [37, 38]. He named it "monacolin K" and it is found in the dietary supplement red yeast rice extract (RYR). This was later isolated and is now known to be of the same structure as lovastatin, the first marketed statin. Thus, RYR could also be considered one of the first statins used in medical history.

RYR favorably competes with lovastatin, pravastatin and simvastatin in terms of potency, and is now considered an alternative for statin intolerant patients [39–41]. RYR has demonstrated a significant reduction in cardiovascular events (primary endpoint) in a randomized controlled trial of almost 5000 participants followed for a median of 4.5 years (Chinese Coronary Secondary Prevention Group study) [42].

RYR is a traditional Chinese herbal medicine first mentioned in 800 AD in the Tang Dynasty for blood circulation [43, 44]. It is produced by the fermentation of the fungal strain Monascus purpureus Went (red yeast) over moist and sterile rice. RYR is also actually a common dietary compound and food colorant utilized in numerous Asian countries. In China, Japan, and several other countries it is utilized as an additive and preservative for fish and meat. It has a vibrant red color, flavor, and aroma, thus it is also utilized as a flavoring agent in a number of Chinese recipes and dishes, and it is even used for brewing red rice wine. RYR is also known by multiple synonyms as a food product including: Hong Qu, Hung-Chu, Ang-kak, Ankak rice, Red Mold Rice, and Beni-Koji.

It is now known that RYR contains ten different compounds known as "monacolins" (statin-like compounds) that block the rate-limiting enzyme for cholesterol synthesis [45]. These are listed in Table 4.5. Of these, again monacolin K is likely most responsible for the primary LDL reduction associated with RYR.

RYR overall lipid and clinical efficacy

A meta-analysis of over 9600 patients in 93 randomized trials involving three different commercial variants of RYR has summarized this extensive experience [46]. The mean reduction in total cholesterol, LDL, triglyceride, and increase in

Table 4.5 Monacolin compounds that can be detected in red yeast rice (RYR) [45]	Monacolin compounds in RYR
	Dihydromonacolin K
	Monacolin J
	Monacolin JA
	Monacolin K (lovastatin equivalent)
	Monacolin KA
	Monacolin L
	Monacolin LA
	Monacolin M
	Monacolin X
	Monacolin XA
	Total monacolin content (sum of the ten detectable monacolins)

HDL was the following: -35 mg/dl (-0.91 mmol/L), -28 mg/dl (-0.73 mmol/L), -36 mg/dl (-0.41 mmol/L), and $+6$ mg/dl ($+0.15$ mmol/L).

Xuezhikang is a commercial RYR product evaluated in a large, randomized, placebo-controlled clinical trial with robust endpoints [42, 47]. The China Coronary Secondary Prevention Study (CCSPS) enrolled 4870 participants (3986 men, 884 women) with a previous myocardial infarction (MI), and a baseline mean total cholesterol, LDL, triglyceride, and HDL of approximately 208 mg/dl (5.38 mmol/L), 129 mg/dl (3.34 mmol/L), 165 mg/dl (1.85 mmol/L), and 46 mg/dl (1.19 mmol/L). Participants received RYR 600 mg twice daily (1200 mg total, monacolin K 2.5–3.2 mg/capsule) or matching placebo and followed for 4.5 years. The trial was conducted from May 1996 to December 2003 in 65 hospitals in China. The primary endpoint was nonfatal MI or death from coronary or cardiac causes. Secondary endpoints included total mortality from CV disease, total all-cause mortality, need for coronary revascularization procedure, and change in lipid levels. Fasting blood samples were drawn at baseline, 6–8 weeks after randomization, and at 6-month intervals. There were two interim analyses, and the second one demonstrated a significant difference for the primary endpoint. The study was stopped in June 2003. A total of 98 % of the participants completed the study and mean BMI was 24–25 (normal weight). It is of interest that a plethora of these endpoints were significantly reduced with the exception of a nonsignificant reduction in fatal MI. Cancer mortality and all-cause mortality were reduced. Lipids were also modestly and significantly reduced. No serious adverse events were observed during this trial. Total adverse events and treatment cessation numbers were similar for RYR and placebo. The number needed to treat (NNT) to prevent a primary end-point over the 4.5 year duration of the trial is 21, which favorably compares to the NNT range (19–56) observed in previous secondary prevention trials [48]. Subsequent subgroup evaluations from the CCSPS trial have found equivalent benefits with RYR among diabetics [49], elderly (mean age 69 years) [50], and hypertensive participants [51]. Potential anticancer benefits found in the overall trial with RYR were also found among the elderly

Table 4.6 Lipid results from the intervention group versus placebo in the largest randomized trial (CCSPS) of RYR [42, 47]

Lipid value	Change with RYR compared to placebo (%)	p Value
Total cholesterol	−11	<0.001
LDL cholesterol	−18	<0.001
Triglycerides	−15	<0.001
HDL cholesterol	+4.2	<0.001

Table 4.7 Multiple clinical endpoint observations in the largest randomized trial (CCSPS) of RYR versus placebo [47]

Clinical endpoints	Risk reduction with RYR compared to placebo (%)	p Value
Nonfatal myocardial infarction (MI)	−62	<0.001
Coronary disease death	−31	0.005
Fatal MI	−33	0.19
Fatal stroke	−9	0.85
Revascularization	−36	0.004
CVD death	−30	0.005
Cancer death	−56	0.014
Total or overall deaths	−33	0.0003

(significant reduction in cancer deaths) [42, 50], and included a 51 % reduction in cancer incidence [50]. Thus, the data has been consistent that RYR reduces lipid parameters, especially LDL [52–54], and appears to have a favorable impact on clinical endpoints [42]. The summary of the lipid results compared to placebo and of the clinical endpoints results for the CCSPS are listed in Tables 4.6 and 4.7.

Other clinical trials conducted continue to support the lipid lowering impacts and safety of RYR. A randomized trial of 74 dyslipidemia patients comparing 40 mg/day of simvastatin to a high potency RYR (2.53 mg monacolin K per capsule, total monacolins, 5.3 mg/capsule) and lifestyle changes with fish oil found that the LDL reductions between both groups were similar after 12 weeks (−40 % for simvastatin, −42 % for RYR) [45]. Participants consuming RYR needed to consume 4–6 capsules (2400–3600 mg RYR total) per day compared to one pill per day for the prescription drug group. No dropouts occurred, and there was no difference in adverse events reported. In the simvastatin arm three patients experienced musculoskeletal symptoms with one having elevated liver function tests (LFTs). RYR group had one patient with elevated creatine kinase numbers. This abnormality may have been caused by excessive exercise.

Another trial (n = 62) by the same principal author utilized a less potent RYR (1.02 mg monacolin K per capsule, total monacolins, 2.16 mg/capsule) at a dose of six capsules (3600 mg total RYR) per day compared to placebo for statin-intolerant (myalgia induced) patients for 24 weeks and found a significant (p = 0.01) LDL reduction of −21.3 % [39]. It should also be of interest that 93 % of the subjects on RYR in this trial with a history of statin-intolerance were able to tolerate this supplement without myalgia.

Another group of 43 statin-intolerant adults with dyslipidemia were randomized in a separate trial to prescription pravastatin at 20 mg (40 mg total) or RYR 2400 mg twice daily (4800 mg total, monacolin K at 1.245 mg per capsule, eight capsules per day), and both groups were asked to adhere to weekly healthy lifestyle educational sessions [41]. After 12 weeks a 30 % reduction in LDL was observed for RYR and a 27 % reduction for pravastatin. Only one of 21 in the RYR (5 %) and two of 22 (9 %) participants in the pravastatin group discontinued because of myalgia recurrence. Mean pain severity, and muscle strength at week 4, 8, and 12 did not differ. Other recent publications report similar results [40, 55]. A recently published crossover study of children (aged 8–16 years) with heterozygous Familial hypercholesterolemia ($n=24$), and Familial Combined Hyperlipidemia ($n=16$) found that a RYR supplement significantly ($p<0.001$) reduced LDL by 25 % [56]. There were no adverse events in terms of liver or muscle enzyme abnormalities over the 8-week treatment period.

Multiple reasons can be proffered for a low rate of toxicity with RYR overall in the literature (none proven): the diluted monacolin K in a supplement that contains mostly other ingredients, lower dose and potency of monacolin K (lovastatin) compared to the previous statin utilized, multiple capsules during the day compared to one bolus at one specific time, which reduces the risk of excessive blood concentrations or impact with CYP3A4 inhibitors, other compounds that may deter myalgia in RYR (coenzyme Q-like effects), lack of aggressive monitoring, the desire to report less side effects from patients on a supplement compared to a drug, etc. Regardless of the reason, RYR with an appropriate standardized amount of monacolin K is a viable alternative for statin intolerant patients.

RYR and cancer

Laboratory studies of RYR in some tumor types including hormonally driven cancers are preliminarily impressive. For example, RYR has direct effects on androgen-dependent LNCaP cells (prostate cancer) and androgen-independent cells over expressing androgen receptor [57]. RYR inhibited prostate cancer growth compared to a prescription statin (lovastatin). Whole RYR inhibited proliferation to a greater extent than monacolin K and pigment-enriched fractions isolated from RYR ($p<0.001$). These results suggested that intact RYR, beyond the monacolin content, may favorably inhibit androgen-dependent and -independent prostate cancer growth. Another study showed that RYR significantly reduced androgen-dependent and -independent xenograft tumors in SCID mice ($p<0.05$) [58]. Intact whole RYR again provided more inhibition than monacolin K alone. RYR also significantly ($p<0.05$) reduced gene expression of several androgen-synthesizing enzymes (AKR1C3, HSD3B2, and SRD5A1) in both androgen dependent and independent tumors. A significant ($p<0.001$) association was seen between tumor volume and serum cholesterol. Similar findings have been demonstrated in colon cancer cell lines [59].

Other studies have demonstrated that RYR has pleiotropic actions on a variety of pathways and markers beyond lipid lowering [60–63], which could have an impact on cancer proliferation and progression similar to what has been demonstrated with statin drugs [64–66].

Surprisingly, RYR has received minimal attention in breast cancer. A small clinical trial of tumor free breast cancer patients on hormone therapy is of some interest. This study utilized with a daily single table use of RYR (200 mg equivalent to 3 mg monacolins) over 3-months and demonstrated a 19 % reduction in LDL beyond dietary changes [67].

Limitations of RYR (duration, toxicity, food, grapefruit, FDA, …)

Quality control (QC) with RYR, an over the counter product in the USA is an issue [68–71]. Different Commercial products of RYR have different concentrations of monacolins. Some contain a potentially harmful by-product of yeast fermentation known as "citrinin" (a nephrotoxin) [71]. And despite recent trials and meta-analysis continuing to demonstrate minimal toxicity many of these studies were only of a short duration [72, 73], thus RYR still requires medical oversight. Case reports of hepatotoxicity [74, 75], myopathy [76–81], rhabdomyolysis [82], and a case report of the potential of a negative interaction (peripheral neuropathy) with one cancer drug (imatinib) have been reported [83]. The contraindications for RYR should be similar to the drug lovastatin [84], including hepatic or renal impairment, and allergies to yeast or fungus [32]. RYR should be taken with or especially after meals [32, 85], since lovastatin absorption is significantly improved under these circumstances, but only as long as pectin or oat bran (high fiber) is not consumed simultaneously because these products specifically reduce absorption [86–88]. There has been no consistent mention of the interaction of RYR and food in the medical literature or data relating to RYR specifically, and only the drug lovastatin carries these concerns. However, since the chemical structure of monacolin K and lovastatin are similar then grapefruit should not be consumed with or around the time of RYR. Again, this is another reason to monitor patients utilizing RYR.

A final serious limitation of RYR, especially in the USA involves standardization of the active ingredient "monacolin K" the lovastatin mimic [89, 90]. Currently, because of past litigation and current FDA monitoring RYR is not allowed to standardize the cholesterol-lowering ingredient, monacolin K. This is nonsensical because it only punishes the consumer and health care professional seeking a viable statin alternative [89]. In my opinion, either ban the supplement in the USA or allow for a standardization of monacolin K because any other option only confuses the clinical picture and forces the patient into a risky and costly guinea pig scenario where they test various brands to determine which one might have sufficient monacolin K at the moment. How does this make any sense? In the meantime, companies continue to recall products for having standardized ingredients [91]. Some patients and clinicians will simply not want to engage in this nebulous milieu and opt for other ways to deal with cholesterol lowering and statin intolerance. And one point that must be reiterated is that prescription generic statins are now less costly than many RYR supplements.

Statin/RYR induced myopathy (SIM)

The incidence and prevalence of CVD in general, and in those diagnosed and treated for breast cancer along with recent alteration in cholesterol treatment guidelines dramatically increases the potential number of statin candidates [92, 93]. And the ongoing data that suggests pleiotropic actions of these agents for the potential prevention of other highly prevalent medical conditions such as Alzheimer disease will also arguably continue to maintain interest in statin utilization [94]. Yet one overt issue is not only the number of individuals that cannot tolerate statins in general because of statin induced myopathy (SIM) but also due to a higher prevalence of musculoskeletal issues with several standard breast cancer drugs such as the aromatase inhibitors [95–97]. One option, perhaps the most attractive but not always the most realistic, is to exercise more and to further educate patients on dietary changes to lower cholesterol so again the lowest statin dosage possible is achieved. Prospective research is beginning to demonstrate that statin compliance and improved fitness has a synergistic and profound ability to reduce all-cause mortality significantly (up to 70 %) beyond what the drug can provide [98]. Regardless of BMI, fitness can improve overall health and in some cases negate the effects of excess weight [99].

Still, muscle pain is the primary reason for statin cessation [100–105]. This main concerning side effect of statin treatment is in reality known as "myalgia" (muscle ache, pain or weakness) without an abnormal blood creatine kinase (CK) levels, and this rate of)muscle problems is not low because it is reported in about 10 % of statin users and it might be higher (up to 33 %). Aging increases the prevalence of muscle aches and pain and confuses the situation. Myalgia more commonly occurs when starting treatment or within the first 6 months, but there are a minority of people that can develop it years after taking statins. The risk of muscle pain from statins is usually dose-dependent, and this is another reason to incorporate lifestyle changes to lower the dose. Research suggests going to half the recommended dose via lifestyle changes appears to reduce your risk of muscle problems similar to a placebo for many individuals.

"Myopathy" is a general term that describes any disease of the muscles, which includes myalgia [100–105]. "Myositis" is muscle symptoms with increased CK levels and myopathy includes myalgia or myositis, or even rhabdomyolysis, which is a CK increase above 10,000 U/L or a situation that usually results in a CK ten times the upper limit of normal and brown urine, products from muscle tissue spilling in the urine, blood creatinine (test of kidney health) increases and kidney function abnormalities or kidney failure can occur. The good news is that severe statin toxicity is extremely rare today (rarely observed in clinical trials). Still, If the CK test is high a urine myoglobin test (product of muscle tissue spilling into the urine) or even a muscle biopsy in really rare cases could assist in identifying statin toxicity.

Patients should never just deal with the pain or taking a supplement to solve SIM first, but to determine the cause and do something different apart from taking more medication to eliminate the pain. This is what gets missed often with SIM because there are so many reasons or causes for it and it needs to be identified. Here is the partial list of risk factors for SIM or what can increase the risk of SIM [89, 100–105]:

– Age (older than 70 years increases risk)
– Alcohol abuse

- Asian ethnicity (Chinese or Japanese) for those on the drug rosuvastatin
- Carnitine deficiency syndromes
- Diabetes
- Exercise (excessive exercise can raise CK levels above normal-review exercise patterns such as frequency and intensity with a high CK level)
- Female
- Genetics
- Grapefruit/Grapefruit juice (it and perhaps even pomegranate juice can cause large increases in statin drug blood concentrations. Atorvastatin, lovastatin, and simvastatin are impacted the most by grapefruit. Statin drugs NOT IMPACTED by grapefruit includes: fluvastatin, pitavastatin, pravastatin, and rosuvastatin)
- Hereditary muscle problem
- High blood potassium levels
- High statin dose or Dose-Dependent (higher chance of muscle pain on higher dosages)
- High triglycerides
- Hypertension (some medications can increase risk like amiodarone or other drugs like verapamil or diltiazem and you may need to change to another drug like amlodipine or just review with your doctor)
- Infection
- Interactions with other medications (drugs, supplements and even grapefruit juice and some other juices and compounds)
- Kidney problems (low glomerular filtration rate or high creatinine levels)
- Liver problems (fatty liver, hepatitis, high liver enzymes, …)
- Low thyroid levels (untreated hypothyroidism, ask for the TSH blood test)
- Low vitamin B12
- Low vitamin D
- Medications (other cholesterol lowering meds such as gemfibrozil can increase stain dose)
- McArdle's disease
- Muscle pain previously on statins
- Small body frame or low body mass index
- Substance abuse (amphetamines, cocaine, heroin, …)
- Surgery

Prevention and treatment of SIM: Conventional and integrative
Diet
Obviously, multiple dietary options can be proffered to reduce LDL cholesterol and statin dosage [89]. One interesting diet known as the "dietary portfolio" which originated from Toronto (for example St Michaels Hospital and other Canadian researchers) demonstrated higher intakes of plant sterols, soy protein (11–15 g/day), soluble fiber (5–10 g), nuts and seeds, more veggies, less beef, poultry, fish, and eggs, and on average experienced 10–15 % reduction in LDL [106]. Also, please see Chap. 3 on lifestyle changes for the plethora of dietary methods to reduce LDL.

Fiber

Reduce the statin dose slightly and add 5–15 g of psyllium fiber powder or another soluble fiber product [107–109]. An older study from the Robert Wood Johnson Medical School in New Jersey found the LDL cholesterol drop was the same with 10 mg simvastatin and 15 g of psyllium (Metamucil) fiber compared to just taking 20 mg of simvastatin with no fiber [109].

Statin dose and frequency change

Reduce the statin dose or frequency or stop statin for several weeks and start again [89, 100–105].

Statin dose and/or frequency and add ezetimibe

Reduce your statin dose and/or frequency and add the dietary cholesterol absorption inhibitor ezetimibe at 10 or even 20 mg/day (also known as "Zetia®"). The potential for an extra 10 % reduction in LDL exists with two pills a day of ezetimibe compared to the already 15–25 % reduction with one pill of ezetimibe [110].

Change statin and/or dose and/or frequency

Use a different statin with a longer half-life (atorvastatin, pitavastatin, or rosuvastatin) so it is ingested less frequently [100–105]. Rosuvastatin (Crestor®) at the lowest dose (5 mg or split dose to 2.5 mg) once a week [111, 112], twice weekly, or every other day or perhaps even once every 10 days in the worst-case scenario are all options. Another option is rosuvastatin once a week and also daily 10 mg of ezetimibe (Zetia). Atorvastatin (generic) three times weekly, and remember that it is now generic. Also there is the option of adding daily ezetimibe, or simply pitavastatin (Livalo®) three times weekly alone or adding daily 10 mg ezetimibe.

Ezetimibe (Zetia®) alone once or twice/day and IMPROVE-IT

Just Use ezetimibe alone or another non-statin drug [100–105]. Ezetimibe blocks the absorption of cholesterol from food/intestines. Again, the potential for an extra 10 % reduction in LDL exists with two pills a day of ezetimibe compared to the already 15–25 % reduction with one pill of ezetimibe [110]. Some doctors use drugs called "bile acid sequestrants" but these can increase the risk of gastrointestinal problems so it is not high on the list but an option. More recent long-term (9-years) clinical trial data (IMPROVE-IT) with statins have actually demonstrated a moderate positive impact on clinical endpoints and not just lipid values with ezetimibe [113]. This should increase the use of ezetimibe immediately in those patients with SIM and reignite the discussion of a "lower is better" philosophy because in high-risk CVD patients ezetimibe and simvastatin lowered LDL to almost 53 mg/dl compared to approximately 70 mg/dl in simvastatin only participants.

The IMPROVE-IT trial was more specifically a double-blind, randomized trial of 18,144 patients from 1147 medical centers in 39 countries who had been hospitalized for an acute coronary syndrome (acute myocardial infarction, or high-risk unstable angina) within the previous 10 days [113]. The combination of simvastatin (use to be known as Zocor) at 40 mg and ezetimibe at 10 mg was compared to simvastatin (40 mg) and placebo. The primary endpoint of this trial was the combined endpoint of cardiovascular death, nonfatal myocardial infarction, unstable angina needing rehospitalization, coronary revascularization (procedure 30 or more days after randomized in the trial), or nonfatal stroke. The average age of the participants was 63–64 years of age (50 years or older to be eligible), 76 % were male, 84 % were Caucasian, 61 % had hypertension, 27 % had diabetes, and 33 % were current smokers! Additionally the mean BMI was 28, which is overweight, and the mean LDL was 84 mg/dl before they the trial started. The median follow-up was 6 years and the LDL cholesterol average 54 mg/dl in the combination statin-ezetimibe group and 69.5 mg/day in the statin only group. The rate of the primary endpoint at 7 years was 32.7 % in the combination group and 34.7 % in the statin only group, which is only an absolute difference of 2 percentage points but this was still significant ($p=0.02$). Muscle, gallbladder, and liver side effects and cancer were similar between the two groups. Discontinuation of the medication in either group because of side effects was approximately 10–11 % in both groups (again no difference). However, in reality compliance was a big issue throughout the trial because 42 % of the participants in IMPROVE-IT (combination or statin alone group) stopped their study medication prematurely (for any reason), which is about 7 % per year, which actually closely resembles what has been observed in other trials!

Thus, adding ezetimibe lowered LDL by 24 %. It should be kept in mind that no differences between the groups were found for death from cardiovascular disease or death from any cause (cancer …), but significant reductions were found in the combination group for the rates of myocardial infarction and ischemic stroke [113]. This is a credible finding since the differences began to emerge after 1-year and the trial was only conducted for an average of 6 years. Thus, overall it represents a moment where a non-statin therapy to reduce LDL can also reduce cardiovascular outcomes (something missing with niacin, and others). It appears that lower is better and had these patients started with higher LDL levels arguably even better results would have been observed. It is also interesting that in the combination group the reduction in the inflammatory blood marker hs-CRP was also significantly reduced compared to the statin only group. This is part of the reason I believe ezetimibe should continued to be studied against breast and prostate cancer because of the reduction in this inflammatory marker.

Still, the IMPROVE-IT trial offers important new evidence for the "LDL Hypothesis" that lowering of this blood marker is the primary driver of what changes cardiovascular risk (after the first year of the study the LDL was 53 mg/dl in the combination group and 70 mg/dl in the statin only group) [113]. Despite just a 2 % difference in the primary endpoint in favor of the combination group this is almost identical to what would have been predicted from past trials based on the LDL difference! Again, offering more evidence for the LDL hypothesis. Additionally, this represents new options or hope for those that cannot achieve their target LDL with diet, exercise and statins. This also offers hope for new medications such as "PCSK9 inhibitors" that reduce LDL via reducing LDL-receptor removal to allow for more LDL to be cleared from the circulation, and these agents have the ability to lower LDL as much as 60 %. However, the problem with these drugs is that they are supposed to be given by subcutaneous injection once every 2–4 weeks, and with compliance overall in the IMPROVE-IT trial not very good then this is not a good sign of future drug compliance if PCSK9 blockers work. Interestingly, an FDA committee recommended approval of a PCSK9 inhibitor at the time of this book submission, so this should get very interesting soon. And at least the IMPROVE-IT trial should maintain interest in plant sterol/stanol dietary supplements or alternative methods of reducing cholesterol and perhaps even better to reduce the risk of cardiovascular and other diseases.

RYR

Red yeast rice (RYR) extract dietary supplements (usually 2–4 pills a day) at dosages as low as 600 mg (one pill) on up to 1800 mg in some studies, 2400 mg in other studies can lower LDL (bad cholesterol) 10–30 % and 3600 mg in other very rare circumstances can also provide benefits [84]. Also, please keep in mind that monacolin K has a similar structure to the drug lovastatin, so it should be taken with food and you should avoid grapefruit and its juice and perhaps pomegranate juice when on this supplement.

CoQ10 (placebo?) Myalgia and/or diabetes reduction

Statins and RYR block the ability of the liver to make cholesterol, but part of what is produced in the process of constructing cholesterol in the liver is the building block for CoQ10, the fat-soluble antioxidant that is needed in every single cell of the human body [89]. Thus, statins or RYR usually significantly reduce CoQ10 blood and potentially tissue levels [80]. For example, atorvastatin (previous trade name of Lipitor) causes a significant reduction in CoQ10 within 2 weeks, and a 40–50 % reduction in CoQ10 levels in the blood in just 30 days that is maintained during statin use [114, 115]. Since CoQ10 is needed in every cell by the mitochondria (power house or energy producers) to produce energy it could impact muscle tissue causing pain when muscle tissue levels are low.

The rationale for using CoQ10 with statins was so convincing that Merck and Co., Inc the pharmaceutical company sought and was awarded two patents (Merck & Co., Inc.: US933165 and US929437, 1990) for a combination statin and CoQ10 product that might reduce muscle and liver abnormalities issues [116]. Yet this ultimately was not included in the product. Today, CoQ10 has the most human research completed for lowering the risk of muscle problems compared to any other dietary supplement. However, the results are mixed with about half the studies showing some benefit and the other half no benefit. In fact, recent studies and a meta-analysis question whether the benefit is significant beyond a placebo [117, 118]. Another issue, as mentioned earlier, is the diverse and multiple etiologies of muscle abnormalities, which means it is unlikely there will be any dietary supplement or drug that will ever be found that will prevent or reduce SIM in most individuals. Most studies have participants taking dietary supplement CoQ10 at 100–400 mg per day to prevent or reduce myalgia. One of the biggest side effects of CoQ10 is the cost!. It is for this reason I do not have patients start CoQ10 when on initiating a statin because not only is this costly but it only encourages the use of more pills and pill dependence when in fact most patients on statins do not need CoQ10.

If CoQ10 is NOT working within 4 weeks increase the dose and if it not working at the maximum dosage (300 or even 400 mg per day) then it is time to discontinue it or use it for another potential benefit. For example, in those that exercise regularly, there is some preliminary research to suggest an improved muscle performance and a small increase in strength [119]. Since statin intolerance is usually resolved by multiple methods (changing drug, dose, frequency, …), again the use of CoQ10 should be a last resort and not a first step. Another option is to continue to watch the research on statins especially in high dosages and the risk of type 2 diabetes because it is plausible based on the ongoing research that CoQ10 could play a role in reducing this risk. Therefore, patients could theoretically utilize CoQ10 for the prevention of statin-induced diabetes but again this is very embryonic research but has captured my attention. Again, this is another reason to encourage moderate diet and exercise to lower the needed statin dose in any patient on higher dosages.

Side effects are rare with CoQ10 but gastrointestinal side effects and allergic rash have been reported [120]. CoQ10 has antiplatelet effects so one needs to be careful on blood thinning drugs (like clopidogrel), but ironically it also acts like vitamin K and may reduce the efficacy of the blood thinner warfarin. CoQ10 is best taken with a meal (fat-soluble) that has some fat in it for better absorption and although there are a plethora of companies that promote a better absorbing CoQ10 compared to the plain old less costly ones that has been used in most studies, I do not believe the more expensive brands should be purchased unless they change tangible or clinical endpoints. Some doctors like to determine blood levels of CoQ10 but research continues to suggest that even when the blood level of CoQ10 is high, it does not reflect muscle tissue concentrations and vice versa. So, this is a controversial test (like numerous nutritional antioxidant blood tests).

Creatine monophosphate

Preliminary research from the Annals of Internal Medicine journal suggests taking 5–10 g of the powdered dietary supplement creatine monophosphate daily with water to reduce myalgia [121]. Participants ingest a loading dose of 10 g for the first 5 days with no statin drug (glass of water with each dose), and then switch to 5 g a day and are reintroduced to the statin that caused problems or a new statin, and it can help some individuals reduce or eliminate their myalgia after 2–3 months. Use creatine powder and not the pills because you have to take too many for equivalence. Creatine monophosphate inside muscle tissue helps produce energy [122], so it helps some individuals improve their workouts, especially weight lifting. Some individuals experience a decrease in creatine when taking a statin and other drugs, which could cause muscle pain. Many folks use creatine to enhance their workouts, and it is already a commonly recommended supplement for athletic or exercise enhancement. Creatine failed to demonstrate efficacy in a large phase 3 US trial in Parkinson disease despite some past positive data and overall safety [123, 124], which implies something similar with SIM that until more and larger trials are conducted whether or not it works better than a placebo is not known.

l-carnitine dietary supplements

There is an unusually high level of carnitine metabolizing issues in the general population and those on statins [116, 125, 126]. Genetics have caused some individuals to be deficient in the amino acid carnitine. For example heterozygous carriers for the carnitine palmitoyltransferase-2 (CPT2) deficiency and other conditions that cause this problem are treated in multiple ways including with L-carnitine dietary supplements to prevent muscle problems. Thus, it is not uncommon for individuals with carnitine metabolizing abnormalities to suffer from SIM. Dosages of 1000–2000 mg/day (with or without food) of cheap L-carnitine (acetyl-L-carnitine for example) is a preliminary option and I have not observed more expensive types like propionyl L-carnitine to have better initial data.

Vitamin D blood levels/supplementation (negative acute phase reactant?)

Numerous preliminary investigations, especially retrospective have found a lower level of vitamin D in patients with myopathy and even myalgia from aromatase inhibitors [127–130]. However, what has not been resolved is whether or not the low vitamin D level is the result or the cause of SIM. There appears to be no harm in attempting to raise vitamin D (25-OH vitamin D) status with moderate amounts of vitamin D, for example 1000–2000 IU per day to determine if it resolves this situation over several months. Still, there is excellent preliminary evidence to suggest that vitamin D appears to be acting as a negative acute phase reactant and is not the cause of many medical conditions but the result of them [131, 132], which may help to explain why it has now failed multiple major clinical trials in a variety of disease categories [89].

Plant sterol/stanol dietary supplements/diet

Phytosterols block the uptake of cholesterol from dietary and bile sources in the intestinal tract. LDL cholesterol is reduced by phytosterols, and HDL and triglycerides are not impacted. Over 100 clinical trials utilizing phytosterols themselves have been conducted [133, 134]. Plant sterols have been shown to reduce LDL by approximately 10–15 % (average of 10–12 %) when approximately 2000–3000 mg per day is ingested. Plant sterols may also reduce the absorption of some fat-soluble vitamins, so a multivitamin should be used daily. Plant sterols are just weaker or less potent copycats of the drug ezetimibe (Zetia®), which can reduce LDL by approximately 20 % with 10 mg dose.

Plant stanol/sterol esters (2 g/day) are a therapeutic option to enhance LDL cholesterol lowering. This can be done by ingesting one or two caplets two times a day with a glass of water right before your largest one or two meals of the day (so you can block cholesterol absorption).

Non-options for SIM

Fish Oil

This is arguably one of the biggest errors I witness by health care professionals and patients. Fish oil can increase LDL as you increase the fish oil dosage especially when the marine omega-3 compound DHA is present! [135, 136]. Some experts discount this LDL increase and think it is a non-issue because the particle size change in LDL appears positive but this has not been demonstrated with hard clinical endpoints as a guide. Fish oil or the active ingredients EPA and DHA are FDA approved to lower triglycerides (not LDL). There is no data to suggest it can prevent or reduce existing myopathy whether from the prescription or over the counter option.

Niacin or no-flush niacin

Niacin dietary supplements can only add to the toxicity of a statin [137]. And then there is no-flush niacin (inositol hexaniacinate) that does not cause the flushing facial reaction that niacin causes but it also has no impact on lipid levels, so it has not worked better than a placebo [138].

Vitamin E

Some publications have noted a lower vitamin E level for patients on statins and the hypothesis that increasing vitamin E with supplementation could be of benefit [139], but this has not been the case [140]. Vitamin E at dosages of 400 IU have not reduce myalgia and have been associated with toxicity (increased risk of prostate cancer and internal bleeding) in healthy individuals from two major randomized trials (PHSII, and SELECT) [89, 141, 142].

Selenium

Selenium supplements at 200 μg/day have not worked either to reduce SIM [143, 144]. In addition, at these dosages there have been reports of a higher level of type 2 diabetes [145], recurrent skin cancer [146], and prostate cancer [147], especially in patients already replete in selenium from dietary sources from two major randomized trials (NPC and SELECT) [89].

Conclusion

Cholesterol plays a role in breast cancer but severity of its impact will continue to evolve with further research [148]. For example, a cholesterol metabolite, 27-hydroxycholesterol (27HC) could mimic estrogen and increase the risk of breast cancer and heart disease [149, 150]. There does appear to also be preliminary evidence that statins may lower the risk of breast cancer recurrence as mentioned earlier, and perhaps even a higher LDL may increase disease progression [151]. Regardless, of whether the role of cholesterol is dramatic or minuscule it is difficult to argue with the fact that CVD has been the number one cause of mortality in women for 114 or the last 115 years. Thus, it has become paramount to discuss cholesterol and other CVD risk factors in women with and without a breast cancer diagnosis and statins and other "natural" options for lipid improvement should be a part of the discussion, as should SIM and how to prevent and treat it. And the ongoing debate over the PCSK9 inhibitor drugs or other options and methods apart from statin use will also be of enormous future interest in other diseases such as breast and prostate cancer.

Interestingly, at the time of this chapter's submission data from two noteworthy studies were presented [152, 153]. The first was a Case Western Reserve University of 267 breast cancer patients (mean age 60 years and mean BMI was 30) [152]. In the hormone negative sub-cohort, both total cholesterol ($p=0.01$) and LDL cholesterol correlated ($p=0.01$) with larger tumors at presentation (surgical resection/ diagnosis), and these correlations were still statistically significant after age and BMI adjustment. This is arguably the first reported correlation of an increased LDL and tumor size. The next study was from the noteworthy Women's Health Initiative (WHI) clinical trial, which was also released at the annual American Society of Clinical Oncology (ASCO) meeting [153]. The study enrolled women aged 50–79 from 1993 to 1998 at 40 US clinical centers. There were a total of 146,326 participants with a median follow-up of 14.6 years. A total of 23,067 incident cancers and

3152 cancer deaths were observed. Numerous confounding variables were adjusted for and compared with never users statin utilization was associated with a significant 22 % reduction in cancer mortality. The reduction in cancer death was not associated with statin potency, duration or lipophilicity or hydrophilicity of the medication itself. Current statin use was associated with significantly reduced mortality of numerous cancer types, including breast, colorectal, ovarian, digestive, and bone/connective tissue cancer deaths. Interestingly, statin use was not associated with a decrease in cancer incidence despite its impact on mortality. The conclusion of the study was as follows: "In a cohort of postmenopausal women, regular use of statins or other lipid-lowering medications may decrease cancer mortality, regardless of the type, duration, or potency of statin medications used." Thus, in the worst case scenario if cholesterol lowering does not alter the course of breast cancer and continues to only lower the risk of morbidity and mortality in women then this is still a worst case scenario with ample merit; don't you agree?

References

1. Go AS, Mozaffarian D, Roger VL, Benjamin EJ, Berry JD, Blaha MJ, et al., American Heart Association Statistics Committee and Stroke Statistics Subcommittee. Heart disease and stroke statistics—2014 update: a report from the American Heart Association. Circulation 2014;129:e28–292.
2. Taylor FC, Huffman M, Ebrahim S. Statin therapy for primary prevention of cardiovascular disease. JAMA. 2013;310:2151–452.
3. Taylor F, Huffman MD, Macedo AF, et al. Statins for the primary prevention of cardiovascular disease. Cochrane Database Syst Rev. 2013;1:CD004816.
4. Golomb BA, Evans MA, Dimsdale JE, White HL. Effects of statins on energy and fatigue with exertion. Arch Intern Med. 2012;172:1180–2.
5. Stone NJ, Robinson J, Lichtenstein AH, Bairey Merz CN, Blum CB, Eckel RH, et al. 2013 ACC/AHA guideline on the treatment of blood cholesterol to reduce atherosclerotic cardiovascular risk in adults. Circulation. 2014;129(25 Suppl 2):S1–45.
6. Downs JR, Clearfield M, Weis S, Whitney E, Shapiro DR, Beere PA, et al., for the AFCAPS/TexCAPS Research Group. Primary prevention of acute coronary events with lovastatin in men and women with average cholesterol levels: results of AFCAPS/TEXCAPS. JAMA 1998;279:1615–22.
7. Nakamura H, Arakawa K, Itakura H, et al., MEGA Study Group. Primary prevention of cardiovascular disease with pravastatin in Japan (MEGA Study); a prospective randomized controlled trial. Lancet 2006;368:1155–63.
8. Ridker PM, Danielson E, Fonseca FA, et al., JUPITER Study Group. Rosuvastatin to prevent vascular events in men and women with elevated C-reactive protein. N Engl J Med 2008;359:2195–207.
9. Robinson JG. Accumulating evidence for statins in primary prevention. JAMA. 2013;310:2405–6.
10. Ridker PM, Pradhan A, MacFadyen JG, Libby P, Glynn RJ. Cardiovascular benefits and diabetes risks of statin therapy in primary prevention: an analysis from the JUPITER trial. Lancet. 2012;380:565–71.
11. Preiss D, Seshasai SRK, Welsh P, et al. Risk of incident diabetes with intensive-dose compared with moderate-dose statin therapy: a meta-analysis. JAMA. 2011;305:2556–64.

12. Aiman U, Najmi A, Khan RA. Statin induced diabetes and its clinical implications. J Pharmacol Pharmacother. 2014;5:181–5.
13. Henrikbo BD, Lau TC, Cavallari JF, Denou E, Chi W, Lally JS, et al. Fluvastatin causes NLRP3 inflammasome-mediated adipose insulin resistance. Diabetes. 2014;63:3742–7.
14. Naci H, Ioannidis JP. Comparative effectiveness of exercise and drug interventions on mortality outcomes: metaepidemiological study. BMJ. 2013;347:f5577.
15. Phan BP, Toh PP. Dyslipidemia in women: etiology and management. Int J Womens Health. 2014;6:185–94.
16. Undela K, Srikanth V, Bansal D. Statin use and risk of breast cancer: a meta-analysis of observational studies. Breast Cancer Res Treat. 2012;35:261–9.
17. Nielsen SF, Nordestgaard BG, Bojesen SE. Statin use and reduced cancer-related mortality. N Engl J Med. 2012;367:1792–802.
18. Sestak I, Cuzick J. Update on breast cancer risk prediction and prevention. Curr Opin Obstet Gynecol. 2015;27:92–7.
19. Ahern TP, Lash TL, Damkier P, Christiansen PM, Cronin-Fenton DP. Statins and breast cancer prognosis: evidence and opportunities. Lancet Oncol. 2014;15:e461–8.
20. Kwan ML, Habel LA, Flick ED, Quesenberry CP, Caan B. Post-diagnosis statin use and breast cancer recurrence in a prospective cohort study of early stage breast cancer survivors. Breast Cancer Res Treat. 2008;109:573–9.
21. Ahern TP, Pedersen L, Tarp M, Cronin-Fenton DP, Game JP, Sillman RA, et al. Statin prescriptions and breast cancer recurrence risk: a Danish nationwide prospective cohort study. J Natl Cancer Inst. 2011;103:1461–8.
22. Chae YK, Valsecchi ME, Kim J, Bianchi AL, Khemasuwan D. Reduced risk of breast cancer recurrence in patients using ACE inhibitors, ARBs, and/or statins. Cancer Invest. 2011;29:585–93.
23. Nickels S, Vrieling A, Seibold P, Heinz J, Obi N, Flesch-Janys D, et al. Mortality and recurrence risk in relation to the use of lipid-lowering drugs in a prospective breast cancer patient cohort. PLoS One. 2013;8:e75088.
24. Boudreau DM, Yu O, Chubak J, Wirtz HS, Bowles EJ, Fujii M, et al. Comparative safety of cardiovascular medication use and breast cancer outcomes among women with early stage breast cancer. Breast Cancer Res Treat. 2014;144:405–16.
25. Murtola TJ, Visvanathan K, Artama M, Vainio H, Pukkala E. Statin use and breast cancer survival: a nationwide cohort study from Finland. PLoS One. 2014;9:e110231.
26. Garwood ER, Kumar AS, Baehner FL, Moore DH, Au A, Hylton N, et al. Fluvastatin reduces proliferation and increases apoptosis in women with high grade breast cancer. Breast Cancer Res Treat. 2010;119:137–44.
27. Bjarnadottir O, Romero Q, Bendahl PO, Jirstrom K, Ryden L, Loman N, et al. Targeting HMG-CoA reductase with statins in a window-of-opportunity breast cancer trial. Breast Cancer Res Treat. 2013;138:499–508.
28. Stamm JA, Ornstein DL. The role of statins in cancer prevention and treatment. Oncology (Williston Park). 2005;19:739–50.
29. Osmak M. Statins and cancer: current and future prospects. Cancer Lett. 2012;324:1–12.
30. Koyuturk M, Ersoz M, Altiok N. Simvastatin induces apoptosis in human breast cancer cells: p53 and estrogen receptor independent pathway requiring signaling through JNK. Cancer Lett. 2007;250:220–8.
31. Higgins MJ, Prowell TM, Blackford AL, Byrne C, Khouri NF, et al. A short-term biomarker modulation study of simvastatin in women at increased risk of a new breast cancer. Breast Cancer Res Treat. 2012;131:915–24.
32. Schachter M. Chemical, pharmacokinetic and pharmacodynamics properties of statins: an update. Fundam Clin Pharmacol. 2005;19:117–25.
33. Hu M, Tomlinson B. Evaluation of the pharmacokinetics and drug interactions of the two recently developed statins, rosuvastatin and pitavastatin. Expert Opin Drug Metab Toxicol. 2014;10:51–65.

34. Naci H, Dias S, Ades AE. Industry sponsorship bias in research findings: a network meta-analysis of LDL cholesterol reduction in randomized trials of statins. BMJ. 2014;349:g5741. Epub ahead of print.
35. Naci H, Dias S, Ades T. No evidence of industry sponsorship bias in statin trials. BMJ. 2014;349:g6579. Epub ahead of print.
36. Landers P. Stalking cholesterol. How one scientist intrigued by molds found first statin. Feat of Japan's Dr. Endo led to heart-care revolution but brought him nothing. Nature as a drug laboratory. Wall Street Journal, Monday, 9 Jan 2006, p. A1, A8. Published by Dow Jones & Company, New York, NY.
37. Endo A. A historical perspective on the discovery of statins. Proc Jpn Acad Ser B Phys Biol Sci. 2010;86:484–93.
38. Endo A. Monacolin K, a new hypocholesterolemic agent produced by a Monascus species. J Antibiot (Tokyo). 1979;32:852–4.
39. Becker DJ, Gordon RY, Halbert SC, et al. Red yeast rice for dyslipidemia in statin-intolerant patients: a randomized trial. Ann Intern Med. 2009;150:830–9.
40. Venero CV, Venero JV, Wortham DC, Thompson PD. Lipid-lowering efficacy of red yeast rice in a population intolerant to statins. Am J Cardiol. 2010;105:664–6.
41. Halbert SC, French B, Gordon RY, et al. Tolerability of red yeast rice (2400 mg twice daily) versus pravastatin (20 mg twice daily) in patients with previous statin intolerance. Am J Cardiol. 2010;105:198–204.
42. Lu Z, Kou W, Du B, et al., for the Chinese Coronary Secondary Prevention Group. Effects of Xuezhikang, an extract from red yeast Chinese rice, on coronary events in a Chinese population with previous myocardial infarction. Am J Cardiol 2008;101:1689–93.
43. Li C, Zhu Y, Wang Y, et al. Monascus purpureus fermented rice (red yeast rice): a natural food product that lowers blood cholesterol in animal models of hypercholesterolemia. Nutr Res. 1998;18:71–81.
44. Lin Y-L, Wang T-H, Lee M-H, Su N-W. Biologically active components and nutraceuticals in the Monascus-fermented rice: a review. Appl Microbiol Biotechnol. 2008;77:965–73.
45. Becker DJ, Gordon RY, Morris PB, et al. Simvastatin vs therapeutic lifestyle changes and supplements: randomized primary prevention trial. Mayo Clin Proc. 2008;83:758–64.
46. Liu J, Zhang J, Shi Y, et al. Chinese red yeast rice (Monascus purpureus) for primary hyperlipidemia: a meta-analysis of randomized controlled trials. Chin Med. 2006;1:4.
47. China Coronary Secondary Prevention Study Group. China coronary secondary prevention study (CCSPS)—lipid regulating therapy with xuezhikang for secondary prevention of coronary heart disease. Chin J Cardiol (Chin). 2005;33:109–15.
48. Ong HT. The statin studies: from targeting hypercholesterolemia to targeting the high risk patient. QJM. 2005;98:599–614.
49. Zhao SP, Lu ZL, Du BM, et al., for the China Coronary Secondary Prevention Study. Xuezhikang, an extract of cholestin, reduces cardiovascular events in type 2 diabetes patients with coronary heart disease: subgroup analysis of patients with type 2 diabetes from China coronary secondary prevention study (CCSPS). J Cardiovasc Pharmacol 2007;49:81–4.
50. Ye P, Lu ZL, Du BM, et al., for the CCSPS Investigators. Effects of xuezhikang on cardiovascular events and mortality in elderly patients with a history of myocardial infarction: a subgroup analysis of elderly subjects from China coronary secondary prevention study. J Am Geriatr Soc 2007;55:1015–22.
51. Li JJ, Lu ZL, Kou WR, et al., for the Chinese Coronary Secondary Prevention Study (CCSPS) Group. Long-term effects of Xuezhikang on blood pressure in hypertensive patients with previous myocardial infarction: data from the Chinese Coronary Secondary Prevention Study (CCSPS). Clin Exp Hypertens 2010;32(8):491–8.
52. Huang CF, Li TC, Lin CC, et al. Efficacy of Monascus purpureus Went rice on lowering lipid ratios in hypercholesterolemic patients. Eur J Cardiovasc Prev Rehabil. 2007;14:438–40.
53. Lin CC, Li TC, Lai MM. Efficacy and safety of Monascus purpureus Went rice in subjects with hyperlipidemia. Eur J Endocrinol. 2005;153:679–86.

54. Heber D, Yip I, Ashley JM, et al. Cholesterol-lowering effects of a proprietary Chinese red-yeast-rice dietary supplement. Am J Clin Nutr. 1999;69:231–6.
55. Bogsrud MP, Ose L, Langslet G, et al. HypoCol (red yeast rice) lowers plasma cholesterol—a randomized placebo controlled study. Scand Cardiovasc J. 2010;44:197–200.
56. Guardamagna O, Abello F, Baracco V, Stasiowska B, Martino F. The treatment of hypercholesterolemic children: efficacy and safety of a combination of red yeast rice extract and policosanols. Nutr Metab Cardiovasc Dis. 2011;21(6):424–9. Epub 12 Feb 2010.
57. Hong MY, Seeram NP, Zhang Y, Heber D. Chinese red yeast rice versus lovastatin effects on prostate cancer cells with and without androgen receptor overexpression. J Med Food. 2008;11:657–66.
58. Hong MY, Henning S, Moro A, et al. Chinese red yeast rice inhibition of prostate tumor growth in SCID mice. Cancer Prev Res (Phila). 2011;4:608–15.
59. Hong MY, Seeram NP, Zhang Y, Heber D. Anticancer effects of Chinese red yeast rice versus monacolin K alone on colon cancer cells. J Nutr Biochem. 2008;19:448–58.
60. Ma KY, Zhang ZS, Zhao SX, et al. Red yeast increases excretion of bile acids in hamsters. Biomed Environ Sci. 2009;22:269–77.
61. Li JJ, Hu SS, Fang CH, et al. Effects of xuezhikang, an extract of cholestin, on lipid profile and C-reactive protein: a short-term time course study in patients with stable angina. Clin Chim Acta. 2005;352:217–24.
62. Zhao SP, Liu L, Cheng YC, et al. Xuezhikang, an extract of cholestin, protects endothelial function through anti-inflammatory and lipid-lowering mechanisms in patients with coronary heart disease. Circulation. 2004;110:915–20.
63. Liu L, Zhao SP, Cheng YC, Li YL. Xuezhikang decreases serum lipoprotein(a) and C-reactive protein concentrations in patients with coronary heart disease. Clin Chem. 2003;49:1347–52.
64. Eisberger B, Lankston L, McMillan DC, Underwood MA, Edwards J. Presence of tumoural C-reactive protein correlates with progressive prostate cancer. Prostate Cancer Prostatic Dis. 2011;14(2):122–8. Epub 1 Mar 2011.
65. Lehrer S, Diamond EJ, Mamkine B, et al. C-reactive protein is significantly associated with prostate-specific antigen and metastatic disease in prostate cancer. BJU Int. 2005;95:961–2.
66. Solomon KR, Pelton K, Boucher K, et al. Ezetimibe is an inhibitor if tumor angiogenesis. Am J Pathol. 2009;174:1017–26.
67. Zanardi M, Quirico E, Benvenuti C, Pezzana A. Use of a lipid-lowering food supplement in patients on hormone therapy following breast cancer. Minerva Ginecol. 2012;64:431–5.
68. Gordon RY, Cooperman T, Obermeyer W, Becker DJ. Marked variability of monacolin levels in commercial red yeast rice products: buyer beware. Arch Intern Med. 2010;170:1722–7.
69. Harding A. Contamination common in red yeast rice products. New York: Thompson Reuters; 2008. www.reuters.com/article/healthNews/idUSCOL97022820080709. Accessed 25 Apr 2011.
70. Klimek M, Wang S, Ogunkanmi A. Safety and efficacy of red yeast rice (Monascus purpureus) as an alternative therapy for hyperlipidemia. P T. 2009;34:313–27.
71. Heber D, Lembertas A, Lu QY, Bowerman S, Go VL. An analysis of nine proprietary Chinese red yeast rice dietary supplements: implications of variability in chemical profile and contents. J Altern Complement Med. 2001;7:133–9.
72. Moriarty PM, Roth EM, Karns A, Ye P, Zhao SP, Liao Y, et al. Effects of Xuezhikang in patients with dyslipidemia: a multicenter, randomized, placebo-controlled study. J Clin Lipidol. 2014;8:568–75.
73. Li Y, Jlang L, Jia Z, Xin W, Yang S, Yang Q, Wang L, et al. A meta-analysis of red yeast rice: an effective and relatively safe alternative approach for dyslipidemia. PLoS One. 2014;9:e98611.
74. Roselle H, Ekatan A, Tzeng J, Sapienza M, Kocher J. Symptomatic hepatitis associated with the use of herbal red yeast rice [Letter]. Ann Intern Med. 2008;149:516–7.
75. Grieco A, Miele L, Pompili M, et al. Acute hepatitis caused by a natural lipid-lowering product: when "alternative" medicine is no "alternative" at all. J Hepatol. 2009;50:1273–7.

76. Polsani VR, Jones PH, Ballantyne CM, Nambi V. A case report of myopathy from consumption of red yeast rice. J Clin Lipidol. 2008;2:60–2.
77. Lapi F, Gallo E, Bernasconi S, et al. Myopathies associated with red yeast rice and liquorice: spontaneous reports from the Italian Surveillance System of Natural Health Products [Letter]. Br J Clin Pharmacol. 2008;66:572–4.
78. Mueller PS. Symptomatic myopathy due to red yeast rice [Letter]. Ann Intern Med. 2006;145:474–5.
79. Smith DJ, Olive KE. Chinese red rice-induced myopathy. South Med J. 2003;96:1265–7.
80. Vercelli L, Mongini T, Olivero N, et al. Chinese red rice depletes muscle coenzyme Q10 and maintains muscle damage after discontinuation of statin treatment [Letter]. J Am Geriatr Soc. 2006;54:718–20.
81. Cartin-Ceba R, Lu LB, Kolpakchi A. A "natural" threat [Letter]. Am J Med. 2007;120:e3–4.
82. Prasad GV, Wong T, Meliton G, Bhaloo S. Rhabdomyolysis due to red yeast rice (Monascus purpureus) in a renal transplant recipient. Transplantation. 2002;74:1200–1.
83. Kumari S, Sherriff JM, Spooner D, Beckett R. Peripheral neuropathy induced by red yeast rice in a patient with a known small bowel gastrointestinal tumor. BMJ Case Rep 2013, Epub ahead of print.
84. Moyad MA, Klotz LH. Statin clinical trial (REALITY) for prostate cancer: an over 15-year wait is finally over thanks to a dietary supplement. Urol Clin North Am. 2011;38:325–31.
85. Schmidt LE, Dalhoff K. Food-drug interactions. Drugs. 2002;62:1481–502.
86. Garnett WR. Interactions with hydroxymethylglutaryl-coenzyme A reductase inhibitors. Am J Health Syst Pharm. 1995;52:1639–45.
87. Sirtori CR. The pharmacology of statins. Pharmacol Res. 2014;88:3–11.
88. Moghadasian MH. Clinical pharmacology of 3-hydroxy-3-methylglutaryl coenzyme A reductase inhibitors. Life Sci. 1999;65:1329–37.
89. Moyad MA. The supplement handbook: A trusted expert's guide to what works and what is worthless for more than 100 conditions. NY: Rodale Publishing; 2014.
90. National Center for Complementary and Integrative Health. Red yeast rice: an introduction. https://nccih.nih.gov/health/redyeastrice. Accessed 1 Feb 2015.
91. Doctor's best issues voluntary nationwide recall of red yeast rice due to undeclared lovastatin. www.fda.gov/Safety/Recalls/ucm402584.htm. Accessed 1 Feb 2015.
92. de Sousa-e-Silva EP, Conde DM, Costa-Paiva L, Martinez EZ, Pinto-Neto AM. Cardiovascular risk in middle-aged breast cancer survivors: a comparison between two risk models. Rev Bras Ginecol Obstet. 2014;36:157–62.
93. Darby SC, Ewertz M, McGale P, Bennet AM, Blom-Goldman U, Bronnum D, et al. Risk of ischemic heart disease in women after radiotherapy for breast cancer. N Engl J Med. 2013;368:987–98.
94. Barone E, Di Domenico F, Butterfield DA. Statins more than cholesterol lowering agents in Alzheimer disease: their pleiotropic functions as potential therapeutic targets. Biochem Pharmacol. 2014;88:605–16.
95. Loaiza-Bonilla A, Socola F, Gluck S. Clinical utility of aromatase inhibitors as adjuvant treatment in postmenopausal early breast cancer. Clin Med Insights Womens Health. 2013;6:1–11.
96. Younus M, Kissner M, Reich L, Wallis N. Putting the cardiovascular safety of aromatase inhibitors in patients with early breast cancer into perspective: a systematic review of the literature. Drug Saf. 2011;34:1125–49.
97. Khan QJ, O'Dea AP, Sharma P. Musculoskeletal adverse events associated with adjuvant aromatase inhibitors. J Oncol 2010, Epub ahead of print.
98. Kokkinos PF, Faselis C, Myers J, Panagiotakos D, Doumas M. Interactive effects of fitness and statin treatment on mortality risk in veterans with dyslipidemia: a cohort study. Lancet. 2013;381:394–9.
99. Barry VW, Baruth M, Beets MW, Durstine JL, Liu J, Blair SN. Fitness vs. fatness on all-cause mortality: a meta-analysis. Prog Cardiovasc Dis. 2014;56:382–90.

100. Ganga HV, Slim HB, Thompson PD. A systematic review of statin-induced muscle problems in clinical trials. Am Heart J. 2014;168:6–15.
101. Ahmad Z. Statin intolerance. Am J Cardiol. 2014;113:1765–71.
102. Harris LJ, Thapa R, Brown M, Pabbathi S, Childress RD, Helmberg M, et al. Clinical and laboratory phenotype of patients experiencing statin intolerance attributable to myalgia. J Clin Lipidol. 2011;5:299–307.
103. Tomaszewski M, Stepien KM, Tomaszewska J, Czuczwar SJ. Statin-induced myopathies. Pharmacol Rep. 2011;63:859–66.
104. Sikka P, Kapoor S, Bindra VK, Sharma M, Vishwakarma P, Saxena KK. Statin intolerance: now a solved problem. J Postgrad Med. 2011;57:321–8.
105. Reinhart KM, Woods JA. Strategies to preserve the use of statins in patients with previous muscular adverse effects. Am J Health Syst Pharm. 2012;69:291–300.
106. Jenkins DJ, Kendall CW, Marchie A, Faulkner D, Vidgen E, Lapsley KG, et al. The effect of combining plant sterols, soy protein, viscous fibers, and almonds in treating hypercholesterolemia. Metabolism. 2003;52:1478–83.
107. Jayaram S, Prasad HB, Sovani VB, Langade DG, Mane PR. Randomized study to compare the efficacy and safety of isapgol plus atorvastatin versus atorvastatin alone in subjects with hypercholesterolaemia. J Indian Med Assoc. 2007;105:142–5.
108. Agrawal AR, Tandon M, Sharma PL. Effect of combining viscous fibre with lovastatin on serum lipids in normal human subjects. Int J Clin Pract. 2007;61:1812–8.
109. Moreyra AE, Wilson AC, Koraym A. Effect of combining psyllium fiber with simvastatin in lowering cholesterol. Arch Intern Med. 2005;165:1161–6.
110. Zlada A, Schwarz UI, DeGorter MK, Tirona RG, Ban MR, Kim RB, et al. Incremental lowering of low-density lipoprotein cholesterol with ezetimibe 20 mg vs 10 mg daily in patients receiving concomitant statin therapy. Can J Cardiol. 2013;29:1395–9.
111. Ruisinger JF, Backes JM, Gibson CA, Moriarty PM. Once-a-week rosuvastatin (2.5 to 20 mg) in patients with a previous statin intolerance. Am J Cardiol. 2009;103:393–4.
112. Macaulay D. Once weekly rosuvastatin is useful in statin intolerance. BMJ. 2012;345:e7457.
113. Cannon CP, Blazing MA, Giugliano RP, McCagg A, White JA, Theroux P, et al., for the IMPROVE-IT Investigators. Ezetimibe added to statin therapy after acute coronary syndromes. N Engl J Med. 2015;372(25):2387–97, Epub ahead of print.
114. Rundek T, Naini A, Sacco R, Coates K, DiMauro S. Atorvastatin decreases the coenzyme Q10 level in the blood of patients at risk for cardiovascular disease and stroke. Arch Neurol. 2004;61:889–92.
115. Mabuchi H, Nohara A, Kobayashi J, Kawashiri MA, Katsuda S, Inazu A, et al. Effects of CoQ10 supplementation on plasma lipoprotein lipid, CoQ10 and liver and muscle enzyme levels in hypercholesterolemic patients treated with atorvastatin: a randomized double-blind study. Atherosclerosis. 2007;195:e182–9.
116. DiNicolantonio JJ. CoQ10 and L-carnitine for statin myalgia? Expert Rev Cardiovasc Ther. 2012;10:1329–33.
117. Taylor BA, Lorson L, White CM, Thompson PD. A randomized trial of coenzyme Q10 in patients with confirmed statin myopathy. Atherosclerosis. 2015;238:329–35.
118. Banach M, Serban C, Sahebkar A, Ursoniu S, Rysz J, Muntner P, et al. Effects of coenzyme Q10 on statin-induced myopathy: a meta-analysis of randomized controlled trials. Mayo Clin Proc. 2015;90:24–34.
119. Deichmann RE, Lavie CJ, Dornelles AC. Impact of coenzyme Q-10 on parameters of cardio-respiratory fitness and muscle performance in older athletes taking statins. Phys Sportsmed. 2012;40:88–95.
120. Wyman M, Leonard M, Morledge T. Coenzyme Q10: a therapy for hypertension and statin-induced myalgia? Cleve Clin J Med. 2010;77:435–42.
121. Shewmon DA, Craig JM. Creatine supplementation prevents statin-induced muscle toxicity. Ann Intern Med. 2010;153:690–2.

122. Jager R, Purpura M, Shao A, Inoue T, Kreider RB. Analysis of the efficacy, safety, and regulatory status of novel forms of creatine. Amino Acids. 2011;40:1369–83.
123. Athauda D, Foltynie T. The ongoing pursuit of neuroprotective therapies in Parkinson disease. Nat Rev Neurol. 2015;11:25–40.
124. Hass CJ, Collins MA, Juncos JL. Resistance training with creatine monohydrate improves upper-body strength in patients with Parkinson disease: a randomized trial. Neurorehabil Neural Repair. 2007;21:107–15.
125. La Guardia PG, Alberici LC, Ravagnani FG, Catharino RR, Vercesi AE. Protection of rat skeletal muscle fibers by either L-carnitine or coenzyme Q10 against statins toxicity mediated by mitochondrial reactive oxygen generation. Front Physiol. 2013;4:103.
126. Hori T, Fukao T, Kobayashi H, Teramoto T, Takayanagi M, Hasegawa Y, et al. Carnitine palmitoyltransferase 2 deficiency: the time-course of blood and urinary acylcarnitine levels during initial L-carnitine supplementation. Tohoku J Exp Med. 2010;221:191–5.
127. Mergenhagen K, Ott M, Heckman K, Rubin LM, Kellick K. Low vitamin D as a risk factor for the development of myalgia in patients taking high-dose simvastatin: a retrospective review. Clin Ther. 2014;36:770–7.
128. Palamaner Subash Shantha G, Ramos J, Thomas-Hemak L, Pancholy SB. Association of vitamin D and incident statin induced myalgia-a retrospective cohort study. PLoS One. 2014;9:e88877.
129. Eisen A, Lev E, Lakobishvilli Z, Porter A, Brosh D, Hasdai D, et al. Low plasma vitamin D levels and muscle-related adverse effects in statin users. Isr Med Assoc J. 2014;16:42–5.
130. Singer O, Cigler T, Moore AB, Levine AB, Do HT, Mandi LA. Hypovitaminosis D is a predictor of aromatase inhibitor musculoskeletal symptoms. Breast J. 2014;20:174–9.
131. Waldron JL, Ashby HL, Cornes MP, Bechervaise J, Razavi C, Thomas OL, et al. Vitamin D: a negative acute phase reactant. J Clin Pathol. 2013;66:620–2.
132. Mangin M, Sinha R, Fincher K. Inflammation and vitamin D: the infection connection. Inflamm Res. 2014;63:803–19.
133. Amir Shaghaghi M, Abumweis SS, Jones PJ. Cholesterol-lowering efficacy of plant sterols/ stanols provided in capsule and tablet formats: results of a systematic review and meta-analysis. J Acad Nutr Diet. 2013;113:1494–503.
134. Ras RT, Geleijnse JM, Trautwein EA. LDL-cholesterol-lowering effect of plant sterols and stanols across different dose ranges: a meta-analysis of randomized controlled trials. Br J Nutr. 2014;112:214–9.
135. Nelson SD, Munger MA. Icosapent ethyl for treatment of elevated triglycerides. Ann Pharmacother. 2013;47:1517–23.
136. Fares H, Lavie CJ, DiNicolantonio JJ, O'Keefe JH, Miliani RV. Icosapent ethyl for the treatment of severe hypertriglyceridemia. Ther Clin Risk Manag. 2014;10:485–92.
137. Lloyd-Jones DM. Niacin and HDL cholesterol-time to face facts. N Engl J Med. 2014;371:271–3.
138. Backes JM, Padley RJ, Moriarty PM. Important considerations for treatment with dietary supplement versus prescription niacin products. Postgrad Med. 2011;123:70–83.
139. Galli F, Iuliano L. Do statins cause myopathy by lowering vitamin E levels? Med Hypotheses. 2010;74:707–9.
140. Caso G, Kelly P, McNurian MA, Lawson WE. Effect of coenzyme Q10 on myopathic symptoms in patients treated with statins. Am J Cardiol. 2007;99:1409–12.
141. Sesso HD, Buring JE, Christen WG, Kurth T, Belanger C, MacFadyen J, et al. Vitamins E and C in the prevention of cardiovascular disease in men: the Physicians' Health Study II randomized controlled trial. JAMA. 2008;300:2123–33.
142. Klein EA, Thompson Jr IM, Tangen CM, Crowley JJ, Lucia MS, Goodman PJ, et al. Vitamin E and the risk of prostate cancer: the Selenium and Vitamin E Cancer Prevention Trial (SELECT). JAMA. 2011;306:1549–56.
143. Bogsrud MP, Langslet G, Ose L, Amesen KE, Sm Stuen MC, Mait UF, et al. No effect of combined coenzyme Q10 and selenium supplementation on atorvastatin-induced myopathy. Scand Cardiovasc J. 2013;47:80–7.

144. Fedacko J, Pella D, Fedackova P, Hanninen O, Tuomainen P, Jarcuska P, et al. Coenzyme Q(10) and selenium in statin-associated myopathy treatment. Can J Physiol Pharmacol. 2013;91:165–70.

145. Stranges S, Marshall JR, Natarajan R, Donahue RP, Trevisan M, Combs GF, et al. Effects of long-term selenium supplementation on the incidence of type 2 diabetes: a randomized trial. Ann Intern Med. 2007;147:217–23.

146. Duffield-Lillico AJ, Slate EH, Reid ME, Turnbull BW, Wilkins PA, Combs Jr GF, et al. Selenium supplementation and secondary prevention of nonmelanoma skin cancer in a randomized trial. J Natl Cancer Inst. 2003;95:1477–81.

147. Kristal AR, Darke AK, Morris JS, Tangen CM, Goodman PJ, Thompson IM, et al. Baseline selenium status and effects of selenium and vitamin e supplementation on prostate cancer risk. J Natl Cancer Inst. 2014;106:djt456. Epub 22 Feb 2014.

148. Nelson ER, Chang CY, McDonnell DP. Cholesterol and breast cancer pathophysiology. Trends Endocrinol Metab. 2014;25:649–55.

149. Umetani M, Ghosh P, Ishikawa T, Umetani J, Ahmed M, Mineo C, et al. The cholesterol metabolite 27-hydroxycholesterol promotes atherosclerosis via proinflammatory processes mediated by estrogen receptor alpha. Cell Metab. 2014;20:172–82.

150. Wu Q, Ishikawa T, Sirianni R, Tang H, McDonald JG, Yuhanna IS, et al. 27-Hydroxycholesterol promotes cell-autonomous, ER-positive breast cancer growth. Cell Rep. 2013;5:637–45.

151. Rodrigues Dos Santos C, Fonseca I, Dias S, Mendes de Almeida JC. Plasma level of LDL-cholesterol at diagnosis is a predictor factor of breast tumor progression. BMC Cancer. 2014;14:132.

152. Bruno DS, White PS, Thompson CL, Adebisi M, Berger NA. Lipid profile and breast cancer characteristics: a retrospective correlational study. J Clin Oncol 2015;33(Suppl; abstr e12659).

153. Wang A, Aragaki AK, Tang JY, Kurian AW, Manson JE, Chlebowski RT, et al. Statin use and all-cancer mortality: prospective results from the Women's Health Initiative. J Clin Oncol 2015;33(Suppl; abstr 1506).

Chapter 5
S.A.M. and Breast Cancer—Focus on Aspirin and Other Integrative Aspirin-Like Medicines: The Real "Natural" Options

Introduction

Ischemic heart disease and stroke are the number 1 and 2 causes of death in the world [1]. Any well-tested, generic, and low-cost option utilized for primary and secondary prevention in the area of cardiovascular disease (CVD) should also receive attention in the area of breast cancer prevention and as an ancillary method to reduce the risk of recurrence. S.A.M. (Statins, Aspirin, and/or Metformin) helps to discern the true evidence-based off-label products from those without the evidence and reemphasizes the need to reduce the risk of CVD is as close to zero as possible in all patients via lifestyle and some medications [2]. Reducing the risk of CVD allows patients to not only reduce their risk of all-cause morbidity and mortality (and arguably the number 2 or number 1 cause of death in breast cancer patients) but the exact same recommendations that allow patients to reduce CVD risk are identical to the recommendations to reduce the risk of breast cancer or the recurrence of this disease. In this chapter, the "A" in S.A.M. or aspirin is discussed.

Remarkable history of aspirin

Extracts of some plants, such as white willow (*Salix alba*), myrtle, meadowsweet (*Filipendula ulmaria*), and poplar have a high concentration of "salicylates" and have been used throughout history to treat a variety of human medical conditions [3–6]. Medicinal recipes from the third Millennium BC in Egypt discussed the infusion of dried myrtle leaves for reducing the pain of rheumatism and back problems. The use of willow tree bark and leaves for medicinal reasons were also referenced by the Assyrians, Babylonians, and Chinese. Hippocrates in the fifth century BC utilized the bark and leaves of the willow tree ("salicin"—a precursor to aspirin) to treat fever and reduce pain. The Reverend Edward Stone in 1763 informed the Royal Society that willow bark contained compounds the reduced the symptoms of "ague," which was probably malarial fever.

"Salicylic acid," the active ingredient from willow and meadowsweet was isolated and purified in the first half of the nineteenth century, and in 1860 was chemically

© Springer International Publishing Switzerland 2016
M.A. Moyad, *Integrative Medicine for Breast Cancer*,
DOI 10.1007/978-3-319-23422-9_5

synthesized by the carboxylation of sodium phenoxide. Salicylic acid was deemed the overall better salicin derivative. Salicin is really a prodrug that experiences hydrolysis in the gastrointestinal tract and is converted to saligenin and glucose. Next, saligenin is oxidized to salicylic acid. Now, back to the story.

Dr. Thomas John MacLagan, a physician from Dundee, Scotland, completed arguably the first documented controlled trial of salicylic acid and suggested in 1876 that this compound had antipyretic, analgesic, and anti-inflammatory properties [3–6]. Salicylic acid, although bitter tasting, was then routinely used to treat fever, pain. and inflammation. *However, in an attempt to reduce the bitter taste and serious side effect of vomiting and ulceration of the stomach, salicylic acid was acetylated.* Arguably, this new synthesized compound was derived from the meadowsweet (the old botanical name was "*Spiraea ulmaria*" — member of the rose family) and not the white willow. Regardless, this compound was clinically introduced in 1899, under the trademark Aspirin or "acetylsalicylic acid" and it is the most commonly used drug in the world.

In one of the most fascinating medical historical observations this author has ever come across, it was the acetylation of aspirin with the purpose of reducing its bitterness and improve palatability, which was actually responsible for its unique antiplatelet or blood thinning effect [3–6]! The acetyl group could now be transferred to the serine residue (position 529) in the active site of the enzyme cyclooxygenase (COX), which then irreversibly blocks its function (permanently in platelets because they have no nucleus) and prevents the production of key prostaglandins. In other words, without the acetylation there is no effective blood thinning potential! A truly remarkable moment of serendipity! Regardless of the acetylation, aspirin is also really a prodrug because it is rapidly deacetylated after it is absorbed from the stomach and small intestine and much of its activity, except for antiplatelet effects, are due to the salicylic acid.

Aspirin (really "salicylic acid" or 2-hydroxybenzoic acid) in Food?

Salicylic acid (2-hydroxybenzoic acid) is widely produced and found throughout the plant kingdom, and it appears that it has many functions especially as part of the plant defense system against pathogen invasion and attack, and even from environmental stress [7, 8]. However, because fruits and vegetables contain "salicylic acid" there is the thought that this may be one of the mechanisms whereby these and other foods lower disease risk. There is also the thought that salicylic acid should be called "Vitamin S" because it is arguably an essential vitamin, and that salicylic acid deficiency should be a recognized health problem.

The first published or noted estimate of the salicylic content of a food is documented as a letter in the journal Lancet in 1903 [9]. It was an anonymous contribution and suggested salicylic acid can be found in strawberries and other fruits in small amounts. Today it is known that salicylic acid is found in a diversity of foods [7, 8]. The content varies though based on the testing method, growing conditions, time of the year, storage, and cooking method. For example, the salicylate concentration of five brands of orange juice tested ranged from 0.47 to 3.02 mg/l. A variety of studies suggest in a moderately health diet a daily salicylic acid intake of anywhere from less than 1 to approximately 4 mg/day. Interestingly, some of the major dietary sources of salicylates are:

- Alcoholic beverages,
- Herbs and spices,
- Fruits and vegetables, and
- Nonalcoholic beverages (fruit juice and tomato-based sauces).

Herbs and spices can contain a large amount of salicylates [7, 8]. As an example, a standard South Indian vegetarian diet (mint chutney, vada, sambar/lentil based vegetable stew, ...) can contain over 10 mg of salicylic acid per day. Table 5.1 is a brief summary of some of the median amounts of total salicylates found in some

Table 5.1 Preliminary median concentration of salicylates in fresh products or dried herbs/spices [7, 8]

Fruits—Median Amount of Salicylates (mg/kg)
Grapes red (4.71)
Cherry (4.43)
Peach (2.96)
Lemon (2.50)
Pear (1.46)
Raspberries (0.90)
Nectarine (0.87)
Blackberries (0.81)
Strawberry (0.63)
Blueberries (0.57)
Mango (0.57)
Green Apple (0.55)
Grapefruit (0.44)
Banana (0.40)
Kiwi Fruit (0.31)
Vegetables—Median Amount of Salicylates (mg/kg)
Peppers-green (6.01)
Broccoli (3.25)
Asparagus (1.35)
Mushroom (1.27)
Onion (1.20)
Green beans (0.59)
Carrot (0.50)
Tomato (0.36)
Cucumber (0.24)
Spices—Top Sources of Salicylates (mg/kg)
Cumin (450)
Turmeric (392)
Garam masala (340)
Cardamon black or green (132–173)
Fenugreek (61.5)

(continued)

Table 5.1 (continued)

Pepper black (34)
Paprika (28)
Black cumin (25.05)
Cinnamon (23.8)
Chili Powder (13)
Garlic (1.0)
Drinks or Miscellaneous—Median Amount of Salicylates (mg/kg)
Pineapple (4.06)
Beer (1.63)
Coffee-instant (1.8)
Tomato (1.32)
Tea (1.06)
Cranberry (0.99)
Apple (0.83)
Orange (0.68)
Red wine (0.50)
White wine (0.44)
Lentil soup (0.21)
Grapefruit (0.10)

common fruits, vegetables, spices, and juices [7, 8]. It should be kept in mind that this is based on preliminary findings of accepted testing methods and arguably these levels vary widely over time and with further research, changing environmental conditions and geographic areas and seasons.

It is interesting that fruits and vegetables appear to account for 25 % of the total intake of salicylates [7, 8]. And fruits and vegetables are also good sources of fiber and nutrients including potassium (low in sodium) and a variety of vitamins and minerals. Spices appear to also be responsible for 10–15 % of the total salicylate intake in men and women. This has led some to theorize that lower rates of colorectal cancer incidence in some Indian populations could be partially due to the higher intake of food salicylates from spices. On the other hand, populations that consume more alcohol, a known carcinogen, could be offsetting the positive effect of salicylates from food. It also appears that total serum and urinary salicylate concentrations of vegetarians are greater than omnivores and in some rare cases could compare with individuals that use low dose aspirin regularly. However, more research is needed in this area because in aspirin users of 75 mg/day the median concentration of salicylic acid is 10.03 µmol/L (range 0.23–25) versus South Indian and vegetarians, which are 0.26 µmol/L (range 0.05–0.64) and 0.11 µmol/L (range 0.04–2.47) from preliminary clinical studies.

Secondary and Then Primary Cardiovascular Disease/Events (CVD) Prevention with Aspirin

The prolonged anticoagulant effect of aspirin actually occurs for several days, even after one dose, and until sufficient numbers of new platelets are produced [10].

Regardless, the use of aspirin for CVD prevention is a matter of the individualized benefit-to-risk scenario. Although aspirin reduces the risk of myocardial infarction and stroke, and potentially venous thrombotic events and cancer, the risk of serious gastrointestinal bleeding and hemorrhagic stroke suggests the greater the risk of vascular events the greater the benefit of aspirin. It is for this reason it is well accepted to utilize aspirin in a secondary prevention setting [10, 11]. The ISIS-2 trial found daily aspirin in the setting of acute myocardial infarction reduced the risk of vascular death by over 20 % [12], and it has also been shown to be effective with acute ischemic stroke, thus it is a primary early therapy with acute coronary syndromes and stroke. Pooled data of approximately 200 clinical trials again demonstrates a risk reduction of more than 20 % with higher dosages but without additional benefit and an increased risk of bleeding events [10, 11]. Currently, the standard practice is to recommend 75–100 mg/day of aspirin for long-term secondary prevention of cardiovascular events, and it is now being utilized to reduce the risk of restenosis after percutaneous coronary procedures [10]. Therefore, with this type of background the next logical step was to determine the impact of aspirin on the primary prevention of CVD.

In the early 1980s multiple large-scale trials were initiated to address the primary prevention question from the British Doctors Trial and the Physicians Health Study have demonstrated modest reductions versus the secondary prevention trials (12 % versus 22 %) [10]. However, the overall the risk of CVD events were extremely low in many of these trials. Additionally, primary prevention trials are not easy to complete or even initiate because of the greater use of multiple prevention measures in subjects today from diet and exercise to blood pressure, cholesterol-lowering and even glucose controlling medication such as metformin with some inherent cardiovascular or metabolic parameter benefits. Additionally, as blood pressure and lipids are improved, along with some inflammatory markers such as hs-CRP, the need for aspirin is reduced based on risk calculators such as Framingham risk score or Reynolds Risk score (this risk score also utilizes hs-CRP).

Current and Future Primary Prevention Trials of Aspirin

Again, most populations studied for primary prevention of cardiovascular events have had very low risk [10]. Thus, this has clouded the picture of the best candidate for aspirin in this setting. Therefore, individuals at higher than average risk are being studied in three ongoing clinical trials of aspirin in primary prevention and include the following:

– ASCEND (A Study of Cardiovascular Events in Diabetes) Study includes patients 40 years and older with type 1 or 2 diabetes and 100 mg of aspirin, which is also being tested with and without a 1000 mg/day omega-3-acid Ethyl Esters product and/or placebo [13].
– ARRIVE (A Study to Assess the Efficacy and Safety of Enteric-Coated Acetylsalicylic Acid in Patients at Moderate Risk of Cardiovascular Disease) Study includes middle-aged and older patients at higher risk of CVD (55 years or more with 2–4 risk factors) utilizing 100 mg of enteric-coated aspirin versus placebo [14].

- ASPREE (Aspirin in Reducing Events in the Elderly) Study includes those older than 65 years of age and will utilize 100 mg of enteric-coated aspirin versus placebo [15].

Buffered or Enteric-Coated Aspirin? As good and safer compared to immediate release/regular/uncoated/plain aspirin and what about probiotics? Aspirin Resistance?

The upregulation of cyclooxygenase-2 (COX-2) in the stomach with aspirin increases the risk of dyspepsia, gastrointestinal ulcers and bleeding [3]. Aspirin induced gastrointestinal injury is dose-dependent, so in an attempt to reduce the risk of gastrointestinal damage causes by regular aspirin, there were two other types developed, buffered and enteric-coated aspirin. *Buffered aspirin contains calcium carbonate, magnesium oxide, magnesium carbonate, or other compounds, which reduce the hydrogen ion concentration of aspirin* [16]. And the reduced hydrogen ion concentration increases the gastric solubility of aspirin, which further reduces the contact time between the gastric mucosa and aspirin. *Enteric-coated aspirin was designed to pass through the stomach before dissolving thus also potentially reducing gastric damage.* Despite the agreement that higher dosages of aspirin have less gastrointestinal toxicity when using alternative forms of aspirin this has not been demonstrated at the low-dose level. For example, enteric-coated aspirin dissolves in the small bowel and could pose a higher risk of small bowel ulcers compared to other types of aspirin including uncoated and buffered aspirin. Although the initial time to antiplatelet response is more rapid with a full dose aspirin (325 mg/day) versus low-dose (81 mg/day) in an emergent setting, prophylactically low-dose aspirin appears as effective.

Small past studies have consistently demonstrated the benefit of uncoated aspirin on bleeding times compared to enteric-coated aspirin and some experts have recommended that uncoated aspirin should be the primary recommended form in the setting of acute MI, unstable angina, or after angioplasty [17]. One small study found that 80 % of the uncoated aspirin group developed abnormal bleeding times versus only 10 % of the enteric-coated group ($p < 0.01$).

In a recent large cohort comparing buffered aspirin (100 mg) to plain aspirin there was no difference found in the reported rates of gastrointestinal symptoms (27 % in both groups) [18, 19]. And the authors suggested plain aspirin as the first choice because of the considerable cost savings compared to other forms of aspirin and the use of a proton pump inhibitor (PPI) if gastrointestinal symptoms occur, and if this does not work then shift to a buffered option. It is important to note that in some countries the cost of these specialty aspirins such as buffered can be twice as much plain aspirin.

The Japanese Primary Prevention Project (JPPP) was an open-label, multicenter, randomized parallel-group trial of 14,464 participants aged 60–85 years with hypertension, dyslipidemia, or diabetes recruited by primary physicians at over 1000 clinics in Japan [20]. Patients were randomized to 100 mg/day enteric-coated aspirin or no aspirin. The study was terminated after a median follow-up of 5 years because of futility or unlikely it would reach a significant reduction, which was death from cardiovascular causes (at the time of termination 56 fatal events occurred in both groups) and nonfatal myocardial infarction and nonfatal stroke (composite outcome). Although aspirin significantly reduced the incidence of nonfatal myocardial infarction and transient ischemic attack, it also significantly increased the risk of extracranial hemorrhage requiring transfusion or hospitalization.

There is a suggestion that the reason some enteric-coated aspirin studies have failed including the JPPP could be due to what is known as "pseudoresistance" [21]. In other words, this was highlighted in a recent study of healthy volunteers screened for their response to a single dose of 325-mg immediate release or enteric-coated aspirin [22]. No case of aspirin resistance was noted, but a delayed and reduced drug absorption was found in up to 49 % of the enteric-coated group but 0 % with plain aspirin. Thus, the term "pseudoresistance" with enteric-coated aspirin is a potential possibility that needs further investigation.

It is interesting that preliminary small human and laboratory studies of probiotics to prevent gastrointestinal toxicity of aspirin, or NSAIDs for example Lactobacillus casei has shown some initial promise [23]. Perhaps the anti-inflammatory effects of lactic acid may be a future option. However, more well-done trials are needed because in the past for example vitamin C was preliminarily investigated to reduce aspirin toxicity but this seems to have stalled from the lack of long-term data [24].

The ultimate question is that the true benefits and limitations of the different forms of aspirin is not sufficiently lucid, including which ones, if any, have more substantial anticancer effects. Again it should be reiterated that most of the cardiovascular clinical trials have utilized plain aspirin for efficacy and the secondary anticancer end points also appear to be primarily from plain aspirin. Still, the question remains.

Aspirin (aka "Salicin") in Dietary Supplements? Be Careful!

On a fairly regular basis a patient may inquire about a dietary supplement that appears to be reducing a painful condition better than any other product on the market. For example, I have found this to be true especially in the area of osteoarthritis. However, these miracle-like products appear to cost patients an excessive amount of money in many circumstances (50 or more dollars a month). When I peruse the bottle label I am often surprised to find that one of the primary ingredients is "salicin." It should be reiterated that salicin was derived from white willow bark and leaves to help create or synthetically produce aspirin. In my opinion, many of these patients are simply paying 50 dollars a month for aspirin and do not know it. This would explain the satisfactory pain relief but it does not of course explain the exorbitant price, and thus I warn patients about this on a regular basis.

It needs to be reiterated that research has suggested that upon ingestion, a large percentage of the salicin in willow bark is absorbed and is metabolized via intestinal flora to saligenin, which is then absorbed and metabolized by the liver to produce salicylic acid [3]. This is exactly what acetylsalicylic acid is converted to with metabolism (salicylic acid), thus unless someone can prove in a head-to-head comparison that salicin is superior to aspirin then there is some skepticism. Still, if any benefit I can theoretically surmise from salicin occurs over aspirin it may be in a minority of individuals that simply do not want the blood thinning effects of aspirin to occur, but still desire the analgesic, antipyretic, and anti-inflammatory effects.

Minimal research has been completed on the safest dosage or percentage (15 %, 20 %, 50 %?) of salicin in a dietary supplement. Further information on salicin can be found from some recent reviews of the subject that provide good background or foundational knowledge [25]. Interestingly, a Cochrane review of herbal treatments of acute low back pain found some evidence that 120 or 240 mg salicin is probably greater than placebo for short-term improvements in pain (two trials with 261 participants and moderate quality evidence) [26]. Again, no head-to-head quality trial against low cost or comparable aspirin dosages has been conducted.

Aspirin and Anticancer Mechanisms of Action

There are two broad mechanisms of anticancer action in aspirin [27–30]:

1. *Cyclo-oxygenase (COX)-dependent effects:*

   – Aspirin is an irreversible inhibitor of both the cyclooxygenase (COX)-1 and -2 isoenzymes. Low daily doses of aspirin blocks COX-1 activity, which results in reduced production of thromboxane A_2 (potent stimulant of platelet aggregation and vasoconstriction). Yet, with COX-2 activity intact, endothelium-derived prostacyclin (prostaglandin I_2), a platelet inhibitor and vasodilator is still produced. The decrease in thromboxane A_2 and production of prostaglandin I_2 allows low-dose aspirin the ability to prevent arterial thrombosis, myocardial infarction and stroke. Still, the inhibition of the COX-1 isoenzyme also reduces the production of other prostaglandins needed for the adequate protection of the gastrointestinal mucosa.

   – Cyclooxygenase is also known as "prostaglandin endoperoxide synthase (PTSG)," which is a primary enzyme in the synthesis of prostaglandins, which have a role in increasing cellular proliferation, migrations, invasiveness and encourages angiogenesis. In the past, the preventive impacts of aspirin were primarily observed in colorectal, esophageal, and gastric cancers. Since aspirin inhibits the pro-inflammatory enzymes COX-1 and COX-2, and aspirin irreversibly binds COX-1 on platelets, preventing aggregation, and platelets adhesiveness may have a role in invasion and metastases.

   – The simple reduction in chronic inflammation may also be the key to its potential anticancer effects. Additionally COX-2 itself is expressed in many cancers and inhibiting this pathway may allow for apoptosis, angiogenesis, and immune modulation.

2. *COX independent effects including:*

   – Inhibition of nuclear factor kB
   – wnt signaling
   – B-catenin
   – Tumor necrosis factor
   – Downregulation of survivin
   – Caspase 9
   – p38 MAP kinase
   – Mitochondrial cytochrome c pathway
   – Ceramide pathway
   – Hormonal changes/reduction in estrogenic effects

Cardiovascular and other Trials and Overall Cancer Risk and Death (Colorectal = Yes, High-Risk Colorectal = Yes, and Other Cancers = maybe)

One of the largest reviews of data from randomized trials of daily aspirin versus no aspirin for the prevention of vascular events (51 randomized trials) has only increased the interest in the anticancer effects of aspirin [31]. Aspirin appeared to reduce the risk of cancer deaths by 15 % ($p=0.008$; 34 trials, 69,224 participants) especially when utilized for 5 or more years (37 % reduction; $p=0.0005$). In six trials of daily low-dose aspirin in primary prevention utilizing 35,535 participants, aspirin reduced cancer incidence from 3 years onward by 24 % ($p=0.0003$) and this significant reduction occurred in women and men. The researchers also found that fatality cases from major extracranial bleeds was significantly lower on aspirin compared to controls (68 % reduction, 8 of 203 and 15 of 132; $p=0.009$).

Researchers have also analyzed observational studies and the overall estimates of the impact of aspirin on individual cancers in case-control studies were closely correlated with randomized data ($r(2)=0.71$, $p=0.0006$) [32]. For example, not just for colorectal cancer but consistent reductions in the risk of esophageal, gastric, biliary and breast cancer was found. Additionally, aspirin appeared to significantly reduce the risk of finding cancers with distant metastasis, which is again consistent with randomized data.

Regardless, it should be kept in mind that gastrointestinal cancer risk reduction and potentially death from this cancer has the most consistent data when it comes to aspirin utilization. Data from over 150 case-control studies and 50 cohort studies have published consistent correlations between regular use of aspirin and a reduced risk of colorectal, esophageal, and stomach cancer.

Aspirin shows even potential greater impacts in those at high-risk of colorectal cancer [33–35]. For example, the in the Colorectal Adenoma/Carcinoma Prevention Programme 1 (CAPP1) 600 mg/day in 200 adolescent FAP (familial adenomatous polyposis) carriers reduced polyp number and a significant reduction in polyp size occurred for those patients utilizing aspirin for more than 1 year. The same intervention was utilized in CAPP2, which was a randomized trial of 600 mg aspirin daily in Lynch syndrome carriers ($n=937$) and a 63 % reduction ($p=0.008$) in incidence was found for those completing at least 2 years of treatment. However, patients with shorter follow-up there were no significant difference [33, 34]. It appears that currently individuals at high risk for colorectal cancer are now potential candidates for aspirin prophylaxis [35]. Gastrointestinal toxicity and compliance was similar between groups during the trial but was not accessed during full follow-up. CAPP3 is an ongoing double-blind trial of 100, 300, or 600 mg daily aspirin in 3000 high-risk patients.

Women's Health Study (WHS) Randomized Trial—The Game Changer?

The Women's Health Study (WHS) could be a game changer but not because of its primary endpoint, but because of the impact on colorectal cancer and perhaps advanced cancers. This was a randomized trial of approximately 10 years of treatment with 100 mg of every other day aspirin versus placebo in middle-aged women to prevent vascular events and cancer was a pre-study outcome [36]. This is arguably the first reliable data in women of aspirin and cancer risk. A total of 19,934 women at least 45 years of age and without previous cardiovascular disease were randomized to aspirin and 19,942 were given placebo. There was no significant reduction in the risk of major cardiovascular events, or death from cardiovascular causes (primary endpoint), but there was a reduction in stroke with aspirin (RR=0.83; p=0.02) with an average use of 10.1 years. Subgroup analysis demonstrated a significant reduction in major cardiovascular events, ischemic stroke, and myocardial infarction for women 65 years and older. Overall gastrointestinal bleeding requiring transfusion was also 40 % significantly higher in the aspirin group compared to placebo arm (p=0.02).

The results of the 18-year follow-up of the Women's Health Study (WHS) have now been published, and the overall data on cancer risk is now available [37, 38]. A reduction in colorectal cancer risk emerged in the aspirin group after 10-years of follow-up. In fact, colorectal cancer risk after this period was reduced by 49 % (p<0.001), which appeared to be primarily due to a larger reduction in proximal colon cancer risk (55 % reduction; p=0.001). The prospective rates of colonoscopy and adenomas were balanced across the treatment groups during and after the study. However, the WHS showed no reduction in the incidence of other cancers including breast cancer. Metastatic cancer was nonsignificantly reduced by 12 % (p=0.055), but there were significant reductions in post-trial metastatic adenocarcinoma (27 % reduction; p=0.03) and Duke stage C or D colorectal cancer (56 % reduction; p=0.004), which appear somewhat similar to past aspirin studies. *This may suggest more of a role to reduce overall and colorectal cancer aggressiveness versus incidence and may also suggest using aspirin in an adjuvant cancer study, whether it is breast or other forms may be more intriguing.* Still, cancer of the colon, esophagus and stomach together represented only 8 % of cancer cases in the WHS compared to 23 % of all cancer deaths in men in the clinical trials of daily aspirin. Thus, aspirin prophylaxis and the benefits and risks need to be considered separately in women and men. And as of the time of this publication all-cause and cancer mortality were not significantly reduced compared to placebo, but there was a significant increase risk in peptic ulcers and gastrointestinal bleeding in the aspirin group. And the issue of daily versus alternate day dosing will always be a question since preliminary data suggests that platelet inhibition is more consistent with daily dosing [39].

Aspirin and overall cancer risk—Bottom Line

It now appears a variety of cancers could be prevented and/or progression slowed based on secondary data from aspirin randomized trials. For example, pancreatic, brain, prostate and a variety of others may also be reduced. Interestingly, benefit was not related to the dose of aspirin or gender, but it did increase with age [40].

More recent bottom line summary data from a publication authored by European and US experts suggests the somewhat surprising (compared to just a decade ago) following conclusions when using aspirin in the general average risk population [41]:

- Long-term aspirin use outweighs the potential risks—primarily hemorrhagic stroke and gastrointestinal bleeding for a large proportion of the middle-aged population.

- "For average-risk individuals aged 50–65 years taking aspirin for 10 years, there would be a relative reduction of between 7 % (women) and 9 % (men) in the number of cancer, myocardial infarction or stroke events over a 15-year period and an overall 4 % relative reduction in all deaths over a 20-year period."
- Prophylactic aspirin utilization for at least 5 years at a dosage of 75–325 mg/day appears to favorable benefit over risk and longer utilization could have greater benefits.
- It is known that it provides some cardiovascular event reductions, but the drug's increasing value against some cancers is noteworthy now.
- Aspirin protects against colorectal, esophageal, and stomach cancer and all but three of the 15 authors concluded that decreases in breast, prostate, and lung cancer were significant enough to also mention as benefits of the drug. It should be noted that colorectal cancer screening in the USA is less than 50 % of those that are eligible—so this should also be emphasized.
- Impact of aspirin on cancer is not apparent until at least 3 years of use.
- Some benefits can still be procured several years after stopping aspirin in long-term users.
- Higher doses in the average population do not appear to demonstrate far greater benefits but only increased toxicity.
- Excess bleeding is the primary concern with aspirin and this risk generally increases with age.
- Some of the authors reminded readers that definitive data is lacking on aspirin and these conclusions and most of the data is derived from secondary analysis of randomized trials or observational data.

Prostate Cancer

It would be noteworthy if aspirin demonstrated some consistent impact with hormone driven cancers other than breast cancer, for example prostate cancer. One of the largest meta-analyses ever conducted on aspirin and prostate cancer (PCa) concluded the following after reviewing 20 case–control and 19 cohort studies and 108,136 prostate cancer cases: "The present meta-analysis provides support for the hypothesis that aspirin use is inversely related to PCa incidence and PCa-specific mortality [42]." The association was actually preliminarily stronger and significant for advanced prostate cancer versus non-advanced disease and the use of aspirin for 4 or more years appeared to provide more of a beneficial effect. And the effects for COX-2 inhibitors and other NSAIDs were not significant.

Breast Cancer (post-diagnosis but not pre-diagnosis benefits and a potential reduction in invasive breast cancer risk)

"NSAIDS and aspirin after but not before diagnosis were associated with improved breast cancer survival, including breast-cancer-specific mortality, all-cause mortality, and relapse/metastasis [43]." This was the conclusion of one of the first meta-analysis ever conducted and a recent review on this topic (aspirin and breast cancer survival). In addition, the authors stated "Our results indicated that the survival benefit of aspirin, a nonselective NSAID that inhibits COX-1 and COX-2, was greater than that of non-aspirin NSAIDS (including many selective NSAIDS that inhibit COX-2 only) in breast cancer." A total of over 4900 studies were identified and over 4500 were excluded because they were not directly relevant to answering the question of aspirin and breast cancer mortality. Another 356 studies were excluded for their lack of complete data or were redundant studies. Finally, a total of 16 (11 cohort and five case–control) studies were included (ten included only aspirin), and aspirin use after diagnosis was significantly associated with a lower breast-cancer-specific mortality (HR = 0.69) and relapse/metastasis (HR = 0.75), and a nonsignificant trend toward an improvement in all-cause mortality (HR = 0.79). However, utilizing cohort studies only yielded similar results except a significant improvement in all-cause mortality was obtained (HR = 0.72).

The only other meta-analysis on aspirin use and mortality in breast cancer was also recently published and included eight cohort and two nested case–control studies (approximately 26,900 post-diagnosis aspirin users and 673,450 pre-diagnosis aspirin users) [44]. Patients using aspirin after diagnosis had a significant ($p = 0.04$) 27 % reduction in breast cancer-specific mortality and a nonsignificant reduction in all-cause mortality (−16 %; 95 % CI = 0.63–1.12, $p = 0.24$). No impact was observed for pre-diagnosis aspirin use similar to the previous analysis [43]. Interestingly, another meta-analysis of 49 publications addressing the question of risk or incidence found the potential for aspirin to reduce the risk of invasive breast cancer by 20 %, which was primarily related to hormone positive tumors [45].

There is the possibility that anticancer effects of NSAIDs may not just include COX-2 inhibition effects but also COX-1-dependent effects [46–48]. For example, breast cancer has been shown to overexpress COX-1 in stromal cells in the vicinity of tumors, and COX-1 could be involved in tumor progression. COX-1 and -2 inhibition appears to be synergistic in providing greater inhibition of breast cancer cells compared to either pathway alone. And as mentioned earlier in the chapter a variety of COX-independent effects have also been proposed not just for a variety of cancers but also in breast cancer [27–30].

Risk factors for bleeding

Since bleeding events are the biggest concern with aspirin [49, 50] a summary of risk factors for an increased risk of bleeding while on this drug are listed in Table 5.2.

Reynolds Risk Score versus Other Risk Scores (Overestimation?)

For high-risk breast cancer patients or those diagnosed and treated another helpful decision tool on the benefits and risk of aspirin is derived from one of the only cardiovascular prediction tools that have a plethora of female data and is current. *It is called the "Reynolds Risk Score" and can be found at www.reynoldsriskscore. org, and can be utilized for healthy individuals without diabetes* [51]. *It was designed to predict an individual's risk of having a future cardiovascular event such as a heart attack, stroke or other major heart disease in the next 10 years and it takes into account 8 factors, which are listed in Table 5.3.*

This Risk score takes seconds to complete and then a percentage risk is calculated, and the result should be shared by the patient with her or his cardiologist or primary care provider. In my experience with cancer patients, if the percentage risk shows that the benefit of aspirin would outweigh the risk (for example a risk of 10 % or higher) and there are no significant bleeding or gastrointestinal risks then the

Table 5.2 Risk factors for bleeding while on aspirin [49, 50]

Alcohol consumption
Diabetes
Dietary supplements with blood thinning potential (Ginkgo biloba, fish oil, …)
H. pylori infection
Hypertension
Overweight or Obese (can also create an increased risk of hypercoagulability)
Previous bleeding episodes/tendencies
Peptic ulcer
Increasing age
Male sex
Smoking (smoking also increases the risk of hypercoagulability)

Note: Bleeding events can include extracranial or nonfatal gastrointestinal bleeding and not just hemorrhagic stroke

Table 5.3 The eight Risk Factors accessed by Reynolds Risk Score (www.reynoldsriskscore.org)—one of the best predictors of 10-year cardiovascular event (heart and stroke) risk for women and men and utilized to determine aspirin benefit-versus-risk [51]

Gender
Age
Smoking Status
Systolic Blood Pressure
Total Cholesterol
HDL or "Good" Cholesterol
High Sensitivity C-reactive protein (hs-CRP)—also known as "cardiac CRP"
Whether or not your mother or father had a heart attack before the age of 60

Note: The addition of hs-CRP blood test and family history information to this risk score along with updated clinical data in women and men is arguably now the most accurate risk calculator on this topic

patient could start 81 mg or low-dose aspirin. However, again the benefit to risk ratio should stem from the overall cardiovascular risk as the primary driver in my opinion so there is a clear "first do no harm" policy. Additionally, there is no test patients can utilize with aspirin to predict their risk of a future bleeding event or ulcer if they are otherwise healthy. This differs from statins and metformin where occasional monitoring of liver and kidney function can reliably predict the potential for ongoing or future serious toxicity. *In other words, when it comes to aspirin the benefit should grossly outweigh the risk.*

Interestingly, in a recent study of the five more popular prediction tools that doctors rely on to predict a cardiovascular event in otherwise healthy individuals, four of them had major issues and overestimated risk [52]! Overestimation in men was as high as 154 % and in women as high as 67 %. *The only risk score that appeared to be in the neighborhood of predicting risk in women (underestimated by 21 %) and men (overestimated by 9 %) was the Reynolds Risk Score.* It was the least flawed of the 5, which also included the famous Framingham Risk score, and the new American Heart Association risk score. However, the fact that it underestimated risk in women should be kept in mind compared to other risk score that can grossly overestimate risk. The problem with many risk scores is they are based on single time points or questions from decades ago rather than following individuals over time and monitoring lifestyle and medication changes. Reynolds risk was based on data from a more recent group of patients compared with other calculators or risk scores, which may explain why it had the best accuracy.

Additionally, it must also be accepted that the threshold for risk to initiate aspirin therapy is not definitive. Reynolds risk score aids in the decision but there are many opinions based on the same set of data. Multiple organizations have different thresholds for aspirin use in primary prevention and some of the more notable are found in Table 5.4 [53]. This should provide an even more objective overview of patients that may qualify for aspirin based on their breast cancer risk or situation; again applying overall cardiovascular risk first strategy. Notable other extensive reviews can also be incorporated in the decision making process [54, 55].

Conclusion

Aspirin continues to garner a remarkable amount of primarily positive attention in a diversity of health and prevention settings from cardiovascular event risk to colorectal cancer and other cancer risk, to a more recent recommendation by the US Preventive Service Task Force for preventing morbidity and mortality from preeclampsia in high-risk women at a dosage of 60–150 mg/day after the first trimester of pregnancy (may also reduce preterm birth, IUGR, and perinatal mortality) [56].

What is fascinating is the potential for aspirin to have a current application for the prevention of breast cancer or the prevention of the recurrence of this disease even at low dosages. This data is primarily derived from indirect or secondary information gleaned from clinical trials and from observational studies. Patients that qualify for aspirin primarily based on their cardiovascular risk utilizing multiple tools (Reynolds Risk Score ...) and clinical assessment may get a secondary benefit from aspirin. It is interesting that aspirin, one of the heart healthiest and generic drugs that was derived from natural sources (willow bark and meadowsweet), appears to have more data compared to any other dietary supplement in regard to anti-breast cancer effects. Therefore, it is the "A" component in S.A.M. that are the three primary off-label pills that should be discussed with individuals concerned about breast cancer (see Table 5.5).

Table 5.4 Summary of some of the guidelines utilized by various authoritative groups for aspirin use in a primary prevention setting [53, 54]

Authoritative guideline group	Cardiovascular disease (CVD) risk	Gender	Age	Dosage
American Heart Association (AHA)/American Stroke Association	Higher coronary heart disease (CHD) risk—especially for those with 10-year CHD risk≥10%	None specified	None specified	75–160 mg/day
American College of Chest Physicians (CHEST)	Individuals aged≥50 years without symptomatic CVD	None specified	≥50 years	75–100 mg/day
Canadian Cardiovascular Society (CCS)	Not recommended regardless of CVD risk	Does not apply	Does not apply	Does not apply
European Society of Cardiology (ESC)	10-year risk score of CVD>10% and blood pressure is controlled	None specified	None specified	75 mg/day
US Preventive Services Task Force (USPSTF)-Women and stroke risk primarily	– 10-year stroke risk≥3%	– Women	– 55–59 years of age	– No recommendation
	– 10-year stroke risk≥8%	– Women	– 60–69 years of age	– No recommendation
	– 10-year stroke risk≥11%	– Women	– 70–79 years of age	– No recommendation
US Preventive Services Task Force (USPSTF)—Men and myocardial infarction risk primarily	– 10-year CHD risk≥4%	– Men	– 45–59 years of age	– No recommendation
	– 10-year CHD risk≥9%	– Men	– 60–69 years of age	– No recommendation
	– 10-year CHD risk≥12%	– Men	– 70–79 years of age	– No recommendation

Note: The American Diabetes Association (ADA) recommends low-dose aspirin (75–162 mg/day) for adults with diabetes and no prior history of vascular disease but who have a 10-year risk of cardiovascular disease events greater than 10 % and who do not have an increased risk for bleeding events

Table 5.5 Overview of the diversity of direct and indirect clinically relevant observations noted with aspirin

Aspirin from A to Z	Commentary
Aspirin	Also known as "acetyl-salicylic acid" which is then quickly metabolized to salicylic acid, which is responsible for most of its effects. However, the acetyl group is also immediately removed after absorption in the stomach and small intestine and transferred to platelets for example that causes the blood thinning effects!
Buffered versus Enteric versus Immediate-Release (plain, uncoated, regular, …) Aspirin (*Note*: Enteric-coated aspirin could also be responsible for "pseudoresistance" to aspirin observed in some small clinical studies where there is delayed and reduced aspirin absorption with this alternative form)	– During a cardiovascular event the use of immediate release aspirin is needed and this form has the most clinical trials with evidence – Buffered aspirin contains calcium carbonate, magnesium oxide, magnesium carbonate, or other compounds, which reduce the hydrogen ion concentration of aspirin and increases the gastric solubility of aspirin, which further reduces the contact time between the gastric mucosa and aspirin. This was designed to reduce further damage to the stomach – Enteric-coated aspirin was designed to pass through the stomach before dissolving and being absorbed in the small intestine thus also potentially reducing gastric damage – However, these alternative forms (buffered and enteric-coated) are more expensive and the clinical endpoint evidence long-term of whether they truly reduce gastrointestinal and other toxicity, especially at lower dosages, while maintaining the same clinical benefits of immediate-release aspirin is controversial – In terms of regular versus low-dose aspirin, the initial time to antiplatelet response is more rapid with a full dose aspirin (325 mg/day) versus low-dose (81 mg/day) in an emergent setting, bur prophylactically low-dose aspirin appears as effective
Bleeding Events	The number one consistent risk factor that occurs with aspirin regardless of dosage and can disqualify a patient for aspirin prophylaxis
Breast Cancer Risk/Recurrence	Preliminary secondary evidence from aspirin clinical trials and observational studies suggest aspirin may reduce the risk of breast cancer and more consistent data suggests a reduction in breast cancer recurrence after treatment – Arguably, adjuvant treatment with aspirin appears to be one of the most interesting potential clinical trials in breast cancer based on this past research of the potential for predictable benefit
Cancer Risk	A variety of cancers appeared to be reduced or advanced disease and death from cancer appears to also be reduced with aspirin use from secondary analysis of clinical trials or post hoc analysis or observational studies. Gastrointestinal cancers primarily but also brain, breast, esophageal, lung, pancreatic, prostate, and others. This does not prove cause and effect and numbers of events were small and there is the increased risk of bleeding that must be critically accessed
Cardiovascular Clinical Facts	– Aspirin for primary prevention is controversial and based primarily on 10-year cardiovascular event risk versus risk of bleeding (generally 10 % or higher risk increase likelihood of greater benefit) – Aspirin reduces the risk of nonfatal myocardial infarction – Aspirin reduces the risk of nonfatal stroke – When used within 24 h of onset of symptoms it reduces the risk of nonfatal MI, stroke, or death (similar to magnitude of streptokinase) – When used in stable angina it reduces risk of MI or death and now used after CVD procedures in many cases

Aspirin from A to Z	Commentary
Colorectal Cancer Risk	The most evidence in cancer prevention with aspirin. High-risk colorectal cancer patients (Lynch syndrome, FAP, …) should be offered aspirin as a potential definitive chemopreventive drug
COX-1 and COX-2 (cyclooxygenase or COX)	COX-1 blocked by low dosages of aspirin but COX-2 require higher dosages
Fast Facts (History)	– 1904 Aspirin was introduced for widespread public use – Aspirin is the most widely used drug in medicine-approximately 20 % of adults in the USA use it regularly (daily or every other day), and almost 50 % 65 years and older utilize it regularly
Gastrointestinal Cancer Risk	Aspirin has the most clinical research for this body system (esophageal, stomach, colorectal, …) compared to any other in terms of cancer risk
Half-Life on average	Less than 30 min (however half-life of the primary or principal metabolite salicyclic acid is several hours)
Lowest Dose that inhibits platelet action	Dosages as low as 30 mg/day can effectively reduce platelet aggregation
Major Medical Authoritative Groups Opinion on Aspirin use for Primary Prevention of cardiovascular events (AHA, CHEST, CCS, ESC, USPSTF, …)	All groups recommended aspirin prevention when benefit outweighs the risk except the Canadian Cardiovascular Society (CCS) that does not recommend aspirin for women or men in a primary prevention setting
Mechanism of Action	Irreversibly cyclooxygenase (COX) inhibition and suppression of prostaglandin production. Antithrombotic effects of aspirin are the result of acetylation of COX in platelets (not discovered until 1971 and later publications)
Metabolism	Aspirin has three compounds within the same molecule. Salicylic acid and the acetyl moiety are released within minutes of ingestion. Acetyl group binds to serine (530) in platelets and inactivates COX-1, which prevents arachidonic acid access and irreversibly blocks prostaglandin synthesis (blood thinning effect in platelets)
Natural versus Synthetic Salicylates	Subject of a JAMA editorial in 1913 and no difference could be demonstrated
Pain, Fever, and Inflammation Reduction (PFI)	The classic triad for aspirin–salicin and salicylic acid—all reduce the occurrence of these three issues
Prostate Cancer Risk/ Recurrence	Preliminary secondary evidence from aspirin clinical trials and observational studies suggest aspirin may reduce the risk of aggressive prostate cancer and prostate cancer recurrence after treatment
Resistance to aspirin effects	This is controversial and could be due to genetics, intake of other NSAIDs, stress, metabolic syndrome, and patient noncompliance. Also recent concern that enteric-coated aspirin is some patients could be less effective and explain part of "resistance"

(continued)

Table 5.5 (continued)

Aspirin from A to Z	Commentary
Reynolds Risk Score (*Note*: Utilizes eight factors in the following order: Gender, Age, Smoking Status, Systolic BP, Total Cholesterol, HDL, hs-CRP blood test results, and whether your mother or father had a heart attack before the age of 60)	Arguably the most recent and accurate risk score/estimate for future heart attack and stroke in women and men that should be used for any patient considering aspirin prophylaxis
Salicin (aspirin precursor)	– One active ingredient in willow bark, and also found in meadowsweet – A prodrug that is metabolized to glucose and "saligenin" in the gastrointestinal tract. Saligenin is then oxidized to Salicylic Acid! Salicylic acid was isolated after salicin and found to be more potent – Some costly "natural" or dietary supplement pain relievers or other related products such as osteoarthritis supplements utilize salicin as one of its primary ingredients, which is arguably no different than aspirin except salicin has minimal to no blood thinning potential – Hippocrates in the fifth century BC utilized the bark and leaves of the willow tree ("salicin"—a precursor to aspirin) to treat fever and reduce pain
Salicylic Acid (2-hydroxybenzoic acid) (also called "vitamin S") (the deacetylated metabolism of aspirin in the body) (aka biologically active component of aspirin) (first derived from *Spirea ulmaria*— member of the Rose family) *Note*: The bitter taste of salicylic acid is what led researchers to create a potential less bitter acetyl-salicylic acid ("aspirin") and this small change was responsible for its now famous blood thinning ability (acetyl group goes to platelet serine residue and blocking COX ... leading to blood thinning)!	– Most of the properties of aspirin come from salicylic acid (except antiplatelet effects). Aspirin is a prodrug and is rapidly deacetylated after it is absorbed in stomach and small intestine. Half-life of salicylic acid is several hours! A 75 mg dose of aspirin = approximately 66 mg of salicylic acid – Salicylic acid is also a widely distributed compound throughout the plant kingdom (arguably first found in strawberries). It is a plant secondary metabolite generated to prevent and contain pathogen invasion and environmental stress. It may also be involved in stomatal closure, ion uptake through roots and a stimulus for flowering – Some bacteria also synthesize salicylic acid. It was isolated and purified from willow and meadowsweet in the first half of the 1800s – Dr. John MacLagan, a physician from Dundee, Scotland, established in 1876 that salicylic acid had anti-fever, analgesic, and ant-inflammatory properties – When synthetically acetylated by humans in the laboratory, salicylic acid is now basically called "Aspirin" (which now adds blood thinning properties to aspirin) – Salicylic acid can be detected in blood and urine of individuals not using aspirin but utilizing foods and beverages (fruits, veggies, spices, ...) with salicylic acid

Aspirin from A to Z	Commentary
Side Effects	– Intracranial and gastrointestinal (GI) bleeding can occur at any dose. Dosages as low as 10 mg/day can cause GI bleeding. Hypertension and gastrointestinal or kidney toxicity are generally dose-related – Rarely excessive dosages can cause tinnitus
Willow Tree Bark (Salix alba) (Salix = willow)	One of the primary sources of the precursor to aspirin dating back to Hippocrates and Galen. Ground dried bark from the English willow tree was used in the first recorded clinical trial in 1758 (Reverend Edward Stone of the Royal Society of London) for treating the symptoms of malaria
Women's Health Study (WHS)	One of the largest primary prevention trials of aspirin and largest in the world in women. Approximately 40,000 women aged 45 years and older utilizing 100 mg aspirin *every other day* had a significant reduction in stroke (primarily in women 65+ years of age) and colorectal cancer (−20 % and with post-trial reduction of −42 %) that emerged after 10 years. Aspirin was primarily responsible for lowering proximal colon cancer risk (−27 %). A significant increase in gastrointestinal bleeding and peptic ulcers occurred with aspirin. Additionally, aspirin may have reduced the risk of metastatic cancer but overall cancer mortality and breast cancer was not reduced at the time of the most recent publication. Women that have not smoked and had a recent negative screening colonoscopy may not need aspirin for colorectal or lung cancer prophylaxis

I also find it interesting that of the hundreds of supplements I have discussed over the past 30 years with cancer patients, few patients or clinicians realize that S.A.M. including aspirin has exponentially greater positive data against cancer compared to the supplement that they want to primarily discuss at that moment. It is gratifying to know that even if aspirin does not reduce the risk of breast cancer or especially recurrence that it still might reduce the risk of stroke, heart attack and even colorectal or other cancers with hopefully a minimal impact on the risk of bleeding.

References

1. The top 10 causes of death. World Health Organization website. http://www.who.int/media-centre/factsheets/fs310/en/. Accessed 1 Feb 2015.
2. Moyad MA, Vogelzang NJ. Heart healthy equals prostate healthy and statins, aspirin, and/or metformin (S.A.M.) are the ideal recommendations for prostate cancer prevention. Asian J Androl 2015, Epub ahead of print.
3. Wick JY. Aspirin: a history, a love story. Consult Pharm. 2012;27:322–9.
4. Mahdi JG, Mahdi AJ, Mahdi AJ, Bowen ID. The historical analysis of aspirin discovery, its relation to the willow tree and anti-proliferative and anticancer potential. Cell Prolif. 2006;39:147–55.
5. Fuster V, Sweeny JM. Aspirin: a historical and contemporary therapeutic overview. Circulation. 2011;123:768–78.

6. Elwood PC. Aspirin: past, present and future. Clin Med. 2001;1:132–7.
7. Wood A, Baxter G, Thies F, Kyle J, Duthie G. A systematic review of salicylates in foods: estimated daily intake of a Scottish population. Mol Nutr Food Res. 2011;55:S7–14.
8. Duthie GG, Wood AD. Natural salicylates: foods, functions and disease prevention. Food Funct. 2011;2:515–20.
9. Anonymous. Salicylic acid in strawberries. Lancet 1903;162:1187.
10. Gaziano JM, Greenland P. When should aspirin be used for prevention of cardiovascular events? JAMA. 2014;312:2503–4.
11. Antithrombotic Trialists' Collaboration. Collaborative meta-analysis of randomized trials of antiplatelet therapy for prevention of death, myocardial infarction, and stroke in high-risk patients. BMJ. 2002;324:71–86.
12. Second International Study of Infarct Survival Collaborative Group (ISIS-2). Randomized trial of intravenous streptokinase, oral aspirin, both, or neither among 17,187 cases of suspected acute myocardial infarction. Lancet. 1988;349:360.
13. ASCEND (A Study of Cardiovascular Events in Diabetes) Study. https://clinicaltrials.gov/ct2/show/NCT00135226?term=ascend+aspirin&rank=1. Accessed 1 June 2015.
14. ARRIVE (A Study to Assess the Efficacy and Safety of Enteric-Coated Acetylsalicylic Acid in Patients at Moderate Risk of Cardiovascular Disease) Study. https://clinicaltrials.gov/ct2/show/NCT00501059?term=ARRIVE+aspirin&rank=1. Accessed 1 June 2015.
15. ASPREE (Aspirin in Reducing Events in the Elderly) Study. https://clinicaltrials.gov/ct2/show/NCT01038583?term=ASPREE+aspirin&rank=2. Accessed 1 June 2015.
16. Endo H, Sakai E, Kato T, Umezawa S, Higurashi T, Ohkubo H, et al. Small bowel injury in low-dose aspirin users. J Gastroenterol. 2015;50:378–86.
17. Gantt AJ, Gantt S. Comparison of enteric-coated aspirin and uncoated aspirin effect on bleeding time. Cathet Cardiovasc Diagn. 1998;45:396–9.
18. Jaspers Focks J, Tielemans MM, van Rossum LG, Elkendal T, Brouwer MA, Jansen JB, et al. Gastrointestinal symptoms in low-dose aspirin users: a comparison between plain and buffered aspirin. Neth Heart J. 2014;22:107–12.
19. Pre BC, van Laake LW. Buffered aspirin: what is your gut feeling? Neth Heart J. 2014;22:105–6.
20. Ikeda Y, Shimada K, Teramoto T, Uchiyama S, Yamazaki T, Oikawa S, et al. Low-dose aspirin for primary prevention of cardiovascular events in Japanese patients 60 years or older with atherosclerotic risk factors: a randomized clinical trial. JAMA. 2014;12(312):2510–20.
21. Spence JD. Aspirin for the prevention of cardiovascular events in older Japanese patients. JAMA. 2015;313:1473.
22. Grosser T, Fries S, Lawson JA, Kapoor SC, Grant GR, Fitzgerald GA. Drug resistance and pseudoresistance: an unintended consequence of enteric coated aspirin. Circulation. 2013;127:377–85.
23. Endo H, Higurashi T, Hosono K, Sakai E, Sekino Y, Iida H, et al. Efficacy of Lactobacillus casei treatment on small bowel injury in chronic low-dose aspirin users: a pilot randomized controlled study. J Gastroenterol. 2011;46:894–905.
24. Patel V, Fisher M, Voelker M, Gessner U. Gastrointestinal effects of the addition of ascorbic acid to aspirin. Pain Pract. 2012;12:476–84.
25. Shara M, Stohs SJ. Efficacy and safety of white willow bark (Salix alba) extracts. Phytother Res. 2015;29(8):1112–6. Epub 22 May 2015.
26. Oltean H, Robbins C, van Tulder MW, Berman BM, Bombardier C, Gagnier JJ. Herbal medicine for low-back pain. Cochrane Database Syst Rev. 2014;12:CD004504.
27. Thorat MA, Cuzick J. Role of aspirin in cancer prevention. Curr Oncol Rep. 2013;15:533–40.
28. Usman MW, Luo F, Cheng H, Zhao JJ, Liu P. Chemopreventive effects of aspirin at a glance. Biochim Biophys Acta. 1855;2015:254–63.
29. Phillips I, Langley R, Gilbert D, Ring A. Aspirin as a treatment for cancer. Clin Oncol. 2013;25:333–5.
30. Farag M. Can aspirin and cancer prevention be ageless companions? J Clin Diagn Res. 2015;9(1):XE01–03. Epub ahead of print.

31. Rothwell PM, Price JF, Fowkes FG, Zanchetti A, Roncaglioni MC, Tognoni G, et al. Short-term effects of daily aspirin on cancer incidence, mortality, and non-vascular death: analysis of the time course of risks and benefits in 51 randomized controlled trial. Lancet. 2012;379:1602–12.

32. Algra AM, Rothwell PM. Effects of regular aspirin on long-term cancer incidence and metastasis: a systematic comparison of evidence from observational versus randomized trials. Lancet Oncol. 2012;13:518–27.

33. Burn J, Bishop DT, Mecklin JP, et al. Effect of aspirin or resistant starch on colorectal neoplasia in the Lynch syndrome. N Engl J Med. 2008;359:2567–78.

34. Burn J, Gerdes A-M, Macrae F, et al. Long-term effect of aspirin on cancer risk in carriers of hereditary colorectal cancer: an analysis from the CAPP2 randomized controlled trial. Lancet. 2011;378:2081–7.

35. Burn J, Mathers JC, Bishop DT. Chemoprevention in Lynch syndrome. Fam Cancer. 2013;12:707–18.

36. Ridker PM, Cook NR, Lee IM, Gordon D, Gaziano JM, Manson JE, et al. A randomized trial of low-dose aspirin in the primary prevention of cardiovascular disease in women. N Engl J Med. 2005;352:1293–304.

37. Cook NR, Lee IM, Zhang SM, Moorthy MV, Buring JE. Alternate-day, low-dose aspirin and cancer risk: long-term observational follow-up of a randomized trial. Ann Intern Med. 2013;159:77–85.

38. Rothwell PM. Alternate-day, low-dose aspirin and cancer risk. Ann Intern Med. 2013; 159:148–50.

39. Swalm L, Hillman RS. Aspirin administered to women at 100 mg every other day produces less platelet inhibition than aspirin administered at 81 mg per day: implications for interpreting the women's health study. J Thromb Thrombolysis. 2009;28:94–100.

40. Rothwell PM, Fowkes FG, Belch JF, Ogawa H, Warlow CP, Meade TW. Effect of daily aspirin on long-term risk of death due to cancer: analysis of individual patient data from randomized trials. Lancet. 2011;377:31–41.

41. Cuzick J, Thorat MA, Bosetti C, Brown PH, Burn J, Cook NR, et al. Estimates of benefits and harms of prophylactic use of aspirin in the general population. Ann Oncol. 2015;26:47–57.

42. Liu Y, Chen J-Q, Xie L, Wang J, Li T, Yu H, et al. Effect of aspirin and other non-steroidal anti-inflammatory drugs on prostate cancer incidence and mortality: a systematic review and meta-analysis. BMC Med. 2014;12:55.

43. Huang XZ, Gao P, Sun JX, Song YX, Tsai CC, Liu J, et al. Aspirin and nonsteroidal anti-inflammatory drugs after but not before diagnosis are associated with improved breast cancer survival: a meta-analysis. Cancer Causes Control. 2015;26(4):589–600. Epub 21 Feb 2015.

44. Zhong S, Zhang X, Chen L, Ma T, Tang J, Zhao J. Association between aspirin use and mortality in breast cancer patients: a meta-analysis of observational studies. Breast Cancer Res Treat. 2015;150:199–207.

45. de Pedro M, Baeza S, Escudero M-T, Dierssen-Sotos T, Gomez-Acebo I, Pollan M, et al. Effect of COX-2 inhibitors and other non-steroidal inflammatory drugs on breast cancer risk: a meta-analysis. Breast Cancer Res Treat. 2015;149:525–36.

46. Hwang D, Scollard D, Byrne J, Levine E. Expression of cyclooxygenase-1 and cyclooxygenase-2 in human breast cancer. J Natl Cancer Inst. 1998;90:455–60.

47. Jeong HS, Kim JH, Choi HY, Lee ER, Cho SG. Induction of cell growth arrest and apoptotic cell death in human breast cancer MCF-7 cells by the COX-1 inhibitor FR122047. Oncol Rep. 2010;24:351–6.

48. McFadden DW, Riggs DR, Jackson BJ, Cunningham C. Additive effects of Cox-1 and Cox-2 inhibition on breast cancer in vitro. Int J Oncol. 2006;29:1019–23.

49. Baigent C, Blackwell L, Collins R, Emberson J, Godwin J, Peto R, et al. Aspirin in the primary and secondary prevention of vascular disease: collaborative meta-analysis of individual participant data from randomized trials. Lancet. 2009;373:1849–60.

50. Moyad MA. The supplement handbook. New York, NY: Rodale Publishing; 2015.

51. Reynolds risk score: calculating heart and stroke risk for women and men. www.reynolds riskscore.org. Accessed 1 June 2015.
52. DeFillipis AP, Young R, Carrubba CJ, McEvoy JW, Budoff MJ, Blumenthal RS, et al. An analysis of calibration and discrimination among multiple cardiovascular risk scores in a modern multiethnic cohort. Ann Intern Med. 2015;162:266–75.
53. Nemerovski CW, Salinitri FD, Morbitzer KA, Moser LR. Aspirin for primary prevention of cardiovascular disease events. Pharmacotherapy. 2012;32:1020–35.
54. Ittaman SV, VanWormer JJ, Rezkalla SH. The role of aspirin in the prevention of cardiovascular disease. Clin Med Res. 2014;12:147–54.
55. Sutcliffe P, Connock M, Gurung T, Freeman K, Johnson S, Kandala NB, et al. Aspirin for prophylactic use in the primary prevention of cardiovascular disease and cancer: a systematic review and overview of reviews. Health Technol Assess. 2013;17:1–253.
56. Henderson JT, Whitlock EP, O'Conner E, Senger CA, Thompson JH, Rowland MG. Low-dose aspirin for the prevention of morbidity and mortality from preeclampsia: a systematic evidence review for the US Preventive Services Task Force. Rockville (MD): Agency for Healthcare Research and Quality (US); 2014 Apr. Report No.: 14-05207-EF-1. US Preventive Services Task Force Evidence Syntheses, formerly Systematic Evidence Reviews.

Chapter 6
S.A.M. and Breast Cancer—Focus on Metformin and Other Integrative Metformin-Mimic Medicines: The Real "Natural" Options

Introduction—Basic and Interesting Facts About Metformin

History of Metformin

Metformin is a biguanide drug (also known as N′,N′-dimethylbiguanide or 1,1-dimethyl-biguanide) and the number one prescribed insulin-sensitizing drug in the world [1–5]. Metformin is primarily available as a generic medication and it was originally derived from a "natural source"—the French Lilac or *Galega officinalis*. This is the herbal prototype of the biguanides and also is known by the names "goat's rue" or "Italian fitch" or "professor-weed." Galega officinalis derives from "gale" (milk) and "ega" (to bring on) because Galega has been utilized as a galacta-gogue in small domestic animals, which is how the name "goat's rue" originated.

Metformin has actually been available in Europe since the 1950s but was not approved by the US FDA until December 30, 1994 [1–5]. An extended release (XR metformin) version was approved in October 2000. Metformin was actually first synthesized and found to lower blood sugar in rabbits in the 1920s, and then put aside for decades because of an increase in insulin synthesizing/utilization research based on the discovery of insulin. A 1957 published clinical trial of diabetes (by French physician Jean Sterne—who coined the name of metformin as the glucose eater or "Glucophage") was then completed and the UK introduced it in 1958, and Canada in 1972.

Metformin is somewhat similar in structure to the drug "phenformin" (phenethylbiguanide), which in 1977 was removed from the US market because of an increased risk of lactic acidosis [1–5]. And it is also similar to the drug "buformin" (synthesized as an oral antidiabetic in 1957), which was withdrawn from the market in many countries because of an increased risk of lactic acidosis. It was never sold in the USA and still sells in some countries such as Romania.

Metformin is now considered a first-line pharmacological treatment along with diet and exercise for adult and pediatric patients with type 2 mellitus because of its favorable overall profile (glucose control, weight loss, and low risk of hypoglycemia) [6, 7].

© Springer International Publishing Switzerland 2016
M.A. Moyad, *Integrative Medicine for Breast Cancer*,
DOI 10.1007/978-3-319-23422-9_6

It is arguably the only drug proven to prevent prediabetes (high-risk diabetes patients) from becoming diabetes and is a primary treatment in patients with metabolic syndrome. Overall, few drugs in medicine cost less with such a long-term safety profile and even added potential heart health benefits [6].

Mechanism of Action
Metformin works by reducing hepatic glucose production (inhibiting gluconeogenesis) and increasing skeletal muscle tissue uptake of glucose [1–5]. Metformin suppresses gluconeogenesis by 0.6 mg/kg per minute, which essentially leads to a maximum 75 % reduction in liver glucose production. It also reduces blood insulin levels (not directly), increases insulin sensitivity, suppresses synthesis of proteins, fatty acids and cholesterol, and increases the utilization of free fatty acids. Metformin has also demonstrated some evidence of reduced intestinal glucose absorption. Metformin increases insulin sensitivity by activating hepatic and muscle AMP-activated protein kinase (AMPK—"metabolic master switch"), which results in reduction of fatty acid synthesis and stimulation of fatty acid oxidation in the liver and increase in muscle glucose absorption.

Dosage Options and Half-Life
Metformin is generally available in 500-, 850-, and 1000-mg tablets [1–5]. The starting dose is 500 mg BID or 850 QD, given with meals. The recommended maximum daily dose is 2550 mg (using 850 mg tablets) or 2500 mg/day (using 500 mg tablets) divided and given three times daily [1–5]. For example, the dosage utilized in the United Kingdom Prospective Diabetes Study (UKPDS) was 850 mg TID [8, 9]. The most common dosage utilized in the Diabetes Prevention Program (DPP) was 850 mg BID [10, 11]. In general, clinical experience suggests 500 mg QD with a meal and increasing dose in 500 mg increments every 2–4 weeks until maximum dosage is achieved. Metformin XR can be prohibitively expensive and available in 500- and 750-mg tablets utilized with the evening meal. The maximum recommended dosage is 2000 mg QD [1, 2, 12].

The half-life of metformin is on average 5–6-h in plasma (longer retention in red blood cells or blood—up to 18 h), which suggests 94 % of the drug is removed by the body in 24 h [1–5]. This short half-life emphasizes the need for daily compliance whether it is for patients or when measuring glucose and other parameters in clinical trials.

Side Effects/Adverse Events (from GI to vitamin B12 deficiency)
Metformin is limited by gastrointestinal complications (soft stool, diarrhea, flatulence, abdominal pain, and more rarely nausea and vomiting) in up to 50 % of patients, but these adverse effects are usually transient and resolve within days to weeks of initiating treatment [1–5]. Additionally, GI side effects are reduced greatly by titrating increasing dosages of the drug every 2–4 weeks (for example 500 or 850 QD for 2 weeks and then 500 mg additional) and when it is consumed with food. Although food has been reported to reduce the rate and extent of metformin absorption by increasing the time to peak plasma concentration by approximately 40 min, but this appears to be a small issue especially compared to the overall

importance of long-term compliance. Less than 5 % of patients in clinical trial are not able to tolerate the drug due to side effects. Extended-release (XR) metformin appears to improve gastrointestinal tolerability and can be given once a day but is more expensive [12].

Metformin can reduce vitamin B12 and/or potentially magnesium levels so these should be monitored in patients [13, 14]. It has been known that this drug interferes with B12 absorption in the distal ileum and can lower B12 in 10–30 % of patients [13]. The reduction of B12 by metformin appears to dose-dependent. The clinical significance of this change is unknown since megaloblastic anemia has been rarely reported. Metformin increases the risk of vitamin B12 deficiency (serum level <150 pmol/L) and borderline-deficient vitamin B12 (serum level 150–220 pmol/L). Patients should use one multivitamin pill a day with the current recommended daily allowance of B12 (2.4 µg/day for individuals beyond 14 years of age). Abnormally high serum levels of homocysteine and methylmalonic acid (MMA) are also utilized to indicate a B12 deficiency. The impact on magnesium is a more controversial issue in the literature [14], but metformin is at least associated with lower blood magnesium levels and should still be monitored since this could also impact cardiovascular disease status.

Rarely, patients complain of a "metallic taste" with the drug, which has been more commonly found with similar medications such as buformin [1–5]. Regardless, "metallic taste" has been reported in clinical trials in approximately 3–11 % of patients. It also appears to be self-limiting with only 0.5 % of patients complain of metallic taste after 3 months of treatment. Regardless, a reduction in dose (again my clinical experience) appears to resolve this issue almost immediately in patients distressed by this issue.

The most serious concerning adverse event with metformin is lactic acidosis, where a low pH in body tissues and blood (acidosis) along with increases in lactate is problematic [1–5]. This situation usually occurs when cells are exposed to minimal amounts of oxygen (hypoxia), and then cells metabolize glucose anaerobically, which increases lactate levels. Increased lactate is symbolic of tissue damage from hypoxia and hypoperfusion. Liver lactate uptake is reduced with metformin because lactate is a substrate for hepatic gluconeogenesis, which is blocked by metformin. In healthy individuals this slight increase in lactate is simply cleared by healthy kidneys and no increase in blood lactate is observed. However, any condition that exacerbates lactic acidosis is a contraindication of the use of metformin including: alcoholism, heart failure, and/or respiratory disease (inadequate oxygenation of tissues), and the most common cause is kidney disease.

Lactic Acidosis Revisited—Not without controversy
The overall incidence of lactic acidosis on metformin has been estimated to be 0–0.08 per 1000 patient years [15]. A Cochrane review of 347 trials and observational studies found no greater risk of lactic acidosis with metformin compared to other type 2 diabetic drugs [16]. Again, phenformin (another biguanide) was withdrawn in 1977 because of the risk of lactic acidosis [1–5]. And it is also similar to the drug "buformin" (synthesized as an oral antidiabetic in 1957), which was

withdrawn from the market in many countries because of an increased risk of lactic acidosis, but it was never sold in the USA.

Metformin is excreted by the kidneys, and it theoretically could accumulate with reduced renal function and increase the risk of lactic acidosis. Metformin was approved in 1994 and the FDA established strict prescribing criteria based on kidney function which remains today and includes the following: Metformin is contraindicated in those with renal issues as suggested by serum creatinine levels of 1.5 mg/dl or greater in males and 1.4 mg/dl or greater in females and should not be used in patients 80 years or older unless creatinine clearance reveals that renal function is not reduced [17].

"The overall incidence of lactic acidosis in metformin users varies across studies from approximately 3 per 100,000 person-years to 10 per 100,000 person-years and is generally indistinguishable from the background rate in the overall population with diabetes" [18]. Still, metformin is contraindicated in some individuals because of impaired kidney function and the potential concerns of lactic acidosis. Yet recent research from a systematic review of 65 past studies suggest despite metformin being renally cleared, drug concentrations usually remain within the therapeutic range and lactate concentrations are not significantly changed when utilized in patients with mild to moderate chronic kidney disease (CKD) (estimated glomerular filtration rates, 30–60 mL/min per 1.73 m^2) [18]. These authors suggested individuals with chronic kidney disease (CKD) stage 1 (90 or higher eGFR mL/min) and stage 2 (60–90 eGFR) can receive a maximum dose of 2550 mg of metformin a day for example. And stage 3A (45–<60) or 3B (30–<45) CKD could also receive 2000 or 1000 mg metformin depending on stable CKD. And stage 4 (15–<30) and stage 5 (<15) should not receive metformin. These were only suggestions based on their analyses but are still intriguing and evidence-based.

Imaging Contrast Precautions with Metformin
Intravascular iodinated contrast media administration could result in lactic acidosis in a patient utilizing metformin [19–21]. However, this rare adverse effect occurs if the contrast causes renal failure. Metformin is excreted primarily by the kidneys so continued utilization of metformin after the initiation of renal failure causes toxic concentrations of the drug and subsequent lactic acidosis. In order to avoid this complication metformin should be withheld after the administration of contrast agent for 48 h, and if renal function is normal after 48 h from receiving contrast then metformin can be reinitiated. However, despite what the package insert recommends, which is also to withhold metformin 48 h before contrast medium is given, others have argued there is no justification for this before and then after procedure (for 48 h). Interestingly, large variations exist for metformin and contrast administration from five international guidelines, which is due to a low amount of evidence within the guidelines themselves [20]. Overall, most guidelines suggest that a patient with normal creatinine and renal function (estimated glomerular filtration rate or eGFR greater than 60 mL/min/1.73 m^2) and without comorbidities can continue metformin use after receiving contrast medium. Yet despite a lack of good evidence it also seems prudent to stop metformin 2 days before and after contrast in

Table 6.1 Some of the contraindications to metformin treatment

– Creatinine clearance <60 mL/min (keep in mind that aging is associated with reduced renal function)
– Renal disease or dysfunction-serum creatinine ≥1.5 mg/dl for men and ≥1.4 mg/dl for women
– Excessive alcohol intake (potentiates the effect of metformin on lactate metabolism and increases blood flow to endocrine pancreatic area which increases insulin secretion and subsequently increases risk of hypoglycemia)
– Congestive heart failure (CHF) requiring pharmacologic treatment or other conditions characterized by hypoxemia such as acute myocardial infarction
– Acute or chronic metabolic acidosis (includes diabetic ketoacidosis with or without coma)
– Imaging studies involving the utilization of intravenous iodinated contrast media-metformin should be stopped before or at the time of the scan, withheld for 48 h, and restarted only after renal function has been evaluated and fount to be normal
– Surgical procedures-metformin should be discontinued temporarily before all surgical procedures with the exception of minor procedures not associated with restricted intake of fluids and food
– Severe liver dysfunction or severe COPD (increase acidic status and lactic acidosis despite normal creatinine)
– Known hypersensitivity to metformin

any patient with a hint of renal insufficiency simply because the benefit exceeds the risk in my opinion, even though in many patients with mild to moderate chronic kidney disease it has been shown to be safe to take metformin.

Regardless, for a good overview or summary of the contraindications to metformin treatment please refer to Table 6.1. It should be reiterated to patients that even alcohol consumption should be minimized on metformin treatment because it has the potential to create insulin surges and potentiate hypoglycemia [1–5], and one mechanism it accomplishes this task appears to be a direct shift in pancreatic microcirculation from exocrine to the endocrine cells with an increase in nitric oxide concentrations and vagal stimuli [22]. Additionally, the caloric content of alcohol and not just insulin alterations can often result in weight gain and inhibit the metabolic benefits of metformin.

Drug and Supplement Interactions (not emphasized in the literature)
Drug and supplement interactions are minimal with metformin because it is not protein bound (negligible binding to plasma proteins), not metabolized hepatically, and accumulates in the gastrointestinal tract, salivary glands and kidneys [1–5]. Metformin is eventually excreted unchanged in the urine. Since metformin is excreted primarily via renal tubular secretion medications that compete with this pathway or interfere with renal function should not be used with metformin. Cationic drugs such as: amiloride, cimetidine, digoxin, morphine, procainamide, quinidine, quinine, ranitidine, triamterene, trimethoprim, and vancomycin are discarded via this renal tubular pathway. However, only cimetidine and metformin has been adequately accessed where a 50 % increase in plasma levels (AUC) of metformin and a 27 % reduction in the 24-h renal excretion of metformin occurred in healthy volunteers [3]. Interestingly, phenformin undergoes hepatic aromatic

Table 6.2 A partial list of dietary supplements with the potential to cause glucose and/or insulin alterations

Alpha Lipoic Acid (may also activate AMPK-partial metformin mimic)
Berberine (may also activate AMPK-partial metformin mimic)
Branched Chain Amino Acid Supplementation (Leucine, Iso-leucine, and Valine)
Carnitine
Chromium
Chromium picolinate + Biotin
Cinnamon
Coenzyme Q10
Fenugreek (a fiber source)
Fiber supplementation (guar gum, pectin, psyllium, …)
Ginkgo biloba (could increase metabolism of glucose medications)
Ginseng (American or *Panax quinquefolius*)
Gymnema sylvestre
Magnesium
Resveratrol
Selenium (*note*: may increase insulin resistance in large doses—200 µg …)
Vanadium
Zinc

hydroxylation, which could lead to increased concentration of the drug in those with minimal hydroxylation ability. This is one method whereby phenformin may increase lactic acidosis.

One dietary fiber supplement, guar gum has been preliminarily found to potentially reduce plasma levels of metformin [3, 23]. Still, it is theoretically possible that most fiber supplements would have a similar impact and could also potentiate the glucose lowering effects of this drug. There is a growing list of glucose reducing and/or insulin sensitizing supplements that should either not be combined with metformin or the patient should be monitored more closely when utilizing them initially and these include fiber dietary supplements. A partial listing of these supplements can be found in Table 6.2 [24, 25]. For example, there is some evidence that psyllium fiber (one of the most popular commercial sources in the world) may synergistically reduce glucose levels in diabetics but in my opinion should be taken several hours before or after metformin ideally to prevent absorption or bioavailability issues with the drug.

Metformin—The first and only heart healthy and mentally healthy weight loss drug?

The history of dietary supplements and prescription weight loss medications has been fraught with controversy and removal of products from around the globe, but it still provides an important teachable moment. This is primarily because despite helping individuals lose weight the weight loss medications also increased the risk of cardiovascular disease, cardiovascular events and even death [25]. When a drug or supplement dramatically increases metabolism the downstream implications could result in heart rate, heart rhythm, and blood pressure increases. Fenfluramine, and sibutramine were removed due to an increase in cardiovascular disease (CVD) risk, while a cannabinoid type 1 (CB1) receptor agonist, rimonabant, was removed because of serious psychiatric issues [26]. Currently, almost all of the multiple weight loss drugs and supplements on the markets appear to have some tangible controversy in terms of short and long-term safety, which could partially explain their disappointing sales numbers compared to original projections [25].

Cardiovascular disease (CVD) is the leading cause of morbidity and mortality in diabetics, which only further emphasizes the need for a "heart Healthy" drug or supplement to be used in this population. And CVD is the number one cause of death in men and women overall and this has been the situation in the USA for over 100 years. Thus, the desire to find a medication that improves weight loss and heart health while simultaneously maintaining or improving mental health status should be paramount but could appear to be unrealistic. This is not necessarily the case.

Again, the primary mechanism whereby metformin reduces glucose and insulin is via AMP-activated protein kinase (AMPK) activation, through activation of the upstream kinase liver-kinase B1 (LKB1), and this results in gluconeogenesis inhibition [1–5, 25]. AMPK is the so-called "master metabolic switch" or central cellular energy sensor which responds to increases in the adenosine monophosphate (AMP)/adenosine triphosphate (ATP) ratio (cellular stress). Nutrient deprivation activates AMPK for example leading to blockage of energy-consuming processes and stimulation of pathways that generate energy, which results in increases in ATP supply. Inadequate activity of AMPK permits uncontrolled cell growth and may also accelerate the cellular aging process. Again AMPK is activated by cellular stress, which results in the restoration of energy levels via regulation of growth and metabolism. A variety of direct and indirect (with weight loss primarily adipose tissue for example) heart healthy markers are improved with metformin. Reduced food consumption with this drug has been documented and not just the potential for an anorectic effect. Improvements in glucose and lipids, but also a reduction in inflammatory markers has occurred with metformin. Endothelial dysfunction improves via improved blood flow and normoglycemia is associated with restoration of normal platelet function. Additionally, there appears to be little to no change in mental health status in patients on metformin, but B12 levels should be monitored because deficient levels could cause cognitive changes.

The impact of metformin on cardiovascular outcomes or endpoints of patients with type 2 diabetes has been studied in two randomized trials [27–29]. In the UKPDS, a 39 % lower risk of myocardial infarction over 10 years was observed in overweight patients versus patients on conventional dietary therapy [27], and post-trial follow-up continues to demonstrate positive effects [28]. The second study, the HOME trial, included 390 patients with type 2 diabetes on insulin found metformin reduced the composite cardiovascular endpoint by 40 % [29]. Overall, there appears to be a reduction in all-cause mortality with metformin versus other type 2 diabetes treatment regimens, especially in regards to patients with stable coronary disease, following acute coronary syndrome, and in CHF [30, 31]. Indeed an older systematic review of 40 publications found metformin was associated with a reduced risk of cardiovascular mortality (OR=0.74) compared with placebo or any other oral diabetes drug [32].

The limitation with metformin and CVD is little is the lack of long-term data of the cardiovascular preventive effects of this drug in the nondiabetic population. Still, a recent small randomized trial examining the effects of metformin (850 mg BID with morning and evening meals, $n=173$) on progression of mean carotid intima–media thickness (cIMT) or carotid plaque score in nondiabetics with coronary heart disease and an average BMI and waist circumference of 30–31 and 105 cm found no difference compared to placebo [33]. Regardless, the metabolic effects were impressive overall and safety issues were predictable. This single-center study (Glasgow, UK) known as "CAMERA" (Carotid Atherosclerosis: MEtformin for insulin ResistAnce) was only 18 months with participants also utilizing statins. Metformin did significantly reduce all parameters of adiposity including bodyweight, body fat, BMI, and waist circumference at 18 months ($p<0.0001$ for all). Mean weight loss in the metformin group was 3.2 kg versus 0.0 kg in the placebo group after 18 months. Interestingly, 7 % ($n=6$) of placebo group developed new-onset diabetes and 2 % ($n=2$) with metformin. Tissue plasminogen nonsignificantly dropped with metformin, which is consistent with past studies, which suggests that another one of its cardioprotective properties could result from a decrease in prothrombotic potential. Although 21 % ($n=18$) of patients experienced diarrhea compared to 5 % ($n=4$) with placebo. And 12 % ($n=10$) of patients experienced nausea or vomiting versus 1 % ($n=1$) with placebo. Metformin caused a significant reduction in vitamin B12 levels (-62 pmol/L; $p<0.0001$) by 18 months. Interestingly, gamma-glutamyltransferase (GGT) levels also dropped in the participants on metformin versus placebo ($p=0.0002$) but there were no significant changes in alanine aminotransferase (ALT).

In the near future a better understanding of CVD prevention from metformin will occur. For example, there is the GLINT trial, which is a double-blind randomized trial of approximately 12,000 nondiabetic hyperglycemic and increased cardiovascular risk individuals [34]. Participants will be on metformin or placebo for 5 years. Another fascinating trial with be GIPS-III which will access left ventricular ejection fraction for 4 months after acute myocardial infarction in nondiabetic patients (NCT01217307). And the MetCAB (Metformin in Coronary Artery Bypass grafting) study will also examine the impact of metformin on cardiac injury in the setting of bypass grafting (NCT01438723). Preliminary laboratory studies suggest metformin could limit myocardial infarct size and damage.

In order to appreciate the overall heart healthy changes attributed to metformin from a variety of clinical trials Table 6.3 is provided, which are the metabolic parameter benefits of metformin [1–5].

Additionally, an appreciation of the diabetes prevention ability of metformin and/or lifestyle changes has arrived via phase-3 evidence and this is the subject of the next two sections of this chapter.

Table 6.3 Partial summary of metabolic parameter advantages of metformin

Clinically reported metabolic markers	Numerical range	Percentage change from baseline in studies
Blood Glucose (fasting)	−2 to 4 mmol/L	−20 to 30 %
Postprandial Blood Glucose	−3 to 6 mmol/L	−30 to 40 %
Hemoglobin A1c	−1 to 2 %	−10 to 25 %
Fasting Plasma Insulin	−0 to 3.5 uU/mL	−0 to 20 %
LDL Cholesterol	−0 to 1.00 mmol/L	−0 to 25 %
HDL Cholesterol	+0 to 0.16 mmol/L	+0 to 17 %
Triglycerides	−0 to 1.67 mmol/L	−0 to 50 %
Blood Pressure	No change	No change
Body Weight	−0 to 4 kg	−0 to 6 %
Serious Hypoglycemia	Negligible	Negligible
Other novel markers: CRP, Fibrinogen, IGF-1, Leptin, PAI-1 antigen,	Reduced (preliminary studies)	Reduced (preliminary studies)

Landmark NIH "Diabetes Prevention Program (DPP) Research Group" Randomized Trial (changed metformin utilization but exercise and weight loss beat metformin)

This landmark trial was published on February 7, 2002 in the New England Journal of Medicine [10]. This trial consisted of 3234 nondiabetic individuals with elevated fasting blood glucose (mean of 106 mg/dl and hemoglobin A1c of 5.9 % and 67 % with a fasting glucose of 95–109 mg/dl and 33 % with 110–125 mg/dl) were assigned to placebo, 850 mg metformin twice daily (850 mg for first month then 850 mg BID thereafter), or lifestyle changes with a goal of at least 7 % weight loss (via low-fat low caloric diet) with 150 min of physical activity per week. Mean age and BMI was 51 years and 34 with 68 % women, 45 % members of a minority group and 20 % 60 years of age or older. However, almost 33 % of the participants had a baseline BMI of 22–29! Approximately 70 % of the participants had a family history of diabetes and 16 % of the women had a history of gestational diabetes. *The average follow-up was only 2.8 years and compared to placebo the group utilizing metformin reduced the risk of diabetes by 31 % (95 % CI 17–43) and the lifestyle intervention reduced the incidence by 58 %. In addition, and one of the key findings of this landmark publication was the "lifestyle intervention was significantly more effective than metformin." In fact, the number needed to treat (NNT), or to prevent one-case of diabetes over 3-years for metformin was 13.9 persons for metformin and 6.9 for lifestyle-intervention. Regardless of BMI group (22–<30, 30–35 or >35) metformin or lifestyle was beneficial in reducing the incidence of diabetes regardless of gender and race or ethnic group, but metformin appeared to have a greater impact in those with a BMI of 35 or more. Overall, treatment effects did not significantly differ by gender or race or ethnic group. Daily caloric intake was reduced by 249 kcal in the placebo group, 296 in the metformin group, and 450 kcal in the lifestyle group (p < 0.001). The average weight loss was 0.1, 2.1, and 5.6 kg in the* *placebo, metformin, and lifestyle groups (p < 0.001).* Interestingly, side effects with metformin were significantly ($p < 0.02$) greater than placebo in terms of gastrointestinal symptoms (diarrhea, flatulence, nausea, and vomiting), but were significantly ($p < 0.02$) lower with lifestyle changes compared to placebo.

10-Year Follow-Up of Diabetes Prevention Program Outcomes Study (DPPOS) Trial

In 2009, the Diabetes Prevention Program Research Group published their 10-year follow-up or outcomes study in the journal Lancet (known as "DPPOS") [35]. A total of 88 % of the participants (2766 of 3150) enrolled for an additional follow-up of 5.7 years. On the basis of the original findings all three groups were offered lifestyle support. During the 10-year follow-up since randomization to DPP the modest weight loss with metformin was maintained but some weight gain occurred in the lifestyle group. Regardless, diabetes incidence in the 10 years since DPP randomization was reduced by 34 % in the lifestyle group and 18 % in the metformin group versus placebo. Interestingly, during this follow-up period the incidences of diabetes in the former placebo and metformin groups was reduced to those in the former lifestyle group, but overall and cumulatively the diabetes incidence continued to be lowest in the lifestyle intervention group. Further analysis of this study has found that diabetes risk was 56 % lower for subjects who had their glucose return to the normal range compared to those that consistently experienced prediabetes (HR = 0.44, $p < 0.0001$) [11]. Regardless, this follow-up demonstrated that lifestyle interventions or metformin can prevent or delay diabetes for at least 10 years [35]! Interestingly, lipid and blood pressure medication use was less in the lifestyle group and the impact on long-term cardiovascular disease risk parameters were similar for metformin and lifestyle intervention [36].

The American Diabetes Association (ADA) Risk Score

Clinically, now that so much preventive data has been documented from a variety of studies it is of interest to utilize the this type 2 diabetes risk score in clinical practice and patients can easily go on line and complete this test in less than 1 min [37, 38].

American Diabetes Risk Score consists of seven questions:

1. How old are you?
   (40–49 years = 1 point, 50–59 years = 2 points, and 60 years or older = 3 points)
2. Are you a male of female?
   (male = 1 point and female = 0 points)
3. If female, have you ever been diagnosed with gestational diabetes?
   (Yes = 1 point, No = 0 points)
4. Do you have a mother, father, sister, or brother with diabetes?
   (Yes = 1 point, No = 0 points)
5. Have you ever been diagnosed with high blood pressure (hypertension)?
6. Are you physically active?
   (Yes = 0 points, No = 1 point)
7. What is your weight status?
   (Point value assigned from chart at www.diabetes.org, for example if you are 5′5″ and you weigh 150–179 = 1 point, 180–239 = 2 points, and 240+ = 3 points,

and if you weigh less than the lowest amount in the column=0 points—149 or less from this example)

Total Score=_____?

Note: If you scored 5 or higher you are at increased risk for having type 2 diabetes.

Metformin—Miscellaneous (Autoimmune, Bone Health, Cancer, Dementia, NASH, PCOS, ...)

Metformin is utilized as one standard of care for many patients with PCOS (polycystic ovary syndrome) [39], and still utilized in some patients with nonalcoholic steatohepatitis (NASH) [40]. Metformin in the laboratory and observationally has exhibited bone protective properties and a neutral or reduced risk of bone fractures [41]. Insulin resistance is also associated with cognitive decline and dementia and preliminary evidence suggests a reduction in this risk with metformin in type 2 diabetes patients [42, 43]. Mental health status is not significantly impacted by metformin except a profound reduction in cobalamin or B12 can occur with this drug, which can increase the risk of depression [44]. Thus, again monitoring of B12 levels is critical with long-term metformin usage. And metformin is known as a drug that down regulates inflammatory cytokines and is also being studied against a variety of other disease including autoimmune conditions [45].

Type 2 diabetes is associated with insulin resistance or increased insulin levels which can itself act as a cellular growth factor or mitogen. This is perhaps one of the reasons that there is a higher cancer risk and cancer-related mortality in diabetics, which includes breast cancer [46, 47]. Regardless, countless epidemiologic data has now suggested a reduced risk of cancer and cancer mortality in diabetics utilizing metformin.

Preliminary Anticancer Human Studies and Metformin
(Reducing risk, recurrence, mortality, and/or side effects of conventional treatment?)

Metformin is currently in well over 100 human clinical trials with and without conventional treatment for various forms of cancer [48]. It has shown an ability to not only potentially prevent various forms of cancer, slow progression, act synergistically with some conventional agents, and has already demonstrated a reduction in some conventional treatment side effects (for example weight gain from hormone suppressive medications) [6, 47–49]. A rapid appreciation of the potential role for metformin in cancer can be derived from a diversity of completed studies and their conclusions. It could simply be argued that by preventing diabetes metformin has already demonstrated an ability to prevent cancer.

Breast, Cervical, Endometrial, and Ovarian Cancer (Gynecologic Cancers)

After a review of 18 publications: "Our analysis support a protective effect of metformin on breast cancer risk among postmenopausal women with diabetes [50]," although not just for prevention, but as an ancillary treatment in breast, endometrial, and ovarian cancer appears promising [51, 52]. Additionally, recent laboratory evidence suggests a potential anti-cervical cancer effect [53].

Colorectal Cancer (CRC)

"Patients with CRC and diabetes treated with metformin appear to have an improved survival outcome." This was the conclusion of a meta-analysis of six cohort studies [54].

Head and Neck Cancer

"Metformin reportedly improves the overall survival of HNSCC (head and neck squamous cell carcinoma) patients [55]."

Hepatocellular Carcinoma (HCC)

A total of seven studies (three cohort and four case–control) studies found "Metformin treatment was associated with reduced risk of HCC in diabetic patients [56]."

Lung Cancer

Data from the Surveillance, Epidemiology, and End Results registry linked to Medicare claims identified 750 patients with diabetes 65–80 years of age diagnosed with stage IV NSCLC. Researchers found the following: "Metformin is associated with improved survival among patients with diabetes with stage IV NSCLC, suggesting a potential anticancer effect [57]."

Multiple Myeloma (MM)

A retrospective review of 1240 MM patients from MD Anderson found metformin is associated with improved clinical outcomes [58].

Pancreatic Cancer

After a review of 13 studies including 10 cohort and three case controls, "use of metformin appears to be associated with a reduced risk of pancreatic cancer in patients with type 2 diabetes mellitus [59]."

Prostate Cancer

Metformin appears to be associated with a lower incidence of prostate cancer and a reduced risk of recurrence after a meta-analysis of 21 observational studies was conducted [60]. Another rigorous systematic review and meta-analysis of 230 citations and only nine studies meeting the inclusion criteria also found the potential for a reduced risk of recurrence [61].

Anticancer Mechanism of Action of Metformin

There are a plethora of potential anticancer mechanisms of action attributed to metformin and a brief review is presented here [6, 62, 63]:

- Metabolic changes (weight loss, glucose and insulin control, CRP reduction, leptin reduction, ...) that have indirect and direct antitumor effects.
- Cell growth inhibition.
- Reduces IGF-1 levels and downstream signaling (activation of AMPK in liver, muscle, adipose tissue, and pancreas reduces insulin and IGF-1).
- Reduces HER-2 protein expression and inhibits HER-2 protein kinase activation (reduced signaling downstream).
- Angiogenesis (reduces VEGF ...) and/or inflammation inhibition.
- Apoptosis induction via p53-dependent or -independent mechanisms.

- Induction of cell cycle arrest (via reduced cyclin D1 expression).
- Induction of a cellular energy deficit via ATP reduction, which inhibits lipogenesis and other pathways.
- Vitamin B12 deficiency initiation.
- Direct antitumor effects require the presence of organic cation transporters (OCTs) on the surface of tumor cells for direct uptake of the drug [64].
- Inhibition of mitochondrial respiratory chain leading to AMPK activation (metabolic master switch) with downstream mTOR inhibition or inactivation (limits mTOR signaling) [65–67].
- Reductions in markers of cell proliferation (Ki-67) [62].
- Increases in markers of apoptosis (TUNEL) [68].
- Direct cytotoxicity to cancer cells especially cancer stem cells (CSCs) which are usually chemoresistant and radioresistant [69, 70].
- Sensitizes cancer cells to radiation [69, 70].

The number of breast cancer clinical trials now utilizing metformin at all stages of this disease from prevention to advanced carcinoma is impressive and many of these trials are summarized in Table 6.4 [71].

Metformin and Breast Cancer and the NCIC CTG MA.32 Clinical Trial (Clinical Trials.gov identifier: NCT01101438) and already interesting findings from the Metabolic Substudy!

Perhaps, the most observed and truly landmark event is an ongoing phase 3 trial being conducted in North America, the UK, and Switzerland and it has already completed enrollment of 3649 nondiabetic women receiving conventional treatment for T1-3, N0-3, M0 breast cancer diagnosed during the previous 12 months [62]. Interestingly, patients needed to have a fasting glucose of less than or equal to 126 mg/dl (7.0 mmol/L), which is the threshold for diabetes diagnosis, but essentially enrolls only prediabetics or those with euglycemia. Women with a history of lactic acidosis, current use of diabetes drugs, previous or recurrent breast cancer, greater than moderate intake of alcohol, or "marked" liver, kidney, or cardiac abnormalities were excluded. Subjects were randomized to metformin 850 mg oral caplet twice a day for 5 years, which included a 4-week initial metformin acclimatization period of 850 mg a day for 4 weeks and then the addition of another 850 mg/day.

Interestingly, this study also included a metabolic substudy that has now been completed [62]. The first 492 individuals with fasting blood samples at baseline and after 6-months were included. Mean age, BMI, and glucose of participants in the substudy was 52 years, 27–28, and 95 mg/day or 5.3 mmol/L (range 88–101 mg/dl or 4.9–5.6 mmol/L). The results from this substudy were impressive because the results below "did not vary by baseline BMI or fasting insulin" including the following:

- Weight reduced 1.7 kg or −2.3 % with metformin and increased 0.5 kg or +0.7 % with placebo ($p < 0.001$). BMI change versus placebo also was significant ($p < 0.001$).
- Glucose reduced 1.9 % with metformin and increased 1.9 % with placebo ($p = 0.002$)

Table 6.4 Metformin human randomized clinical trials and breast cancer

Sampling of current Metformin and Breast Cancer Prevention or Treatment Randomized Trials	Commentary
NCT01101438-Phase 3 (Treatment in adjuvant setting)	Metformin versus Placebo Premenopausal and postmenopausal women with early breast cancer. Preliminary results have at least demonstrated weight loss, glucose, insulin, leptin, and CRP reduction in an interim analysis of a subset of patients
NCT01905046-Phase 3 (Prevention Trial)	Metformin versus Placebo for 24 months Premenopausal women at increased risk of breast cancer from atypical hyperplasia or in situ breast cancer
NCT01885013-Phase 2 (Treatment in advanced setting)	Metformin with chemotherapy combination Premenopausal and postmenopausal HER2-negative metastatic breast cancer patients
NCT01310231-Phase 2 (Treatment in advanced setting)	Metformin with chemotherapy Premenopausal and postmenopausal breast cancer receiving first or second line chemotherapy utilizing anthracyclines, platinum, taxanes, or capecitabine
NCT01042379-Phase 2 (Treatment in neo-adjuvant setting)	Metformin with a chemotherapy combination Premenopausal and postmenopausal women with locally advanced breast cancer
NCT01929811-Phase 2 (Treatment in neo-adjuvant setting)	Metformin with a chemotherapy combination. Premenopausal and postmenopausal women with locally advanced breast cancer
NCT01566799-Phase 2 (Treatment in neoadjuvant setting)	Metformin with a chemotherapy combination Premenopausal and postmenopausal ER+ or PR+, HER2 negative breast cancer
NCT01589367-Phase 2 (Treatment in neoadjuvant setting)	Metformin + letrozole ER-positive post-menopausal breast cancer
NCT02028221-Phase 2 (Prevention in high-risk setting)	Metformin versus placebo. Overweight/obese premenopausal women with metabolic syndrome
NCT01340300-Phase 2 (Prevention of recurrence)	Metformin versus metformin and exercise (I love this thought process in a clinical trial and study-just an FYI) Colorectal and breast cancer survivors
NCT0909506-Phase 2 (Prevention of recurrence)	Metformin versus placebo Operable breast cancer patients with BMI greater than or equal to 23 or fasting blood sugar of 100–125 mg/dl

Note: More details and metformin clinical trials are available for viewing at www.clinicaltrials.gov

- Insulin reduced 11.1 % with metformin and did not change with placebo ($p = 0.002$).
- hs-CRP was unchanged with metformin and increased 6.7 % with placebo ($p = 0.002$).
- Leptin reduced 9.5 % with metformin and increased 10.7 % with placebo ($p < 0.001$).

Interestingly, members of this research group had found previously that higher insulin levels in breast cancer were associated with two times the risk of distant recurrence and three times the risk of death [72, 73]. The results of this and other trials should be available soon and regardless of outcome at least the metabolic changes in nondiabetic women with breast cancer have clinical significance.

Metformin Dietary Supplement Mini-mimics (Alpha-Lipoic Acid and/or Berberine?)

Alpha-Lipoic Acid (thioctic acid)

Alpha-lipoic acid has initial noteworthy data for reducing/treating peripheral neuropathy in diabetics at 600 mg/day [74], and could have some potential for preventing this same condition as a result of chemotherapy. Alpha-lipoic acid is a dietary supplement in the USA and is treated as a drug in numerous other countries and even can be ordered in some hospitals in Europe as an IV drug. Weight loss is another potential option with this oral intervention at higher dosages [75, 76]. It is of interest that one mechanism of action for weight loss could be activation of AMPK (adenosine monophosphate-activated protein kinase) [75–86], which is similar to what is described for metformin [1–5].

Two major clinical trials with almost 1500 participants, one placebo controlled and published in a reputable US medical journal (American Journal of Medicine), which is highly unusual for a weight loss supplement, suggests that alpha lipoic acid at a dosage of 800–1800 mg a day (ideally 1800 mg/day) could significantly assist with weight loss versus placebo (discussed later in this chapter) [75, 76]. Other clinical and laboratory investigations support this finding, and suggest a fairly safe mechanism of action similar to metformin, but less effective.

An unusually large observational clinical study of 1127 individuals, 445 men and 682 women, ages 18–60 were included and consisted of nonsmokers, and DEXA scanning was utilized to assist in supporting the observational study. A total of 43 % of the subjects were pre-obese (overweight, $n=480$) and 53 % were obese ($n=595$) [75]. Individuals (mean age 43–45) were treated for 4 months with 800 mg of alpha-lipoic acid (Liponax, Segix Italia, S.r.l. 00040 Pomezia, Italy). Significant ($p<0.001$) reductions in weight (8 % in both men and women), BMI (−2 points), blood pressure, and belly fat/abdominal circumference (males −7 cm, female −6 cm) were found in the pre-obese group. And in the obese group, significant ($p<0.001$) reductions in weight (9 % in both men and women), BMI (males −4 points, female −3 points), blood pressure, and belly fat/abdominal circumference (male −11 cm, female −9 cm) were found. Additionally, participants received the SNAQ, which is the Simplified Nutritional Appetite Questionnaire, which found a significant reduction in the appetite of participants over the 4-month period of time. The issue with this clinical study is again the observational nature and lack of a placebo or comparative arm.

A second large study of racemic alpha-lipoic acid (only the R-isomer is produced naturally, but chemical synthesis is a 50/50 racemic mixture of two optical isomers or R- and S-alpha-lipoic acid) was recently published in a major US clinical journal (The American Journal of Medicine) that was a randomized, double-blind, placebo-controlled, 20-week trial of 360 individuals (mean age 40–42, range 18–64 years, mean BMI of 33, but as low as BMI 27 was accepted) [76]. There was a 4-week run in phase during which all participants received placebo (three tablets 30 min before each meal for a total of nine pills per day) to demonstrate those with good compliance. Participants were also instructed with the goal of reducing daily caloric intake by 600 calories/day (with a minimum intake of 1200 calories/day and general diet instructions were 55–65 % carbohydrates, 20–25 % fat, and 15–20 % protein). Participants took three tablets 30 min before each meal (nine tablets daily) and ingested three meals a day. Many of the participants (120 in each group) either had high cholesterol (21 % in 1800 mg group) or high blood pressure (27 % in 1800 mg) or diabetes (28 %) and 23 % appeared to have no comorbidities, The average blood pressure was 133/82, LDL of 108–114 mg/dl, triglyceride of 144–150, fasting glucose range was 108–144 mg/dl (diabetes was defined as fasting glucose greater than or equal to 126 mg/dl on two separate occasions or the use of hypoglycemic agents). In both the 1200 mg and 1800 mg group average weight decreased significantly from baseline, starting as early as 4-weeks. The 1800 mg alpha-lipoic acid group lost significantly more weight compared to placebo ($p < 0.05$). In addition, analyses of both the intent-to-treat and per-protocol completion populations found that weight loss at 20 weeks was significantly greater in the 1800 mg compared to the placebo group. Also significant reductions occurred in waist circumference in the 1800 mg per protocol compared to placebo, and so was the percentage of subjects that achieved a greater or equal to 5 % reduction in baseline body weight (21.6 % versus 10.0 %, $p < 0.01$). "When responders were compared with non-responders (<5 % loss), we observed no significant differences in initial clinical or laboratory parameters. Even in the group with BMI of 27–30 (overweight), there was a significant reduction in body weight in the 1800 mg group compared to placebo." Side effects were not significantly different except in the alpha-lipoic acid group that was a higher number of individuals with "itching sensation" compared to placebo (13 events to 3 in the 1800 mg group) that led to 1 withdrawal. There appeared to be no relationship with these side effects and actual efficacy of this dietary supplement. In my clinical experience, itching and temporary rash, and are more common than reported in the literature and tends to occur on the extremities and should be monitored by the patient and the health care professional during the weight loss regimen. Although there appears to be no correlation with these side effects and other more serious toxicity (see Hirata disease below) there have not been enough rigorous trials to understand the full spectrum and severity of adverse events associated with this supplement (as is the case with most dietary supplements on the market). Additionally, malodorous urine (from what I theorize to be a sulfur reaction similar to asparagus consumption) appears to be another side effect that does not receive enough attention in the literature and although it appears to be harmless it should be monitored more often in clinical trials. The capsules of alpha-lipoic acid should never be opened and utilized as a dissolvable liquid powder because of the acidity or caustic nature of the product and the risk of esophageal irritation.

Interestingly, a past published open-label trial of six patients on antipsychotic drugs for schizophrenia that had caused weight gain (10 % or more) found that 1200 mg/day of alpha-lipoic Acid over 12 weeks significantly reduced weight [77]. Mean weight loss was significant at the end of 12-weeks (3.16 kg, $p = 0.04$), and

BMI was significantly reduced ($p = 0.03$). And two patients now followed for 9 and 6 months had weight reductions of 16.4 and 12.5 kg. This and other studies have led to the interest and initiating of larger randomized clinical trial utilizing this supplement versus placebo to prevent weight gain on antipsychotic medications.

Recent clinical reviews [78] and laboratory studies continue to suggest that alpha lipoic acid can cause weight loss. In rodent experimental models, alpha-lipoic acid has been shown to cause weight loss and prevent weight gain by encouraging satiation, increasing energy expenditure, reducing hyperglycemia and reduce insulin resistance. For example, a study of ovariectomized rats treated with 2000 mg/kg of alpha lipoic acid for 3–10 weeks after surgery compared to control rats demonstrated a significant reduction in appetite and fat accumulation potentially via the regulation of central and peripheral AMPK activities [79]. Another recent mouse study of alpha lipoic acid found that it stimulated AMP-activated protein kinase and multiple other weight control enzymes and "dramatically" reduced body weight and visceral fat content (despite mice given a high fat diet) [80]. Another study that involved aged mice found that with alpha-lipoic acid (0.75 % in drinking water) there was an improvement in body composition, glucose tolerance, and energy expenditure compared to mice not supplemented with lipoic acid [81]. Researchers concluded by stating: "LA may be a promising supplement for treatment of obesity and/or insulin resistance in older patients." Other animal studies suggest that alpha-lipoic acid may work by reducing insulin resistance [82–84], or again through weight control mechanisms [85, 86].

A final note on alpha-lipoic acid should receive more attention and this is the rare side effect (not described as of yet in the USA) of insulin autoimmune syndrome (IAS or Hirata disease) [87, 88]. Drugs with sulfhydryl groups (like alpha-lipoic acid) have the ability to cause spontaneous hypoglycemia from high insulin levels caused by high concentrations of autoantibodies against intrinsic insulin receptors. In Japanese individuals IAS is associated with human leucocyte antigens (HLA-DRB1*04:06 allele) and again occurs from exposure to sulfhydryl-harboring medications [88]. Only one case had been reported in Caucasians but more recently six cases were reported in European Caucasians and hypoglycemic symptoms occurred within 4 months of ingesting alpha-lipoic acid. The supplement was discontinued and patients were treated with oral or IV glucose and prednisone (12.5–25 mg/day) and HLA analysis found HLA-DRB1*04:03 in five of the six patients and HLA-DRB1*04:06 present in the other patient.

Berberine

Berberine is a plant alkaloid used for 3000 years in Ayurvedic and Chinese medicine. It is actually found in the root, rhizome, and stem bark of numerous plants [89–92]. For example, *Berberis aquifolium* (Oregon grape), *Berberis vulgaris* (barberry), *Berberis aristata* (Tree Turmeric). Berberine is also manufactured synthetically today and it appears to partially mimic metformin via AMPK activation [89, 90]. Again, AMP-activated kinase (AMPK) turns on or increases when the ratio of cell AMP+ADP/ATP increases (metabolic stress occurs), and thus it functions to be a barometer of cell fuel deficiency or a metabolic master switch. It has been implicated in antiaging processes from caloric restriction to metformin use and it appears this mechanism of action of turning a cell into a primarily catabolic position, and not anabolic, thus could combat metabolic disorders.

A meta-analysis of 11 randomized clinical trials of berberine ($n=874$) found a minimal to no toxicity and a potential ability to significantly lower LDL (mean difference −25 mg/dl or −0.65 mmol/L) and triglycerides (−44 mg/dl or −0.5 mmol/L) and potentially increase HDL (2 mg/dl or 0.05 mmol/L) [93]. Another meta-analysis of 27 randomized controlled trials ($n=2569$) found berberine to be as efficient as oral hypoglycemic and some medications to lower cholesterol and improve blood pressure with minimal to no toxicity [94]. For example, Berberine at 500 mg three times a day (1500 mg total) has demonstrated some efficacy on par with 1500 mg of metformin in preliminary research [95, 96]. Although promising it is easy to become slightly skeptical when a supplement/drug apparently carries no overt side effects. One clear caveat is that the methodologies of many past studies were of a low quality [95]. And there appears to be a suggestion from some studies of bitter taste, diarrhea, flatulence, and abdominal pain with berberine, which also occurs with metformin [96]. Regardless, because of this history of preliminary clinical efficacy in diabetes and via its impact on other proliferative pathways there is some interest in studying the anti-breast cancer effects of this supplement [97].

Conclusion

Indeed, direct and indirect observations and knowledge about metformin abound and are summarized in Table 6.5. Most of these observations were derived from this chapter.

One could argue that even if metformin is not found to reduce the risk of breast cancer or slow the progression of this disease or even provide a breast cancer mortality benefit that it has already demonstrated an anti-breast cancer effects. Why? Since this "natural," low-cost, generic, and heart healthy medication has already shown the ability to significantly lower diabetes risk and improve metabolic parameters it is essentially reducing cancer risk. Whether this suggests incidence or morbidity or mortality alterations in breast cancer this medication is one of the first win-win preventive drugs. For example, it only serves to reduce side effects of breast cancer treatment than the patient still wins regardless of outcome.

The story of metformin in breast cancer is fascinating and whether or not it proves to have a definitive consistent anti-breast cancer effect is not currently known. However, metformin should serve as a reminder to health care professionals and patients that heart healthy changes are tantamount to breast healthy and overall salubrious changes and this has been known for some time [98], regardless of whether these interventions are derived from lifestyle modifications (weight loss, exercise, diet, ...) and/or low-cost, generic medications from the French Lilac.

Table 6.5 Overview of a diversity of direct and indirect interesting observations with metformin

Metformin from A to Z	Commentary
Alpha-Lipoic Acid (a dietary supplement in the USA and a prescription in some other countries) *Note*: Alpha-lipoic acid is also known in the medical literature as "thioctic acid" because it is contains a sulfur group (actually two bonded sulfur groups), and it is created by the human body to maintain aerobic metabolism and assist in other physiologic processes including production of glutathione	– Is utilized as an oral and IV drug in many countries but in the USA it is a common oral dietary supplement. It also has a history of being utilized as a medication to prevent and treat diabetic peripheral neuropathy from multiple clinical trials (especially for prevention of neuropathy) – Has some preliminary metformin like activity as a dietary supplement, including an impact on AMPK, and should not be used together with metformin without closer supervision and it is arguably less effective than metformin – A well-done 5-month randomized trial of 1800 mg/day (600 mg TID 30 min before meal time) found the potential for significant benefit (small studies with efficacy have utilized even lower dosages). However, rashes and itching are a fairly common side effect at higher dosages and occasional malodorous urine can occur arguably from a reaction similar in nature to what occurs with the consumption of asparagus – In very rare circumstances insulin autoimmune syndrome (IAS or Hirata disease) with profound hypoglycemia caused by insulin autoantibodies could occur, as it is known to also occur with some drugs containing sulfhydryl compounds – It should not be used together with metformin without closer supervision and is arguably less effective than metformin
Berberine (it is synthetically produced, but can also be found in a variety of plants)	– A potential dietary supplement with metformin-like potential including glucose and lipid control, weight loss and an impact on AMPK. Commonly utilized dosage is 500 mg three times a day around meal-time (somewhat similar to metformin) – Side effects have not been well described but appear to be similar to metformin in terms of diarrhea, abdominal pain, flatulence and taste change in some patients – It should not be used together with metformin without closer supervision and is arguably less effective than metformin
Biguanide Class of Medications	Generally refers to the oral antihyperglycemic drugs utilized for prediabetes and diabetes and includes the drugs Buformin (butyl derivative of biguanide), Metformin (dimethylbiguanide), and Phenformin (phenethylated biguanide)
Bone Mineral Density (BMD)	– Metformin has primarily a neutral or minimally positive effect on BMD, and neutral or preliminary reduction in fracture risk via slight enhancement of osteoblastic differentiation and negative effect on osteoclast differentiation

(continued)

Table 6.5 (continued)

Metformin from A to Z	Commentary
Buformin (1-butylbiguanide)	– Oral antidiabetic drug of the biguanide class (synthesized in 1957), structurally related to metformin and phenformin. Buformin is marketed by a German pharmaceutical company Grunenthal as "Silubin" – It is also available as a sustained release and still sold in some countries (Romania). It was withdrawn from market in many countries because of an increased risk of lactic acidosis. It also has some anticancer properties
Caloric Reduction (another mechanism of action of metformin)	In the famous Diabetes Prevention Program (DPP) trial (first published February 7, 2002 in the New England Journal of Medicine) metformin reduced caloric intake by approximately 300 kcal/day versus 250 kcal/day with placebo and 450 kcal/day with lifestyle interventions (150 min/week of exercise) and low-fat diet with 7 % weight loss
Cardiovascular Disease (CVD) Risk	Metformin appears to reduce CVD risk in diabetics and potentially after a myocardial infarction to reduce infarct size, and is being tested in nondiabetics to reduce CVD risk
Cancer Prevention and Treatment	Metformin is currently in over 100 clinical trials from cancer prevention to treatment at all cancer stages with conventional medications. It has also been shown to reduce side effects such as weight gain caused by some hormone suppressive medications (good clinical evidence in breast and prostate cancer)
Cognition and/or Depression	Preliminary evidence suggests metformin may improve cognitive function, which then can result in recovery from depression. Regardless, metformin appears to be a mentally neutral or healthy weight loss drug. In the DPP trial metformin did not increase or decrease depression status
Contrast Agents	This is a controversial contraindication to metformin use and suggested to be stopped for 48 h after contrast is given and renal function is proven normal. Some experts suggest 48 h before and after contrast. Overall minimal risk in those with normal renal function
CRP	Recent studies suggest a reduction or at least stabilization of this inflammatory marker with metformin
Diabetic Confounding/Catch in Cancer	It must be kept in mind that a good deal of the positive anticancer data with metformin is in diabetic patients and may primarily benefit this group compared to nondiabetics or simply reflect the fact that type 2 diabetics on metformin reflect less serious diabetic disease and hence lower risk of cancer morbidity and mortality

(continued)

Table 6.5 (continued)

Metformin from A to Z	Commentary
Diabetes Prevention Program (DPP) and Diabetes Prevention Program Outcomes Study (DPPOS)	– Landmark phase 3 clinical trial of 850 mg bid metformin (Glucophage), which was conducted at 27 medical centers (baseline fasting glucose was 95–125 mg/dl) and it demonstrated a reduction in diabetes risk in high-risk patients in less than 3 years versus placebo – This trial was remarkable based on participant diversity-approximately 66 % of the individuals were female and 50 % minority race/ethnicity – However, the third arm of the trial was 7 % weight loss via exercise (150 min a week) and caloric reduction (low-fat diet) and it reduced diabetes risk greater than placebo and metformin (even after 10 years of follow-up)! Metformin reduced diabetes risk by 31 % and lifestyle intervention reduced risk by 58 % compared to placebo and it was found to be safer versus the drug. Caloric reduction was approximately 250 kcal/day with placebo, 300 kcal/day with metformin and 450 kcal/day with the lifestyle intervention
Diarrhea/Soft Stool	A fairly common side effect of metformin but it is reduced when the drug is utilized with a meal
Fiber Supplementation (Psyllium …)	Some fiber supplements such as psyllium could synergistically further control or lower blood sugar and HgbA1c when used with metformin. Arguably, the fiber supplement should be used several hours before or after metformin ingestion to reduce the chances of a reduction in metformin absorption and bioavailability. One study showed better tolerance to metformin and glucose control when psyllium was utilized at approximately 10 g/day
French Lilac (*Galega officinalis*)	– Also known as "Goat's Rue." Guanidine is the active ingredient in the French Lilac and was found to have hypoglycemic activity in 1918. Guanidine's utilization in was limited by adverse effect including: hypotension, atrial fibrillation, tremor, ataxia, and seizures – Biguanides were developed from guanidine and studied for the treatment of diabetes in the 1920s, but interest in these compounds decreased with the discovery of insulin in 1921
Gestational Diabetes mellitus (GDM)	Up to 14 % of all pregnancies are complicated by GDM. Metformin does not cause weight gain or hypoglycemia (like insulin treatment) but it crosses the placenta. Still, new research suggests it may a role in GDM and preliminary human evidence suggests it may be safe and reduce malformations but more studies are needed
Glucophage (from Bristol-Myers Squibb)	Arguably the most well known patented immediate release metformin, which is now generic and it was used in the famous DPP trial
Glucose/Insulin	Reduced with metformin (insulin can be reduced by as much as 75 %)
Growth Factors	Reduced with metformin (especially IGF-1 pathway)

(continued)

Table 6.5 (continued)

Metformin from A to Z	Commentary
Half-Life	Only 18 h maximum in the blood (includes retention in red blood cells), but only 5–6-h official maximum half-life in plasma, which suggests 94 % of the drug is removed by the body in 24 h. Metformin requires drug compliance even until blood measurements are completed (especially in clinical studies because markers can change dramatically with even 1 or 2 missed medication days)
Lactic Acidosis	Not in excess of three cases per 100,000 patients treated. Cochrane review of 347 clinical trials and observational studies found no greater risk of lactic acidosis compared with other type 2 diabetes treatments
Leptin (hormone that helps in the control of hunger and feeling of satiation)	Preliminarily reduced with metformin, which actually suggests an increased sensitization to this hormone versus previous desensitization with excessive weight gain
Lifestyle Interventions!!! (please never forget to tell patients and health care professionals)	Always keep in mind that in the landmark DPP trial aggressive lifestyle intervention (7 % weight loss-150 min of exercise per week and low-fat/caloric restriction of 450 calories/day) significantly beat metformin in terms of type 2 diabetes reduction (−58 % versus −31 %) and weight loss (−12.3 pounds versus −4.6 pounds)
Magnesium	Reduced with metformin or lower magnesium levels are at least associated with metformin
Meals or After Meals	Metformin gastrointestinal side effects are reduced with the use of this medication with meals or right after a meal is consumed. All patients utilizing metformin should be informed of this fact
Mechanism of Action	Reduce hepatic glucose production and increase glucose uptake in muscle tissue (via AMPK activation). May also block absorption of glucose from gastrointestinal tract and appears to also reduce appetite and overall caloric intake
Metallic Taste	Increased risk with metformin and usually transient when starting therapy
Metformin XR (extended release or also known as Glucophage XR)	Tends to be more expensive than generic immediate release metformin but also tends to have less gastrointestinal side effects and allows for once daily dosing and better potential compliance in appropriate patients. It also is absorbed slower than regular metformin and takes several more hours to reach maximum plasma concentration
NCT01101438-Phase 3 Trial (Treatment in adjuvant setting) (Conducted in North America, the UK, and Switzerland)	Metformin (850 mg BID) versus Placebo for 5-years in a Phase 3 landmark trial. Premenopausal and postmenopausal nondiabetic women with early breast cancer were recruited, and the enrollment is completed. Preliminary results have at least demonstrated weight loss, glucose, insulin, leptin, and CRP reduction in an interim analysis of a subset of patients
Nonalcoholic Fatty Liver Disease (NAFLD)/Nonalcoholic Steatohepatitis (NASH)	Metformin may help in the treatment of prediabetics and diabetics that have NAFLD or NASH

(continued)

Table 6.5 (continued)

Metformin from A to Z	Commentary
Prediabetes (aka high risk for diabetes)	Metformin is arguably the only drug ever proven to reduce the risk of type II diabetes in prediabetes
Phenformin (phenethylbiguanide) *Note*: Metabolized via cytochrome P450 2D6 in the liver and individual differences in the activity of this enzyme system (CYP2D6 polymorphisms) can further increase toxicity. Metformin is not metabolized by the liver and eliminated unchanged by kidneys	– Antidiabetic oral drug from the biguanide class (along with buformin and metformin). Half-life of the drug is 7–15 h and it is metabolized by the liver and eliminated by kidneys (versus 1.5–6 h half-life with metformin) – Introduced in the USA in 1957 (marketed by Ciba-Geigy) to treat type 2 diabetes and withdrawn from the USA and European markets in 1977 because of a high incidence (and fatalities) of lactic acidosis occurring at standard treatment dosages (average lactic acidosis causing dosage was 123 mg/day). It has been estimated that one in 4000 patients utilizing phenformin develops lactic acidosis versus one in 40,000–80,000 with buformin or metformin (approximately 10–20 times lower). In a past review of 330 cases of biguanide related lactic acidosis (285 cases from phenformin) approximately 50 % of the patients died (50 % mortality rate!) – There are appeared to be an increased cardiovascular risk with phenformin versus a potential reduced cardiovascular risk with metformin – Standard dosages utilized were much lower for phenformin (50–200 mg/day) versus metformin (850 mg BID)
Polycystic Ovary Syndrome (PCOS)	Metformin has become one of the medications that are standard of care in this situation. It has the potential to be an effective ovulation induction agent for some women with PCOS, and it could be an alternative to the oral contraceptive pill (OCP) for the treatment of hyperandrogenic symptoms including hirsutism and acne and may increase pregnancy rates
Pregnancy	Metformin is classified as a FDA category B drug for use during pregnancy, which suggests that animal studies have not demonstrated any risk to the fetus, but there are no appropriate and well-controlled studies in pregnant women Preliminary evidence suggests it may be safe in pregnancy but more studies are needed. Metformin clearance increases during pregnancy due to enhanced renal elimination
Side Effects	Common side effects from clinical trials and personal observations include: soft stool, diarrhea, gastrointestinal upset, metallic taste, carbohydrate cravings, vitamin B12 and magnesium reductions. Many of the GI side effects are reduced by increasing dose titration every 2–4 weeks and consuming pills with meals and dividing drug dosages throughout the day
Titration to full dose	Metformin should only be utilized as one pill per 2–4 weeks and then next pill or dose can be added. For example, in DPP 850 mg was the starting dose and at 1 month the dose was increased to 850 mg twice daily, unless gastrointestinal symptoms occurred that required a longer titration period

(continued)

Table 6.5 (continued)

Metformin from A to Z	Commentary
Tissue Plasminogen Activator (TPA)	Consistently reduced in studies with metformin and suggests it may also reduce pro-thrombotic potential
United Kingdom Prospective Diabetes Study (UKPDS) (*Note*: It was a 20-year study involving 23 medical centers in the UK and more than 5000 patients with type 2 diabetes were recruited. First published in Lancet in 1998)	– UKPDS observed that improving blood glucose or blood pressure in newly diagnosed diabetes reduced the risk of major diabetic eye disease, serious reduction in vision, early kidney damage, strokes, and deaths from diabetes-related causes (Lancet 1998) – This was another landmark trial for metformin (along with DPP above) that utilized newly diagnosed type 2 diabetes patients and placed them on dietary restrictions (increase carbohydrates to 50 % and more fiber and less saturated fat and calories) or intensive therapy with medications, one of which was metformin that was utilized in overweight/obese patients (BMI of 31–32). In the metformin group even after a decade of follow-up significant reductions in myocardial infarction (33 %, $p=0.005$), and death from any cause (27 %, $p=0.002$) occurred. This study essentially proved that even after 10-years of follow-up serious medical complications in overweight patients could be significantly improved with metformin (N Engl J Med 2008) – It is interesting in this study that treatment started with one 850 mg tablet/day, then 850 mg twice daily, and then 1700 mg in the morning and 850 mg with the evening meal (maximum dose-2550 mg). If on any specific dose diarrhea or nausea occurred then patients were asked to reduce the dose to the previous dose that did not cause these issues
Vitamin B12	Metformin increases the risk of vitamin B12 deficiency (serum level <150 pmol/L) and borderline-deficient vitamin B12 (serum level 150–220 pmol/L). The drug increases the risk of vitamin B12 malabsorption and/or a reduction in intrinsic factor secretion
Weight Loss	Metformin is arguably the only medication proven to consistently assist with weight loss and is heart and mentally healthy

References

1. Setter SM, Iltz JL, Thams J, Campbell RK. Metformin hydrochloride in the treatment of type 2 diabetes mellitus: a clinical review with a focus on dual therapy. Clin Ther. 2003;25:2991–3026.
2. Graham GC, Punt J, Arora M, Day RO, Doogue MP, Duong JK, et al. Clinical pharmacokinetics of metformin. Clin Pharmacokinet. 2011;50:81–98.
3. Scheen AJ. Clinical pharmacokinetics of metformin. Clin Pharmacokinet. 1996;30:359–71.
4. Dunn CJ, Peters DH. Metformin. A review of its pharmacological properties and therapeutic use in non-insulin-dependent diabetes mellitus. Drugs. 1995;49:721–9.
5. Campbell RK, White Jr JR, Saulie BA. Metformin: a new oral biguanide. Clin Ther. 1996;18:360–71.

6. Moyad MA, Vogelzang NJ. Heart healthy equals prostate healthy and statins, aspirin, and/or metformin (S.A.M.) are the ideal recommendations for prostate cancer prevention. Asian J Androl 2015, Epub ahead of print.

7. Onge ES, Miller SA, Motycka C, DeBerry A. A review of the treatment of type 2 diabetes in children. J Pediatr Pharmacol Ther. 2015;20:4–16.

8. United Kingdom Prospective Diabetes Study Group. United Kingdom Prospective Diabetes Study 24: a 6-year, randomized, controlled trial comparing sulfonylurea, insulin, and metformin therapy in patients with newly diagnosed type 2 diabetes that could not be controlled with diet therapy. Ann Intern Med. 1998;128:165–75.

9. United Kingdom Prospective Diabetes Study Group. United Kingdom Prospective Diabetes Study (UKPDS). 13: Relative efficacy of randomly allocated diet, sulfonylurea, insulin, or metformin in patients with newly diagnosed non-insulin dependent diabetes followed for three years. BMJ. 1995;310:83–8.

10. Diabetes Prevention Program Research Group. Reduction in the incidence of type 2 diabetes with lifestyle intervention or metformin. N Engl J Med. 2002;346:393–403.

11. Diabetes Prevention Program Research Group. Effect of regression from prediabetes to normal glucose regulation on long-term reduction in diabetes risk: results from the Diabetes Prevention Program Outcomes Study. Lancet. 2012;379:2243–51.

12. Jabbour S, Ziring B. Advantages of extended-release metformin in patients with type 2 diabetes mellitus. Postgrad Med. 2011;123:15–23.

13. Liu Q, Li S, Quan H, Li J. Vitamin B12 status in metformin treated patients: systematic review. PLoS One. 2014;9:e100379.

14. Peters KE, Chubb SA, Davis WA, Davis TM. The relationship between hypomagnesemia, metformin therapy and cardiovascular disease complicating type 2 diabetes: the Fremantle Diabetes Study. PLoS One. 2013;8:e74355.

15. Rose Jr T, Choi J. Intravenous imaging contrast media complications: the basics that every clinician needs to know. Am J Med 2015, Epub ahead of print.

16. Salpeter SR, Greyber E, Pasternak GA, Salpeter EE. Risk of fatal and nonfatal lactic acidosis with metformin use in type 2 diabetes. Cochrane Database Syst Rev 2010;(4):CD002967.

17. Glucophage (metformin hydrochloride) [final printed labeling]. US Food and Drug Administration website. http://www.accessdata.fda.gov/drugsatfda.doc/nda/2000/20357S019_Glucophage_prntibl.pdf. Accessed 1 June 2015.

18. Inzucchi SE, Lipska KJ, Mayo H, Bailey CJ, McGuire DK. Metformin in patients with type 2 diabetes and kidney disease: a systematic review. JAMA. 2014;312:2668–75.

19. Rasuli P, Hammond DI. Metformin and contrast media: where is the conflict? Can Assoc Radiol J. 1998;49:161–6.

20. Goergen SK, Rumbold G, Compton G, Harris C. Systematic review of current guidelines, and their evidence base, on risk of lactic acidosis after administration of contrast medium for patients receiving metformin. Radiology. 2010;254:261–9.

21. Thomsen HS, Morcos SK, Almen T, Aspelin P, Bellin MF, Clement O, et al. Metformin and contrast media. Radiology. 2010;256:672–3.

22. Huang Z, Sjoholm A. Ethanol acutely stimulates islet blood flow, amplifies insulin secretion, and induces hypoglycemia via nitric oxide and vagally mediated mechanisms. Endocrinology. 2008;149:232–6.

23. Gin H, Orgerie MB, Aubertin J. The influence of guar gum on absorption of metformin from the gut in healthy volunteers. Horm Metab Res. 1989;21:81–3.

24. Abdall D, Samson SE, Grover AK. How effective are antioxidant supplements in obesity and diabetes? Med Princ Pract. 2015;24(3):201–15. Epub 14 Mar 2015.

25. Moyad MA. The supplement handbook: a trusted experts guide to what works & what's worthless for more than 100 conditions. New York, NY: Rodale Publishing; 2014.

26. Comerma-Steffensen S, Grann M, Andersen CU, Rungby J, Simonsen U. Cardiovascular effects of current and future anti-obesity drugs. Curr Vasc Pharmacol. 2014;12:493–504.

27. UK Prospective Diabetes Study (UKPDS) Group. Effect of intensive blood-glucose control with metformin on complications in overweight patients with type 2 diabetes (UKPDS 34). Lancet. 1998;352:854–65.

28. Holman RR, Paul SK, Bethel MA, Matthews DR, Neil HA. 10-Year follow-up of intensive glucose control in type 2 diabetes. N Engl J Med. 2008;359:1577–89.
29. Kooy A, de Jger J, Lehert P, et al. Long-term effects of metformin on metabolism and micro-vascular and macrovascular disease in patients with type 2 diabetes mellitus. Arch Intern Med. 2009;169:616–25.
30. Scheen AJ, Paquot N. Metformin revisited: a critical review of the benefit-risk balance in at-risk patients with type 2 diabetes. Diabetes Metab. 2013;39:179–90.
31. Azimova K, San Juan Z, Mukherjee D. Cardiovascular safety profile of currently available diabetic drugs. Ochsner J. 2014;14:616–32.
32. Selvin E, Bolen S, Yeh HC, Wiley C, Wilson LM, Marinopoulos SS, et al. Cardiovascular outcomes in trials of oral diabetes medications: a systematic review. Arch Intern Med. 2008;168:2070–80.
33. Preiss D, Lloyd SM, Ford I, McMurray JJ, Holman RR, Welsh P, et al. Metformin for non-diabetic patients with coronary heart disease (the CAMERA study): a randomized controlled trial. Lancet Diabetes Endocrinol. 2014;2:116–24.
34. Riksen NP. It takes more than one CAMERA to study cardiovascular protection by metformin. Lancet Diabetes Endocrinol. 2014;2:105–6.
35. Diabetes Prevention Program Research Group. 10-Year follow-up of diabetes incidence and weight loss in the Diabetes Prevention Program Outcomes Study. Lancet. 2009;374:1677–86.
36. Diabetes Prevention Program Outcomes Study Research Group. Long-term effects of the Diabetes Prevention Program interventions on cardiovascular risk factors: a report from the DPP Outcomes Study. Diabet Med. 2013;30:46–55.
37. Bang H, Edwards AM, Bomback AS, Ballantyne CM, Brillion D, Callahan MA, et al. Development and validation of a patient self-assessment score for diabetes risk. Ann Intern Med. 2009;151:775–83.
38. American Diabetes Association web-site. www.diabetes.org/are-you-at-risk/diabetes-risk-test/. Accessed 1 June 2015.
39. Johnson NP. Metformin use in women with polycystic ovary syndrome. Ann Transl Med. 2014;2:56.
40. Gitto S, Vitale G, Villa E, Andreone P. Treatment of nonalcoholic steatohepatitis in adults: present and future. Gastroenterol Res Pract. 2015;2015:732870. Epub 18 Mar 2015.
41. Meier C, Schwartz AV, Egger A, Lecka-Czernik B. Effects of diabetes drugs on the skeleton. Bone 2015, Epub ahead of print.
42. Ng TP, Feng L, Yap KB, Lee TS, Tan CH, Winblad B. Long-term metformin usage and cogni-tive function among older adults with diabetes. J Alzheimers Dis. 2014;41:61–8.
43. Cheng C, Lin CH, Tsai YW, Tsai CJ, Chou PH, Lan TH. Type 2 diabetes and antidiabetic medications in relation to dementia. J Gerontol A Biol Sci Med Sci. 2014;69:1299–305.
44. Biemans E, Hart HE, Rutten GE, Cuellar Renteria VG, Kooijman-Buiting AM, Beulens JW. Cobalamin status and its relation with depression, cognition and neuropathy in patients with type 2 diabetes. Acta Diabetol. 2015;52:383–93.
45. Son HJ, Lee J, Lee SY, Kim EK, Park MJ, Kim KW, et al. Metformin attenuates experimental autoimmune arthritis through reciprocal regulation of Th17/Treg balance and osteoclastogen-esis. Mediators Inflamm. 2014;2014:973986.
46. Zhou Y, Zhang X, Gu C, Xia J. Diabetes mellitus is associated with breast cancer: systematic review, meta-analysis, and in silico reproduction. Panminerva Med. 2015;57:101–8.
47. Gardini S, Puntoni M, Heckman-Stoddard BM, Dunn BK, Ford L, DeCensi A, et al. Metformin and cancer risk and mortality: a systematic review and meta-analysis taking into account biases and confounders. Cancer Prev Res (Phila). 2014;7:867–85.
48. U.S. National Institutes of Health (NIH). www.clinicaltrials.gov. Accessed 1 June 2015.
49. Nobes JP, Langley SE, Klopper T, Russell-Jones D, Laing RW. A prospective, randomized pilot study evaluating the effects of metformin and lifestyle intervention on patients with pros-tate cancer receiving androgen deprivation therapy. BJU Int. 2012;109:1495–502.
50. Col NF, Ochs L, Springmann V, Aragaki AK, Chlebowski RT. Metformin and breast cancer risk: a meta-analysis and critical literature review. Breast Cancer Res Treat. 2012;135:639–46.

51. Stine JE, Bae-Jump V. Metformin and gynecologic cancers. Obstet Gynecol Surv. 2014;69:477–89.
52. Febbraro T, Lengyel E, Romero IL. Old drug, new trick: repurposing metformin for gynecologic cancers? Gynecol Oncol. 2014;135:614–21.
53. Yung MM, Chan DW, Liu VW, Yao KM, Ngan HY. Activation of AMPK inhibits cervical cancer cell growth through AKT/FOXO3a/FOXM1 signaling cascade. BMC Cancer. 2013;13:327.
54. Mei ZB, Zhang ZJ, Liu CY, Liu Y, Cui A, Liang ZL, et al. Survival benefits of metformin for colorectal cancer patients with diabetes: a systematic review and meta-analysis. PLoS One. 2014;9:e91818.
55. Rego DF, Pavan LM, Elias ST, De Luca Canto G, Guerra EN. Effects of metformin on head and neck cancer: a systematic review. Oral Oncol. 2015;51:416–22.
56. Zhang H, Gao C, Fang L, Zhao HC, Yao SK. Metformin and reduced risk of hepatocellular carcinoma in diabetic patients: a meta-analysis. Scand J Gastroenterol. 2013;48:78–87.
57. Lin JJ, Gallagher EJ, Sigel K, Mhango G, Galsky MD, Smith CB, et al. Survival of patients with stage IV lung cancer with diabetes treated with metformin. Am J Respir Crit Care Med. 2015;191:448–54.
58. Wu W, Merriman K, Nabaah A, Seval N, Seval D, Lin H, et al. The association of diabetes and anti-diabetic medications with clinical outcomes in multiple myeloma. Br J Cancer. 2014;111:628–36.
59. Wang Z, Lai ST, Xie L, Zhao JD, Ma NY, Zhu J, et al. Metformin is associated with reduced risk of pancreatic cancer in patients with type 2 diabetes mellitus: a systematic review and meta-analysis. Diabetes Res Clin Pract. 2014;106:19–26.
60. Yu H, Yin L, Jiang X, Sun X, Wu J, Tian H, et al. Effect of metformin on cancer risk and treatment outcome of prostate cancer: a meta-analysis of epidemiological observational studies. PLoS One. 2014;9:e116327.
61. Raval AD, Thakker D, Vyas A, Salkini M, Madhavan S, Sambamoorthi U. Impact of metformin on clinical outcomes among men with prostate cancer: a systematic review and meta-analysis. Prostate Cancer Prostatic Dis. 2015;18(2):110–21. Epub 10 Feb 2015.
62. Goodwin PJ, Parulekar WR, Gelmon KA, Shepherd LE, Ligibel JA, Hershman DL, et al. Effect of metformin vs placebo on weight and metabolic factors in NCIC CTG MA.32. J Natl Cancer Inst 2015;107, Epub ahead of print.
63. Jalving M, Gietema JA, Lefrandt JD, de Jong S, Reyners AK, Gans RO, et al. Metformin: taking away the cancer for cancer? Eur J Cancer. 2010;46:2369–80.
64. Shu Y, Brown C, Castro BA, et al. Effect of genetic variation in the organic cation transporter 1, OCT1, on metformin pharmacokinetics. Clin Pharmacol Ther. 2008;83:273–80.
65. Kahn BB, Alquier T, Carling D, Hardie DG. AMP-activated protein kinase: ancient energy gauge provides clues to modern understanding of metabolism. Cell Metabolism. 2005;108: 1167–74.
66. Zhou G, Myers R, Li Y, et al. Role of AMP-activated protein kinase in mechanism of metformin action. J Clin Invest. 2001;108:1167–74.
67. El-Mir MY, Nogueira V, Fontaine E, Averet N, Rigoulet M, Leverve X. Dimethylbiguanide inhibits cell respiration via an indirect effect on the respiratory chain complex 1. J Biol Chem. 2000;275:223–8.
68. Niraula S, Dowling RJ, Ennis M, et al. Metformin in early breast cancer: a prospective window of opportunity neoadjuvant study. Breast Cancer Res Treat. 2012;135:821–30.
69. Song CW, Lee H, Dings RP, Williams B, Powers J, Santos TD, et al. Metformin kills and radiosensitizes cancer cells and preferentially kills cancer stem cells. Sci Rep. 2012;2:362.
70. Lee H, Park HJ, Park CS, Oh ET, Choi BH, Williams B, et al. Response of breast cancer cells and cancer stem cells to metformin and hyperthermia alone or combined. PLoS One. 2014;9:e87979.
71. Pizzuti L, Vici P, Di Lauro L, Sergi D, Della Giulia M, Marchetti P, et al. Metformin and breast cancer: basic knowledge in clinical context. Cancer Treat Rev. 2015;41(5):441–7. Epub 17 Mar 2015.

72. Goodwin PJ, Ennis M, Pritchard KI, et al. Fasting insulin and outcome in early-stage breast: results of a prospective cohort study. J Clin Oncol. 2002;20:42–51.
73. Goodwin PJ, Ennis M, Pritchard KI, et al. Insulin- and obesity-related variables in early-stage breast cancer: correlations and time course of prognostic associations. J Clin Oncol. 2012;30:164–71.
74. Mijnhout GS, Kollen BJ, Alkhalaf A, Kleefstra N, Bilo HJ. Alpha lipoic acid for symptomatic peripheral neuropathy in patients with diabetes: a meta-analysis of randomized controlled trials. Int J Endocrinol. 2012;2012:456279.
75. Carbonelli MG, Di Renzo L, Bigioni M, Di Daniele N, De Lorenzo A, et al. Alpha-lipoic acid supplementation: a tool for obesity therapy? Curr Pharm Des. 2010;16:840–6.
76. Koh EH, Lee WJ, Lee SA, Kim EH, Cho EH, Jeong E, et al. Effects of alpha-lipoic acid on body weight in obese subjects. Am J Med. 2011;124:85e1–8.
77. Kim E, Park D-W, Choi S-H, Kim J-J, Cho H-S. A preliminary investigation of alpha-lipoic acid treatment of antipsychotic drug-induced weight gain in patients with schizophrenia. J Clin Psychopharmacol. 2008;28:138–46.
78. Pershadsingh HA. Alpha-lipoic acid: physiologic mechanisms and indications for the treatment of metabolic syndrome. Expert Opin Investig Drugs. 2007;16:291–302.
79. Cheng PY, Lee YM, Yen MH, Peng JC, Lam KK. Reciprocal effects of alpha-lipoic acid on adenosine monophosphate-activated protein kinase activity in obesity induced by ovariectomy in rats. Menopause. 2011;18:1010–7.
80. Chen WL, Kang CH, Wang SG, Lee HM. Alpha-lipoic acid regulates lipid metabolism through induction of sirtulin 1 (SIRT1) and activation of AMP-activated protein kinase. Diabetologia. 2012;55(6):1824–35. Epub 30 Mar 2012.
81. Wang Y, Ki X, Guo Y, Chan L, Guan X. Alpha-lipoic acid increases energy expenditure by enhancing adenosine monophosphate-activated protein kinase-peroxisome proliferator-activated receptor-gamma coactivator-1alpha signaling in the skeletal muscle of aged mice. Metabolism. 2010;59:967–76.
82. Thirunavukkarasu V, Anitha Nandhini AT, Anuradha CV. Lipoic acid attenuates hypertension and improves insulin sensitivity, kallikrein activity and nitrite levels in high fructose fed rats. J Comp Physiol B. 2004;174:587–92.
83. Vasdev S, Ford CA, Parai S, Longerich L, Gadag V. Dietary lipoic acid supplementation prevents fructose-induced hypertension in rats. Nutr Metab Cardiovasc Dis. 2000;10:339–46.
84. Lee WJ, Song KH, Koh EH, Won JC, Kim HS, Park HS, et al. Alpha-lipoic acid increases insulin sensitivity by activating AMPK in skeletal muscle. Biochem Biophys Res Commun. 2005;332:885–91.
85. Lee WJ, Lee IK, Kim HS, Kim YM, Koh EH, Won JC, et al. Alpha-lipoic acid prevents endothelial dysfunction in obese rats via activation of AMP-activated protein kinase. Arterioscler Thromb Vasc Biol. 2005;25:2488–94.
86. Kim MS, Park JY, Namkoong C, Jang PG, Ryu JW, Song HS, et al. Anti-obesity effects of alpha-lipoic acid mediated by suppression of hypothalamic AMP-activated protein kinase. Nat Med. 2004;10:727–33.
87. Gullo D, Evans JL, Sortino G, Goldfine ID, Vigneri R. Insulin autoimmune syndrome (Hirata Disease) in European Caucasians taking alpha-lipoic acid. Clin Endocrinol (Oxf). 2014;81:204–9.
88. Uchigata Y, Hirata Y, Iwamoto Y. Drug-induced insulin autoimmune syndrome. Diabetes Res Clin Pract. 2009;83:e19–20.
89. Kumar A, Ekavali, Chopra K, Mukherjee M, Pottabathini R, Dhull DK. Current knowledge and pharmacological profile of berberine: an update. Eur J Pharmacol. 2015;761:288–97. Epub ahead of print.
90. Pang B, Zhao LH, Zhou Q, Zhao TY, Wang H, Gu CJ, et al. Application of berberine on treating type 2 diabetes. Int J Endocrinol. 2015;2015:905749. Epub 11 Mar 2015.
91. McCarty MF. AMPK activation—protean potential for boosting healthspan. Age (Dordr). 2014;36:641–63.

92. Hardie DG. AMP-activated protein kinase: a cellular energy sensor with a key role in metabolic disorders and in cancer. Biochem Soc Trans. 2011;39:1–13.
93. Dong H, Zhao Y, Zhao L, Lu F. The effects of berberine on blood lipids: a systemic review and meta-analysis of randomized controlled trials. Planta Med. 2013;79:437–46.
94. Lan J, Zhao Y, Dong F, Yan Z, Zheng W, Fan J, et al. Meta-analysis of the effect and safety of berberine in the treatment of type 2 diabetes mellitus, hyperlipidemia and hypertension. J Ethnopharmacol. 2015;161:69–81.
95. Dong H, Wang N, Zhao L, Lu F. Berberine in the treatment of type 2 diabetes mellitus: a systemic review and meta-analysis. Evid Based Complement Alternat Med. 2012;2012:591654.
96. Wei W, Zhao H, Wang A, Sui M, Liang K, Deng H, et al. A clinical study on the short-term effect of berberine in comparison to metformin on the metabolic characteristics of women with polycystic ovary syndrome. Eur J Endocrinol. 2012;166:99–105.
97. Jabbarzadeh Kaboli P, Rahmat A, Ismail P, Ling KH. Targets and mechanisms of berberine, a natural drug with potential to treat cancer with potential special focus on breast cancer. Eur J Pharmacol. 2014;740:584–95.
98. Eyre H, Kahn R, Robertson RM, Clark NG, Doyle C, Hong Y, et al. Preventing cancer, cardiovascular disease, and diabetes: a common agenda for the American Cancer Society, American Diabetes Association, and the American Heart Association. Stroke. 2004;35:1999–2010.

Chapter 7
Rapid Review of Breast Cancer Treatment Side Effects and Dietary Supplement/ Integrative Options from A to Z: What Helps, Harms, or Does Nothing?

Introduction

It is critical to keep in mind, especially in this chapter that multiple lifestyle options exists that can improve or actually not improve and even exacerbate side effects from cancer treatments. And there are many integrative medicines, especially dietary supplements that can improve, have no impact or actually cause a side effect from cancer treatment to become worse! The purpose of this chapter just like the rest of this book is to cover all of those integrative medicines that work, have no effect or are worthless for multiple cancer treatment side effects. When applicable prescription drug treatments are mentioned and reviewed. Still, this chapter and the book is not intended to provide a summary or exhaustive list of the conventional prescription treatment options for these side effects from A to Z because it would not only create an unreadable voluminous text, but this also would not serve the purpose of this text—to simply provide a non-biased and objective review of the medical research in the area of breast cancer and integrative medicines, especially in regard to lifestyle changes and dietary supplements. This is the area of oncology that appears to have arguably the greatest current needs for more objective and educational attention to this issue.

• Anemia from hormone manipulation therapy/chemotherapy and/or neutropenia (Vitamin B12, folate, iron, copper, wheat grass juice)?
A. B12, folate, iron, copper
In prostate cancer when a man receives hormone suppressive treatment then a mild asymptomatic normochromic normocytic anemia can occur in 90 % of patients (acutely or chronically) and it is usually asymptomatic [1, 2]. This is due to testosterone being reduced to almost undetectable levels and this hormone is needed for red blood cell production. Thus, these cancer patients do not usually need iron, B12 or folic acid to improve anemia because it is not macrocytic or microcytic. It should be mentioned that the shape and size of the cells being produced are normal but the

© Springer International Publishing Switzerland 2016
M.A. Moyad, *Integrative Medicine for Breast Cancer*,
DOI 10.1007/978-3-319-23422-9_7

rate at which these cells are being produced is not maximum or normal. I often give the example of a factory producing widgets and the factory is producing or creating them correctly but it is not able to produce enough of them without some testosterone. And again, few dietary supplements are able to correct anemia in cancer patients unless it is more overt and caused by some rare situation of deficiency or because of a medication induced deficiency (e.g., acid reflux or metformin medications and B12 deficiency) [3].

In women with breast cancer on aromatase inhibitors these drugs prevent the conversion of androstenedione and testosterone to estrogen, and there is arguably a chance of erythrocytosis/polycythemia (similar to that observed with exogenous androgens), albeit small, that has been described in some case studies that resolved with drug cessation [4]. And there is a concern with erythrocytosis when aromatase inhibitors are utilized in other medical settings [5].

Patients and health care professionals often inquire about the need for dietary supplements to ameliorate anemia associated with breast cancer treatments. However, similar to what was mentioned earlier a supplement can rarely provide a benefit for these treatment-based anemias unless a deficiency was caused by medication or another lucid situation. For example, a breast cancer patient on a chronic proton pump inhibitor (PPI) could theoretically increase the risk of vitamin B12 deficiency and/or iron absorption issues [6]. The drug metformin can also cause vitamin B12 deficiency [3]. Additionally, weight gain and obesity are associated with a reduction in iron from the generalized inflammatory reaction caused by adipose tissue and an increased hepcidin concentration, which can impair duodenal iron absorption [7]. Chronic use of high-dose zinc can also create a copper deficiency that can result in a sideroblastic anemia and neutropenia [8]. And it is not unusual today for some cancer patients to be ingesting high-doses of zinc (along with other standardized compounds) as part of their macular degeneration supplement because this regimen has shown an ability to prevent vision loss in randomized controlled trials (AREDS), but patients should also seek a product with 2 mg of copper in these eye health products to prevent this issue.

B. Wheat grass juice (mini-multivitamin but with nausea and allergies)?

Thus, despite a paucity of data to ingest dietary supplements when experiencing anemia from cancer treatment itself and occasional small publication can invoke enormous interest among patients and alternative medicine enthusiasts. For example a pilot study of 60 cc (2 fluid ounces) of wheat grass (*Triticum aestivum*) juice daily versus a control group in breast cancer patients during the first three cycles of chemotherapy showed some promise [9]. This was based on a significantly lower rate ($p=0.01$) of 5 "censoring events" (premature termination of chemotherapy, dose reduction or initiating GCSF or epoetin) versus 15 in the control arm. The effect of wheat grass appeared to have a greater impact on reducing hematologic toxicity (17 % versus 37 %, $p=0.04$) with reductions in neutropenic fever events or neutropenic infections. The authors suggested "apigenin" (bioflavonoid) might inhibit the adhesion of white blood cells to endothelial cells. Another theory is "chlorophyll" (highly concentrated in wheat grass) resembles hemoglobin and has antioxidant activity, as well as other nutrients in wheat grass, which could provide some benefits. Although 73 % of the patients (22 out of 30) in the wheat grass arm had difficulty ingesting the juice because the pungent grassy taste and six patients had worsening nausea. A total of 20 % of the patients could not complete 9 weeks of wheat grass ingestion due to progressive nausea. And this increased incidence of nausea has been reported in another study of patients with inflammatory bowel disease [10]. Thus, wheat grass juice itself is not benign in cancer patients and the statistical clinical outcome difference, which has not received further publications in the past decade may be partially explained by the lack of a placebo group so there was no true blinding. Additionally, wheat grass juice has somewhat of a mini-multivitamin or liquid nutritional support feature to it. Again, it contains chlorophyll (majority of the solid content), but also 18 amino acids and the following vitamins and minerals and dosage per 100 ml or 100 cc:

- Vitamin C (25 mg)
- Vitamin E (8 mg)
- Carotene (2 mg)
- Potassium (57 mg)
- Phosphorous (8 mg)
- Calcium (2 mg)
- Sulfur (2 mg)
- Magnesium (2 mg)
- Sodium (1 mg)
- Aluminum (0.3 mg)
- Zinc (0.02 mg)
- Copper (0.007 mg)

An older observational study of wheat grass juice also displayed some potential benefits for a lower rate of transfusion, which some experts again credit to chlorophyll having a structural similarity to heme so that production of hemoglobin can occur at a faster rate [11, 12]. There is also some mixed evidence with thalassemia major that wheat grass (tablets in some cases) may reduce transfusions [12–14], but in a 1-year study no clinically significant benefit was documented [13]. The preliminary research sounds interesting but again little has been done recently on this alternative medicine and the mechanism of action has not been thoroughly explored. If a patient wanted to consume 60–90 cc (2–3 ounces) of wheat grass juice the nutrient profile is diverse and low enough in its inherent concentration that it would be somewhat similar to ingesting a children's multivitamin. It should be kept in mind that wheat grass allergies are also not uncommon and if nausea is already an issue this should be completely avoided. Regardless, diet and dietary supplements have a minimal role in preventing anemia or neutropenia caused by conventional breast cancer treatment and this should be explained to patients to save them time, effort, money and increase safety.

• Aromatase inhibitor arthralgia (AIA) and/or aromatase inhibitor associated musculoskeletal symptoms (AIMSS)

Arthralgia, which is defined as pain and/or stiffness in the joints, is experienced by 50 % of breast cancer patients treated with aromatase inhibitors (AIs), and it is the number one reason for poor compliance on these medications [15].

A. Exercise = HOPE (aerobic, resistance, tai chi, yoga, others ... acupuncture ...)

It appears that estrogen deprivation appears to be the cause of arthralgia, but there is also a notably higher risk of general joint issues with aging. It is theorized and plausible that exercise increases perfusion to tissues and increase maximum oxygen utilization, reduces fatigue, and improves mood and range of motion [16–18]. And the preliminary impact of exercise on AIA is profound. For example a randomized 1-year trial of 121 breast cancer survivors were assigned to exercise or 150 min per week of aerobic exercise and supervised resistance training twice a week or usual care [16]. This was one of the first such trials to address this issue in terms of physical activity and it was known as the HOPE (Hormones and Physical Exercise) study. Worst pain scores were reduced by 29 % (1.6 points) at 1-year with exercise versus a 3 % increase (3 %) among those with usual care ($p < 0.001$). Pain severity and interference and Disabilities of the Arm, Shoulder and Hand (DASH) and the Western Ontario and McMaster Universities Osteoarthritis (WOMAC) index were also reduced significantly in the exercise group versus usual care (all $p < 0.001$). On average, pain scores in women were reduced from moderate at baseline to mild at the end of the exercise program and additional benefits included an increase in fitness, upper- and lower-body strength and weight loss. Interestingly, some benefit was found after 3 months but maximum benefit was observed after 1-year and these patients did have a past history of inactivity. The aerobic exercise intervention involved primarily brisk walking or similar intensity exercises such as stationary bicycling. Exercise was initiated at 50 % of maximal heart rate and increased over the first month to 60–80 % of maximal heart rate for the rest of the study. The resistance protocol consisted of six exercises (8–12 repetitions for three sets and if an individual could lift the same weight 12 times during each set then the weight was increased to the next smallest increment) including three upper- and three lower body activities:

– Bench press
– Latissimus pull down
– Seated row
– Leg press
– Leg extension
– Leg curl

Several other clinical studies and even home-based programs continue to demonstrate benefit against arthralgia including a simple 5-day a week 30 min a day walking program [17, 18]. Since weight gain or obesity has the potential to exacerbate joint pain, another benefit of exercise is simply weight loss, which reduces stress on the joint itself. Regardless, numerous other types of exercise including yoga and tai chi are also promising [19]. One trial of acupuncture demonstrated a 50 % reduction in pain versus no change in the sham arm [20], but more trials are needed because other studies demonstrating no benefit have also been published [21] and most studies include only a small number of evaluable patients. Thus, a large multicenter randomized trial is being conducted by SWOG to provide more clarity on the impact of acupuncture in this setting.

B. Glucosamine-sulfate (up to 1500 mg/day, usually derived from shellfish) + Chondroitin-sulfate (up to 1200 mg/day, usually derived from bovine sources) = GAIT, LEGS, MOVES, ...

Glucosamine and chondroitin are both naturally found in human cartilage and both of these compounds are believed to have multiple benefits including local anti-inflammatory effects within joints and even increase production of other joint supportive compounds [3]. Glucosamine is a hexosamine sugar (amino acid sugar or aminomonosaccharide) and a basic building block for the production of glycosaminoglycans (GAG) and proteoglycans that are important parts of articular cartilage and synovial fluid. It is naturally produced by the body and widely distributed in connective tissue, including cartilage. Glucosamine supplements are generally derived from crab shells or shells of sea creatures but there are now some sources of glucosamine that are vegetarian friendly that can be derived from corn for example. Patients with a shellfish allergy should avoid taking it unless it comes from a non-shellfish source. It may help with osteoarthritis joint pain and it now also comes in a liquid low-calorie form. Doses of 500–1500 mg/day of glucosamine sulfate versus placebo may be associated with a reduction in pain and an improvement in function versus placebo. Some experts believe that even if glucosamine does not help with pain it may improve cartilage structure. The potential side effects of glucosamine are unknown at this time, but individual reports of blood thinning (do not combine with warfarin), stomach upset and excess gas have been reported in some cases. Check for the amount of sodium in the glucosamine supplement because it is a high source of sodium but even the cheapest glucosamine supplements are able to reduce the amount and many only contain 20–50 mg of sodium per 1–2 capsules.

Chondroitin sulfate (CS) is a GAG found in proteoglycans of articular cartilage or extracellular matrix of connective tissue [3]. It is a complex carbohydrate molecule that helps retain water in cartilage. The supplements are generally produced from shark, pig, or cow (bovine) cartilage, but now there are some potential algae or fermentation derived non-animal sources coming to market (the problem in the past and currently is the cost of producing a line of these non-animal based alternatives). It may increase proteoglycan synthesis in the chondrocytes (cells) of articular cartilage. Doses of 800–1200 mg a day have provided some pain relief by itself or when combined with Glucosamine. Some have argued that the dosage should be divided over 2–3 different times during the day but this is controversial. In fact, more recent studies and longer studies of chondroitin sulfate have found the potential for this supplement to reduce cartilage volume loss. Hand and knee pain appear to have more data compared to lower back issues.

Two recent randomized clinical trials (LEGS and MOVES) and a surprising objective extensive analysis need to be reviewed for the reader, and again provides an excellent background to at least extend the testing of these supplements with AIA [22–24]. The first known as "LEGS" (Long-term Evaluation of Glucosamine Sulfate) was a double-blind randomized placebo-controlled trial in over 600 patients reporting chronic knee pain and evidence of medial tibio-femoral compartment narrowing [22]. Patients were assigned glucosamine sulfate (source not immediately specified) 1500 mg, chondroitin sulfate 800 mg (bovine-derived), both or placebo over 2 years (product was provided by Sanofi-Aventis Consumer Healthcare). Although there were no statistically significant symptomatic advantages at the end of the trial, the group utilizing glucosamine and chondroitin in combination experienced a significant ($p = 0.05$) reduction in joint space narrowing after 2 years versus placebo (mean difference 0.10 mm). This would suggest that this supplement combination has the potential of slowing the osteoarthritis process at least from imaging studies. No differences in side effects were observed between the groups.

Additionally, a recent double-blind multicenter randomized trial of over 600 patients found 1500 mg of Glucosamine hydrochloride and 1200 mg of chondroitin sulfate (Droglican, Bioiberica, S.A., Barcelona, Spain) to be of comparable efficacy to prescription 200 mg daily celecoxib in decreasing pain, stiffness, functional limitation and joint effusion after 6 months in participants with painful knee osteoarthritis and with a similar side effect profile (known as the "MOVES" trial or Multicentre Osteoarthritis Intervention trial with SYSADOA) [23].

A recent Cochrane Database review also found adequate support of efficacy for chondroitin in osteoarthritis and a low risk of toxicity after reviewing 43 past randomized clinical trials with over 4900 participants given this supplement versus over 4100 utilizing a placebo or comparison product [24]. Many of these trials were of low quality so the manuscript was a cautionary endorsement of this supplement except more recent higher quality trials such as LEGS and MOVES should add more quality evidence to these objective clinical reviews. One of the more notable controversial clinical trials of these supplements was the "GAIT" trial (Glucosamine/chondroitin Arthritis Intervention Trial), which reported no impact with these supplements at 24 weeks when the data was analyzed. However, when examining the subgroup of patients with moderate to severe pain at baseline the actual response rate was significantly higher with glucosamine and chondroitin together versus placebo (79.2 % versus 54.3 %, $p = 0.002$) [25]. Thus, with this as background it appears logical to believe that these agents could have some preliminary efficacy against AIA assuming there are some related mechanisms of action.

Glucosamine sulfate (1500 mg/day from a shellfish source) and chondroitin sulfate (1200 mg/day from a bovine source; both supplements from Thorne Research-Sandpoint, ID) utilized for 24 weeks in postmenopausal women experiencing pain from AI participated in a single-arm, open-label phase 2 study [26]. This group demonstrated a significant ($p < 0.05$) improvement in pain and function, and 50 % of the patients experienced 20 % or more improvement in pain, stiffness, and function. Additionally, statistical and clinical improvements in arthralgias and myalgias were reported at 12 and 24 weeks (all $p < 0.05$). There were no changes in estradiol levels and the most common side effects were headache (28 %), dyspepsia (15 %), and nausea (17 %). However, at baseline 47 % of the participants used pain medications and there were no reported differences in medication use from baseline to 12 or week 24. There was a 30 % dropout rate partially due to the high number of capsules needed for daily use (six capsules per day, each containing 250 mg of glucosamine and 200 mg chondroitin). Patients could use a glucosamine/chondroitin liquid that could replace pills/capsules, but comparative attention should be paid to the caloric content and cost of these newer liquid options. Other novel options include powders or packets that are portable and can be mixed with water produced by numerous companies (Emergen-C® Joint Health …). Pill count is indeed an issue from my experience with glucosamine and chondroitin as well as omega-3 fatty acids that could be resolved with the latitude in delivery methods now available in the supplement industry.

C. Omega-3 fatty acids (SWOG S0927 = power of the placebo)
Omega-3 fatty acids, especially EPA and DHA have preliminary evidence to suggest they may help patients with AIA [27, 28]. For example, mechanistically they can block the conversion of arachidonic acid to prostaglandin and leukotrienes, which can cause decreases in inflammation. It is of interest that perhaps even an autoimmune-like component or etiology of AIA is plausible based on animal models where aromatase is eliminated and symptoms similar to Sjogrens syndrome occurs. And the preliminary research for omega-3 and even -6 products to reduce dry eye (not dry mouth) for example is intriguing [3]. An older meta-analysis found significant changes in pain, stiffness, painful/tender joints, and NSAID usage with omega-3 supplementation for inflammatory joint pain (not AIA specific but of interest) [27].

A well-done 24-week randomized multicenter placebo-controlled trial (known as "SWOG S0927") of 240 patients found a 50 % reduction in pain/stiffness in both the 3360 mg/day omega-3 fatty acid group as well as the placebo group (soybean/corn oil) [29]. Triglyceride levels were significantly reduced (-22.1 mg/dl) in the omega-3 group versus no change in the placebo arm ($p = 0.01$). Patients utilized six capsules per day and each omega-3 capsule contained 560 mg of EPA plus DHA in a 40-to-20 ratio (Ocean Nutrition, Dartmouth, Nova Scotia, Canada). However, why no difference could be found may also have to do with the choice of a potential anti-inflammatory placebo or simply lack of efficacy of omega-3. Regardless, the question needs to be raised that a 50 % improvement may still be an option with these supplements but the choice of six capsules a day appears excessive in my opinion and patients could use a children's flavored omega-3 liquid that only requires multiple teaspoons a day or 1–2 tablespoons and no pills/capsules. Again, it would be of interest for future clinical trials to utilize more realistic and easier to ingest delivery systems in the future since they are available to the consumer and clinician now.

Thus, plain old cheap fish oil (from sardines and anchovies and/or mackerel) with the two active ingredients (EPA and DHA) have preliminary positive data for overall joint health, but so does Krill oil now and even New Zealand Green Lipped Mussel [3]. And all these companies claim that their omega-3 product is somehow different than the competitors but in my opinion this is not based on strong evidence! Omega-3 compounds from anchovies, krill or green-lipped muscle (Perna Canaliculus) are going to be structurally similar and maybe some may require higher or slightly lower dosages or smaller pills. I tell patients to first purchase the lowest cost product and see if it helps. Most companies that sell cheap fish oil have been able to concentrate their pills so all you need is 1–2/day or if you cannot take a fish oil pill buy a flavored children's liquid supplement as mentioned earlier. In fact, about one teaspoon (5 ml) per day will give you over 1000 mg of the active ingredients (EPA and DHA) in fish oil in many cases. So, fish oil at 1000–2000 mg/day of the active ingredients (EPA and DHA) has preliminary evidence in the veterinary and human world that it may reduce aches and pains in the joints. Higher doses might even work better but this should receive more research. Some Krill oil enthusiasts would argue that one tiny Krill oil pill also has "phospholipids" and some data to suggest that are as bioavailable as a much higher dose of fish oil so the price difference works out to be the same. This sounds interesting but until a head-to-head longer study with relevant clinical endpoints is made, it is more theory compared to fact. If a patient has a shellfish allergy keep in mind that Krill is also a shellfish folks. Prescription omega-3 oil in my opinion is of questionable value compared to over the counter brands. This is due to the general use of tiny fish such as anchovies and sardines that do not live a long life and have plenty of omega-3 then they are going to have little to no mercury and most other contaminants (many of those are water soluble are not carried with the final oil product)! So, in this case the smartest business move for the fish oil business turned to provide an unexpected quality control advantage for the consumer! Additionally, in another area of arthritis known as "rheumatoid arthritis" that is a chronic inflammatory disease of the joints and bones there has been a consistent modest benefit for fish oil on pain and joint swelling, morning stiffness, and the ability to reduce the amount of conventional pain medication usage. It is this kind of track record that has to allow for the benefit of the doubt when it comes to this supplement for arthritic pain and as a potential option for some AI patients. If a patient is experiencing gastrointestinal problems (like nausea, diarrhea, or discomfort) or any skin abnormalities (itching, eruptions, allergies) or easy bleeding then your fish oil dose it either too high and switching to an enteric-coated option (if primarily GI issues) or a different product should be considered.

D. Vitamin D (Definitive association but causation? Negative acute phase reactant? VITAL? Deficiency and dosing issues?)
The vitamin D deficiency theory, or even the potential suggestion that vitamin D could significantly improve joint or muscle issued from AIs is intriguing, and has indirect but not consistent direct clinical evidence [28, 30]. Vitamin D deficiency and insufficiency is common in women taking AIs. Proximal muscle strength could improve with vitamin D, estrogen increases the conversion of inactive to active vitamin D and activates the vitamin D receptor. Preliminary research suggests higher blood levels of vitamin D with or without supplementation are associated with a lower risk of joint pain from Ais [30, 31].

And in the still yet to be published (since the publication of this text) randomized VITAL trial (Vitamin D for Arthralgias from Letrozole), 160 postmenopausal women with a blood vitamin D level less than 40 ng/ml received 30,000 IU oral vitamin D3 weekly for 24 weeks or placebo. Approximately 38 % of the women on vitamin D reported an increase in pain compared to 61 % of the controls ($p=0.008$) [32]. Still, peer review and more rigorous investigation are needed to prove absolute cause and effect. The good news for patients is that these vitamin D interventions can be attempted to improve AI compliance in some benefits with the benefit exceeding the risk for most.

Vitamin D3 has been suggested as a treatment for AIMSS, but again no rigorous trials of more moderate dosages of vitamin D have been conducted until recently (US study—Minneapolis and Washington, DC) [33]. A total of 113 postmenopausal women ingesting 600 IU D3 ($n=56$) or 4000 IU D3 ($n=57$) for 6 months was conducted and after this time the 25-OH vitamin D test was 33.8 ng/ml for the low-dose versus 46 ng/ml for the high-dose group. And no difference was found for AIMSS or other measures such as pain or stiffness between groups.

What appeared to be complicating matters are several issues including the potential for 25-OH vitamin D to potentially function as a negative acute phase reactant [34]. A recent systematic review of eight relevant studies found that six demonstrated a drop in blood levels of vitamin D with an initial inflammatory insult and in another study there was a suggestion of hemodilution with no impact on inflammation [35]. Regardless, there is sufficient preliminary data to suggest 25-OH vitamin D can act as a negative acute phase reactant and could also be reduced with multiple other patient parameters such as weight gain. Thus, the question remains—does vitamin D really ameliorate AIA or do individuals with greater health parameters and a higher probability of having a sufficient vitamin D level (with or without supplementation) give the perception that vitamin D is effective when in reality it is the health status of the patient that really determines outcome (not vitamin D supplementation)?! This needs to be addressed and may explain some of the negative findings in other clinical trials outside of breast cancer.

It is of interest in osteoarthritis that in a 2-year randomized trial of a moderate dosage (2000 IU/day increased serum levels 16 mg/dl) of vitamin D in individuals with a baseline BMI of 30 and 25-OH vitamin D of 22 ng/ml was not helpful [36]. Higher dosages, especially in overtly deficient patients (10 ng/ml or less for example) are needed to resolve some of the issues as to who are the best (if any) candidates for vitamin D supplementation in regards to joint and muscle issues.

E. Miscellaneous (capsaicin, curcumin, SAM-e, ...)
There are a plethora of osteoarthritis dietary supplements that theoretically could be tested and utilized for AIA, but have not received adequate attention in this area [3, 37].

F. Capsaicin (topical OTC and Rx looks good but no research in AIA?)
Over the counter joint creams or gels such as capsaicin (ingredient from the hot pepper plant that makes it "hot") seem to work real well for hand arthritis, and for the knee, but not very well on the hip because that joint is too deep in the body to be

impacted by the topical cream. In at least five double-blind randomized clinical trials participants used 0.025 % capsaicin four times daily for 4–12 weeks. In other trials 0.015 % capsaicin was applied once per day for 6 weeks and 0.075 % four times daily for 4 weeks. In all of these clinical trials (*especially 0.025–0.075 % up to four times a day*) capsaicin was found to be significantly more effective in improving pain compared to placebo. It appears that the longer the study, the greater the reduction in pain severity and benefit. Redness and burning sensation are common because of the way this herbal topical works and it should be applied with gloves to the site of concern and that area covered if possible to preventing spreading of this substance to sensitive areas (especially eyes, mouth, …). Capsaicin has also become a well-documented conventional option for painful diabetic peripheral neuropathy [38], and even can be obtained as a higher strength (8 %) prescription patch option that has efficacy against HIV neuropathy and post-herpetic neuralgia [39]. Thus, with all of this background and evidence with over the counter or prescription strength capsaicin where is the research on AIA? There is even some preliminary evidence for topical capsaicin to improve post-mastectomy pain syndrome at a concentration of 0.025–0.075 % [40, 41]. And there appears to be far greater interest in the potential antitumor effects of capsaicin (via apoptosis induction) [42] versus AIS. Capsaicin may have some of its own aromatase inhibitory potential from preliminary basic science research [43]. Still, most AI-related symptoms or arthralgia appear to impact the joints close to the skin such as wrist/hands, ankles/feet, elbows, and knees more often [44], which is precisely where topical capsaicin could provide the most benefit. It would be of interest even if a case study or case series could be published to help resolve this issue and whether it could be helpful or harmful. Unfortunately no initiated or ongoing clinical trials of capsaicin and breast cancer could be found at the clinical trials.gov website. Capsaicin dietary supplement pills are also available now but have no adequate research in the area of arthralgia.

G. Curcumin (needs more research with joint pain)
Curcumin (diferuloylmethane) is a yellow coloring agent/pigment that is derived from turmeric (*Curcuma longa*), and it is a spice commonly found in curry powders, and appears to have been crowned the king or queen of anti-inflammatory agents by so many pseudo experts. What it needs, are more clinical trials ASAP [3]. Of course I am excited about the preliminary data that curcumin can reduce the pain of OA [45, 46], but with such a crowded field of potentially beneficial supplements "you have to earn your way into this crowd" if what I often cite to patients. And very high doses of curcumin in some studies have the ability to create abdominal fullness and pain, and the bioavailability of this supplement is not good and needs assistance (another molecule attached to it for increased absorption) [3]. It is for this reason an even cursory view of the medical literature will suggest that a variety of commercialized highly bioavailable curcumin powders mixed with other ingredients might have efficacy against arthritis or joint issues.

Curcumin has received some phase I research as a potential synergistic agent with chemotherapy for breast cancer and it also receives numerous clinical reviews [47, 48], but it is in need of effective clinical trials. Perhaps, most of the interesting work thus far has been published in pancreatic cancer where higher doses have been utilized (8 g) with chemotherapy and no patients, among 18 in one trial, experienced a partial or complete response but it appeared that median survival time could have been increased compared to retrospective controls so more study is needed [49]. Another small study of advanced pancreatic patients ($n = 17$) needed to lower the 8-g curcumin dose to 4 g because of abdominal complaints and efficacy appeared "modest" with only one potential partial response [50]. Another issue here is simply the sheer number of pills (16 or more) used in these clinical trials. This needs to be resolved for research to realistically continue along with some more impressive clinical data.

H. SAM-e (another missed opportunity for AIA?)
S-adenosylmethionine (SAM-e) is a nutritional supplement that has received a lot of attention recently in the USA because it is widely used in Europe for a variety of conditions especially osteoarthritis and depression (see depression section) [3]. SAM-e is a naturally occurring sulfur-containing compound produced from the amino acid L-methionine and adenosine triphosphate (ATP). Researchers are not sure how it can control pain but it does play a primary role in several pathways in the body including transmethylation, transsulfuration, and aminopropylation, which basically suggests it could impact multiple physiologic locations where it can help to ameliorate pain. SAM-e was actually brought into the USA in 1999 as a dietary supplement to improve joint health. In Europe it is a prescription drug in some countries and it is also given as an IV drug.

A recent review of numerous clinical trials of SAM-e compared to placebo or NSAIDs (most over the counter pain relievers and some prescription anti-inflammatory medications including Celebrex) concluded that the existing evidence points toward at least an equal efficacy of this supplement for osteoarthritis compared to NSAIDs and with a lower rate of side effects—in fact those taking SAM-e were almost 60 % less likely to experience a side effect compared to NSAIDs [51, 52]. SAM-e appears to have a slower onset of action for pain reduction but by the end of the first or second month of use the efficacy is again similar to over the counter and many popular pain medication.

SAM-e may help to build one component of cartilage based on some laboratory (not human) studies [3, 51]. More clinical studies are always needed especially again popular prescription medication and a placebo. The effective dosages have ranged from 600 mg to 1200 mg/day for at least 30–90 days usually on an empty stomach. Lower dosages of SAM-e did not use pills but were given IV (400 mg) in other countries. The amount of time SAM-e was tested in clinical trials was from 10 days to 3 months. The most common duration of treatment was 30 days, which means that overall SAM-e has not been tested in a long-term study (6–12 months). The average amount of time individuals were suffering from OA before receiving SAM-e was almost 6 years. SAM-e may reduce morning stiffness, swelling, pain at rest and in motion, and improving range of motion and walking ability and could even reduce the popping or cracking sounds associated with OA. More safety data are needed with these supplements and they are not low-cost. An older concern with SAM-e is that it may increase blood levels of homocysteine, which may be an indirect marker of cardiovascular risk and some doctors recommend taking B-vitamins (B6, B12, folate) with SAM-e but recent studies show this is not as much of an issue and maybe a non-issue [3].

Taking both NSAIDs and SAM-e is a possibility based on safety but has not really been studied. SAM-e has been studied primarily for knee osteoarthritis and some studies of hip and spine osteoarthritis but whether or not pain reduction in other locations can occur with SAM-e is not known. Finally, the biggest side effect of SAM-e in my experience is prohibitive cost because SAM-e can be more expensive than most over the counter pain medications. A review of lower cost retail sources (national pharmacies and shopping chains) could provide a more realistically priced SAM-e. Thus, the consistent preliminary efficacy of SAM-e in osteoarthritis would suggest this could have some efficacy in other areas such AIS, especially since there are anecdotal reports of NSAIDs providing benefits for some patients [30].

• **Bone loss and sarcopenia (muscle loss)**

A. Weight gain (no longer an advantage?)

Obesity appears to increase bone mineral density (via greater aromatization and increased estrogen) which is a quantitative observation [53], but what about the qualitative aspects of bone health? Recent evidence suggests a challenging novel and now evidence-based theory that weight gain could be detrimental to bone health (not beneficial because of increased aromatase conversion to create more estrogen). For example, a review 8833 abdominal or thoracic CT scans in patients aged 18–65 years old from one major health system found adipose tissue appeared to infiltrate into muscle and bones [54]. Even when these results were adjusted for age, sex, and BMI there were significant correlation between visceral adipose tissue and lower bone and muscle quality. It is possible that weight gain at an early or older age is associated with poor bone quality and less bone formation. This also supports the notion that obesity may be associated with an increased risk of bone fracture. Muscle also surrounded by fat tissue appears to also lower muscle quality.

B. Weight loss = more vitamin D?

What are some other benefits of weight loss apart from the potential to increase the qualitative aspects of bone? It appears that despite weight gain being associated with lower blood levels of vitamin D, weight loss could "naturally" increase vitamin D levels. A total of 439 overweight and obese postmenopausal women (mean age 58 years) were assigned to one of four groups: diet change, exercise, diet and exercise, or control. Diet change consisted of caloric reduction (total intake of 1200–2000 calories/day), and exercise consisted of 45 min of moderate to more high intense aerobic activity 5 days a week [55]. Vitamin D levels were measured at the beginning and after 12 months. Individuals that lost <5 %, 5–9.9 %, 10–14.9 %, or ≥15 % of their initial weight experienced significant increases in vitamin D blood levels of 2.1, 2.7, 3.3, and 7.7 ng/ml. Lower or higher baseline blood levels did not have an impact on the effectiveness of the interventions for weight loss. So, the researchers concluded that weight loss via caloric restriction or exercise could potentially increase vitamin D levels without ingesting more of this supplement.

C. Aerobic + resistance exercise = stops bone loss? Improves muscle mass, Reduces Falls ... AI muscle advantages with testosterone?

A 1-year randomized trial of aerobic and resistance activity three times a week (45–60 min) in breast cancer survivors, including 40 % on aromatase inhibitors (AI), preserved bone mineral density (BMD) at the lumbar spine versus controls (0.47 versus −2.13 %; $p=0.001$) [56]. Interestingly, the increases in lean mass were actually higher in women on AI versus controls not on AI ($p=0.01$). One theory is higher free testosterone found in women on AI could improve muscle response. A previous smaller 6-month randomized trial found that 150 min per week of exercise that included brisk walking could also maintain BMD in post-menopausal breast cancer survivors [57]. Clinicians should emphasize some form of upper- and lower-body resistance activity to enhance bone and muscle effects. A series of exercises from a variety of past studies in breast and prostate cancer effective trials were culled and placed in 178 [1, 3]. Table 7.1 is not intended to have a patient following this specific program 2–3 days a week but rather review the diverse upper- and lower-body exercises used in past studies. Whether or not a patient and clinician choose 2 or 3 upper- and lower-body exercises from the list (as I recommend) is between the patient and clinician. Again, the list is not intended to be the exercises conducted at one time but rather to include a few of these in an individualized regimen.

Table 7.1 A collection of upper and lower resistance exercises that have been utilized in some permutation in breast and prostate cancer studies [1, 3]

Weight-lifting exercise	Initial repetition (the lowest weight with which you are comfortable)	Additional repetition (plus 2–5 pounds or 1–2 kg of weight)
Biceps curl	12–15	8–10
Chest press	12–15	8–10
Latissimus pull-down	12–15	8–10
Modified curl-ups	12–15	8–10
Overhead press	12–15	8–10
Triceps extension	12–15	8–10
Calf raises	12–15	8–10
Leg curl	12–15	8–10
Leg extension	12–15	8–10
Spine bone building exercise[a]	8–12 modified push-ups	8–12 modified push-ups

[a]Some doctors or trainers also like to include a back lift in order to strengthen the spine. A small or low weight that is shaped like a small sac, cushion, bag, or pillow (just a few pounds or kilograms) is placed on the upper back between the shoulder blades. While lying on your stomach, do 8–12 modified push-ups (stomach stays on the floor, hands clasped together behind your head, and lift your upper body up then down, up and down). This places resistance on the spine and may improve bone mineral density in this area

D. Normal intakes of calcium and vitamin D (Calcium normalization for bone/muscle health and vitamin D for muscle health/fall prevention and calcium + vitamin D to enhance prescription osteoporosis medications)

The Women's Health Initiative (WHI) was a double-blind, placebo-controlled clinical trial and the largest to address the issue of calcium and vitamin D supplementation [58, 59]. This trial included 36,282 postmenopausal US women to 1000 mg elemental calcium carbonate plus 400 IU of vitamin D3 (OsCal®, GSK) or placebo for 7 years. The mean BMI was 29 and there were a greater number of obese versus overweight women in the trial, which interestingly appears to reflect the current US population. The primary endpoint was the reduction in hip fractures, and secondarily total fracture and colorectal cancer. Calcium and vitamin D supplementation significantly increased hip and total bone mineral density (BMD) versus placebo ($p < 0.01$), but there was no overall evidence to suggest a reduction in hip or total fracture risk. However, among women compliant with the supplements (80 % or more utilization) there was a 29 % reduction in hip fracture risk, but this relationship cannot be accepted as solid evidence compared to an intention-to-treat analysis. In addition, further analysis found those not taking personal calcium or vitamin D supplements at baseline experienced a significant reduction in the risk of hip fracture (−38 %). There was an increased in kidney stone risk and there were no impacts on cardiovascular event or colorectal cancer risk but there was a suggestion of a reduction in breast cancer risk and total invasive cancer risk. This largest study of its kind continues to suggest that normalization or increased calcium and vitamin D supplementation could improve bone mineral density and reduce hip fracture risk [60].

A recent extensive analysis of the calcium and vitamin D supplementation data from the US Preventive Services Task Force found treatment of vitamin D deficiency in some asymptomatic person might prevent falls (not fractures) [61, 62]. And concluded their other findings the following way:

"Treatment with vitamin D, with or without calcium, may be associated with decreased risk for mortality and falls in older or institutionalized adults. Vitamin D treatment did not reduce fracture risk …" This is a critical initial finding from the research, which in my opinion also suggests breast cancer patients should normalize their calcium and vitamin D intakes to maximize the benefits of bone loss prevention and especially falls, which could lead to an increased risk of fractures. And there is enough evidence from these past reviews of the data that calcium and vitamin D are also integral for muscle health and coordination.

Additionally, most major trials of drug interventions to prevent bone loss and fractures in breast cancer patients, including denosumab and zoledronic acid, utilized some form of calcium (1000 mg/day) and vitamin D supplementation (400 or more IU per day) or normalization of intake to ensure adequate responses to these bone medications [63, 64]. Thus, when these drugs received FDA approval in breast cancer it was due to phase 3 trial evidence of the drug and calcium and vitamin D in combination (not by itself).

Table 7.2 The most popular forms of calcium supplements on the market and the benefits and limitations of each of them [1, 3]. Keep in mind that many of these supplements also can be utilized as a liquid supplemental option if needed

Type of calcium supplement	Elemental calcium by weight	Comments
Calcium carbonate (*Note*: this is the same compound used in over the counter antacid or heartburn supplements like TUMS or Rolaids)	40 % (fewer pills to take to achieve your goal when pill has a greater percentage or content of elemental calcium)	– Most clinically tested (WHI used OsCal supplements …) by itself and/or with prescription osteoporosis medications – Requires fewest pills/day – Can also be used as an acid reflux or heartburn/antacid drug – Least expensive – Should be taken with food because you need some stomach acid to absorb these supplements, in general – Can increase the risk of constipation and kidney stones
Calcium citrate (*Note*: More generic options continue to enter the market and price is beginning to decrease especially if comparing different brands)	21 % (the least concentrated of the major brands which is why the label needs to be read carefully to determine actual number of pills needed per day)	– Better latitude for absorption, especially in a low-acid stomach environment so it can be taken with or without food – More expensive and more pills needed daily, so long-term compliance is an issue – Can increase the risk of constipation but appears to reduce the risk of kidney stones (calcium binds oxalate and citrate reduces stone formation in the urinary tract)
Calcium phosphate (*Note*: this form is also added to some multivitamins and fortified beverages)	38 % or 31 % (pills are approximately the size of calcium carbonate pills but cannot be also used as an antacid—not effective as calcium carbonate for this side benefit)	– Fewer pills to take, in general (for example Tricalcium or dicalcium phosphate) – Best if taken with food – Simplicity and price getting closer to calcium carbonate – Needs many more clinical trials before they will be recommended on a regular basis – Should assume it also increases the risk of constipation and kidney stones

Note: Most of the above supplements may also contain vitamin D, which increases capsule/tablet minimally (not noticeable) since vitamin D IU is really reflective of millionths of a gram. For example 25 µg = 1000 IU of vitamin D

E. Calcium (Carbonate, citrate, and phosphate and vitamin D2 versus D3 similarities and differences)

There are a variety of types of calcium supplements on the market if truly needed. It must first again be kept in mind that countless foods and beverages are now fortified with more calcium than milk (some almond milks have 455 mg per 8 ounces for example) [3]. Thus, it is easier than ever to reduce or eliminate calcium supplements. However, if a calcium supplement is needed it is important to understand the benefits and limitations of each when deciding on the right one. Table 7.2 is a summary of those benefits and limitations [1, 3].

Table 7.3 Vitamin D2 compared to vitamin D3 and a diversity of observations to aid in the decision of which form to utilize for the individual patient [3, 65–72]

– Vitamin D2 and D3 are both cost-effective
– Vitamin D2 is derived from plant-based sources and most (some novel costly exceptions recently) vitamin D3 is derived from sheep lanolin so vegans and vegetarians should be informed of this issue
– Vitamin D3 is the form synthesized by humans when ultraviolet B light comes in contact with the skin
– Vitamin D3 has been utilized in the majority of the osteoporosis prevention clinical trials and in those that included cancer patients
– Vitamin D2 has appeared equally (especially in the conversion to 1,25-dihydroxy vitamin D via the kidney) or slightly less effective versus D3 in clinical trials in terms of raising 25-OH vitamin D but fracture comparative data or stronger endpoint data does not exist
– Vitamin D2 does have a clinical history as part of the protocol to cure rickets and it has been safely given for decades as a prescription
– Wild fish such as salmon tend to harbor D3 and at greater concentrations versus D2, which is found in farmed salmon. Cod liver oil contains vitamin D3 for example
– Vitamin D2 is utilized to fortify many products today including nondairy milk alternatives (some almond milks for example)
– Vitamin D3 has more clinical trial latitude and effects not only from bone health studies but even in studies of burn, kidney disease and other patients with morbidity
– If supplementation is even needed compliance is still the bigger issue over the form of vitamin D
– Most blood tests for 25-OH vitamin D are able to detect D2 and D3
– More nutritional and supplement companies are adding vitamin D2 and D3 to their products, which could soon require minimal to no added pills needed similar to what has occurred with calcium recently

Vitamin D2 (ergocalciferol) versus Vitamin D3 (cholecalciferol) also appears to be debated by experts on a regular basis. However, there are a few critical thoughts and observations in order to decide the appropriate personal choice and these are found in Table 7.3 [3, 65–72].

F. Moyad Dream Clinical Trial—Normalization of Calcium and Vitamin D + Aggressive Lifestyle Changes versus Osteoporosis Drug Treatment—Lessons from Prostate Cancer and SEFIB Trial (Exercise also reduces injurious falls and is superior to supplements)

One large randomized trial can highlight the change in philosophy that should occur with integrative medicine and hormone suppressive bone loss. A large 3-year trial of denosumab given every 6 months ($n=734$) compared to placebo ($n=734$) in men receiving androgen deprivation therapy (ADT) for non-metastatic prostate cancer was published [73]. Participants were instructed to utilize 1000 mg or more of calcium and 400 IU of vitamin D. This represents one of the first long-term randomized studies to provide the placebo arm with realistic and relevant dietary supplementation options. Median serum vitamin D levels at baseline were approximately 24–25 ng/ml, and increased to 31 ng/ml (normal range) after 36 months. Only 14–15 % of participants began the trial with osteoporosis (T score below −2.5) at any site, and the median time on ADT at baseline was 20–21 months. The primary endpoint was the percent change in BMD at the lumbar spine at 24 months, and secondary endpoints included percent change in BMD at the femoral neck and total hip at 24 months and at all three anatomic locations at 36 months, along with incidence of new fractures. After 24 months there was a significant loss in lumbar spine BMD at 24 months in the placebo group, but this loss was just 1 %, and minimally changed at 36 months. There were also significant reductions in femoral neck and total hip, but this loss was only 2–3 % at 36 months. The largest percentage of bone loss occurred in the distal radius. Fracture at any anatomic location was lower with denosumab compared to placebo, but the difference was not found to be statistically significant at 36 months. No significant differences were found in the time period to first fracture (non-vertebral or vertebral) between the groups. The authors reported that more than one fracture at any location occurred in significantly more patients on placebo compared to denosumab, and a significantly higher rate of vertebral fractures. Yet these were secondary endpoints, and more participants in the placebo group had a history of vertebral fracture (+2.6 %) and a history of osteoporotic fracture (+4.5 %) at baseline. The 36-month clinical difference of 2.4 % more new vertebral fractures (3.9 % versus 1.5 %) in the placebo group cannot be due to the intervention alone, but may also have been due to the slight inequality between groups as it related to vertebral and overall fractures at baseline in favor of denosumab. The difference between most clinical endpoints for the calcium and vitamin D group compared to pharmacologic treatment was minimal at 36 months. Furthermore, a less than 4 % total fracture percentage in the placebo arm (versus 1.9 %) over 3 years is low considering that no aggressive lifestyle and supplemental preventive therapy before ADT was initiated. How much difference would have existed if the placebo group were also assigned to regular resistance and aerobic exercises during this study period or before initiating ADT? Denosumab appears to be an option for accelerated spinal and hip bone loss despite aggressive supplemental intervention, and perhaps for those men that cannot adequately maintain distal radius density with aggressive lifestyle changes. Regardless, a clinical trial of non-metastatic patients on hormone suppression from breast and prostate cancer treatment with adequate calcium and vitamin D status with aerobic and resistance exercise may compare favorably to pharmacologic intervention over 1-year or more. Yet a long-term and more lifestyle and supplement balanced trial has not been conducted. In my clinical experience I have not observed significant differences between breast and prostate cancer patients adopting aggressive lifestyle and supplement measures versus prescription medications for osteoporosis unless the patients was also on steroid treatment. Again, this has not been tested in a clinical trial.

Interestingly, an 18-month randomized trial of 180 healthy men aged 50–79 years allocated to exercise (resistance training 3 days a week) with and without fortified milk (1000 mg calcium and 800 IU of vitamin D) consumed daily was conducted [74]. Exercise increased femoral neck 2.1 % and improved lumbar spine (LS) trabecular BMD 2.2 % with no effect on mid-femur or mid-tibia BMD. No primary effects of fortified milk occurred at any skeletal site, which suggests exercise alone could have profound effects in excess of what supplementation provides. The results of this unique trial in men with baseline calcium intakes of 1000 mg/day and vitamin D blood levels of approximately 35 ng/ml suggests that individuals replete with this nutrients may allow for an optimal skeletal response to exercise as noted by the authors.

Of even greater interest for women was a similar multicomponent 19-month randomized trial in women 65 years and older ($n=246$) observed significant 1–2 % benefit at the femoral neck and lumbar spine and a reduced risk of falls [75]! All participants were provided with 1500 mg of calcium and 500 IU of vitamin D3 supplements per day (Opfermann Arzneimittel, Wiehl, Germany). This trial was known as the Senior Fitness and Prevention (SEFIP) study.

A recent 2-year randomized trial of placebo, 800 IU of vitamin D3 (provided by Oy Verman Ab-Kerava, Finland), exercise, and vitamin D and exercise (4-arms trial) in Finland of 70–80 year old home-dwelling women ($n=409$) found that the rate of "injurious falls and injured fallers" was reduced by 50 % with strength and balance training while 800 IU of vitamin D daily alone despite not impacting the rate of falls maintained femoral neck BMD and modestly increased tibial trabecular density [76]. The baseline intake of calcium and vitamin D was approximately 1100 mg/day and 400 IU and 25-OH vitamin D baseline was 27 ng/ml suggesting that women in this trial were already replete with calcium and replete or almost replete with vitamin D.

And a past 10-month trial in Chinese postmenopausal women with low calcium intakes (less than 275 mg/day) when given 800 mg/day of calcium supplementation improved the impact of resistance bearing exercise on femoral neck BMD [77]! Again, suggesting the optimal benefits of exercise or synergy occur with normalization of calcium and vitamin D status (not excessive intakes).

The preliminary cumulative observation provides part of the reasoning of a "dream" trial in breast cancer with aggressive lifestyle changes and supplements versus prescription medications to prevent osteoporosis. Additionally, the cardiovascular, metabolic, psychological, and overall qualify of life benefits would arguably be far more impressive than the comparative pharmacologic intervention, and if needed would only serve to enhance the pharmacological product (3–4 arm trial ideally). Another unique trial utilizing a vibratory plate should only further increase the interest in exercise for bone health for patients.

G. Power Plate versus lifestyle?
Several few years ago I began to notice what looked like a large circular metal plate that you are suppose to stand on and it vibrates at various speeds in order to improve your bones or BMD and reduce your risk of osteoporosis. And after a few more months I began to see these "whole-body vibration (WBV)" therapy machines in most very high-end (aka "expensive") health clubs. The idea behind these machines seems logical, since the skeletal system similar to the rest of our bodies operate on a "use it or lose it" scale.

Whole body vibration machines are costly (thousands of dollars), thus evidence was needed to justify cost. Some machines allow for more vibration compared to others, so that the intensity of WBV is expressed by vibration frequency (1 Hz = 1 oscillation/s). A research group from Toronto set up a 1-year randomized control trial of low-magnitude WBV at two frequencies (30 Hz and 90 Hz) compared to no WBV [78]. A total of 202 healthy postmenopausal women (average age of 60 years, 95 % of women did not smoke) with osteopenia and not receiving prescription bone drugs for osteoporosis were included in this study. Participants were placed in one of three groups that allowed them to stand on WBV platform for 20 min daily at one of two frequencies (first two groups), or not use the WBV device at all (group 3—control group). All of the groups were requested to utilize calcium and vitamin D supplements, so that their total daily intake from diet and supplements was approximately 1200 mg calcium and 1000 IU of vitamin D daily. This is important because many past studies of WBV did not have participants take calcium and vitamin D. However, after 12 months there was no difference in bone density changes between the WBV groups (high or low frequency) compared to the control group at any bone site measured in the body, which included the spine, hips, legs, and wrist. In fact, the group that just took calcium and vitamin D supplements had a similar outcome to the WBV groups! Interestingly, there were no differences in side effects reported among the groups, but three participants stopped WBV therapy within 60 days because of dizziness at night, shin pain, and foot pain. Other mild and temporary side effects reported included pain, numbness of feet, or weakness at different leg sites (five participants in WBV) group; nausea (two participants in WBV); worsening of headaches, bladder discomfort, inner ear sensitivity, or neck pain (one participant in WBV). The researchers also did an analysis on lower leg bone (tibial trabecular area) structure and found that some women seemed to achieve a slightly worse outcome with the WBV. However, in all fairness, overall the results were not different and the side effect rates were similar. It appears that the WBV groups in my opinion did not fare better compared to the control groups because these postmenopausal women were healthy in terms of overall lifestyle (mean BMI of 24, minimal alcohol intake, 380+ calories expended per day from exercise, non-smokers primarily, 1350 mg calcium and 800 IU vitamin D baseline intake, …). Perhaps WBV will have more success in those with spinal cord injury and elderly frail individual or even specific children in need of this assistance [79]. Additionally, data in breast cancer is minimal [80], but it would be more optimal to test this therapy for lymphedema because patients have mentioned over time it appears to be of some benefit but this has not been studied. Regardless, when maximizing lifestyle changes it is not easy to provide results from a device or intervention that are far superior to these methods.

H. Miscellaneous dietary supplements (Omega-3, strontium, vitamin K, whey protein powder, …)
There are many dietary supplements that are touted to work better or as effectively as calcium and vitamin D [3]. However, since calcium and vitamin D are not needed in excessive dosages and can now be derived primarily in realistic quantities from food/beverage and multivitamin sources what else is really needed apart from lifestyle options and pharmacologic interventions if really needed? Omega-3 supplements

have a randomized trial being initiated in breast cancer patients to determine if they can improve lean body mass (LBM, for example MODEL study) and even preserve BMD, so there is not enough evidence to suggest a benefit or not at this point.

Strontium citrate supplements have been touted and it appears based on the results with the prescription oral drug strontium ranelate they could provide some benefit. However, the drug strontium ranelate is now being questioned because of an increased potential risk of cardiovascular events including a 60 % increased risk of myocardial infarction [81, 82]. Since strontium citrate and ranelate could theoretically have overlapping mechanisms of action [83], it would be prudent to not recommend strontium citrate or any strontium dietary supplements for bone loss or to breast cancer patients.

The only other dietary supplements that theoretically could provide some value currently and is being tested are vitamin K1 and K2 supplements. The overall data on bone markers and fracture risk is still embryonic and inconsistent [84]. And the long-term safety issues of ingesting high-dosages of vitamin K have not been established. For example, K2 is recommended in dosages as high as 45 μg and dosages as low as 10 μg could offset the effect of vitamin K antagonist prescription anticoagulation [85]. Increasing rates of cardiovascular disease (CVD) with age and those placed on prescription anticoagulants suggest a clear benefit over risk needs to be established with vitamin K1 or K2 in women and men before it could be considered as an adjunct to bone loss prevention. Thus, it would appear prudent to continue to follow the research before recommending large dosages of vitamin K for osteoporosis and fracture prevention.

I. Whey protein—Whey not? Plant protein powders? Chocolate milk? Caffeine?
Whey protein and other powders are the most concentrated protein sources available commercially with little to no sugar and aid with weight loss, and muscle development [3]. A protein powder with no sugar, no lactose, and over 20 g of protein for about 100–125 calories easily surpasses what could be found nutritionally in most protein bars. Compliance with protein intake is more important than time of day of ingestion and 14 randomized trials (n=626) reviewed have found the ability of whey protein to enhance or act synergistically with muscle protein synthesis produced from resistance exercise and to act as a weight loss supplement [86]. Body weight in eligible studies was reduced by −4.20 kg and body fat by −3.74 kg when within group analysis was conducted and the increase in lean body mass was 2.24 kg (all significant). However, this meta-analysis does not appear to support this form of protein powder over others, and I agree [3]. Ongoing and recent trials continue to demonstrate benefits [87], although a large trial in breast cancer patients is needed.

The current maximum intake of protein per day is body weight in pounds divided in half to equal maximum intake (150 pound person should get a maximum intake of 75 g of protein per day), which is not an easy task and protein powder can assist with this goal [3]. It appears that all types of animal-based (whey, casein, egg white, ...) and plant-based (soy, pea, brown rice, hemp, ...) could all be effective but apart from soy protein powder the plant based protein powder have suboptimal taste when mixed with water unlike animal based protein powders and this could cause a compliance issue.

Chocolate milk can contain 200 calories or more while whey or soy is about 100 calories. And chocolate milk has less than 10 g of protein while whey/soy contains around 20–25 g of protein! Chocolate milk has about 30 g of carbohydrate and simple sugars (27 g in one serving—in many cases as much as a full calorie soda) and whey and soy isolate have little to no carbohydrates and fat and a low sodium content and can function as an appetite suppressant. Thus, for the average exerciser trying to combat weight loss it does not appear to be the best option. However, the 4:1 carbohydrate to protein ratio (identical to commercial athletic beverages) is a good option for endurance workouts or high-intensity regimens where muscle glycogen concentrations are compromised and adequate muscle recovery from fatigue is required on a regular basis [88]. Arguably, another common compound, caffeine, utilized in moderate dosages (coffee, tea, other beverages) has increasing evidence as a compound that improves glycogen storage potential, reduces muscle fatigue and enhances exercise regimens so I often mention this in a consult ("few sips of a beverage before, during and after a workout") [3].

Creatine monohydrate has minimal long-term data in elderly individuals but it appears to be synergistic with resistance exercise from dosages as high as 20 g/day by improving lean muscle mass and function [89]. A small meta-analysis of older adults ($n = 357$, mean age 56–70 years, dosages generally from 3 to 5 g/day) from ten studies found that it could significantly increase fat-free mass and increase the performance of some resistance exercises [90].

- **Cardiovascular issues (dyslipidemia, glucose, blood pressure, …)**

Note: Please see Chaps. 3, 4, 5, and 6 (statins, aspirin, and metformin) for detailed information on the preferred options.

- **Constipation (and diarrhea)**

Note: Please see Chap. 3 on lifestyle changes and the different forms of fiber and please see the hot flash section of this chapter and the results with magnesium dietary supplements. In addition, diarrhea was not treated as a separate topic since the conventional options with this side effect from cancer treatment should be the primary option. In the future, the data with antibiotic associated diarrhea (AAD) and probiotics (Lactobacillus, Saccharomyces, …) could be an option in cancer patients but the majority of the data now has been for *Helicobacter pylori* eradication [3]. There have been some rare causes of sepsis from probiotics (bacteremia/fungus/positive blood cultures …) that must be addressed and benefit needs to greatly exceed risk for this medical condition.

- **Depression (major depressive disorder or MDD)**

A. *Exercise and/or medication, UPBEAT study, breast cancer?*

Unfortunately, exercise is often advocated as having mild or moderate changes in those with depression from the clinical research, or there appears to be a tone of indifference when reviewing the entire research. For example, in an extensive review of 39 clinical trials involving 2326 participants exercise was found to be "moderately more effective than a control intervention" and in more robust trials only "a smaller effect in favor of exercise" [91]. Still, in this same publication the authors point out that "exercise appears to be no more effective" compared to pharmacologic or psychological therapies! The consistent findings with exercise even as a potential treatment option is what is most striking and it is an intervention that combats overall disease morbidity and mortality.

Recently, it was more lucidly explained that the majority of clinical studies (13 out of 16) with exercise demonstrated a 5-point improvement on average compared to prescription medication for depression with an average of a 2–3 point improvement over placebo [92]. Thus, this is not an indication to abandon conventional medicine in favor of exercise but rather the potential synergism of these two agents. In fact, there are notable past clinical trials where exercise not only enhanced the response of notable FDA approved prescription antidepressants agents and increased the likelihood of remission [93].

Exercise also appears to be as effective as conventional treatment in patients being monitored for different disease conditions that experience a higher rate of depression [94]. And the beneficial effects occur with only three times a week of activity and within the first 4 months. For example this is what was found in the UPBEAT (Understanding the Prognostic Benefits of Exercise and Antidepressant Therapy) study, which included patients with heart disease and depression.

Yet one question that is more pertinent to answer in terms of exercise is the impact of the socialization of exercise versus the isolation of exercise. In other words, in many clinical trials there have been trainers or exercise leaders (supervised) working with patients with major depressive disorder (MDD), thus it could also be argued that this socialization or instruction type exercise has a higher probability of being successful versus isolated work outs. This question and the potential contribution of each form of exercise need to be further researched. Some preliminary clinical trials suggest profound effects even with home-based exercise but placebo responses are also high which suggests multiple factors, including more attention given to patients, could have profound impacts [95].

The data with aerobic or resistance exercise in breast cancer patients appears to be more consistent with an overall improvement in energy levels or a reduction in fatigue than with most other subjective parameters [96, 97].

Regardless, one of the most extensive reviews of this research over 25 years in breast cancer utilizing 51 studies found consistent suggestions of objective benefit for body composition, strength, and cardiorespiratory function and subjective benefits including improvements in fatigue, depression, and overall quality of life [98].

B. Dietary supplements (SAM-e, St. John's wort, Omega-3?)
C. S-adenosyl-l-methionine (SAM-e—why not if in need of more options?)
The most common dosage utilized in clinical trials of major depressive disorder (MDD) was 800–1600 mg a day, or 400–800 mg twice a day. However, there is a lack of good data in breast cancer patients [3]. Regardless, this supplement (actually drug in some countries and also has an IV form) should be reviewed since it has preliminarily impressive data [99, 100]. SAMe is an option with and without conventional antidepressant treatments. SAM-e is a compound that is involved in methylation and improving the creation and utilization of several brain neurotransmitters

including dopamine, epinephrine, and serotonin as well as donating methyl groups to membrane phospholipids, myelin, choline, and other compounds commonly found I brain tissue. It has some features similar and different to prescription medications for depression. The overall impact of SAM-e appears similar to other antidepressants. Past systematic reviews have been positive with seven of seven trials using IV SAM-e and four of five studies using oral doses of 1600 mg/day [99, 100]. It was shown more efficacious than placebo and as efficacious to tricyclic antidepressants in three trials. Overall, there was reduction in Ham-D (Hamilton Rating Scale for Depression) scores in four of the five randomized controlled trials of the oral supplement. Still, more data was needed to determine if it could provide a modern day clinical benefit.

A preliminary Harvard study suggested a benefit of SAM-e at 800 mg twice a day when added to conventional drug treatment (SSRI drugs) in individuals that were not responding to SSRI medications [101]. This 6-week study was funded by the National Institutes of Health and included 73 nonresponders and compared to placebo the HAM-D response (36 % versus 18 %) and remission (18 % versus 12 %) rates, low number needed to treat (1 out of 6–7) and discontinuation rate similar to placebo was interesting. Further trials with this group have also found efficacy similar to some standard antidepressants (escitalopram or Lexapro), and in fact nonsignificantly higher response and equal remission rates. However, the SAM-e dosage utilized was higher (1600–3200 mg/day) and side effects occurred in 20 % of the SAM-e group (stomach upset and diarrhea) and interestingly the FDA approved drug and supplement did not statistically beat placebo in this major trial [102–104]. It also appears that men could have experienced a greater response rate versus women but more research is needed in this area.

There has been a concern that SAM-e raises blood levels of homocysteine (a controversial marker of heart disease) but this has really not occurred in more recent studies but patients should still be followed periodically with this blood test [105].

Side effects like gastrointestinal upset and diarrhea can occur but they are rare when using the standard dosages (up to 1600 mg/day) [99, 100]. Other rare side effects that have been reported are: nausea, dry mouth, headache, mild insomnia, anorexia, sweating, dizziness, nervousness especially at high dosages, and it can make some people with depression feel anxious. SAM-e might lead to toxic reaction when used with cough suppressant dextromethorphan, certain antidepressants, or narcotic pain relievers; could worsen symptoms when taken with Parkinson's drug levodopa.

Regardless, the biggest side effect with SAM-e is the cost (one of the most expensive supplements I have observed in my career for treating a condition), so comparisons on the internet and stores can save a very large amount of money (FYI—in Europe it is a prescription drug that can get covered) [3]. SAM-e also oxidizes quickly in a bottle the expiration date should be reviewed carefully because this is one the only supplements I have observed that really expires at the date is says it expires (pills can change color …), compared to most other pills which you can use up to a year or two after expiration.

Arguably there are two notable preliminary potentially side benefits observed with SAM-e, which is the lack of sexual side effects that commonly occur with many of the conventional prescription antidepressants that did not occur in a recent trial with SAM-e. It appeared to have a positive benefit on male arousal and erectile dysfunction, and further research with women and sexual health should also be investigated from SAM-e depression trials [106]. And again it may be one of the best supplements for pain reduction (600 mg/day) from osteoarthritis (work as well as over the counter pain relievers with less side effects from preliminary studies—see AIA section in this chapter) [3].

D. St. John's wort (SJW; supplement known for drug interactions and efficacy)
SJW or St. John's Wort at 500–1200 mg/day is commonly recommended in authoritative dietary supplement texts and medical reviews [3, 100]. SJW at a dose of 500–1200 mg/d over 4–12 weeks has been moderately effective when used as 2–3 divided doses and extracts standardized to contain 0.3 % hypericin—the active ingredient (the most common dosage in clinical trials was 900 mg/day). SJW is an extract of the plant Hypericum perforatum, which is a yellow-flowering perennial herb found in temperate areas worldwide. It was actually a recorded medicinal compound in ancient Greece and has been used in Europe for depression as an IV and oral medication since the 1980s. The exact mechanism of action has not been elucidated but it appears to block serotonin uptake and alters levels of multiple brain neurotransmitters including dopamine, norepinephrine, and gamma-aminobutyric acid (GABA). Side effects have been low or rare in clinical trials, but critics have mentioned that SJW has the potential to interact or reduce the effectiveness of almost half of the available prescription drugs including the birth control pill and this is true. And SJW should not be combined with prescription antidepressants including SSRIs, Tricyclic antidepressants (TCA), or monoamine oxidase (MAO) inhibitors. It should also be avoided in those individuals on specific drugs such as immunosuppressants, antiretrovirals (anti-HIV drugs), blood thinners like warfarin, oral contraceptives, chemotherapy drugs. Still, SJW is often inappropriately tagged as being the supplement that should rarely be utilized in patients because of its potential drug interactions, especially its ability to induce CYPs and P-glycoprotein, thus reducing the concentration of another drug's active ingredient as mentioned above. Yet it still has a role in clinical medicine [107].

Many individuals and doctors still utilize it as a single agent or monotherapy. A notable past Cochrane review of 29 past trials with approximately 5500 patients found it may work as well as conventional antidepressants and participants were 50–75 % less likely to drop out of a clinical trial compared to a prescription antidepressant and concluded with the following statements that St. John's wort for major depression is [108]:

– Greater than placebo
– As effective as standard antidepressants
– Have fewer side effects than standard antidepressants

Currently, most objective reviews of St. John's wort for depression continue to suggest it is arguably an integrative medicine with perhaps the strongest evidence for depression [109]. *Some alternative "experts" comment that SJW works as well as most conventional drug options for depression and that is not accurate because many of the positive head-to-head clinical trials were with older prescription drugs that are not commonly used today.*

Side Effects of SJW include: Insomnia, vivid dreams, anxiety, dizziness and can cause skin to become sensitive to the sun [3].

Several preliminary clinical trials have demonstrated a potential for benefit in breast cancer survivors even when also utilizing tamoxifen [110]. An ethanolic extract of St. John's wort extract (900 mg three times a day, extract standardized to 0.3 % hypericin extracted in 50 % ethanol and tablets taken at mealtime) versus placebo showed a nonsignificant benefit in a reduction of hot flash frequency and hot flash scores. There were significant benefits observed with menopause-specific quality of life ($p=0.01$) and reduced sleep problems ($p=0.05$) and 26 of the 42 patients were breast cancer survivors. More primary endpoint depression trials with this herb in cancer patients of course are needed. Some cancer drugs are reduced more than others in efficacy such as imatinib and irinotecan, and regardless caution does not be followed when combining this product with any cancer medication [111].

E. Miscellaneous—Omega-3 Supplements have bias, folate or perhaps l-methylfolate at 15 mg/d for SSRI-partial/nonresponders? Chromium? Inositol? Rhodiola? 5-HTP?

Omega-3 supplements have a mixed and modest history at best for preventing or treating major depressive disorder (MDD). A meta-analysis of 13 randomized, placebo-controlled trials of 731 participants and found no significant benefit over placebo [112]. In addition there was significant heterogeneity and publication bias. There was an increasing pattern of omega-3 fatty acid effectiveness in trials of lower methodology, shorter duration trials, greater baseline depression severity trials and trials that did not use intention-to-treat analysis but completers only for data. More recent clinical trials of either 1000 mg EPA or 1000 mg DHA per day for 8 weeks versus placebo in MDD patients ($n=196$, 53 % female) found no benefit over placebo [113]. If omega-3 were to assume some role for depression there appears to be some preliminary recent data to suggest they may augment the response to an SSRI medications [114, 115]. Future better studies to access the impact of these supplements alone or compared to prescription antidepressants are being conducted (for example "The Beyond Ageing Project Phase 2") [116]. In the meantime, the reader should see the section on hot flashes or follow the data on omega-3 in breast cancer for other side effects for treatment because these can provide an additional insight into the cognitive or antidepression effects (or not) of omega-3 supplements. Overall, these effects thus far have been modest at best.

Folate has had minimal effects in past randomized controlled trials (small reduction in HAM-D scores) [100], but the more bioavailable or the active form known as "L-methylfolate" at a dosage of 15 mg/day has shown some preliminary clinical promise (32 % response rate versus 15 % with placebo and similar side effects) in SSRI partial or nonresponders that should receive more investigation [117]. A dosage of 7.5 mg/day of L-methylfolate in this same trial was not effective.

L-methylfolate is also the only form of folate that crosses the blood–brain barrier and it also has a regulatory role for a major cofactor for neurotransmitter production known as "tetrahydrobiopterin" or BH4. And BH4 is also need for several enzyme systems required for the production of the neurotransmitters serotonin, dopamine, and norepinephrine. Thus, low levels of L-methylfolate could theoretically lead to low concentrations of brain neurotransmitters.

Other dietary supplements being investigated for more specific types of depression include chromium for atypical depression and seasonal affective disorder, inositol in combination with mood stabilizers for the treatment of bipolar depression, Rhodiola rosea for lethargic or asthenic depression and in combination with conventional medications could reduce some of their adverse effects, and 5-hydroxytryptophan (5-HTP) to improve the concentration of serotonin in some patients should also receive more attention [118]. Other alternative agents/methods such as acupuncture have not demonstrated consistent efficacy [100].

- **Dry eye/dry mouth/dry skin**
  A. Dry eye (lifestyle, omega-3 and/or omega-6, and oral sea buckthorn oil? Vitamin A drops. Lifestyle changes?)
All of the above medical conditions have minimal to moderate effective sufficient evidence-based options especially in the area of dietary supplements and integrative medicines.

There are arguably some lifestyle options that have some moderate data that should be mentioned [3]. Diets higher in omega-3 fatty acids from fish and plants have shown a potential to reduce the risk of dry eye. Interestingly, consuming fish such as tuna several times weekly has been associated with a lower risk of dry eye. Keep in mind that these were diet studies of preventing dry eye and not treatment. Again, for the most part they support was is supported in the area of dietary supplements. Blinking produces Meibum (secretions) because the ever so tiny muscles squeeze the glands around the eyes. Try full blinks when at the computer for a long time and squeeze eyelids together for several seconds every 15–20 min. Eye movements from side to side and up and down (eye yoga) also helps. Sunglasses protect the eyes especially from wind that can cause tears to evaporate quickly and cause inflammation. Eyeglasses used regularly help to discourage the evaporation of tears and just improve vision. If dry air is a problem so purchase and use a humidifier (40–50 % in your living environment) or do more blinking exercises on airplanes. Avoid smoke, pollutants or anything that can irritate the eyes. Better contact lens care is helpful especially taking a break and wearing glasses every few days, and take your lenses out at night and use a gentler contact solution. Massaging upper and lower eyelids with a cotton swab (small circles around each eyelid). Hot compress helps to loosen and release hardened oil in clogged meibomian glands. So, twice a day wash your face with a cloth then rinse the cloth with warm water and use it as a compress over your closed eyelids for 30 s. Next, clean the lower lids with a dry, tightly wrapped cotton swab. This process removes lid debris that could be disrupting with the tear film, stimulates your own reflex tears, and the meibomian glands release oily secretions into the tear film.

Regardless, the most promising and recent research with omega-3 and/or omega-6 supplementation for dry eye is interesting and several large-scale clinical trials are currently addressing this issue. Interestingly, dry eye is the number one reason people visit the eye doctor [3]. Specific dosages are mentioned below of omega-3 and/or omega-6 supplementation but the clinician and patients should not get caught in the minutiae but instead realize there is good preliminary evidence to support the use of these dietary supplements for dry eye of various etiologies because they may simply just increase tear production and tear volume. And please keep in mind that in many cases omega-3 and omega-6 pills are no longer needed because liquid flavored options that are low in calories offer wonderful non-pills options utilizing several teaspoons or 1–2 tablespoons per day that equate with all the effective pill dosages (for example see Barlean's Omega Swirl® and other non-pill options).

A meta-analysis of seven independent studies ($n = 790$) demonstrates the positive data with omega-3 fatty acid supplements [119]. For example with flaxseed oil at 1000 mg/day divided into three daily doses (total of 3300 mg of plant omega-3 alpha-linolenic acid), or just ingesting 800–1500 mg of the active ingredients in marine or fish oil (EPA and DHA omega-3 fatty acids) has been beneficial (1–2 fish oil pills on average) in preliminary clinical trials [3].

Omega-6 supplementation is controversial because some "experts" have been falsely touting that omega-6 fatty acids create inflammation and are bad for you and this is not accurate and it is a gross generalization. Some omega-6 compounds have anti-inflammatory effects, which is why they are potentially effective for dry eye symptoms and are low cost [120]. For example, an omega-6 compound known as LA (linoleic acid) can be converted in humans to gamma-linolenic acid (GLA) and further converted to another omega-6 known as DGLA (dihomo-gamma-linolenic acid), which can result in an anti-inflammatory effect and may stimulate tear production [3].

LA at 57–224 mg and/or 30–300 mg GLA in studies has been beneficial in reducing symptoms of dry eye. The human study that also relates to my experience with individuals with dry eye from diverse causes including contact lenses (as was the participants of this study) involved using 300 mg of gamma-linolenic acid (GLA) from evening primrose oil (or black current oil can also be used—whatever is cheaper). Evening primrose has the better research taken as capsules but this is cumbersome and could require up to six capsules a day.

Additionally, the combination of omega-3 and omega-6 supplementation could also be effective against dry eye [3, 119–122]. Using at least 750–1000 mg of the active omega-3 ingredients in fish oil (EPA and DHA), and 1000 mg of flaxseed oil daily for 90 days, or using the same dosage of fish oil with 15–82 mg GLA and 126 mg LA showed benefits in multiple small but noteworthy clinical trials. It should also be kept in mind that topical omega-3 and/or omega-6 preparations also have preliminary positive data [121].

Interestingly, other supplements which harbor omega-3 and omega-3 compounds also have preliminary data such as oral sea buckthorn (*Hippophae rhamnoides*) oil

[123, 124]. A study of 2000 mg a day (two capsules twice a day with meals) in 20–75-year-old men and women appeared to improve the tear film and potentially reduce redness and burning in the fall and winter (consumed for 3 months). Again, this study was not provided to promote this oil but to show that omega-3 and/or supplements are promising for dry eye. This oil has a high content of the omega-6 LA, and plant omega-3 and some monounsaturated fat.

A large (*n* = 150) study from Korea that used vitamin A (retinyl palmitate, 0.05 % and polysorbate 80 1 % and preservative free from Vision Pharmaceuticals Inc., Mitchell, South Dakota known as "Viva Drops®") drops four times daily for dry eye and it was found that the vitamin A improved blurred vision, tear film and produced results that appear to be similar to the FDA approved drug cyclosporine A (0.05 %, also known as "Restasis") [125]. The participants of this study were on average 30–40 years old and their dry eye did not respond to conventional suggestions. Both options significantly improved the symptoms of dry eye within 2–3 months. It appears that either of these options worked fine in this study with an artificial tears product. You can find Viva Drops online (www.vivadrops.com).

Check medications (beta-blockers, antidepressants, anticonvulsants, anti-parkinsonian, antihistamines, decongestants, antipsychotics, and even some pain medications, antithyroid, cancer drugs, antiemetic, acid reflux medications, blood pressure meds, urinary incontinence, antiviral, antimalarial, respiratory medications, ... the list is long) and supplements including your topical ones because they could be a problem. For example, niacin supplements have a history of causing eye issues in some individuals including dry eye and blurred vision [126]. One popular line of prescription antiaging skin creams known as "retinoids" (high potency vitamin A derivatives) can cause dryness of the skin as a side effect. These medications reduce sebaceous gland size, which is why they were also tried on acne in the past but can cause dry eye because the meibomian glands are sebaceous glands, and accidentally getting some in the eyes can cause burning sensation and inflammation and potential dry eye.

Although studies of dry eye in breast cancer have received minimal attention, the subject itself from cancer treatment is an issue. For example, preliminary retrospective chart reviews of patients on aromatase inhibitors suggest that dry eye could be more prevalent in this breast cancer population [127]. Estrogen receptors exist in the eye and eye glands and the risk of dry eye does increase with age and lower estrogen levels [128].

B. Dry mouth (Connection to dry eye, acupuncture, chewing gum, and yohimbine?)
Often dry eye and dry mouth can occur together, so integrative medicines that work for one should be tested for the impact on the other. Still, dry mouth has few integrative medical options at this time, especially from cancer treatment. Interventions that appear to reduce this medical condition especially from Sjogrens syndrome and radiotherapy to the head and neck should also provide some clues on how to treat dry mouth from other causes [129]. Few adequate studies have been conducted in this area. However a review of six studies (three randomized and three

prospective) that met more rigorous methodology criteria the following options could be tried [130]:

- Acupuncture
- Artificial saliva
- Chewing gum
- Pilocarpine (Rx drug)

Yohimbine (4 or 6 mg to a maximum of three times a day) could be another option for dry mouth based on preliminary data outside of cancer treatment [131, 132]. Yohimbine comes from the West African Yohimbe tree and can be found as a supplement and a prescription drug (Yocon® etc.) [3]. Whether or not it is consistently effective is controversial, but what is not controversial is that it is a "alpha-2-adrenoreceptor antagonist" (alpha-2-adrenergic agonist), which has increased salivary secretion in animals, healthy volunteers and in some medication-induced and other etiologies of dry mouth. Arguably an intact salivary gland with some functional parasympathetic stimulation is needed for efficacy. Additionally, because of its mechanism of action some of the side effects include: headache, sweating, nausea, dizziness, nervousness/agitation, tremors, sleeplessness, antidiuresis, and elevated blood pressure and heart rate. It cannot be used by individuals with kidney diseases, those on antidepressants, or other mood-altering drugs, and in some individuals with specific cardiovascular, neurological, and psychological issues. Since yohimbine can increase brain norepinephrine, and increased norepinephrine can trigger some hot flashes then caution should also be exercise when dealing with severe hot flashes and dry mouth. Interestingly, clonidine has provided a mild benefit for some women with hot flashes and this drug is an alpha-adrenergic agonist, which can reduce brain norepinephrine.

Many media and other credible sources appear to suggest yohimbine is as an alternative medicine or over the counter dietary supplement, but this is really not the case based on its clinical trial efficacy [3]. And this is the real problem here, which is yohimbine HCL is a prescription drug, but many dietary supplements that mimic this drug have quality control problems and are dangerous (like the drug). Again, yohimbine HCL is the active ingredient found in the bark of a West African tree, but many dietary supplements really sell "yohimbe" which in may cases has little to no or variable quantities of the active ingredient "yohimbine HCL" in it. Again, if there is an interest in yohimbine HCL in the area of dry mouth I believe the prescription drug should be utilized because of quality control issues and because the successful clinical trials throughout medicine primarily utilized this version.

C. Dry skin

Note: Most moisturizer conventional options or lotions that also contain a broad-spectrum sunscreen (UVA and UVB such as Lubriderm and others) are adequate. Replacing the conventional options or acting as an adjunct with integrative medicines without adequate minimal evidence is not advised.

• **Fatigue (Cancer-related fatigue or CRF)**

A. Aerobic and/or resistance exercise = standard of care during and after cancer treatment

A Cochrane review of 56 studies (*n* = 4068) found aerobic exercise to be especially helpful in significantly reducing CRF during and after cancer treatment especially in the area of breast and prostate cancer patients [133]. Resistance activity appeared to be benefit in numerous studies but aerobic exercise had more significant data. The type, intensity and timing of exercise to achieve a benefit were not consistent or clear, but suggest a variety of types of exercise could have profound benefits for patients. Another extensive review of this research over 25 years, but only in breast cancer utilizing 51 studies found consistent suggestions of objective benefit for body composition, strength, and cardiorespiratory function and subjective benefits including improvements in fatigue, depression and overall quality of life [98].

B. American ginseng and perhaps Panax ginseng (why not a primary treatment option for CRF?)

"Nevertheless, for patients who want to try a pharmacologic product and physicians who are early adapters of new promising agents, the pure ground root American ginseng product, as used in the above studies, might be an option to consider" [134].

This was an editorial from some of the top experts in the field of conventional treatments for CRF, which is arguably one of the strongest potential partial endorsements of a dietary supplement to prevent or treat a common cancer treatment side effect.

The reason for such an initial positive reaction for American ginseng (*Panax quinquefolius*) was based on two strong in methodology clinical trials—somewhat similar to a phase 3 trial and also reviewed in Chap. 2 of this text [135, 136]. A total of 364 participants were enrolled from 40 medical centers (clinical trial sites or primarily community cancer centers) and approximately *60 % of the participants were being treated for breast cancer* (the others consisted of colon at 12 %, hematologic 5 %, and prostate 4 %, and then gynecologic and others) and the average age was 55 years [135]. *After approximately 2 months a significant difference (twice the effect at reducing fatigue compared to placebo) was observed and side effects were similar to placebo.* Regardless, in the first month there was a nonsignificant benefit, but again it did not become statistically significant until after 2 months. Participants received 2000 mg of Wisconsin ginseng, which is just a common type of American ginseng or placebo. Ginseng consisted of pure ground root from one production lot and it contained 3 % ginsenosides (theorized active ingredients). Keep in mind that most ginseng products on the market have at least 3 % and some as high as 50 %, but you would need to try ginseng at lower dosages as the potency or concentration of ginsenosides increases. Ideally one should mimic what worked in the clinical trial but this same research group from Mayo Clinic also observed efficacy at 1000 mg/day with a 5 % ginsenoside (Rb1 ginsenoside being the most prevalent) product in a previous clinical trial (*n* = 290) that included 109 breast cancer patients (39 % respectively) [136]. The pure ground root ginseng in these studies was donated by the *Ginseng Board of Wisconsin (Wausau, WI, go to www.ginsengboard.com to find information on the product used in the clinical trial) and was manufactured by Beehive Botanicals (Hayward, WI).* It is also of interest that in these large clinical trials patients appeared to receive greater antifatigue benefits the earlier in the course of treatment the ginseng was utilized as opposed to later or after treatment. In other words, the preventive aspects of this treatment may be greater than simply trying to treat more significant fatigue after it has already occurred.

Another small single arm trial of 800 mg/day of Panax/Asian Ginseng (Indena S.p.A. Milan, Italy) at MD Anderson Cancer Center found a significant reduction in CRF within one month utilizing a 7 % ginsenoside product that needs confirmation in a randomized trial [137]. This supplement also appeared to significantly improve quality of life and this also appeared to improve sleep, appetite, pain, and other issues related to CRF in 30 days.

Thus, the cumulative evidence from the Mayo Clinic directed and MD Anderson Cancer Center studies are arguably sufficient evidence currently to offer ginseng as a primary antifatigue option especially since patients have few options in this area, and some of the more expensive pharmaceutical based products (psychostimulants …) have been disappointing when further studied [134].

Ginseng may be reducing the inflammatory process associated with cancer or chronic fatigue due to inflammation in general [3, 134–137]. Ginseng could reduce cortisol and reduces stress overall and then improve energy levels. Whether or not the primary antifatigue effects are being derived from the ginsenoside and/or poly-saccharides or another compound is a matter of debate and more research. Again, the fact that there were no side effects beyond placebo and American ginseng has been found to have no real strong drug interactions or interfere overtly with drug metabolism is noteworthy. *Ginseng from water extraction or from pure ground root has been associated with the best results and safety, and ginseng extraction methods due to alcohol or methanol based procedures could be less effective and some researchers believe toxic or even estrogenic with long-term use* [135]. Additionally, ginseng (Panax or American ginseng) has a long history of having an ability to improve energy levels in healthy individuals, but again because it worked for more extreme fatigue from cancer treatment it can help with many types of fatigue from my experience. Ginseng can be ingested with or without food, but with a meal could reduce gastrointestinal side effects caused by pill consumption in general.

C. Guarana (Paullinia cupana) 50 mg twice a day (caffeine or 1,3,7-trimethylxanthine mimics) or not more than 40 mg of caffeine derived from these sources per day utilized in the morning or early afternoon. Is it just the caffeine?
Caffeine is found in many products and plants and so recommending a caffeine product is easy based on the proven track record of improving energy and attention levels [3]. Guarana is a plant from the Amazon basin that has been utilized for fatigue because it has caffeine in it, which comprises on average 2.5–5 % of the dry weight (some can be slightly higher), but it also has a high content of saponins and tannins, which suggests it could provide other nutritional properties.

The Bayer company (Consumer Care Division, Basel, Switzerland) sponsored a study of over 222 mg of guarana in a dissolvable tablet in liquid that contained

40 mg of caffeine and found it worked better than placebo in reducing mental fatigue and improving focus and attention to different tasks ($n = 129$ healthy adults ages 18–24 years) [138]. Other clinical studies of 75 mg of Guarana appeared to improve memory in multiple studies. In other words, there is enough preliminary research on caffeine itself along with the fact that guarana contains low doses of other compounds to recommend guarana supplementation to improve energy levels.

Past data was of only a passing interest until preliminary studies have found a potential antifatigue effect from cancer treatment [139]. The guarana standardized extract used in an adequate 21-day study ($n = 75$) was from Cathedral Pharmaceutical Industry (Nova Pampulha, Vespasiano, Minas Gerias, Brazil), and it had a 6.46 % caffeine content and 1.7 % tannin content. This suggests that patients in this study only received approximately 5 mg of caffeine a day from guarana compared to a standard cup of coffee, which is 50–100 mg or more. There was a large reduction in fatigue that approached 50 % in patients in the guarana supplement (50 mg supplement twice a day) compared to placebo group in breast cancer patients experiencing progressive fatigue after their first cycle of chemotherapy. The guarana caffeine content again is fairly low, which is understandable why anxiety and insomnia have not been observed to increase in these clinical trials unlike what one would witness with pure caffeine. Interestingly, a guarana extract (75 mg once a day—similar research group as in the previous study) used in breast cancer patients experiencing post-radiation fatigue did not appear to work as well as a placebo [140], which could suggest that the study was either too small ($n = 36$ total), caffeine content was not high enough or there is no impact in this setting.

Still, the reader should keep one important issue in terms of caffeine and studies, which is when precisely participants stopped drinking coffee or ingesting caffeine. For example, if a washout occurs several weeks before a study the benefits of caffeine look better when reinitiated [3]. This is not what appeared to be the case in these and other studies of guarana, which makes these results even more believable. Keep in mind the half-life of caffeine can vary from a few hours to up to 6–8 h which is why anything with caffeine in it should not be used in the later afternoon or early evening because of its ability to cause insomnia. Yerba mate is another plant with caffeine in it, which is also beginning to show some benefits for improved energy when placed in beverages and arguably may soon be found to work as well as guarana supplements but needs more research right now in terms of safety. Pregnant women should not use guarana because although it is a mild stimulant it is still cannot be considered safe in pregnancy unless it receives more safety research in this area.

Caffeine pills appear tantamount to concentrated energy [3]. I do not mind a single 5-h energy or other similar drinks, but taking more than 2 a day is an excessive amount of concentrated (not diluted like soda, coffee, tea..) caffeine or energy. For example, shots of hard liquor allow a shorter interval to feel inebriated, but more diluted sources of alcohol like light beer require large volumes of the beverage to feel the same effects. I often explain to patients that caffeine is somewhat similar that when you concentrate the amount in a very small volume of liquid it is easy to overdose and produce anxiety, anxiousness, and palpitations (cardiovascular effects). It is for this reason that I am not a caffeine pill advocate for most individuals except for some rare situations where nothing else is working. Another problem with becoming addicted to higher doses of caffeine is tolerance or tachyphylaxis, whereby much larger doses are needed over time to have any effect. Finally, withdrawal from these very high doses of caffeine provided by pills and energy drinks is difficult and often can cause moderate to severe headaches.

D. Miscellaneous supplements for fatigue (Hype but little hope?)
E. B-vitamin injections versus supplements = similar = nothing

– "B-vitamins to support energy metabolism"? Why don't companies that put huge amounts of B-vitamins in their pills just say that it increases energy levels or reduces fatigue? This is due to the lack of evidence that B-vitamins reduce fatigue unless a patient has a rare overt anemia from a deficiency of B-vitamins. The human body needs such minimal amounts of B-vitamins aid in the production of cellular energy and normal functions, so there are no credible studies that show taking B-vitamins as supplements improve metabolism or energy or in reality reduce fatigue. And in past clinical trials the costly B-12 injection does not work any better in raising B-vitamin levels compared to a low-cost high-dose pill (1000–2000 µg for a limited time) unless an overt B-vitamin absorption disease exists [141, 142]. It is also important to note that from a prevention standpoint the *Women's Antioxidant and Folic Acid Cardiovascular Study (WAFACS)* utilizing 2.5 mg of folic acid, 50 mg of vitamin B6, and 1000 µg of B12 (high dosages of B-vitamins) versus placebo ($n = 379$ women) for 7.3 years found no difference between placebo in the risk of cardiovascular disease or cancer [143], but a hint that a significant reduction (30–40 %) in age-related macular degeneration could occur with this supplement from a secondary endpoint [144]. The potential benefit against this eye disease became evident during the second year of the trial and persisted throughout the rest of the study. It is also of interest that the average BMI of these participants was 30.5 (obese) and average age was 63 (21 % were ages 40–54 years). Thus, the initial concern that high-doses of B-vitamin supplements could increase the risk of breast cancer in a short period of time was not supported by this trial.

F. CoQ10 (Remember the QE3 study that failed)
A total of 236 women (Wake Forest Associated Study) with newly diagnosed breast cancer and planed adjuvant chemotherapy were randomized to 300 mg CoQ10 or placebo and each combined with 300 IU of vitamin E divided into three daily dosages and the treatment was continued for 24 weeks [145]. Supplementation caused improvement in plasma CoQ10 but no improvement in fatigue, depression or quality of life. This is arguably equivalent to a phase-3 like clinical trial for CRF and 300 mg of CoQ10 is not a small dose and can be costly. It is also of interest that CoQ10 had promising preliminary data in early Parkinson disease to improve daily function and was elevated to a phase-3 trial called "QE3 Study" and at a dosage of 1200 mg or 2400 mg/day or placebo (all participants received 1200 IU a day of vitamin E) and conducted in 67 medical centers in North America ($n = 600$) and the

trail was stopped after 16 months because of futility [146]. This trial is a reminder of how preliminary extensive data in one area of medicine that does not show any activity in a phase 3 could provide some clue in another seemingly unrelated area of medicine.

G. d-*ribose*

D-ribose is a natural pentose sugar that can be purchased as a powder to place into beverages and can be purchased at health food stores or online. Ribose (also known as "D-ribose") can also be purchased as a pill. There have been a few preliminary studies that suggest that when utilizing 5 g a day with a beverage at breakfast, lunch and dinner (15 g total) that it can help to reduce fatigue from fibromyalgia and chronic fatigue syndrome [147]. The problem is not only preliminary indirect studies demonstrating no impact [148], but the lack of a well-done large study in those with any type of chronic fatigue that proves it can beat a placebo and the lack of any adequate trial of methodology over the last decade.

H. l-*carnitine (mechanism of action without impressive data in a Phase-3 trial)*

L-carnitine is a dietary supplement that had a lot of researchers excited because it just makes sense as to why it might work to reduce fatigue [3]. l-*carnitine is a compound that exists in every cell of the human body to aid in the transport of long-chain fatty acids into the mitochondrion to increase energy (ATP) production.* However, the more sound clinical trials have not followed all the hype and a recent phase-3 trial was a disappointment in multiple ways [149]. There have been a few small studies to suggest that getting 1–2 g (1000–2000 mg)/day of L-carnitine supplements or pills may reduce fatigue in some individuals, but this recent large phase-3 study of 2000 mg/day of L-carnitine over 4 weeks in cancer patients did not show a benefit compared to placebo [149]. Some might argue that the study was not long enough, but no trend in improvement was observed, even in the subgroups. The real limitation of this study was the 25–30 % failure to complete the assessments by the participants, which "weakens the conclusions of the study." A total of 367 patients were included in this trial (conducted by the reputable Eastern Cooperative Oncology Group or ECOG—funded by the National Cancer Institute or NCI) and supplementation caused a significant rise in carnitine plasma level by week 4 in the supplement versus the placebo arm. None of the primary or secondary endpoints using validated instruments for fatigue found a difference between the placebo and no impact on depression and pain. *More importantly, when examining a subset of patients who were actually carnitine-deficient at baseline there was also no significant improvement in fatigue or other outcomes with this supplement.*

Interestingly, a recent preliminary 3000 mg L-carnitine versus placebo per day trial for 2 weeks, followed by a 2-week, open-label phase with the exact same dosage of L-carnitine for all patients was conducted by similar researchers that performed the past phase-3 cancer trial [150]. In this case, patients with terminal HIV/AIDS were included and 18 patients in the treatment arm and 17 in the placebo completed the trial. Significant increases in the total (28–48 nM/L, $p < 0.001$), and free carnitine (24–40 nM/L, $p < 0.001$) occurred with the supplement and there were no changes in these levels in the placebo arm. And the primary outcome, fatigue at the end of the blinded phase, did not improve. Secondary outcomes of function, quality of life, and mood also demonstrated no changes versus placebo. A secondary outcome–serum lactate–was reduced significantly ($p < 0.005$) with L-carnitine (1.45–1.28 nmol/L) and increased (1.38–1.84) in the placebo arm. *And although this is interesting and again statistically significant, it did not translate into any documented clinical significance.*

Some advocates of L-carnitine refer to two studies of combinations of drugs and supplements to suggest L-carnitine has some activity against fatigue, but a closer examination of these investigations does not actually suggest directly that L-CARNITINE by itself has a positive impact [151, 152], so it seems like an exhaustive attempt to find some level of evidence where currently none to minimal exists. Another thought that is often lost in the cacophony or desire of a supplement to work is the observation that L-carnitine is not a low cost product, and it is generally supplied to patients in 500 mg capsules (even though in the phase-3 and HIV/AIDS trial a liquid suspension was utilized—another credit to the sensitivity of the ECOG group). Even if L-carnitine did demonstrate some efficacy patients would be consuming at least 4–6 capsules a day in the best-case scenario and ten or more capsules for those that cannot tolerate the larger sized pills! The accessible and affordable delivery system for any supplement or medication needs to be practical and realistic for compliance regardless of the overall efficacy against the specific medical condition. Therefore, cumulatively the overall evidence currently suggests L-carnitine should not be utilized to improve fatigue.

I. Miscellaneous—Mushrooms …

There are countless dietary supplement options espoused on the internet and even from integrative medicine "experts" in the medical literature. However, as was the case with L-carnitine there is nothing more than a wonderful theory defiled by good clinical trial results. In other words, just because a mechanism of action exists to explain why something will be effective does not always and in many cases translate to real world effectiveness. If a placebo response can occur in one-third to one-half of patients with subjective outcomes then these generally costly supplements and prescription medications need to be rigorously and objectively tested.

For example, *Ganoderma lucidum* ("Reishi" mushroom) spore powder (1000 mg three times a day for 4 weeks) in breast cancer patients ($n = 48$) did appear to reduce fatigue versus a control group, but there were no specific details provided on the placebo arm (no focus or section of description) nor were statistics completed on side effects (even on the placebo) which appeared to be statistically significant for the intervention but dismissed [153]. In other words, in order to elevate the status of some dietary supplements the description or methodology and the peer review of the journal that accepts the article needs to be rigorous enough to convince the reader that the compound really functions greater than a placebo. This and so many well-done studies would receive more objective appreciation if greater transparency or descriptive details were provided. And this is a limitation I find in some dietary supplement and pharmacologic clinical studies. The intervention and study appear sound but the ability to objectively review the evidence is compromised by the written article itself.

CRF and fatigue treatment in general is desperate for more and better studies, and integrative medicine has the potential to provide and is currently first-line evidence-based treatment for this condition, as was recently demonstrated from American ginseng phase-3 trial and past exercise interventions [133–136]. This is a profound moment for integrative medicine and breast cancer especially at a time that pharmacologic treatments have struggled overall to find success in this category as a recent Cochrane Review of 18 drugs, 4696 participants and 1645 publications concluded with the following statement: "Based on limited evidence, we cannot recommend a specific drug for the treatment of fatigue in palliative care patients" [154].

• Hot flashes/flushes/vasomotor symptoms (hot flashes, night and/or cold sweats)
A. Weight gain can exacerbate hot flashes (contrary to popular belief)
Vasomotor symptoms were the number one reason women stopped tamoxifen in the landmark P-1 study and it was more common in the tamoxifen arm. Researchers looked back on this data and found something remarkable when comparing the women of normal BMI to those obese women in the trial [155]. They analyzed data from 11,064 women enrolled at least 3 years before the trial unblinding in May, 1998. It appears that hot flashes, night sweats and cold sweats were significantly worse in obese women and all three symptoms (hot flashes 57 % greater, night sweats 50 % greater, and cold sweats 64 % greater) were more likely to lead to non-adhering to the study medications. Contrary to past belief that obese women have more aromatase activity, arguably from greater estrone concentrations (also conversion of androstenedione to estrone) that should reduce frequency and severity of hot flashes, it appears in menopausal and women with breast cancer hot flashes become more severe with weight gain [156, 157]. A preliminary and interesting observation from a randomized trial of weight loss ($n = 154$) found decreases in weight, BMI, and waist circumference were each correlated with improvements in flushing after 6 months [158]. Potential mechanisms of action proffered include increased adipose insulation against heat dissipation, increased sympathetic neural activity correlated with increased visceral fat, and changes in cytokines such as leptin from adipose tissue that impact thermoregulatory centers. Obesity with more severe or frequent hot flashes could also be a marker for a higher risk of metabolic syndrome and overall cardiovascular risk [159], as well as other comorbidities such as depression that could impact vasomotor symptoms [160], and even breast cancer patients with greater weight/waist size could be responsible for a plethora of negative effects on quality of life [161].

B. Other lifestyle interventions (Benefit ≫ risk)
It appears from this past trial and a Cochrane review of five studies ($n = 733$) that exercise has an inconsistent effect on hot flushes [162]. It has been my clinical experience with hot flashes in cancer patients for decades that some were convinced their exercise regimen cured them and others will find that they exacerbated them. Still, the overall profound impact of exercise on symptoms from sleep quality, reduced insomnia and depression [163–165], should always be discussed with breast cancer survivors. Another option that appears to be espoused by some alternative medicine educational sources is "Paced Respiration" or abdominal breathing exercises at a

slower pace to control hot flash frequency and/or severity and although in theory it appears to make some sense the clinical research to support this activity thus far in menopausal and breast cancer patients is weak [166, 167].

Before a discussion of lifestyle interventions and/or other integrative medicines can commence it must be keep in mind that a personal hot flash diary is critical to utilize for maximum benefit and control of hot flashes. Patients can utilize these diaries (or simply create their own) for 1–2 weeks to determine the average frequency and severity of their hot flashes [1]. A hot flash diary allows the health care practitioner and patient a better method of determining whether or not vasomotor symptoms could also be controlled by lifestyle, and/or supplements, and/or prescription medication. For example the mild to moderate hot flashes are usually controlled through lifestyle/supplements and more severe and very severe or frequent hot flashes that clearly interfere with day-to-day activities and sleep patterns are better controlled through prescription medications. An example of how to score hot flashes themselves is found in Table 7.4 [1].

Overall, lifestyle changes and breast cancer and vasomotor symptoms have minimal data, but there are common sense changes that should be applied where benefit always seemed to outweigh risk and these are found in Table 7.5 [1].

Tough to beat a placebo (Acupuncture, black cohosh, flaxseed, soy, vitamin E, and now magnesium supplements—Soften the stool but no hot flash reductions in breast cancer)

Hot flashes and integrative medicine have a research background unlike arguably anything else tested in the field of supplements for breast cancer. *Multiple phase III clinical trials of popular dietary supplements in breast cancer patients demonstrated that it is difficult to beat a placebo. Thus, although hormonal (estrogen and/ or progesterone based) treatment can reduce hot flashes by 80–90 % and antidepressants and anticonvulsants by 50 %, the dietary supplements appear to reduce*

Table 7.4 Hot flash diary that patients can utilize for 1–2 weeks to determine the average frequency and severity of their hot flashes, which allows a better method of determining whether or not vasomotor symptoms could also be controlled by lifestyle, and/or supplements, and/or prescription medication [1]

Severity	Score	Length/duration	Observations
MILD Hot Flash	1 point	Less than 1 min	Warm and slightly uncomfortable, no perspiration
MODERATE Hot Flash	2 points	Less than 5 min	Warmth involving more of the body, perspiration, taking off some layers of clothing
SEVERE Hot Flash	3 points	Greater than 5 min	Burning warmth, disruption of normal life activities such as sleep or work, excessive perspiration, frequent thermostat changes in your house
VERY SEVERE Hot Flash	4 points	Time is not an issue	Complete disruption of normal activities to the point where it would make you consider discontinuing the hormone-deprivation treatment

Table 7.5 Lifestyle changes associated with a reduction in hot flash frequency and/or severity [1]. Keep in mind that completing a hot flash diary will allow a patient to personally identify the more common and uncommon triggers of vasomotor symptoms

Lifestyle change	Commentary
Keeping a diary	Diary-keeping for just 1–2 weeks can give a patient and clinician the best insight into what impacts hot flashes and how best to treat them
Avoid excess alcohol, caffeine, and hot beverages or spicy food	Many foods or beverages can trigger hot flashes or make them worse
Controlled, deep, slow abdominal breathing (6–8 breaths per minute) for at least 15 min twice daily (morning, midday, and/or evening) or at the beginning of a hot flash	Also known as "paced respiration," it has at least been shown to decrease blood pressure (temporarily), hot flash number and severity in some patients, but not in larger clinical trials. However, this technique needs practice or it may need to be taught to you because it involves moving abdominal muscles in and out
Avoid smoking or breathing secondhand smoke	Tobacco exposure is not just heart unhealthy, but can make hot flashes worse by causing circulatory and temperature changes in the body
Low-impact daily exercise	Exercise has been shown to reduce stress and fatigue, improve mood and sleep, and for some select patients it could reduce vasomotor symptoms. Use a fan or work out in a lower temperature environment
Stress reduction (meditation, relaxation techniques, yoga, etc.)	Relaxation exercises can help with hot flashes in some patients and could also improve other areas of health such as sleep, energy levels, and blood pressure
Use cooling methods—ice-cubes, cool beverages, fan or reducing room temperature, opening a window, chilling pillows and/or pillow coverings	A slight increase in the body's core temperature can trigger a hot flash or the severity of a hot flash
Wear loose-fitting clothing and layer clothing	Helps to keep the body's core temperature slightly lower and prevents clothing from feeling constricting when a hot flash occurs. Layers allow one to easily shed clothing to regulate temperature shifts

them by 20–33 % (similar to placebo). And there is always the possibility that some supplements could make hot flashes worse either because they discourage lifestyle changes or lengthen the time a patient requests more effective pharmacologic treatments from her/his doctor, or they simply may be associated with worsening vasomotor symptoms [168].

C. Acupuncture

A recent meta-analysis of breast cancer patients experiencing menopause symptoms utilized seven studies of 342 patients and found a small benefit to acupuncture except when compared to sham acupuncture the benefit was not statistically significant [169]. A similar finding with arguably one of the largest reviews of acupuncture for cancer patients found minimal to no benefit for hot flashes from a review of 41 randomized clinical trials (2151 publications) but did find some potential benefit for chemotherapy-induced nausea and vomiting [170]. And a similar finding for women dealing with menopausal symptoms was reported for 16 studies that included 1155 women, but eight of these studies compared acupuncture to sham acupuncture and when this occurred found a minimal to no benefit for hot flashes [171].

D. Black Cohosh

Black cohosh (*Cimicifuga racemosa*, or Remifemin® from GSK was unable to be obtained so another product was chosen—Hi-Health Corporation, Scottsdale, Arizona—standardized to contain 1 mg of triterpene glycosides) was utilized in a phase-3 double-blind crossover trial with two 4-week periods, and one 20 mg capsule of this supplement twice a day versus placebo (*n = 132 women with a history of breast cancer from over 10 medical centers*) were the interventions [172]. Patients were included if they had "bothersome" hot flashes, which was defined as 14 or more per week for at least 1 month and desired some intervention. Patients receiving black cohosh reported a reduction of 20 % in the hot flash score versus 27 % reduction with placebo, and mean hot flash frequency was reduced 17 % on black cohosh and 26 % on placebo. Thus, there were no statistically significant differences throughout the trial and on the primary outcomes.

E. Flaxseed (personal favorite despite not better than a placebo, "first do no harm"?)

Postmenopausal women *with breast cancer (50 % of the participants)* and without breast cancer were randomly allocated to consume a flaxseed bar (7.5 g of flaxseed—5 % lignans or 410 mg of lignans, 6 g of protein, 20 % fiber, and 190 calories from Glanbia Nutritionals) for 6-weeks versus a placebo bar (no flaxseed, lignans or soy) [173]. *A total of 188 women from 22 medical centers were included in the trial and mean hot flash score was reduced by 4.9 in the flaxseed group and 3.5 in the placebo arm (p = 0.29).* Approximately one-third of women in both groups experienced a 50 % reduction in hot flash scores (mean 30 % change overall in frequency and score). Grade 1 pruritus was the only side effect more common between groups with 8 % experiencing this event with placebo versus 1 % with flaxseed. Both groups reported gastrointestinal upset arguably related to the fiber content of the bars.

Arguably, this intervention/flaxseed powder continues to be my favorite dietary intervention for women and men dealing with hot flashes from cancer treatment because it appears to work the same or slightly better than placebo, it is low cost, provides a good source of fiber, it is low in calories, and it has been shown to be heart healthy and contains one of the largest sources of plant omega-3 fatty acids [3]. A total of 2–3 tablespoons of flaxseed powder can be applied to diverse sources (cereal, oatmeal, beverages, salad, …) and it discourages expensive dietary supplement pill utilization that can occur with this medical condition. I have found no greater benefit versus risk for any other product currently (except perhaps for soy protein powder [174]) especially when dealing with aging issues (from constipation, hemorrhoids, to glucose and lipid control). Please see Chap. 3 for more information on the heart healthy effects of flaxseed powder in women with breast cancer. And there are numerous high-quality objective reviews of past clinical data on flaxseed for heart health found in the literature, for example a review of 28 studies that found modest LDL lowering benefits for flaxseed (not the oil) especially in postmenopausal women [175].

F. Magnesium (the most recent to succumb to the placebo effect)
An outstanding double-blind, placebo-controlled, randomized arguably phase-3 trial was recently completed that included *289 postmenopausal women from over 20 medical centers with a history of breast cancer* and "bothersome hot flashes" (greater than 28 times per week and of a severity to request intervention) were randomized to [176]:

- 800 mg magnesium oxide daily
- 1200 mg magnesium oxide daily
- Placebo

No differences were found for magnesium or placebo for all endpoints including mean hot flash score (number multiplied by the mean severity) and frequency using a validated hot flash diary, *but an increased incidence of diarrhea at a lower incidence of constipation was found with magnesium* [176]. No other significant differences in side effects or quality of life were found. Approximately a steady reduction over 8-weeks in hot flash score and frequency occurred eventually leading to a 30–35 % reduction in these values over time for all the groups. Thus, despite preliminary non-randomized trials of magnesium observing large reductions in hot flashes [177, 178], it appears the placebo provided a reality check. It is of interest that magnesium is touted for a plethora of health conditions on the internet but many of these conditions have not received high-powered clinical trials such as the one mentioned previously [176], but at least it is well-known now that if a patient suffers from regular constipation and some vasomotor symptoms then magnesium supplements could be an appropriate choice in this specific setting.

G. Omega-3 (promise then failure)
A large 12-week phase-3 like trial of omega-3 supplements ($n = 177$, 1800 mg/day) versus placebo ($n = 178$) in perimenopausal and postmenopausal women for 12 weeks found no improvement in vasomotor symptoms frequency, bother, sleep, or mood versus placebo [179]. One could argue that the dosage was not high enough to observe a response but there was no trend in benefit and ingesting large numbers of capsules for the potential of a modest benefit is not practical. In the future, perhaps a trial of a higher dose liquid product could be conducted to resolve this issue.

H. Red clover (Trifolium pratense) (high cost, hype, minimal effects)
Overall, these supplements touted as high in plant estrogens have failed overall to provide a consistent reduction over placebo in vasomotor symptoms [180, 181]. Some of the more costly and best selling brands were tested in some of these studies. And some past studies that failed to demonstrate a benefit over placebo were 1 year in length [182]. Another 1-year trial ($n = 89$) of 120 mg of red clover demonstrated an impressive 57 % reduction in vasomotor symptoms (black cohosh = −34 %), but the placebo demonstrated a 63 % reduction and 0.625 mg conjugated equine estrogen/2.5 mg medroxyprogesterone acetate group had a 94 % reduction [183]!

I. Sage (also known as "Salvia officinalis," the spice but not the supplement)
Sage, a plant native to Mediterranean Europe has been used in food and folk medicine to treat menopausal symptoms for many years but has no strong methodology clinical studies [1]. There was one open, multicenter clinical trial completed in eight practices in Switzerland [184]. A total of 71 patients with an average age of 56 years, menopausal for at least 12 months, and with a minimum of five hot flushes daily were recruited. There was no placebo arm. Participants were given a hot flash diary and a once-daily tablet of fresh sage leaves for 8 weeks. The average number of hot flushes was significantly reduced within 4 weeks, and they continued to be reduced even further after 8 weeks. Severe and very severe hot flushes were reduced by 79 % and approximately 100 % over 8 weeks. A total of two participants experienced gastrointestinal issues during the study attributed to the sage preparation. Sage is a safe herbal spice that can be added to food. So, perhaps it should be used as a seasoning for tomato sauce, add to morning eggs or omelets, or on a piece of pizza, in salads, and to chicken or fish when cooking so the food will absorb the herbs nice flavor. Sage dietary supplements are generally low cost, but how can one recommend a dose when a trial that can be replicated in the real world has not been published? Currently there is also minimal information on potential drug–supplement interactions in the medical literature. The sheer dearth of overall clinical trials with this supplement is noteworthy and does not allow for a benefit-versus-risk analysis (except more of the spice in food is always an option).

J. Soy (traditional food sources but not supplements)
A total of 177 women in a phase-3 like trial with a history of breast cancer from over ten medical centers were randomized and 149 had complete data over the 9-week study period [185]. Patients utilized soy tablets (600 mg tablets containing 50 mg of soy isoflavones in each tablet—40–45 % genistein, 40–45 % daidzein, and 10–20 % glycitein; one tablet three times a day for 150 mg isoflavones per day, amount similar to three glasses of soy milk, product provided by Pharmavite, Mission Hills, CA) or placebo for 4-weeks and then crossed-over to other regimen. The percentage of patients reporting a greater than 50 % reduction in hot flash score was 38 % with placebo and 35 % with soy, *and 36 % of patients on placebo reported their hot flash frequency reduced to half and 24 % with soy (p = 0.01).* There was no difference found versus placebo and patients preferred the soy supplement 33 % of the time, placebo 37 % of the time, and neither pill 31 % of the time. There were no differences in side effects between the pills. This is does not quell my enthusiasm for recommending soy protein or traditional soy sources (edamame, tofu, …) for heart health and based on the potential benefit in breast cancer for some patients that are comfortable utilizing it as part of a cholesterol and weight loss reducing regimen [181].

K. Vitamin E (safe as a placebo and about as effective)
A total of 120 patients from over ten medical centers with a history of breast cancer were recruited for a 4-week crossover trial of 800 IU of vitamin E succinate daily versus placebo or vice versa [186]. There was a similar reduction in hot flash frequency during the first crossover period (25 % with vitamin E and 22 % with placebo), but a minimal significant decrease in hot flashes (one less per day with

vitamin E versus placebo, $p = 0.05$), but at the end of the study patients did not prefer vitamin E over the placebo (32 % versus 29 %).

L. Miscellaneous—DHEA, 5-HTP (5-hydroxytryptophan), SJW (St. John's wort, sesame seed powder (healthy at least), _____ (insert the name of next potential product here)

DHEA has had inconsistent data and could have androgenic side effects and has unpredictable conversion (patient-to-patient variability) to testosterone and estrogen, but potentially has a role for some women with sexual dysfunction due to adrenal insufficiency [3, 187]. DHEA also has inconsistent effects on lipid parameters and can lower HDL in some patients. 5-HTP has had minimal research against placebo for hot flashes and even at 150 mg/day has not demonstrated preliminary benefit. And SJW has had mixed results, but it is the dietary supplement antidepressant mimics such as these that should receive more research since venlafaxine and other prescription antidepressants with similar mechanisms of action have displayed some success for treating vasomotor symptoms in breast cancer patients. Sesame seed (*Sesamum indicum*) powder has an adequate content of protein and fiber and had some preliminary heart healthy data that would need to be replicated [188–190]. It is also a good sources of lignans (like flaxseed) that could be tested in a hot flash study but based on past hot flash trial with similar products there is little confidence it could provide a significant benefit over placebo.

M. Finding the next American ginseng and fatigue equivalent for hot flashes?

Hot flash frequency and severity in breast cancer and other scenarios is simply daunting and not simple to resolve. If the hot flashes are mild to moderate the placebo response is extremely high and difficult to exceed with any supplement. If the hot flashes are more severe or very severe then pharmacologic interventions or something with a more overt benefit-to-risk ratio needs to be discussed. The idea that a dietary supplement with side effects seemingly similar to placebo could consistently surpass a placebo in a clinical trial or be as effective or more effective than some pharmacologic agents is optimistic. However, I am always hopeful of an exception to the rule (as is the case with American ginseng and cancer-related fatigue or CRF).

• Insomnia/difficulty sleeping

Most patients experience problems falling asleep or maintaining sleep, but a smaller percentage meet the clinical criteria for insomnia (20 %) [191, 192]. Insomnia is associated with reduced quality of life and increased rates of depression. Sleep problems in cancer patients are a real problem with some studies reporting as high as six out of every ten individuals having issues with sleep. Pharmacologic options are not of low cost and have been estimated to cost 50–100 dollars per month but dietary supplements from this chapter run 10 dollars a month maximum in many cases if used daily.

A. Lifestyle changes/exercise/sleep hygiene

Multiple clinical trials continue to demonstrate the impact of light to heavy exercise on sleep quality in breast cancer patients. A Canadian multicenter trial of over 300 breast cancer patients on chemotherapy found that light to moderate aerobic exercise improves sleep but a combination of aerobic and resistance activity 50–60 min three times a week may provide the best results [193]. Some studies suggest the improvement in sleep with exercise is not significant enough, which opens the door to other potential interventions in these patients [194]. Still, multiple exercise options appear promising, for example, yoga in 75 min sessions twice a week over 4 weeks demonstrated significant improvement in multiple aspects of sleep quality including reducing sleep medication among cancer survivors compared to those that did not participate ($n = 410$) [195].

Dietary supplements could play a significant role for insomnia breast cancer patients. It should be kept in mind that the potential out of pocket costs and toxicity of prescription medications again are not insignificant. For example, recently the FDA reduced the daily dosage of prescription eszopiclone because of serious reports of fugue or abnormal changes in behavior and even driving while the patient was not even aware of these actions the next day [196]. And the leading causes of unintentional overdose leading to morbidity and mortality from medications in the USA are opioids, and then antianxiety drug, but in third or fourth position are the insomnia-based prescription medications [197]. Still, first-line of treatment should be lifestyle changes and sleep hygiene options (including behavioral therapy—bedroom is for sleep, no TV, computer, bright lights, …) that receive enormous attention today and are best handled by other reviews on the subject and/or insomnia professional.

B. Melatonin (Why not a potential standard of care in some patients with insomnia? Immediate release and PR-melatonin)

Melatonin is produced from the amino acid tryptophan in the pineal gland of the brain and is released in a circadian pattern [3, 198]. It binds to melatonin receptors and reduces the firing of neurons in the suprachiasmatic nucleus in the hypothalamus (where a high receptor concentration exists), promoting sleep induction or the ability to fall asleep.

Melatonin is actually available over the counter in several forms but the immediate and prolonged release (PR) forms enjoy most of the positive clinical data. Controlled release (CR) melatonin or slow release is basically identical to PR melatonin. Whether or not sustained release (SR) or extended release (ER) works similarly than PR melatonin is not known and when immediate release is not effective then *PR is an option because it has multiple clinical trials and is an improved medication in Europe for the treatment of primary insomnia with poor sleep quality in patients aged 55 years and older.* This is important because age can reduce melatonin production as measured by the primary urinary metabolite 6-sulfatoxymelatonin (6SMT), which is also a test to show the circadian release of this hormone.

Interestingly, the use of PR melatonin has not been associated with a reduction in endogenous melatonin production [198]. It has not been associated with psychomotor effects or memory and driving issues at the most common dosage (2 mg) and had significantly less impairment with prescription medications such as zolpidem. And it has not been associated with dependence, hangover, tolerance, rebound insomnia or withdrawal symptoms and has even shown excellent efficacy and safety in a variety of patient populations, for example Alzheimer's disease. PR melatonin is usually given 1–2 h before bedtime. Alcohol can reduce the efficacy of melatonin. The bioavailability of oral melatonin is only approximately 15 %, and there is significant first pass metabolism and food can also lower the absorption. The half-life of immediate release melatonin is less than 30 min, which is why there is increasing interest in PR melatonin. A 2-mg preparation of PR melatonin known as "Circadin®" was developed by Neurim, Tel Aviv, Israel, and again has been approved by European Medicines Agency (EMEA) since 2007. It has a terminal half-life of 3.5–4 h. Keep in mind the FDA even approved a drug that acts as a melatonin receptor agonist (ramelteon) back in 2005. Numerous reviews, meta-analysis, and recent clinical trials continue to demonstrate the efficacy of melatonin and overall safety profile in a variety of patients from those with cancer to Autism and Alzheimer disease, but at the lowest potential dosage in order to mimic physiologic levels [199–203].

C. Melatonin and breast cancer (3 mg or below, or 2 mg PR melatonin?)
A Dana-Farber Cancer Institute (DFCI, Boston, MA) randomized, double-blind trial of 95 postmenopausal women with a previous history of stage 0–III breast cancers with a mean age of 59 years and BMI of 25 who completed conventional treatment were assigned to 3 mg of oral melatonin or placebo for 4 months [204, 205]. Melatonin was purchased from a single supplier who also guaranteed the composition and purity of these supplements (Rugby Laboratories, a subsidiary of Watson Laboratories—Duluth, GA, USA). Melatonin was ingested at 9 PM each evening because of the potential sedating effects of this supplement. The primary endpoint of the trial was estradiol, IGF-1, or IGF-binding protein-3 and there was no change in these measurements with melatonin. Other endpoints included sleep quality, depression scores, and hot flashes. At baseline, 52 % of participants reported poor sleep in the month before trial enrollment. *Subjects utilizing melatonin had significantly greater improvements in sleep quality (PSQI, Pittsburgh Sleep Quality Index) including domains on sleep quality, daytime dysfunction, and total score.* Melatonin has no impact on depression or hot flashes.

This was arguably the fist randomized placebo-controlled trial of breast cancer survivors to demonstrate melatonin improves subjective sleep quality with no significant adverse effects compared to placebo. Still, headache, fatigue and bad dreams were the most common side effects reported with melatonin. The dosage of 3 mg is still s supra-physiologic level, but returns to normal with minimal hangover effect in morning as shown in insomnia and jet lag. It would be informative to test the 2 mg PR-melatonin (for example the approved product Circadin® in Europe) in breast cancer patients to determine if overall sleep outcomes would improve compared to immediate-release.

Again, melatonin has been well studied in cancer patients as a standalone agent and even with chemotherapy without significant adverse events [3]. Dosages of 0.1–5 mg have been the most commonly tested and exceeded this dosage could favor risk over benefit. In fact, from experience some breast cancer patients have been told to utilize high dosages of melatonin (for example 10–20 mg/day) because of preliminary evidence that it may have anti-breast cancer effects and because of ongoing clinical trial addressing this issue. Not only is this unproven but this is unsafe because of the daytime drowsiness and fatigue can impair quality of life and could be dangerous when driving or operating machinery. This is no different than the recent FDA concern of sleep medication dosages and their ability to create fugue or dysfunction in my opinion. There are some reviews of past clinical studies that suggest melatonin has anticancer effects at higher dosages [206], but until more definitive proof is provided and better methodology in a clinical trial this should not be recommend.

D. Melatonin—The catch?

Apart for the encouragement by some in the integrative medicine world for cancer patients to take excessive dosages, the other concerns from this author are more minor at this time. Melatonin for insomnia and jet lag and has an excellent safety record over a range of dosages and duration of use [3]. Arguably more daytime fatigue and a potential reduction in nocturnal blood pressure are some concerns but these events occur more often with excessive dosages that again should not be recommended. Side effects have been rare—similar to placebo overall at the 3 mg and below dosages.

The impact on melatonin and blood pressure should be reviewed with patients. Melatonin could reduce nocturnal blood pressure in normotensive and even in hypertensive patients, but its impact on heart rate is inconsistent and could be an issue of dosage [207, 208]. An older study of 47 patients found 5 mg melatonin over 4 weeks blunted the effects of the calcium channel blocker nifedipine, which caused significant increases during the daytime in blood pressure and heart rate [209]. A meta-analysis of seven studies ($n = 221$) found no impact of melatonin on blood pressure but subgroup analysis found a significant reduction in nocturnal systolic (−6.0 mmHg) and diastolic (−3.5 mmHg) blood pressure with controlled release melatonin and no impact with immediate- or fast-release melatonin [210]. Safety issues were similar to placebo overall and authors argued that "the safety of melatonin in hypertensive patients is good, and implies that add-on melatonin therapy does not present significant risks of detrimental drug interactions with the main major drugs used to treat hypertension." And even recent randomized trials utilizing sublingual melatonin at 3 mg to reduce anxiety demonstrate no blood pressure effects. It has the potential to be a preoperative anxiolytic that could replace the concerns with Benzodiazepines [211, 212]. Melatonin (1–3 mg immediate-release or 2 mg prolonged release) helps with sleep induction or falling asleep but not necessarily for sleep maintenance in my experience, which also allows some patients to only utilize the immediate release form of melatonin if they awake in the night and can't get to sleep. Otherwise, headache, drowsiness, dizziness, nightmares, and fatigue are more common in my experience but this again appears to be primarily dose-related.

E. Valerian (controversial results but less so in breast cancer after a phase-3 trial?)

Valerian (also known as *Valeriana officinalis* that comes from aqueous or ethanol extracts usually) is actually the dietary supplement that has been moderately effective in some studies for helping someone fall asleep and stay in deeper and more refreshing states of sleep from preliminary studies [3]. Some would argue that this supplement has yet to prove itself or has not worked in some studies, and there is some merit to this argument in regards to objective parameters, but in terms of subjective sleep parameters it has multiple randomized trials demonstrating success and safety (minimally demonstrated drug interactions thus far) [213, 214] . Regardless, this supplement should never be combined with any other type of sleeping pills, or other what is known as "central nervous system depressants" such as strong pain medications, and a review of the latest specific drug interactions with this supplement is always prudent. Some clinical trials have reported diarrhea as a potential side effect in a small percentage of individuals. Valerian should be purchased as a root extract with at least 0.8 % valerenic acids in it (active ingredient), and it could several weeks to become effective (2–4 weeks in the studies). The most well studied dosage has not been determined, but studies that have used 200–600 mg (most common is arguably 600 mg) of Valerian daily have been proven to be safer and more effective in my opinion. The supplement is usually taken 30–60 min before bedtime. Additionally, valerian should be purchased itself and not mixed in with other herbs because most of the well-done studies utilized valerian as a stand along, and the more ingredients added to the effective ingredient only potentially dilutes the effectiveness of a drug or supplement (see Chap. 2). Side effects in clinical studies have been rare with some cases of morning grogginess, headache, and vivid dreams that in some cases were not pleasant.

There was one notable randomized phase 3-like trial that applies to breast cancer patients utilizing valerian conducted at approximately 20+ medical centers [215]. This Mayo clinic led trial consisted of patients undergoing cancer treatment (64 % breast cancer, 25 % other cancers, less than 5 % colon or prostate cancer, mean age 59 years) randomized to 450 mg of valerian or placebo daily for 8 weeks taken 1 h before bedtime. The valerian utilized in this trial was "pure ground, raw root, from one lot and standardized to contain 0.8 % valerenic acid," which were supplied by Hi-Health (Scottsdale, Arizona). The primary endpoint was the Pittsburgh Sleep Quality Index (PSQI), and secondary endpoints several other measures of sleep, fatigue and mood. A total of 227 patients were randomized and 119 evaluated for the primary endpoint (patients were currently being treated for cancer and more dropouts occurred with placebo), which was found to be no different from placebo by the end of the trial. *However, several other secondary measures showed significant difference in favor of valerian including several fatigue endpoints* as measured from Brief Fatigue Inventory (BFI), and Profile of Mood States (POMS) Fatigue-Inertia subscale. Secondary endpoints should be interpreted with some hesitation but in this case the differences were large or usually over 10 points on a 100-point scale suggesting a real effect. Participants reported less trouble with sleep and less drowsiness on valerian. Additionally, other secondary endpoints including the change from baseline related to sleep latency, amount of sleep per night, improvement in sleep problems, and less drowsiness all supported the valerian group performing better than the placebo and similar side effects with valerian compared to placebo. The researchers concluded by stating "Further research with valerian exploring physiologic effects in oncology symptom management may be warranted."

It was noted in the publication that the main impact of valerian in past trials was on sleep latency or the time needed to fall asleep and regardless the 10 dollars a month cost compares favorably with some 50–100 dollar a month pharmacologic sleep aids. This trial was supported in part by Public Health Services grants.

Another randomized trial of 100 postmenopausal women (not breast cancer) aged 50–60 years experiencing insomnia were randomized to 530 mg of concentrated valerian root extract or placebo twice daily (1060 mg/day total) for 4 weeks [216]. Quality of sleep was significantly improved ($p < 0.001$) with valerian over placebo (30 % demonstrated improvement versus 4 %).

F. Miscellaneous dietary supplement/other sleep aids—Massage, or other supplements such as 5-HTP, tryptophan (when all else has failed?)
Massage therapy could also improve sleep quality and should also be discussed based on positive preliminary evidence [217]. Ideally, again finding a non-pill based option (mediation, yoga, other exercises) should always be the first line treatment including any improvements in sleep hygiene [3]. Other dietary supplement sleep aids do not have the evidence to feel confident that the benefit truly outweighs the risk in breast cancer patients. For example, 5-HTP, tryptophan, passionflower, and numerous other herbals that are also utilized for stress and anxiety in some cases have minimal clinical evidence and promoting them for sleep appears no different in my opinion than promoting antistress or antianxiety medication for sleep where toxicity and dependence are major issues. For example, 5-HTP and tryptophan could alter brain neurotransmission significantly at higher dosages and there are not enough long-term safety trials to feel confident utilizing them in cancer patients. It has been known that they also function as sedatives increasing REM (Rapid Eye Movement) sleep in some patients but also reducing NREM (non-REM) or deep sleep [218, 219]. These supplements have a good observational safety record overall (except of course for the L-tryptophan dietary supplement contaminant that cause Eosinophilia Myalgia Syndrome due to a contaminant and removal of the product in 1989) [220, 221], but in my experience the sedative nature and dependency it could create is a reminder of how individuals chronically depend on pharmacologic agents for assistance. Since there are virtually no reliable studies in breast cancer patients with these supplements nor consistent benefit versus risk dosage ranges for sleep promotion it is difficult to recommend these dietary supplements for insomnia unless all else has failed.

• Lymphedema and improvement in range of motion/mobility
A. Lifestyle, complete decongestive therapy (CDT), aerobic and resistance exercise are now supported and do not generally exacerbate this issue and weight loss is arguably just as critical in preventing lymphedema
There is no optimal program to treat lymphedema that can occur in up to 40 % of women treated for breast cancer [222–224]. One standard of care is to utilize complete decongestive therapy (CDT), which includes exercise, manual lymphatic drainage, daily bandaging, skin care and compression over 3-phases. CDT can reduce limb volume and improve overall quality of life, but again provides no clear consistent advantage in other studies and there has been plenty of heterogeneous

comparisons which create further comparative issues. CDT is also costly, time consuming, and could involve lifelong attention or maintenance. Yet there is sufficient evidence to also recommend exercise rehabilitation to improve lymphedema (and shoulder mobility) in breast cancer patients. Strength training is also encouraged and does not appear to improve or exacerbate lymphedema but improves whole body fitness and provides countless benefits for breast cancer patients as observed in this chapter. Resistance training in the impacted lymphedema limb appears to be safest and not exacerbate lymphedema if the condition is stable and has not needed therapy over the past 3 months. Overall, reviews of approximately 20 studies and well as the consistent recent medical literature message suggests that exercise with proper supervision could be safe and generally does not increase the risk of lymphedema or exacerbate symptoms. And since obesity and weight gain in general increases the risk of lymphedema exercise is critical as a preventive method. Each BMI single point increase appears to increase risk 1.11 times versus someone of a single point lower in BMI (30 versus 29 for example). Most of the recommendations for exercise in breast cancer survivors at-risk for lymphedema are similar for the breast cancer survivors with lymphedema. In other words, initiating exercise at lower intensity gradually, low impact aerobic exercises and increased flexibility exercise, adequate warming up and cooling down and compression garments should be worn during exercise especially in those with lymphedema.

B. Dietary supplements (Good data for the prevention of further venous issues such as varicose veins or improving flow but in breast cancer lymphedema?)
Any supplement that appears to reduce the impact of Chronic Venous Insufficiency (CVI) and varicose veins also has the potential to help in the treatment of hemorrhoids [3]. Supplements that can reduce swelling and inflammation of the veins and improve the integrity of the veins can serve other potential purposes and need research, for example especially lymphedema prevention or perhaps even reduction from breast and other cancer treatments. It is for this reason a quick review of supplements in the area of CVI and hemorrhoids will be reviewed.

C. Daflon (also known as MPFF—micronized purified flavonoid fraction—a drug) or 450 mg of Diosmin dietary supplement and 50 mg of other flavonoids, or 500 mg 2–3 times a day for at least 12 weeks. Good for CVI but lymphedema prevention or treatment in breast cancer?
Daflon® (Servier, France) is a well-known semisynthetic prescription drug in France and Europe that is actually 450 mg of Diosmin (a compound found in plant like in citrus fruits) and 50 mg of other flavonoids found from plants primarily hesperidin (and possibly linarin, and isorhoifolin from other similar products) [3, 225, 226]. Daflon can also be known as an MPFF (micronized purified flavonoid fraction), and individuals usually take at least 500 mg twice a day of this product minimally to notice a benefit and some studies used 500 mg three times a day (divided in three doses every 8 h). "Micronized" means that particles were reduced in size to less than 2 μm (real tiny) so that improved its solubility and absorption. It is a drug in other countries but a similar plant product (Diosmin) can be purchased in the USA as a dietary supplement. Most of the studies of Daflon have been from 2 to 6 months.

Keep in mind that it is also possible to purchase MPFF from numerous other companies. MPFF refers to a 90 % diosmin and 10 % hesperidin product, and the product with the most research is Daflon, but again it is a drug in Europe and many supplements can be found that can come close to what is in this drug. In other words, "Diosmin" is the supplement and it is usually combined with Hesperidin in US vein health supplements.

There is evidence that Daflon helps in many ways including prevents endothelial damage, reduces the inflammatory response seen in the microcirculation, improves venous tone and lymph drainage, protects veins from damage, and reduces the calf and ankle swelling and other symptoms of CVI [3, 225–228]. Most of the impressive data from Daflon comes from individuals with more serious CVI such as leg ulcers because of poor circulation so it is believed it can also help with varicose veins or at least preventing more varicose veins. It has also reduced symptoms of pain, heaviness and edema. There is also some preliminary evidence to suggest it can be used with conventional treatments for CVI. Daflon has also been used for the treatment of hemorrhoids, which makes some sense because this is also a problem of increased pressure to an area of the body that contains a concentration of veins. Daflon has not received any good research in the area of potential drug interactions so be careful and do not use in pregnancy or when breast feeding, and it theoretically can affect the metabolism of other drugs but there just have not been enough of these studies. There is also not enough description beyond placebo of potential side effects of diosmin but some clinical trials have reported a higher rate of gastrointestinal side effects. Another concern I have is that I would be careful about combining Diosmin with aspirin or other blood thinning medications only because diosmin can cause a reduction in red blood cells clumping and blood viscosity which means it may increase blood thinning.

Although no supplement is of course endorsed for lymphedema from objective reviews of the literature [229], there was one trial with Daflon (MPFF) 500 mg twice a day and breast cancer lymphedema reported in these reviews and published elsewhere [230, 231]. This was a randomized study of 104 women with upper limb edema following treatment and lymphoscintigraphy was used to evaluate lymph flow at baseline and end of 6-months. And changes in limb volume, measured every 2-months was the other endpoint. Interestingly, a 24-patient subset with severe edema was analyzed separately and demonstrated a significant improvement in the lymphoscintigraphic measurements in the MPFF group. However, overall there were no significant differences found between the lymphoscintigraphy parameters or limb volume of the MPFF and placebo groups at any measured interval of the trial (difference was only in the subset of patients with severe edema). The only parameters where significant differences occurred in the entire group that completed the trial was for symptom analysis. A significant reduction in heaviness symptoms was found for the MPFF ($n=45$) product versus placebo ($n=48$), and a significant decrease in discomfort for both the MPFF ($n=45$) and placebo ($n=48$) groups. It was pointed out that the authors failed to discuss the randomization method, blinding protocol, and no confidence intervals or standard deviations were published. And the study failed to provide information on withdrawals (94 patients completed the study) or side effects, which were reported in eight patients in the MPFF group and six patients in the placebo group.

A previously published pilot study of ten female patients treated for breast cancer utilizing 500 mg of Daflon twice a day for 6 months was also published by the same group of researchers before the larger clinical trial described previously [232]. All patients appeared to have improvement of symptoms and limb volume, and mean reduction in limb volume was 6.80 %, and functional parameters were determined by scintigraphy were significantly improved. Thus, it is understandable why a larger study was then conducted. And it raises the question of the potential for further study and the benefit versus risk scenario for utilizing this in breast cancer patients? How could 20-years have passed with no additional published reports on this compound or the supplement and breast cancer patients with lymphedema? This could be due to unpublished negative data or simply a lack of funding, but it is perplexing that not even a case study or case series has since been published (hint hint).

D. Horse chestnut seed extract 50–75 mg of escin (aescin) 1–2 times a day for 12 weeks for CVI but for lymphedema—not from one small unpublished study?
Horse Chestnut Seed Extract (HCSE or *Aesculus hippocastanum*) has been shown to reduce leg pain, swelling, itching, ankle and calf swelling to a similar extent as compression stockings [3, 233]. The active compound in HCSE is "escin" (complex active triterpenoid saponins, sometimes also referred to as "aescin"), which has been shown to block the activity of the enzyme hyaluronidase, which can degrade proteoglycans or structural support for veins especially when released in higher amounts of legs during CVI because a large number of white blood cells are attracted to these areas. In other words, it blocks the destruction of components in the wall of the smallest blood vessels. However, gastrointestinal upset and dizziness were reported in up to one-third of the individuals in about half of the studies conducted, but other studies reported mild to minimal side effects. Studies are of short duration (4-weeks) so HCSE could be an option for the short-term relief of symptoms or swelling (edema) in individuals that do not receive a benefit or do not like to use compression stockings.

Dosage has been in the range of one capsule twice a day and each capsule was standardized to 50–75 mg of escin (again taken twice a day) and the initial treatment period was at least 12 weeks. Again, this supplement can strengthen the veins, reduce swelling and other issues over a short period of time. Studies of taking over long periods of time have not been done. Still, over seven placebo-controlled trials makes this one of the best dietary supplement options for CVI, which can be used with conventional treatment in many situations. HCSE has not received adequate research in the area of potential drug interactions so be careful and do not use in pregnancy or when breastfeeding and if a patient is on an anticoagulant.

Unfortunately no major published trials of this supplement have occurred to date (only an abstract of interim results). There was one phase-2 trial for lymphedema treatment in breast cancer survivors listed on clinicaltrials.gov and conducted at the University of Wisconsin (NCT00213928) and the study was apparently completed and funded by the Susan G. Komen Breast Cancer Research Foundation [234, 235].

It was a double-blind, randomized, and placebo-controlled study of breast cancer patients with arm lymphedema receiving HCSE (50 mg escins) twice a day for 3 months followed by a 1 month washout or placebo. A total of 25 patients were evaluable at 3 months and 24 patients were at intermediate assessment and although it appeared safe there were no statistically significant differences in lymphedema at 3 months by any of the measured techniques (no objective or subjective improvement).

E. Rutosides (O-beta-hydroxyethyl-rutosides) or Rutin at 1000–2000 mg/day for varicose veins or CVI over 8-weeks, but for breast cancer lymphedema?

The active ingredient is the "rutosides" [3, 229, 236]. It also comes in a topical 2 % gel that can be applied up to three times a day along with taking the supplement. One of the most commonly tested products is "Venoruton" (from Novartis, Basel, Switzerland) is actually a prescription drug in Europe (known as "oxerutins" or "hydroxyethylrutosides"—mixture of semisynthetic flavonoids), but a potential equivalent can be found over the counter in other countries if it cannot be purchased from Europe. "Oxerutins" in head-to-head testing against Daflon for example 2000 mg/day was the most common dose tested. It actually performed better in treating CVI and reducing ankle swelling compared to Daflon in one older head-to-head study. Rutosides appear to protect blood vessel walls from damage, and discouraging cells from adhering to the walls so that they can continue to function normally. Cramps, pain, heavy leg feeling, and swelling have been reduced with this product.

It is also a supplement used for symptoms from hemorrhoids [3, 229, 236]. The side effects of these supplements are rare and include: gastrointestinal (nausea, heartburn, and diarrhea), allergic reaction to the products, and in rare cases headache and hot flashes. The gel and pills can be purchased on reliable sites on line (Amazon etc.) and when in doubt you can also just pick up "rutin" supplements at the local health food store. Rutin is close in molecular structure to rutosides used in these studies so I believe work about as well and is cheaper! Rutin is found in plants like asparagus and buckwheat and in fruits and fruit rinds of limes, lemons, grapefruit, oranges, apples and many others. The chemical structure of rutin is also close to that of the popular supplement "quercetin." Rutins are also known to strengthen capillary walls and despite having very little research it is difficult to ignore that they are almost a mirror reflection of what is working for CVI, leg swelling, and varicose veins—in other words feel free to try them at the same dosage because rutosides can be difficult for some folks to get in some countries.

Additionally there are some rutin like copy cats such as "red grape vine leaf" (folia vitis viniferae) extract contains flavonoids with the primary ones being quercetin-3-O-bea-glucoside and quercetin-3-O-beta-glucuronide. In other words, it shares such similar properties with rutosides and rutins that when it was tested at 360 and 720 mg once daily for 12 weeks in individuals with stage I and II CVI it was found that both dosages reduced lower leg swelling and size to a similar degree as compression stockings [237], and other similar studies also report positive initial findings [238]. Japanese pagoda tree (Styphnolobium japonicum) is also a large source of rutins but searching for rutosides or rutin supplements described above will make purchasing easier.

A review of two publications of randomized, double-blind, crossover, placebo-controlled studies utilizing 3000 mg of hydroxyethylrutosides (HR) per day over 6 months in 48 patients with upper limb lymphedema after breast cancer treatment and 14 with lower limb edema demonstrated preliminary cautionary efficacy [229, 239, 240]. HR appeared to significantly reduce limb volume and circumference, increase limb softness, and reduce increased skin temperature. HR also resulted in significant improvement in limb swelling sensation, heaviness, bursting pain, tension, and mobility. A total of 97 % of the patients of HR reported increased well-being versus 4 % on placebo and 70 % of the patients preferred HR over placebo. Additionally, HR significantly ($p < 0.05$) reduced arm volume by approximately 10 %. The problem with this data report is that it did not have strong methodology from withdrawal information to figure support issues and all original data were derived from graphs. A third trial of utilizing 600 mg of HR in an open study after breast cancer treatment in addition to physiotherapy ($n = 32$) for 4 months resulted in improvement in the signs and symptoms of lymphedema [229], but again this is a pilot study at best. Another trial of 85 patients with metastatic breast cancer utilizing 300 mg of hydroxyethylrutosiden (Venoruton) given orally four times a day or no supplement over a 4-cycle docetaxel treatment to determine its impact on fluid retention (peripheral edema, ascites, pleural or pericardial effusion, or a combination) was published and found not reduction or delay in the incidence and severity of fluid retention caused by docetaxel [241]. Thus, this was more of an indirect study of efficacy and lymphedema. Arguably, there is sufficient preliminary evidence to continue to study these compounds for the prevention and treatment of lymphedema, but again little has been completed in this area since the initially positive publications.

F. Miscellaneous–Pycnogenol conflicts, selenium toxicity, Power Plate, ... (needs testing in breast cancer)

Pycnogenol, a standardized extract from the bark of French maritime pine (*Pinus pinaster* or *Pinus maritima*) is actually found in other areas of the Mediterranean region for example Spain and Portugal, Italy, Morocco, and southern and western France [3]. Pycnogenol contains polyphenols predominantly over 80 % or more oligomeric proanthocyanidins (PCOs) used in studies that appears to be the active ingredient with protective properties. Some supplements now contain 95 % proanthocyanidins. Cramps, pain, heavy leg feeling, and swelling have been reduced in some studies [242]. Pycnogenol is generally utilized at 150–300 mg/day. The active ingredients in pycnogenol (PCOs) are not low cost (this is an issue because it is also proprietary) and other sources of these active compounds can be derived from peanut skin, and grape seed extract [3]. Grape seed extract is a fairly well known supplement but does not have adequate research in the area of lymphedema or CVI. Regardless, a review of 15 diverse clinical trials ($n = 791$), including two studies in CVI ($n = 60$) a review established the following conclusion: "Current evidence is insufficient to support Pycnogenol use for the treatment of any chronic disorder.

Well-designed adequately powered trials are needed to establish the value of this treatment." Past studies have been primarily positive but the methodology and conflict of interest have been questioned enough that this recent conclusion was provided. This has also been my experience that the broad or diverse benefits observed for a plethora of medical conditions (from erectile dysfunction to tinnitus to CVI and more) along with conflict of interest suggests either a groundbreaking supplement or an average product that has been embellished. Regardless, this is an interesting circulatory protective compound and should receive some objective research for breast cancer lymphedema to determine its potential activity (or not).

Selenium supplementation receives some attention as a method to prevent side effects of cancer treatment including lymphedema. However, many of these studies have questionable complete methodology [243], but far more importantly, in light of the potential for selenium toxicity already more clearly documented in phase-3 like trials for other hormone derived cancers (increase risk of prostate cancer, aggressive tumors, and mortality, type 2 diabetes, skin cancer recurrence, ...) [244–248], the risk outweighs the benefit at this time and should not be utilized for the prevention or treatment of lymphedema.

Finally, again I will reiterate commentary in the bone loss and sarcopenia section of this chapter. Some patients have reported whole-body vibration (WBC or Power Plate for example) as providing some relief from their lower leg edema, and even lymphedema. Since this arguably involves a type of circulatory massage it appears relevant to at least objectively test this method in some clinical study. However, it could also be argued that this could exacerbate edema via regional circulatory increases or alterations, but this is why research is needed.

• Nausea and vomiting (Chemotherapy-induced nausea and vomiting or CINV)
A. Lifestyle changes
A plethora of literature exists on dietary changes to prevent and/or treat nausea and these sources along with a discussion with a cancer nutritionist would be advised [1, 3]. Some of these recommendations include:

– Drinking beverages and eating foods that are gentle or easier for the patient to ingest for example when they had the flu such as diet or regular ginger ale, drinks that have lost their fizz or gone flat, bland foods, sour small candy, dry crackers, pickles, ... Also try and eat 5–6 small and more frequent beverage and meals a day compared to 2–3 large meals each day. Cooler in temperature drinks and foods should be easier to tolerate and keep down.
– Try to avoid real spicy, fatty, fried, or very sweet foods. Cooking and freezing several simple meals that you can reheat during times of nausea is a good idea. Eating foods that are colder or at room temperature may be better at controlling nausea compared to the smell from very hot food. Also, try and let someone else prepare food or just order out when feeling nauseated.
– Changing the taste of or blocking the taste of certain drinks and food with another strong taste changer such as lemon or another product has been shown to be beneficial for some individuals.

- Nutritional shakes or liquid nutritional products may be easier to keep down and will help maintain good nutritional levels.
- Keep your mouth clean by brushing at least twice a day and perhaps using mouthwash because even slightly abnormal mouth smells can increase nausea.
- Wear loose fitting clothing and at times go without a belt (nothing that feels too restrictive or puts pressure on your abdominal area).
- Walking or light exercise is usually advised because more vigorous moving or shaking types of exercise or movements can further exacerbate nausea.
- As always and with any side effect from cancer treatment a review of current and future medications/supplements is needed because some supplements for example have a slightly higher risk of stomach upset and nausea (fish oil, iron, …) compared to others.

B. Acupuncture, and/or P6 acupressure (Why not? It should be an opinion)
Interestingly, objective reviews of the role of acupuncture in cancer treatment have found that the area of most positive research although preliminary is in the area of nausea and vomiting prevention and/or reduction [170].

Acupressure wristbands (also known as "P6 acupressure" because this is the point in Traditional Chinese Medicine where nausea is controlled) are newer options that provide some pressure around the wrist area that may help reduce nausea and vomiting [3, 249–251]. Interestingly, most of the better methodology clinical trials (three out of nine) have been completed in breast cancer patients. They can be purchased over the counter. It looks like a wristband with a stud in the middle of the band that pushes down slightly at a point that is located on the anterior surface of the forearm (further pressure can also be applied to the stud), approximately 3-finger width up from the crease of the wrist between the tendons of the palmaris longus and flexor carpi radialis. In general every 2–3 h pushing down on the stud for several minutes has provided anti-nausea benefits for several days after receiving chemotherapy. Wristbands are worn on both forearm areas for maximum potential effectiveness (for example see www.sea-band.com). There are also many devices (for example Comfort Quest Anti-Seasickness Band or ReliefBand) that look like a watch and it is placed on the same P6 area and it delivers a small stimulus to that point while you are feeling nauseous or even while you are trying to prevent nausea (like sea sickness). Multiple mechanisms of action could explain these effects from operating as a distractor and/or releasing compounds that increase threshold for nausea and vomiting in the brain but this has not been well studied, but the current benefits of these options clearly outweigh the risk.

C. Ginger (Zingiber officinale) dietary supplement—Phase-3-like trial (Should be utilized in breast cancer)
A National Cancer Institute (NCI) sponsored Phase-3 like multicenter (23 private practice oncology groups participated) study with cancer patients (total of 744 participants randomized and 576 included in the final analysis) taking 500–1500 mg a day of ginger dietary supplements along with conventional medicines for nausea and vomiting compared to a placebo and conventional medicines had an interesting result [252]. All patients received a 5-HT(3) receptor antagonist drug on Day 1 of

all chemotherapy cycles. This was a 4-arm trial of placebo, 500 mg ginger, 1000 mg ginger and 1500 mg of ginger. Ginger (*Z. officinale*) supplements for chemotherapy-induced nausea and vomiting (CINV) were started 3 days before start of chemotherapy and for 3 days after chemotherapy (total of 6 days). The ginger capsules were also standardized as a purified liquid extract of ginger root "with concentrated 8.5 mg of combined gingerols, zingerone, and shogaol content, equivalent to 250 mg of ginger root, in extra virgin olive oil ..." [252]. *Interestingly, the ginger was manufactured by Aphios Corporation in Woburn, MA, which is now testing their product (called Zindol®) in another phase III clinical trial and should be lauded for this wonderful dedication to research [253, 254]. Again, the difference between an effective drug and supplement is perception and not reality. The ginger product itself can be purchased right now as a dietary supplement (Zindol® DS). In addition, it is critical to mention that the majority of the patients in this clinical trial, approximately 74 %, were breast cancer patients.* The severity of nausea was reported on a 7-point scale (1 = not at all nauseated and 7 = extremely nauseated) by patients on days 1–4 of each cycle. The primary objective was to evaluate whether ginger was more efficacious than placebo at reducing nausea severity on Day 1 of chemotherapy (acute nausea). The analysis from this trial was derived from the 576 patients that provided data that could be evaluated at either study cycle 2 or 3. The mean age of the patients was 53 year and 93 % were female and 91 % were Caucasian. Interestingly, all doses of ginger reduced acute nausea severity significantly versus placebo on Day 1 of chemotherapy ($p = 0.003$). All doses of ginger significantly reduced acute nausea in both study cycles (2 and 3) versus placebo ($p = 0.013$ and 0.003). The greatest or most significant reduction in nausea intensity occurred with 500 mg ($p = 0.017$) and 1000 mg ginger ($p = 0.036$) supplements.

The secondary objectives of this trial included the impact of ginger on delayed nausea, anticipatory nausea, and quality of life in cancer patients receiving chemotherapy [252]. Despite significant reductions in Day 1 acute nausea in all ginger groups versus placebo, the significance was attenuated for Days 2 and 3 (delayed) and Day 4 (follow-up nausea). This suggests patients reported more bouts of severe delayed nausea versus acute nausea. Additionally, no significant differences were found in vomiting or quality of life (FACIT-G) between placebo and the three ginger arms. However, the mean incidence of vomiting was 0.5, so most patients did not report vomiting episodes. The researchers also reported that anticipatory nausea played a primary role in acute chemotherapy-induced nausea ($p < 0.0001$). A total of 24 adverse events were recorded during the trial, and nine events were thought to be associated with the ginger product, and these participants withdrew from the trial. The side effects included gastrointestinal symptoms, for example Grade 2 heartburn, bruising/flushing, and rash.

The ginger trial utilized 3-days before and after the chemotherapy event and this is a similar protocol as they remarked to studies completed for the prevention of motion sickness [252]. Anticipatory nausea (those believing they are susceptible to nausea) in this trial showed that it could promote acute nausea. The researchers also theorized that the anti-inflammatory and antispasmodic effects of ginger could be a reason for the benefit. Ginger can also bind to 5-HT3 receptors to augment antiemetic effects and promote the production of compounds to protect against oxidative tissue injury. And ingesting ginger 3-days before chemotherapy could have "primed" the gastrointestinal tract by binding to and saturating receptors, which could also explain why 1500 mg did not work as well as 1000 mg, which has been observed before in past motion sickness studies. The primary limitations of this trial was not controlling for the higher versus lower nausea and vomiting chemotherapy regimens (patients were enrolled if they reported nausea from a previous chemotherapy cycle), or for the nausea severity level before enrollment. Nausea and vomiting from chemotherapy is more likely in later cycles if experienced in the initial or early cycles. Interestingly patients reported more severe delayed nausea (Day 2 and 3) versus acute nausea (Day 1), which suggested that delayed nausea is a greater problem and this could be another reason for the lack of a significant effect on quality control. Again, this was a large trial, similar to a phase-3 trial (the authors called it a "phase II/III" trial), so it should be encouraged currently to recommended 500–1000 mg of ginger (or ¼ to ½ teaspoon of ground ginger, but ideally the supplements to replicate the trial) daily for several days before and after receiving chemotherapy. Again, it is also interesting that higher doses (1500 mg/day) did not work better compared to the lower doses (500–1000 mg) per day. For individuals that have trouble taking or keeping pills down that are now purified ginger candies, gum and other simple options at most health food stores (including ground ginger mentioned above).

Interestingly, a previous well-done phase 2 clinical trial of 1000 and 2000 mg of a powdered ginger root extract capsule (250 mg per capsule, 15 mg or 5 % total gingerols) versus placebo for CINV in cancer patients ($n = 162$) for 3 days (first dose utilized within 1 h of completing chemotherapy) was not effective and appeared to have interfered with the prescription antiemetic aprepitant (Emend®) [255], and should not be combined with this agent. In addition, a preliminary ginger aromatherapy trial did not find evidence of a reduce risk of nausea and vomiting in breast cancer patients [256], suggesting that capsules continue to have the most effective research. Overall, the data on ginger in cancer chemotherapy and the reduction of nausea has been positive as reviewed in this publication [252] including reductions in significant reductions in acute and delayed nausea and vomiting versus placebo from a trial of 60 young adult patients with sarcoma [257]. *In fact, currently in diverse clinical settings, not just chemotherapy-induced nausea and vomiting (CINV) ginger has now accumulated positive data from morning sickness, postoperative nausea and vomiting, and even antiretroviral-induced nausea and vomiting [258]. Additionally, 5-HT3 receptor antagonistic properties continued to be supported as one potential mechanism of action from these past trials.*

D. Vitamin B6 (pyridoxine)—(Data is for pregnancy and even endorsed by the American College of Obstetrics and Gynecology (ACOG), but for CINV?)
It is also interesting that ginger has really become fairly standard medicine to relieve nausea and vomiting during pregnancy, but so has vitamin B6 (also known as "pyridoxine") based on past clinical trials [259]. *The American College of Obstetrics (ACOG) and Gynecology essentially endorsed this as an option in first trimester of*

pregnancy to prevent and especially treat nausea and vomiting [260]. *The ACOG practice guideline stated under Level A evidence the following: "Treatment of nausea and vomiting of pregnancy with vitamin B6 or B6 plus doxylamine is safe and effective and should be considered first-line pharmacotherapy."* Therefore, if ginger is not effective then vitamin B6 is an option (or vice versa). The doses used in pregnancy have been divided doses at a total of 25–75 mg of vitamin B6 or 10–25 mg three or four times a day. However, other effective clinical studies used approximately 25–40 mg of vitamin B6 (total) a day in divided doses [259–261]. Other objective recent reviews have suggested that vitamin B6 should be stand alone "first-line therapy" for the treatment of nausea and vomiting in pregnancy at 10–25 mg every 8 h because over benefit-versus-risk [262], and arguably due to potential controversial and conflicting safety concerns of using doxylamine with pyridoxine according to some reviews (again controversial) [263]. Regardless, the minimal to moderate benefit of the combination product over B6 monotherapy and the safety history of B6 alone continues to suggest it should be first-line therapy. Other reviews are slightly more cautious in recommending any specific treatment for nausea and vomiting in pregnancy over another without more data, but these reviews fail to consider the benefit-to-risk ratio advantage with B6 alone when considering all the potential options [264]. Side effects of vitamin B6 include paresthesias, headache, and fatigue (uncommon) [262].

It is quite interesting and extraordinary that few published (negative or positive) clinical trials have been conducted in cancer patients with vitamin B6 in an attempt to reduce nausea and vomiting or CINV. One study of 142 ovarian cancer patients utilized an injectable form of vitamin B6 (for 21 days), and when combined with P6 acupuncture was significantly more effective than either intervention alone [265]. Significantly fewer emesis episodes and a greater percentage of emesis-free days versus acupuncture alone or intramuscular B6 injection alone occurred. Excessive doses of vitamin B6 (300 mg or more) for several months or even lower doses for several years, more than 50 mg/day, could cause a sensory neuropathy and are discouraged (as are most cases of mega-supplement intake) [266].

E. Protein powder supplementation? (Someone needs to figure this out)
Adequate protein intake is recommended to cancer patients to maintain body weight and improve nutritional status. And there is some preliminary research to suggest that higher protein intake from meals could reduce the nausea of motion sickness and pregnancy by decreasing gastric dysrhythmias [267]. One small preliminary study of a higher whey protein intake in 28 cancer patients (19 with breast cancer) found that higher supplemental protein intake appeared to produce significant reductions in nausea and need for antiemetic medications versus normal protein intake or control. Patients consumed these products for 3 days beginning after their first day after chemotherapy. A ginger supplement was also utilized in two of the three (control, protein + ginger, high protein + ginger) groups but since the higher-protein group displayed better results the benefit was attributed to the protein quantity and not the ginger. In the authors' words "That the protein group was not different from the control group in terms of the symptoms reported in the diary

while the high protein group reported less nausea suggests that ginger was not critical to the high protein meal's beneficial effects." The normal protein meal (consumed twice a day—morning and late afternoon) consisted of 17 g of whey protein in a beverage (34 g/day) and in the high protein group the 17 g whey protein beverage and an additional 15 g whey protein powder was provided to be added to the beverage (64 g of whey protein per day). Also, five patients in the high protein group tested for gastric myoelectrical activity a significant decrease in gastric dysrhythmia was recorded after ingestion of protein and ginger. This was an interesting study but it was not blinded and thus provides very preliminary results. Regardless, the use of a whey protein or another protein isolate powder with no sugar and no lactose should be tested in a clinical trial since protein powders today have such variety and diverse and excellent nutritional profiles and in many cases improved and satisfying taste or flavor.

Protein powder supplementation to prevent sarcopenia, improve nutritional status and assist in weight loss continues to garner good evidence in the medical literature [3]. It would be of enormous interest to solve this question with protein powder and beverage consumption because it does appear in other high-risk nausea situations (first trimester pregnancy for example) that liquid protein meals reduced gastric dysrhythmias more than solids from preliminary research, and protein appears to provide less nausea compared to carbohydrates and fats [268]. It is also interesting that higher quality protein recommended daily requirements (0.8 g of protein per kg of body weight per day or approximately your total weight in pounds divided by 2 for your maximum daily protein intake—for example a 150 pound person should get 75 g of total protein per day) has been argued to be immediately but gradually increased based on the increasing needs of protein with aging [269].

• **Peripheral neuropathy (PN or chemotherapy-induced peripheral neuropathy or CIPN)**

A. *Introduction—because of this unfamiliar territory for patients*
Side effects of cancer treatment appear to be well known such as the potential for hot flashes or even nausea with some regimens. One fairly common side effect with some chemotherapeutic regimens which appears to surprise some patients is peripheral neuropathy (PN) or chemotherapy-induced peripheral neuropathy (CIPN) because it is not often recognized or discussed or really not experienced in day-to-day life of noncancer patients unless someone is dealing with diabetes. Therefore, I decided to include an introduction to this side effect because I have been asked by patients for years to provide some background to it because it is so unfamiliar to many and is not common with menopause or normal aging or even acute illness. Feel free to photocopy this portion and provide it to patients.

Normally, you should be able to fasten your shirt buttons without difficulty or walk without looking down at your feet, but peripheral neuropathy can make this difficult [1]. This is a nerve problem that can cause of variety of symptoms throughout the body, but mostly in the hands and feet, which is why it is called "peripheral" (on the outside/extremities of the body—like the hands and feet) neuropathy. Many things can cause neuropathy, such as injury, infection, toxic substances, a disease (diabetes is a well known cause), and chemotherapy or other drugs. Neuropathy is caused by injury or damage to the nerves and blood vessels surrounding them. Individuals with diabetes have some of the greatest risks of neuropathy for example because high blood sugar levels damage more than blood vessels but also nerves. One of the most common forms is symmetric distal polyneuropathy, which is a loss of sensation that leads to diabetic foot ulcers.

Symptoms of neuropathy, usually occurs in the hands and feet and include any of the following feelings in these areas of the body [1]:

- Aching
- Burning
- Electric Shock-like
- Heaviness in hands and feet
- Pins and needles touching skin or the area … feels like part of the body falling asleep (known as "paresthesias")
- Increased sensitivity to cold
- Itching
- Loss of reflexes (ankle and knee)
- Needles
- Numbness
- Reduced sensation
- Prickling
- Pain
- Stabbing
- Tenderness
- Tingling
- Throbbing
- Weakness

The symptoms of peripheral neuropathy can result in any (or some) of the following problems that can also be painful or disabling when trying the following [1]:

- Difficulty buttoning a shirt
- Difficulty opening a container such as a jar
- Difficulty picking up small objects such as a pen or loose change
- Difficulty writing
- Difficulty walking like stumbling or tripping
- Trouble going around furniture
- Falling more than usual
- Hugging or holding the wall to walk

Over 100 types of peripheral neuropathy have been identified but there tends to be a focus on three general types in discussions with doctors—let me explain [1]. The motor nerves control movements of all the muscles under conscious control, for example talking, walking, and grasping things. Sensory nerves transmit information about sensory experiences that are going on such as a light touch or brush or even pain resulting from a cut. Autonomic nerves are the controllers or regulators of all the things in the body that you do not control consciously such as breathing, digesting food, heart functions, ... So, there are motor neuropathies, sensory neuropathies, and autonomic neuropathies. These are the three categories of neuropathy that doctors use to help identify the problem. Most neuropathies impact 1 or 2 or can involve both but rarely involve all 3. The problem with diabetes is that it can impact all 3 if it is not aggressively controlled and cancer itself and/or cancer treatment can also impact one or more of these (motor, sensory, and/or autonomic). Most treatments in this chapter are suggested for peripheral neuropathy with a primarily sensory nerve issue. However, the most common form of neuropathy in type 1 and 2 diabetics for example was mentioned earlier and is known as DSPN or Diabetic sensorimotor polyneuropathy, which occurs in 10 % of diabetics within the first year of diagnosis to 50 % after 25 years. Most of the information here applies to folks with nerve pain issues—especially diabetic neuropathy (type 1 and 2 diabetes). Individuals around the world that call me for help with dietary supplements for neuropathy usually have it because of diabetes, cancer chemotherapy drugs, or HIV. The good and bad news is that dietary supplements that help for one of these conditions (like diabetes) appear to help for the others like cancer, but there are also dietary supplements that can exacerbate or make CIPN worse (see below)! Again, many conditions can cause the pain, numbness and tingling of neuropathy and there are so many dietary supplements that are reported to help but very few have any kind of human research that is exciting. Still, the ones that seem to be working have really good short- and long-term research and the ones that do not work or make it worse also have good research. Keep in mind that neuropathy of any kind is a serious condition that should lead to immediate discussion with your doctor or specialist on how to treat it.

A. *Lifestyle changes and PN or CIPN*

Heart health is tantamount to nerve health in general. Anti-inflammatory diet? There has been very little human research on the role of diet and peripheral neuropathy even in those with diabetes, cancer, or HIV [1]. Regardless, it appears that anything that results in reducing the risk of heart disease potentially reduces the risk or occurrence of peripheral neuropathy. So glucose, cholesterol, and blood pressure control, a heart-healthy diet, exercise, and avoiding tobacco are heart and nerve healthy as well as the following quick tips when dealing with PN or CIPN [1]:

- Exercise (aerobic and resistance exercise to improve balance and strength)
- Weight Loss
- Be careful when grasping sharp, hot, or dangerous objects if you have numbness in your fingers because you may not realize you are being injured
- Move carefully and use handrails on the stairs
- Assess the water temperature in the home
- Have someone else test bath water temperature or use a water thermometer
- Turn down water heater temperature
- Use protective gloves when washing dishes
- Use potholders
- Wear cotton socks
- Wear warm socks and gloves in the cold weather

- Wear shoes with rubber soles whenever possible
- Try not to cross your legs on lean on your elbows because it can put pressure on an already damaged nerve
- Make sure rooms have adequate lighting without glare
- Clear walkways and avoid the use of throw rugs and just remove throw rugs entirely
- Create non-skid showers and bathtubs by installing bath mats
- Install handrails in the bath
- Use shower chairs if needed

B. 0.075 % topical capsaicin (standard of care in diabetes and why not CIPN or neuropathic cancer pain/discomfort? Needs Research) Rx 8 % capsaicin patch?
Note: please also see the review on capsaicin found in the aromatase induced arthralgia (AIA) section of this chapter.
Capsaicin cream (active hot ingredient in hot chili peppers) can reduce neuropathic and arthritis pain, so some patients may need to utilize it for neuropathic pain that is near the surface of the skin [1, 270]. However, be careful because the product should be applied with gloves and a Q-tip for example because if capsaicin gets near or into the eyes the burning sensation can be quite painful and potentially harmful. Capsaicin works by reducing levels of a compound in the body called "substance P," which helps to reduce transmit the feeling of pain in the body. When used at 0.075 % concentration up to four times a day it can provide pain relief for some individuals so it is worth a try for at least 1–2 weeks. *The American Association of Neuromuscular and Electrodiagnostic Medicine, the American Academy of Neurology, and the American Academy of Physical Medicine and Rehabilitation recommends capsaicin at 0.075 % as "probably effective and should be considered for treatment of painful Peripheral Diabetic Neuropathy (PDN) …," or Level B evidence* [271]. Still, it also has appears to have some efficacy for CIPN [270], but this needs more immediate research, and this is occurring now with the prescription form of capsaicin. Whether or not clinicians use different concentrations of topical capsaicin for CIPN currently is based on individual and health care professional preferences. The ultimate goal would be to observe some consistent clinical trial benefit that could also reduce the dependence on higher strength opioids for some select patients.

Higher concentrations of capsaicin (up to 8 %) are also now available through a prescription patch placed on the area of pain (for example the drug Qutenza®) [272, 273]. Currently the 8 % capsaicin prescription patch is being used for postherpetic neuralgia, but there is good reason to believe it works with other forms of neuropathic pain (depends on the individuals) and this is the indication for its use in Europe. Side effects have been low and similar to the topical over the counter, but the prescription patch can cause a rare rapid change or increase in blood pressure when it is first applied. Health care practitioners appear to find numerous uses of capsaicin especially as a prescription for multiple types of pain and the side effect profile has been very low [273]. *Additionally, there are clinical trials concluding currently such as ASCEND that will determine the future of prescription capsaicin (and perhaps topical over the counter) for neuropathic cancer pain* [274].

Oral capsaicin dietary supplements are starting to be researched for a variety of conditions but there is no evidence in the area of peripheral neuropathy and there should be some concern about gastrointestinal toxicity using this delivery method [3]. Keep in mind that topical over the counter or prescription patch capsaicin should NOT be combined with anything else that can heat the skin such as a heating pad, hot shower, and direct sunlight because this combined effect can cause the skin to burn and be damaged.

C. Dietary supplements for CIPN (tale of two cities or some make could provide benefit and some could provide harm)
It is important to review this section carefully because unlike some other areas of cancer treatment side effects and dietary supplements, this is a symptom that can worsen or improve CIPN depending on the type of dietary supplement utilized. And the majority of this research in neuropathy with supplements actually applies to diabetic peripheral neuropathy, but cancer patients can experience both diabetic neuropathy and CIPN, which is another reason this chapter reviews the research in diabetes before discussing any research with CIPN.

D. Alpha-lipoic acid (thioctic acid—endorsed for diabetic PN but looking for consistency with CIPN)
Note: This supplement was also reviewed in other areas of this book including Chap. 6
Alpha-lipoic acid is a dietary supplement in the USA but a drug and even an IV drug in other countries around the world. It has become a standard of care for diabetic peripheral neuropathy in these same locations (throughout Europe) that offer an IV form of this compound [1, 3]. Alpha-lipoic acid (ALA) is arguably the only fat and water-soluble antioxidant and it was discovered in 1937 as a potato extract that was required for bacterial growth, and eventually it was realized that it was produced by plants and animals and is needed in every human cell to help with countless functions. Alpha-lipoic acid (ALA, also known as "thioctic acid" or 1,2-dithiolane-3-pentanoic acid) supplements are arguably one of the most common supplements used for diabetic peripheral neuropathy and have interesting and some efficacious human research (human trials such a trial called the "NATHAN 1" trial lasting 4+ years at an oral dose of 600 mg/day in 460 patients) [275]. Part of the reason it probably has received so much research is that this supplement has been a prescription oral and IV drug in many parts of the world. In fact, there have been over 15 randomized trials of giving 300–600 mg/day of ALA for 2–4 weeks as an IV drug in other countries (even covered by insurance as a pill and IV in many of these countries), and it was found to improve nerve conduction and reduce neuropathic symptoms and has a great safety record [276]. In fact, ALA was first used in Europe to treat diabetic neuropathy. However, again ALA in the USA is a dietary supplement.

ALA is usually started at 600 mg/day from clinical studies and results are observed in as little as 2 weeks, and doses as high as 1800 mg/day have been used but have not seemed to work any better than 600 mg/day and higher dosages (except for weight loss—see Chap. 6) increase the risk of gastrointestinal side effects and the risk of a usually minor "itching" effect (feel the need to itch a spot on the body), and many folks will experience malodorous urine or get a smell similar to eating asparagus when they urinate which is common due to the sulfur groups found in ALA or asparagus, and despite being harmless you should still know that it can occur [1, 3, 38, 276, 277]. In fact, as you increase the dosage you not only do not appear to increase the efficacy against neuropathy itself, but increase the risk of gastrointestinal upset and nausea. Thus, it is important to repeat this—for diabetic neuropathy prevention and treatment the dosage of 600 mg/day has the best benefit to risk ratio and it should be tried for at least 5 weeks from past clinical trials. It should be utilized in 2–3 divided doses if side effects occur with the one-time 600 mg dose. Whether or not the supplement is combined with other conventional drugs treatments is not known, but the vast majority of the research on ALA for neuropathy is as monotherapy. And there is no cost comparison of ALA compared to conventional drugs because overall ALA low cost. One more point about adverse effects needs to be mentioned that is covered more adequately in Chap. 6 and this is the risk of a very rare situation of drugs with sulfur groups such as ALA and that is Hirata disease or IAS (Insulin Autoimmune Syndrome), which is a spontaneous hypoglycemia from high serum insulin levels and high titers of autoantibodies against endogenous insulin and although only a handful of cases have been described in Europe and other locations based on HLA characteristics it still should be reviewed occasionally to determine the incidence and any other new information related to this condition [278].

Most individuals do not experience a response to this supplement as treatment for several weeks [1, 3, 38, 276, 277]. And increasing doses can cause side effects such as nausea, vomiting, muscle cramps, headache and vertigo. ALA has shown an ability to especially reduce pain, and in some cases abnormal sensations (paresthesia), and numbness. The R-form of ALA appears to be better absorbed compared to the S-form so look for a dietary supplement that contains the R-form or at least racemic (50/50 mix of R and S). On average 20–40 % of oral racemic ALA is absorbed with R-form reaching higher levels compared to S-form. It is quickly absorbed and utilized which is why many experts think the divided doses throughout the day will eventually be shown to work better compared to single daily doses. Again, maximum blood concentrations are reached within 30–60 min (when given IV half of the compound is eliminated after 30 min). The liver quickly metabolizes this supplement. The safety record has been good enough that it appears that individuals with kidney or liver issues may be able to utilize it. In humans, ALA is actually produced by the liver and several other tissues, and in the diet it can be obtained from plant and animal sources such as organ meats but spinach, broccoli, tomato, Brussels sprouts, garden peas and rice bran are also good sources of R form of ALA. Yet the amounts in diet are small and could never equate to the dosage utilized in clinical trials and with age the ability to produce ALA decreases (similar to many other compounds in the body).

In terms of CIPN there is surprisingly very little adequate research that has been published and especially in breast cancer patients. Since ALA has also been proposed to provide neuroprotective benefits via decreasing oxidative stress from free radicals, the oxidation of platinum chemotherapy could be improved by ALA as was demonstrated in a small open-label pilot investigation when delivered with oxaliplatin (600 mg ALA IV once a week for 3–5 weeks and then *600 mg orally three times a day*) in advanced colorectal cancer patients [279]. In this study there was a decreasing severity of CIPN in eight of 15 patients [279]. The best trial design to address this issue was not able to answer the question [280]. A MD Anderson Cancer Center randomized placebo study of 243 patients with CIPN from cisplatin or oxaliplatin for 24 weeks, *but only 70 patients (29 %) completed the study!* And the dropout was so large that assessments at 36- or 48-weeks could not be conducted. The dosage of oral ALA was *600 mg three times a day (1800 mg total)* and despite the ALA and placebo arm having similar dropout rates there were no statistically significant differences between ALA and placebo for FACT/GOG-Ntx score (Functional Assessment of Cancer Therapy/Gynecologic Oncology Group-Neurotoxicity scale, Brief Pain Inventory (BPI), and patient functional outcomes. The mean age of the members of the trial were 55–57 years and approximately *75 % of the patients were being treated for gastrointestinal cancer*, 12 % for lung cancer, 6 % for genitourinary cancer, and 15 patients for other cancers. So, this study does not directly apply to breast cancer patients and the high dropout rate does not allow definitive conclusions on ALA in this setting as agreed upon by the authors.

The issue in this ALA CIPN trial according to the authors was the dosage and frequency of ALA in the trial (also arguably duration in my opinion) and most of the dropouts/withdrawals (compliance issues) were not able to perceive a benefit-versus-risk ratio that favored their continuation in the trial [280]. This observation has profound implications for future trials with ALA and dietary supplements testing in oncology clinical trials (as argued throughout this text) and countless other medical conditions. The authors have to be commended for this study and the conclusion derived from it. Some of these cancer toxicities and other medical conditions are acute and profound and unless dosages and delivery systems are practical and logical and benevolent (so to speak) then patients will not continue to remain in any study, especially with the knowledge that other perceived options are available immediately for their pain and suffering. Thus, it is not known currently if the positive data observed in diabetes with ALA can be observed in cancer patients with CIPN. Additionally in this trial ALA was stopped 2 days before and 4 days after the delivery of oxaliplatin because of the concern that ALA might protect the tumor from free radical damage (an issue that should be explored with an "antioxidant" supplement) and in the previous study it was given with the chemotherapy drug [279]. This is a difficult decision and must be weighed based on ongoing and future evidence of whether to conduct a trial utilizing the past [279] or current protocol [280]. This is a question without an answer and only speculation. And any implication that ALA has a cancer treatment effect in and of itself is also speculative and without merit. ALA needs more clinical trials in this area of medicine also and currently since it is quickly metabolized other delivery systems may be needed to also really address these future issues adequately [281].

E. Omega-3 fatty acids and paclitaxel-induced peripheral neuropathy (preliminary but interesting)

Although past trials of combining chemotherapy and/or radiation treatment with omega-3 fatty acid supplements have not resulted in worse outcomes overall [282], this is not a reason to encourage the use of omega-3 supplements or any supplements for cancer patients, unless of course it is condition specific (reducing high triglycerides for example with omega-3) [1, 3].

A stand alone trial of a dosage of 640 mg (54 % DHA and 10 % EPA from Mor DHA, Edegem, Belgium) of omega-3 supplement three times a day (total of 1920 mg a day—total dose of just active DHA and EPA was 1244.1 mg/day) in breast cancer patients observed that 70 % did not develop CIPN (actually paclitaxel-induced peripheral neuropathy) versus 40 % in the placebo arm, but this was a small trial of 57 patients [283]. CIPN incidence was significantly reduced ($p = 0.03$) and there was nonsignificant trend in reduced severity in the supplement arm ($p = 0.054$). Severe neuropathy was not observed in the omega-3 fatty acid group. Compliance was documented with increasing blood concentrations of EPA and DHA omega-3 in the intervention versus the placebo arm. The supplement or placebo was given during chemotherapy with paclitaxel and for 1 month after the end of therapy (3-h chemotherapy infusions were delivered every 3 weeks for four cycles). Patients were also instructed to take the "fish oil pearls" with meals and to keep the supplements in a freezer to prevent nausea and gastrointestinal side effects (fish burps, stomach discomfort—all rare in general at this dosage). Omega-3 fatty acids could have neuroprotective properties and needs further research to also ensure that it does not compromise conventional cancer treatment. It is of interest that an omega-3 EPA only supplement has shown some preliminary potential application for diabetic peripheral neuropathy [284]. It is also of interest that the supplements used in this past cancer clinical study consisted primarily of DHA omega-3 [283] and this is also the omega-3 being combined with chemotherapy in some clinical trials to determine if the tumor can receive a greater concentration of this drug with this unique delivery system [285]. Thus, interest in both EPA and DHA for CIPN should continue and more trials should be conducted especially since the current delivery symptoms allow for easy, realistic and flavorful liquid dosing in future trials (for example Omega Swirl by Barlean's and multiple other similar and competitive brands etc) [3, 286].

F. Acetyl-l-carnitine (Should be avoided or discouraged to prevent or treat CIPN because it can make it worse based on a phase-3 like trial and other data!)

Acetyl-l-carnitine (ALC) supplements actually made PN significantly worse in a major study of breast cancer patients taking it to reduce the risk of PN from chemotherapy. This should be concerning to anyone worried about PN because I believe this also suggests it could theoretically make PN worse regardless of the cause of PN. This is actually the first phase-3 like clinical trial to clearly demonstrate an increased risk of PN with a dietary supplement [287].

Acetyl-L-carnitine or ALC (and even L-carnitine) is a dietary supplement that is not low cost and has been touted (not proven) to benefit multiple of medical situations (fatigue, sexual dysfunction, neuropathy, Peyronie's disease, low testosterone, ...) [3]. Yet the problem is it still needed testing in better clinical trials. A 24-week multi-center randomized, double-blind, placebo-controlled clinical trial of 3000 mg (six pills a day initiated at the start of chemotherapy) of ALC compared to placebo daily was conducted in *women undergoing adjuvant taxane-based (docetaxel or paclitaxel) chemotherapy breast cancer treatment (stage I–III)* [287]. The goal was to determine if ALC could impact CIPN as a primary endpoint. A total of 409 patients (median age 50–52) were evaluable in this trial (208 receiving ALC and 201 receiving placebo). Patients receiving ALC had a significantly increased risk of CIPN compared to placebo including severe (grade 3–4) neurotoxicity! It was also interesting in this study fatigue was not impacted by the supplement and functional status on the supplement worsened compared to placebo. And blood levels of carnitine were also measured in patients to prove compliance. The only good news is that there were no differences in dose reductions or treatment delays with the ALC versus placebo supplements. I believe the conclusion of this trial, which was a Columbia University directed study was appropriate:

"There was no evidence that ALC affected CIPN at 12 weeks; however, ALC significantly increased CIPN by 24 weeks. This is the first study to our knowledge showing that a nutritional supplement increased CIPN. Patients should be discouraged from using supplements without proven efficacy."

Another trial conducted in France of 150 patients (98 with ovarian cancer and 52 patients with Castration Resistant Prostate Cancer or CRPC) were given 1000 mg of ALC to prevent sagopilone-induced peripheral neuropathy had results similar to placebo but in a subgroup of the ovarian cancer patients there was significantly less grade 3 or 4 neuropathy versus placebo ovarian cancer patients found with ALC [288]. This should be interpreted with caution because the overall results showed no benefit or difference in incidence and sagopilone is an experimental drug. More recently a study of patients with relapsed and/or refractory multiple myeloma (including those on bortezomib that relapsed) received bortezomib, doxorubicin, and dexamethasone for up to eight cycles ($n = 19$), and the other group received the same chemotherapy and 1500 mg of ALC twice daily (3000 mg total, $n = 13$), and median age was 64 years [289]. And the addition of ALC did not change the incidence or severity of peripheral neuropathy in patients with relapsed multiple myeloma. The cumulative evidence suggests that ALC should not be used to prevent or treat CIPN and simply has minimal to no role currently to prevent or treat conventional cancer treatment side effects, especially in breast cancer.

G. B-vitamin conundrum (rare cause and treatment for neuropathy not caused by CIPN)
Note: Utilization of B12 vitamins for fatigue was also covered in the fatigue section of this chapter.

There is a notable neuropathy caused from alcoholism and other extreme situations such as after bariatric or weight loss surgery in some cases that result from a vitamin B1 deficiency [1, 290, 291]. However, there is recent research to suggest that diabetics may also have low levels or altered metabolism of vitamin B1 or other B-vitamins that when restored through supplementation might provide some benefit against kidney disease or neuropathy [292]. An alternate form (drug called "benfotiamine," a synthetic S-acyl derivative of thiamine) of B1 has been tested with some success at higher dosages so there are some experts that believe vitamin B1 at dosages of anywhere from 25 to 100 mg/day should be offered to those with low levels of vitamin B1 [293]. In the meantime, low levels of vitamin B12 have also been rrely associated with neuropathies because some medications can reduce blood levels of these vitamins (acid reflux medications and metformin reduce B12 levels for example) [6, 294]. Again, these are rare occurrence but testing for a specific B-vitamin deficiency or excess is needed rarely to ensure etiology and the accurate reason for the neuropathy. Even excessive blood levels of some B-vitamins (such as B6) can cause a sensory peripheral neuropathy or in some cases it has also presented with a motor neuropathy component [295].

H. Miscellaneous dietary supplements/integrative options—Acupuncture, glutamine, NAC, vitamin E (Phase-3)...

There appears to be a never ending list of integrative medicines and dietary supplements proposed to assist with CIPN from acupuncture, glutamine, N-acetylcysteine (NAC), vitamin E and on the list continues, but in reality few if any products (including conventional medicines) have been effective when tested in clinical trials with stronger methodology [296, 297]. Acupuncture has a minimal amount of positive controlled randomized trial research [298, 299], but it is always promising for any chronic pain situation especially if it can reduce the amount of pain medication needed.

For example, although preliminary research on vitamin E appeared promising, a phase-3-like, randomized, double-blind, placebo-controlled multicenter clinical trial of 270 patients (*61 % were being treated for breast cancer*) receiving taxanes, cisplatin, carboplatin, oxaliplatin, or combinations with vitamin E (DL-ALPHA-TOCOPHEROL 300 mg twice daily from Hi-Health Corporation, Phoenix, AZ) versus placebo was disappointing [297]. No differences in time to onset of neuropathy, neuropathy induced chemotherapy reductions and no difference in secondary endpoints occurred. There may have been a slight positive effect on the duration of sensory neuropathy with vitamin E (time of onset of grade 2+ neuropathy until resolved to grade 1 or less during chemotherapy), but otherwise no toxicity or no treatment differences. And the efficacy of vitamin E could have been limited to those receiving cisplatin (eight patients) [300], and previous studies suggest vitamin E could have some efficacy against cisplatin toxicity (including ototoxicity) [301]. Arguably, the controversy surrounding an effective dietary supplement will continue, but ultimately it must be "first do no harm," or better stated in the concluding remarks of a comprehensive review of this subject of supplements and CIPN: "Currently no agents has shown solid evidence to be recommended for the treatment or prophylaxis of CIPN. The standard of care for CIPN includes dose reduction and/or discontinuation of chemotherapy treatment" [300].

• Sexual dysfunction (Female sexual dysfunction or FSD)
Note: Male sexual dysfunction and integrative medicine is adequately covered in a previous text [302].

A brief overview of this overall subject is needed for this chapter not because of space commitments, but rather because of the remarkable dearth of research in FSD and cancer, especially breast cancer where the prevalence is higher compared to other female impacted cancers and noncancer groups [303–305]. It appears that relationship satisfaction, body image stigma, vaginal dryness, depression, thyroid dysfunction are just some of the issues that impact sexual function in breast cancer survivors of a variety of ages. Approximately 80 % of women developed new sexual problems (if previously sexually active) and almost 25 % stopped sexual activity with a partner because of these issues after a review of the first 2-years of aromatase inhibitor (AI) use was completed. And long-term FSD is not uncommon based on the diversity of sexual issues that can occur with treatment and/or aging and comorbidities. Additionally, FSD does not cover one domain but multiple (desire, arousal, lubrication, orgasm, satisfaction, pain, …) when utilizing the Female Sexual Functioning Index (FSFI), which is a validated questionnaire of FSD and it could be utilized in breast cancer [306]. Thus, a quick review of at least the preliminary lifestyle and supplement/over the counter (OTC) data in FSD in general is needed to determine what could be potentially be effective in women with breast cancer and FSD (similar to lifestyle and supplement subject instruction in men with sexual dysfunction).

A. Lifestyle changes: Comprehensive approach—Exercise, diet, …
The thought that one isolated type of lifestyle intervention could be effective in FSD from breast cancer treatment has not been supported by the literature, for example just exercise [307]—despite reducing fatigue and other cancer treatment issues. The question remains that if comprehensive lifestyle changes such as a Mediterranean diet pattern or other weight loss reducing regimens have such profound impacts on men's and women's health and male sexual health or erectile dysfunction (ED) [302], then what is potential impact on female sexual dysfunction (FSD)? This question needs immediate research and lags behind male sexual health research and/or cancer treatment. Yet the preliminary evidence is also potentially profound in those with comorbidities [308–311], and the Table 7.6 is a basic review of what is partially involved (apart from more frequent and longer durations of exercise) in the comprehensive lifestyle studies for ED and FSD [308–311]. It should be remembered that the lifestyle changes in Table 7.6 were from randomized trials and the common theme was caloric reduction and exercise for weight loss and improved overall nutritional status from healthy foods along with heart healthy parameter changes: Lower Blood LDL, glucose, blood pressure, some weight/waist loss or maintenance, and improved mood or quality of life. Arguably any comprehensive lifestyle program that could provide these changes could be beneficial [3].

For example, a study of 595 women with type 2 diabetes, ages 35–70 years were analyzed based on adherence to the Mediterranean diet and FSD using the FSFI validated questionnaire [309]. Primarily based on the threshold of 23 as the

Table 7.6 A comprehensive guide to a variety of lifestyle changes that improved female sexual dysfunction (FSD) in patients with comorbidities (diabetes, metabolic syndrome, …)—primarily Mediterranean diet randomized trials

– Reduced caloric intake
– Regular physical activity
– High intake of fruits (3–4 servings/day) and vegetables (2–3 servings/day)
– High intake of monounsaturated-to-saturated fats (ratio of 2 or more)
– Higher intake of olive oil (a monounsaturated fat, used daily)
– Daily intake of cereals (whole grain) and legumes
– Moderate intake of fish and nuts (3–5 servings/week)
– Moderate or no intake of alcohol
– Low intake of red and processed meat (4–5 servings/month)
– Daily intake of low-fat dairy products
– Protein intake of 0.8–1 g per kg body weight (half of body weight in grams of protein maximum—for example 150 pound person would need a maximum of 75 g of total protein per day from foods and supplemental sources)
– Increased Fiber from dietary sources (usually recommended 20–30 g a day)

Note: These were randomized trials and the common theme was caloric reduction and exercise for weight loss and improved overall nutritional status from healthy foods along with heart healthy parameter changes: lower blood LDL, glucose, blood pressure, some weight/waist loss or maintenance, and improved mood or quality of life. Arguably any comprehensive lifestyle program that could provide these changes could be beneficial

cutoff score for FSD with the FSFI, women with greater adherence to the diet had significantly ($p = 0.01$) lower risk of FSD compared to women with lesser adherence after adjusting for confounding variables. Another 2-year randomized trial by this similar research team placed 31 women with metabolic syndrome on a Mediterranean diet compared to 28 in the control group [308]. FSFI significantly ($p = 0.01$) improved in the diet group from a mean of 19.7 to 26.1 at the end of the trial, but were "stable" in the control arm. Two additional findings from this trial did not appear to receive attention but are noteworthy. *First, no single domain of the FSFI (desire, arousal, orgasm, satisfaction, pain) was significantly reduced by the Mediterranean diet, which suggests that multiple minimal to moderate lifestyle changes in diverse areas of sexual health may be cumulative in significantly reducing FSD as a whole.* Second, CRP levels were significantly ($p < 0.02$) reduced in the diet group, which suggests thus far in these studies that men and women may share this as a novel marker for heart disease and sexual dysfunction or improvement from this condition [308].

A clinical trial of obese (mean BMI 43–45) fertile women (ages 18–49 years, mean 36 years) with FSFI-6 scores of 19 or less that were placed in only 16-week intervention programs again highlight the potential for improving FSD with comprehensive lifestyle programs [312]. Women were assigned increased physical activity and reduced caloric intake at a specialized clinical site or at home. Women assigned to the clinic oversight program had significantly higher improvement in sexual activity and FSFI-6, and significant improvements in arousal, lubrication, and satisfaction domain scores (all $p < 0.01$). Significant improvements in insulin sensitivity, endothelial function and weight, BMI, fat mass and percentage of fat mass was also found for the intensive clinic intervention group compared to the home based lifestyle changes group. It should be kept in mind that the intensive at clinic program consisted of: personalized nutrition program designed for the participant with a *reduced caloric intake, protein intake of 0.8–1 g of protein per kilogram of body weight, exercise at 60–70 % of maximum heart rate for an average of 10 h per week*. This trial suggests that morbidly obese women that make profound changes in their lifestyle guided by a multidisciplinary weight loss clinic could result in profound changes (average weight loss of 16 kg or over 35 pounds) or improvement in FSD. It is concerning that the home-based educational group did not experience any significant changes in any parameter. This would suggest that intensive clinic based supervision is far superior to simple education and so-called "do it yourself" self-improvement programs. I would agree with this finding for patients that are in desperate need of more extreme changes based on their current status and past inadequate performance in the area of weight loss for overall and specific health improvements. Yet another intense area of focus for FSD treatment should also be placed on subtle and simplistic changes that could prevent or improve these conditions. FSD appears to be a marker (as does ED) in some women of an associated higher risk of cardiovascular disease. For example, younger women with dyslipidemia are more likely to report worse scores on FSFI diverse domains compared to women of similar age and characteristics that do not have cholesterol issues [313], and this also may be true for multiple heart healthy markers [314]. Additionally, if sexual health benefits in women and men are not adequate from multiple lifestyle changes alone then again it should be an ongoing clinical evaluative marker of the potential need to add other conventional medical/pharmacologic (or non-pharmacologic) treatments for individuals concerned about ED and FSD. It should be reiterated that comprehensive lifestyle changes in breast cancer are simply derived from comorbidities or other situations and the lack of data in this area is the reason for the focus on other programs that could be successful in cancer patients.

B. Lubricants for FSD (Zestra®? l-arginine or l-citrulline? Olive oil lubricant for breast cancer? ...)

Zestra is a female massage oil with some minimal clinical data to suggest it can increase warmth and sensitivity, and increase the probability of arousal when applied to the clitoris, labia, and vaginal opening [315]. This is an over the counter massage oil that is composed of borage seed oil, evening primrose oil, angelica root extract and coleus extract (the estrogenic activity of these herbals appears minimal but check for the latest research). Interestingly, borage seed and evening primrose contain high concentrations of gamma-linolenic acid (GLA) that can be metabolized into dihomo-gamma-linolenic acid (DGLA), and into prostaglandin E1 or E2, which may increase nerve conduction, protection, and blood flow in other medical situations but the impact could be subtle in some cases [316–318]. A small preliminary study of 20 women with sexual arousal disorder and some with normal sexual functioning had significant improvements in the level of arousal, desire, genital sensation, ability to achieve orgasm, and overall sexual pleasure [315]. Mild genital burning in three participants was reported that resolved in 5–30 min were the only reported adverse effects of Zestra. This lubricant has not been adequately tested in breast cancer patients.

The problem with the study of lubricants in general for sexual health and breast cancer is that there is minimal research ever published in this category. There is little doubt that in studies of water or silicon-based lubricants the effectiveness can be clinically significant especially for women experiencing dyspareunia [319, 320]. *Yet it is remarkable that more studies of lubricants to potentially improve other aspects of FSD or even ED have not been attempted or published.* Lubricants are not only commonly used and popular but in general they are associated with greater sexual pleasure and satisfaction during self-stimulation and partnered sexual activity [319, 321]. Hopefully, research on other lubricant ingredients that have the potential to improve arousal or another aspect of FSD such as L-arginine or L-citrulline for blood flow (adequate preliminary research in men) will receive more research (see dietary supplements section below).

Since vaginal lubricants to deter dryness and dyspareunia during sexual activity usually include a discussion of water-based, silicon-based, and petroleum-based options, there are also potential issues with some of them. For example, some water-based products contain higher concentrations of preservatives that could injury sensitive vaginal mucosa, and for example petroleum-based lubricants could increase the risk of vaginal infection. It is for this reason some researchers have suggested *organic olive oil* for longer duration lubrication needs because of its viscosity [322]. *A total of 25 women treated for breast cancer* (mean age of 51 years, range of 37–66 years of age) in a unique study of pelvic floor muscle (PFM) relaxation exercises twice per week to prevent or manage PFM overactivity plus application of a polycarbophil-based vaginal moisturizer three times a week to reduce vaginal dryness, and the use of olive oil as a lubricant for sexual intercourse (follow-up of 26 weeks) found significant ($p < 0.001$) improvements in dyspareunia, sexual function, and quality of life [322]. Non-latex condoms were also provided to those that needed them because they are compatible with olive oil as a lubricant. The maximum benefits of the combination approach were evident at 12 weeks. Women generally rated PFM relaxation exercises (92 %), vaginal moisturizer (88 %), and olive oil (73 %) as acceptable. All of the women in this study (100 %) documented that they would recommend this particular intervention to other breast cancer survivors with similar issues.

C. Dietary supplements for FSD (KRG? l-arginine? Yohimbine? l-citrulline? SAM-e? Combination ingredients-ArginMax, Lady Prelox …)
There is some interesting preliminary basic science and clinical trial data that suggests that *Panax ginseng (Korean Red ginseng or KRG-almost identical to Panax ginseng)* could significantly improve some domains of FSD [323–326]. A crossover trial ($n = 28$ completed the study) of postmenopausal women at a dosage of 3 g/day (approximately 8 % ginsenoside concentration) for 8 weeks demonstrated

a significant improvement in arousal, but not other domains, utilizing the FSFI questionnaire [326]. Mean estradiol levels did not change and side effects were similar to placebo. Two women experienced vaginal bleeding during the trial on ginseng and one of these participants had a significant increase in estradiol (less than 10 pg/ml to 27 pg/ml). There is no current suggestion that ginseng can improve sexual health or FSD in premenopausal women. And ginseng as an FSD supplement has not been studied in breast cancer patients.

Increasing blood flow with a dietary supplement pill may improve sexual function in men [302], but in women this has not been well researched (not even for supplemental lubricants). A preliminary study of a product that contains 200 mg of L-citrulline per tablet (along with 20 mg Pycnogenol, 200 mg L-arginine, and 50 mg of rose hip extract) found improved overall sexual function (FSFI) in women ages 37–45 years ($n = 100$) after 4 and 8 weeks of daily use for their moderate FSD [327]. Another study of healthy postmenopausal women utilizing the same product found significant improvement in the total FSFI versus placebo ($n = 83$), and all domains of FSFI (desire, arousal, lubrication, orgasm, satisfaction, and pain) appeared to respond favorably [328].

l-*citrulline* is usually found in two forms: the free form (just stated as "L-CITRULLINE") on the bottle and "L-citrulline-malate" which is used by many people to enhance their athletic workouts [302]. It is possible that citrulline malate may also help with sexual health but it has not been studied. Keep in mind that since L-citrulline is a vasodilator and arguably the most efficient nitric oxide (NO) producing dietary supplement (as effective as L-arginine at half the dosage), thus it could slightly reduce blood pressure. L-citrulline food sources are few (watermelon rind) so the only method of testing these dosages of L-citrulline is via supplementation. In men with ED supplementation studies up to 1500 mg/day have been preliminarily completed with success over placebo [329], and studies of FSD and women treated with breast cancer and FSD need to be studied. L-Arginine has received minimal attention in FSD and large dosages are usually needed to create nitric oxide. One crossover study of L-arginine glutamate (6 g) + yohimbine HCL (6 mg) or yohimbine HCL (6 mg) alone or placebo alone for arousal disorder did not work significantly better than placebo ($n = 24$) [330]. Again, the need for mega-dosing of L-arginine to create nitric oxide (due to dramatic first pass metabolism and enzymatic metabolism in the gut) and the ability of L-citrulline to be far more effective at a lower dosage suggests future studies utilize L-citrulline only [302].

Lepidium meyenii or "Maca" is an Andean plant that is a part of the brassica family and has been used for centuries in the Andes to enhance fertility and sexual health in humans and animals [331, 332]. Maca may also slightly improved sexual function from a series of recent and past preliminary clinical trials in men, and it does not appear to alter testosterone levels [333, 334]. The data points toward good preliminary safety and a potential enhancement in fertility that should receive attention, but what about FSD?

The potential issues with Maca are threefold: first this product has not been tested beyond preliminary studies with small numbers of individuals, high dosages are required in some studies to observe an impact (2400–3000 mg), and there is a question of what to look for when standardizing the ingredients of Maca. This is also the case in FSD where Maca appeared to significantly increase libido in women in nine women with SSRI-induced FSD when taking 3 g/day compared to seven individuals taking 1.5 g/day, but there was no placebo arm [335]. A past systematic review also agrees that although interesting it is difficult to comment with more certainty whether or not this product can be a stand alone or ancillary option for ED or FSD [336]. *However, a recent 12-week, double-blind, placebo-controlled trial of maca root 3000 mg/day in 45 female outpatients (mean age 41 years, from similar US research group earlier that tested Maca in women) with SSRI/SNRI-induced sexual dysfunction with remission of their depression was published* [337]. The Maca product was obtained from a Peruvian manufacturer and analyzed for a standard consistent macamide content listed in the publication (extensive list). Out of 45 females randomized, 42 were eligible for intention-to-treat analysis (30 premenopausal and 12 postmenopausal). FSD remission rates were higher for MACA versus placebo and greater remission was correlated with postmenopausal status, and could have been due to a significant increase in androgen or testosterone, which significantly improved with sexual function in MACA group ($p = 0.008$, as measured by the Arizona Sexual Experience Scale or ASEX), and the orgasm domain appeared to demonstrated the largest improvement as well as the MGH-SFQ (Massachusetts General Hospital Sexual Functioning Scale) trended toward significance ($p = 0.057$) with MACA. Both the ASEX and MGH-SFQ are 5-item rating scales that evaluate different areas of sexual function (arousal, orgasm, satisfaction, …). No other hormones including estradiol, progesterone, and prolactin changed with the supplement versus placebo. Based on the results of their two preliminary studies this research group is planning a larger clinical trial [335, 337].

My biggest concern is standardization of Maca during a clinical trial because it appears that dried maca roots need to be standardized to a specific amount of the "macamide" and "macaene" (polyunsaturated fatty acids and their amides) amount from a lipidic extract of this herb because these are the proposed potential active ingredients, and macamides for example are a unique class of secondary metabolites not found in another plant species [338, 339]. Therefore, they would be useful markers of not only efficacy, but also quality control. It appears that a product with at least 0.6 % macamides and macaenes should be the minimum quality control marker of standardization from past male studies [340]. However, a comparison of macamides from the more recent clinical study will at least provide a good comparative for future studies [337]. Maca also contains diverse amino acids including almost 100 mg of arginine per gram of Maca [341]. It is a concerning that a large study to determine if Maca really improves sexual desire and other parameters of sexual health in men and women have not been conducted based on the preliminary results with this herbal product, but again is not at least expected in the future with FSD from antidepressant use.

SAM-e (S-adenosyl-methionine) was reviewed in the aromatase inhibitor arthralgia (AIA) and depression sections of this chapter, and a quick reiteration is needed here. Preliminary research also suggests that this supplement used in addition to conventional antidepressants (SSRI) to augment their effect appeared to have a positive significant effect on male arousal and erectile dysfunction (lower arousal and sexual dysfunction), such that scores actually improved in these areas compared to placebo (independent in the improvement in depression) [106]. Why not test SAM-e for women that have antidepressant induced FSD? This type of study should be completed based on the long history and safety of SAM-e. It is also of interest that SAM-e has been used as a prescription drug, given as an IV or an injectable in numerous European countries since the 1970s and its ability to reduce osteoarthritic pain is also notable, well published, and on par with NSAIDs but with less toxicity at dosages of up to 600 mg/day [3].

Combination dietary supplement ingredient products for sexual dysfunction abound, which is why I rarely mention them in terms of research because the product itself tends to piggy back so to speak off of the data of one effective ingredient. However, there may be some rare exceptions (or not) for example Lady Prelox mentioned earlier efficacy could be due to L-citrulline (or not—not tested against it alone) and then there is *ArginMax*®. This supplement utilizes multiple compounds including L-arginine, and ginseng, and appears to have garnered enough data to potentially recommend it to some FSD patients. Two previous placebo-controlled studies published of this combination dietary supplement (L-arginine, *Panax ginseng*, *Ginkgo biloba*, damiana leaf, multiple vitamins and minerals, ...) helped to improve arousal, desire, orgasm, sexual frequency, clitoral sensation, and increased sexual function scores [342, 343]. These preliminary studies ($n = 77$, and $n = 108$, ages 22–73 years) are suggesting that premenopausal, perimenopausal, and postmenopausal women with FSD could benefit. Premenopausal and perimenopausal appeared to derive more diverse benefits whereas desire was primarily increased in postmenopausal women. The more recent clinical study showed a benefit within 4 weeks. This supplement does not appear to have estrogenic enhancement properties, which means that it could be appropriate option for women with breast cancer or those that do not want to use hormone replacement therapy (although this always needs more research). *In fact, to the credit of this company a larger trial in female cancer survivors (median age 49–51, age range 23–72 years) was recently published, which included female cancer survivors* [344]. This was a 12-week, randomized, placebo-controlled trial who were 6 months or more from active treatment and reporting issues with sexual interest, satisfaction, and functioning after therapy. Participants took three capsules of ArginMax (from Daily Wellness Company, Honolulu, HI) or placebo twice daily (six pills per day) and assessments were completed at 4, 8, and 12 weeks. *A total of 78 % of the patients had breast cancer out of the 186 participants enrolled in the trial. At 12-weeks there were no differences between ArginMax and placebo for sexual desire, arousal, lubrication, orgasm, satisfaction, or pain. Although FACT-G (Functional Assessment of Cancer Therapy-General) were significantly better with ArginMax ($p = 0.009$) versus placebo suggesting an improvement in overall quality of life, and side effects were similar to placebo.* One has to commend these researchers and ArginMax for continuing to be involved in some clinical studies. Whether or not this is not enough or enough information to consider utilizing this supplement is a matter of debate and personal preference.

It could also be argued that the benefits of ArginMax could also have occurred from other well-known herbals such as Panax ginseng (improves well-being by reducing fatigue for example) because the concentrations of the active ingredients (ginsenosides) were high (30 %, see Panax or Korean Red ginseng section of this section) [302]. Whether or not L-arginine and/or L-citrulline (improve blood flow) or *Panax ginseng* or other supplements alone could be just as effective as this combination approach has not been tested.

D. The Story and status of DHEA (or androstenedione) for women and men
On January 20, 2005 it became illegal to sell androstenedione dietary supplements in the USA [345, 346]. Androstenedione was considered a "prohormone" supplement that some men and women used in an attempt to build muscle. Some notable US professional athletes utilized it before it was banned, and it created a plethora of controversy. It was a potentially dangerous supplement because it had been associated with significant reductions in "good cholesterol" or HDL and it had potentially other health consequences such as significantly increasing estrogen (estrone and estradiol) in healthy young men (ages 26–32 years) taking 100 mg or 300 mg/day for 7 days, and significantly increasing testosterone levels at 300 mg/day (from 526 to 872 ng/dl on average in one study) [347]. Other studies of young men demonstrated only increases in estrogen with these dosages [348], which is why it would not been surprising that some individual reports of ED from these supplements can also occur because of arguable the suppression of the pituitary and gonadal axis [349]. The individual variability in the response is also what is striking about androstenedione (or DHEA) in men and women, except for the estrogen increases in young and older primarily eugonadal men. Men ages 35–65 years taking 200 mg of androstenedione had significant increases in estrogen but not testosterone over 12 weeks [350]. In postmenopausal women a significant increase in estrone occurred but the individual variability in the response was always notable, which is again part of the problem [351]. Regardless of the population studied the variability or unpredictability of the physiologic response should be mentioned to patients. This has also been my experience that men and women without overt hormone deficiencies have variable results and men experience dramatic increases in estrogen and potentially a small increase in testosterone the more testosterone deficient the male [352].

Therefore, there were so many concerns with these supplements that eventually the FDA and the US government decided to remove almost all of them, including androstenedione, from the market [345]. Other so-called "prohormone" supplements like DHEA were not banned, but are still being allowed for sale. Now, if DHEA is similar to androstenedione in that it has similar effects, than why is this supplement still allowed to be for sale over the counter? This is part of the strange circumstances surrounding some dietary supplements and the inconsistency in the policies that are applied. DHEA supplements enjoy a unique exemption under federal law, because of a bill approved by Congress in late 2004. How did DHEA survive when other similar to identical supplements did not? Sports officials were in favor of an overall ban on steroids and related products, including DHEA. DHEA was banned by the Olympics, the World Anti-Doping Agency, the National

Collegiate Athletics Association, the National Football League, the National Basketball Association, and minor league baseball. The 2005 law that impacts pro-hormone supplements, passed without objection, also gave the Drug Enforcement Administration (DEA) more authority to ban new or novel steroids, with one exemption, DHEA. The term "anabolic steroid" is defined now as any drug or hormonal substance, chemically and pharmacologically related to testosterone (other than estrogens, progestins, corticosteroids, and DHEA). In my opinion, since such a large percentage of Congressional men and women use dietary supplements and some perceived DHEA as unique, the proposal to ban all over the counter pro-hormone supplements in the USA would have not passed Congress if DHEA were included in the proposal. Now, with this pertinent history, what about any new data to support DHEA for women's or men's health or sexual health?

Population studies such as the Massachusetts Male Aging Study have suggested a higher risk of ED with lower blood levels of DHEA-S [353]. Yet what gets missed in referencing these studies is that there were also inverse associations of HDL with ED and a higher risk of ED in those with heart disease, hypertension, smoking and diabetes for example, which is a more tangible and productive conversation. *It should be kept in mind that DHEA levels decrease substantially with aging, and this has been utilized in deceptive advertising in my opinion to encourage men and women to purchase this supplement.* Other studies suggest that a lower level of DHEA and an increase risk of ED is only a weak association [354]. DHEA is produced primarily by the adrenal cortex and in smaller amounts by the testes and the ovaries, and then it is quickly sulfated by sulfotransferases into DHEA-S, which is more stable with a longer half-life and its concentrations stay stable most of the day [355]. DHEA is arguably the most abundant steroid in the human body, thus for this and many other reasons there will always be sufficient physiologic facts to give it some advertising cache. Yet it does not appear to have a role for androgen deficient or insufficient men because it is not predictable.

So, does DHEA appear to be of benefit in men with ED and low DHEA levels or women with FSD and low levels? Small studies of men utilizing 50 mg for 6 months (DHEAS level < 1.5 μmol/L) showed some improvements in function in those with hypertension and ED or those without organic etiology, but not in those with diabetes or neurologic issues [356, 357]. These men were all generally tested with prostaglandin E1 first to ensure that they were capable of having a full erection with pharmacologic intervention.

The problem with DHEA is a lack of large studies with good methodology and no really novel findings with DHEA and ED or in the area of male sexual health. *DHEA-S levels are also not easy to acutely or chronically predict with lifestyle interventions, for example in some studies there is minimal or large changes in this hormonal marker for men and women after large reduction in weight [358–360].* Perhaps this is due to the fact that DHEA levels need to be monitored over many years. Obesity appears to attenuate the association or correlation between higher DHEA and lower morbidity [361].

The problem with DHEA in women is that longer randomized trials in post-menopausal women (26+ weeks) have not shown results better than placebo on sexual desire for example at 50 mg/day [362]. *And more women experienced acne and increased hair growth in the DHEA arm.* Overall the results are so mixed that reviews of past data tend to discourage the use of oral DHEA for sexual health improvements in women with FSD [363], and especially in those with a history of breast cancer (and men with a history of prostate cancer). The good news is that overall the safety of 50 mg of DHEA tends to be excellent in 1-year studies but I still am concerned about reductions in HDL over time with this and higher dosages [364]. Despite some of the criticism with DHEA studies that the dosages utilized are not high enough for efficacy, older studies of higher DHEA dosages (300 mg and more) in small groups of postmenopausal women have suggested a benefit over placebo that could have an impact on mental and physical sexual health and arousal within 60 min of visual sexual stimuli [365]. Yet these are acute dosage studies and the positives and negatives of several days/month high-dose DHEA ingestion have not received adequate attention. For example, a 1600 mg/day for 28 days DHEA supplementation study was published, which showed profound reductions in HDL, and significant increases in testosterone in postmenopausal women (no changes in estrogen) [366].

DHEA is not a promising or predictable option for those that need testosterone replacement therapy (TRT) or postmenopausal FSD, but perhaps those with adrenal or androgen insufficiency might benefit? *Replacement with DHEA in those with androgen or especially "adrenal insufficiency" (adrenal adenectomy, autoimmune, or secondary from pituitary issues for example) appears practical and has some preliminary older data in women* [367, 368], *but the decision of whether or not it has consistent benefits is still very subjective.* For example, a retrospective review (non-placebo) of over 100 women with androgen insufficiency and sexual dysfunction ingesting 50 mg of DHEA on average for 4 months reported a significant reduction in sexual distress, and increases in desire, arousal, lubrication, satisfaction, and orgasm [368]. Women in this study (mean age of 43 years) had testosterone and DHEA-S levels that were in the lower range of normal. Increased facial hair (11 %), weight gain (7 %), acne (5 %), temporary breast tenderness, loss of head hair and skin rash (1 % each) were the most commonly reported side effects. *Thus, there is fairly general agreement that women with androgen or especially adrenal insufficiency are the best potential candidates for DHEA especially is there is a need to increase mood and/or libido* [369]. However, if there is a history of breast cancer again and adrenal issues than this should be discouraged or handled on a case by case basis with blood monitoring to perhaps physiologic levels. Still, all of this is not tantamount to a solid recommendation. Small studies against placebo of women with adrenal insufficiency (AI) for 4 months suggests some benefit of DHEA supplementation of 50 mg/day on general sexual health [370]. Still, this data in patients with AI are controversial and there is always concern about long-term toxicity in these individuals [371]. Additionally, there have been several studies showing no impact on sexual health, which is arguably why one of the only meta-analysis performed on randomized trials for DHEA and quality of life in women with adrenal insufficiency did not recommend it [372]. *This is a classic example of a mixed data situation where the decision to add small amounts of DHEA for women that are androgen or adrenal insufficient should be left to the patient and clinician not this current textbook.*

What about DHEA for specific and general antiaging health purposes? In one of the longest duration clinical trials in the history of DHEA [373], the supplement was given for 2 years at a dose of 75 mg/day in men and 50 mg/day in women, and these researchers decided to look at the impact of this hormone on the body, physical performance, insulin and other factors compared to a placebo. There were a total of 87 men (29 received DHEA, 27 received testosterone, and 31 received placebo) in this study and 57 women (27 received DHEA and 30 received placebo), and the average age of the participants ranged from 66 to 70 years. Men and women in this study were just slightly overweight with a Body Mass Index (BMI) of 26–27. Women that had low levels of DHEA (median value of 0.4 µg/ml or 1.1 mmol/l), and men with low levels of DHEA (median value of 0.7 µg/ml or 1.9 mmol/l) had their levels increased by approximately 3.5 µg/ml or 9.5 mmol/l after taking DHEA. This is a 500 % increase in blood levels of this hormone in some of the patients. This current study showed that quality of life did not change on DHEA, but perhaps a larger study would have provided more clarity in this area. There were no changes in oxygen intake (a measure of metabolism change), muscle strength, or insulin. *The DHEA group experienced an unhealthy drop in HDL or "good" cholesterol, which was a significant 5-point reduction in women,* and an almost significant 3-point reduction in men during the study (US Units). No such HDL drop occurred in the testosterone-receiving group of men during the study. Men receiving testosterone had a slight reduction in fat tissue, and bone mineral density increased at the hip area in men on DHEA and testosterone. *In women, DHEA increased bone mineral density only in the area of the wrist, but not at other sites.* So, again this study leaves open the possibility of testing higher doses of DHEA and testosterone but safety will ultimately also be an issue. Higher doses of DHEA need to be studied, but in the meantime, reversing the signs of aging with hormones has little to no evidence and may have harm.

Why not just give testosterone replacement therapy (TRT) to the men that truly require or qualify for testosterone or smaller amount (10 % or less) to women deficient in androgen? This seems to make more sense as opposed to playing a guessing game with a dietary supplement for general antiaging purposes that also seems to possess safety and quality control issues [345, 346, 374]. And this is also a concern that just because someone purchases DHEA does not necessarily guarantee DHEA is found in the bottle at the reported concentrations [371]. Finally, other areas of health, such as muscle strength and physical function have shown minimal impact with this supplement from short- and long-term studies [375]. Other long-term (2-years) studies of women's health suggest that a significant improvement in spinal bone mineral density (BMD) with 50 mg/day of DHEA in women (ages 65–75) also receiving 650 IU/day of vitamin D and 700 mg/day of calcium versus vitamin D and calcium alone suggests that this may be an area worth pursuing (though not in breast cancer patients arguably) [376].

What does the future hold for DHEA? Vaginally administered DHEA (for example "Prasterone," 0.25–1 % DHEA) appears to provide sexual health benefits (desire, arousal, lubrication, orgasm, and reduced dryness) for women with vaginal atrophy and estrogen deficiency in menopause [363, 377], but I would not consider this a integrative medicine but a prescription drug. It is applied intravaginally with an applicator at bedtime. Vaginal DHEA requires daily application whereas other steroids (estradiol or estriol) require 2–3 times a week dosing and safety has been well established with vaginal estrogen [378]. So, how popular this will be in the future, impact on overall estrogen and androgens in women short- and long-term [379], and whether it has any role in breast cancer is a matter of more research and opinion.

• **Stress and/or anxiety (and cognitive function)**
Note: Stress and anxiety can in some cases also be related to depressive and overall cognitive symptoms (see Chap. 7). Overall, there has been a moderate amount of research on integrative medicines apart from lifestyle changes, and the majority of the supplement research has dealt with stress and anxiety outside of breast cancer, and some of these supplements also have some research in the area of improved cognition. *Thus, a quick review will be provided in the area of dietary supplements that is intended to be more than a cursory approach to this matter and thought for future research in breast cancer since may of these agents appear to have a high benefit-to-risk ratio outside of breast cancer.*

A. Lifestyle changes
Multiple integrative medicines appear to preliminarily provide some consistent benefit against stress and/or anxiety in breast cancer or cancer patients including exercise (aerobic and resistance with 40+ clinical trials in cancer patients) [380], yoga (more than seven randomized trials) [381], Tai chi [382], meditation [383], and massage therapy [384]. *Some form of exercise should be considered a first-line prevention and treatment of stress and/or anxiety for breast cancer patients (along with conventional treatment if needed) during and after breast cancer treatment.* For example, the stress and/or anxiety reduction was also demonstrated when trying to reduce side effects of breast cancer treatment (reconstruction, menopausal symptoms, …). The body responds to being fit by being in an antistress state of mind and body because exercise reduces heart rate, blood pressure, blood sugar, cortisol, and releases endorphins, which are compounds associated with a state of relaxation and improved mood. Remember the so-called "runners high," which is an antistress exercise phenomenon.

Additional stress reducing activities include: joining a support group, journaling, art therapy, guided imagery, hypnosis, music therapy, and horticultural therapy, and many of these opportunities are either low cost or no cost through areas like the Wellness community or even community recreation centers [3]. They not only provide support but family members and spouses can also get help. As one gains control over the stress and/or anxiety, the body can respond by reducing blood pressure, heart rate, stress, and anxiety. Any diet or activity that reduces blood pressure can also theoretically reduce stress and anxiety.

Alcohol, tobacco, and caffeine (can increase blood pressure and heart rate) are often used to "relax" or basically reduce stress temporarily and this is a problem because it can create dependency [3]. In other words, it is a short-term fix that can

Table 7.7 Perceived Stress Scale (one version) abridged or modified (multiple copies can be found online) or PSS. This is the 10-item questionnaire that pertains to experiences over the past month. Each question allows for a 0 (never), 1 (almost never), 2 (sometimes), 3 (fairly often), or a 4-point (very often) answer to each question. Positively worded items (questions 4, 5, 7, and 8) are reversed scored and then all points are added (higher values equal greater perceived stress). Keep in mind that every question starts with the statement "In the past month ..." [385]

Questions—In the past month ... (*Note*: sum all points from questions 1 to 10 and higher values=higher perceived stress)	Point value assigned to the specific question (0=never, 1=almost never, 2=sometimes, 3=fairly often, or 4=very often)
1. How often have you been upset because of something that happened unexpectedly?	
2. How often have you felt unable to control the important things in your life?	
3. How often have you felt nervous or stressed?	
4. How often have you felt confident about your ability to handle personal problems?	(Reverse scored 0=4, 1=3, 2=2, ...)
5. How often have you felt things were going your way?	(Reverse scored 0=4, 1=3, 2=2, ...)
6. How often have you found that you could not cope with all the things you had to do?	
7. How often have you been able to control irritations in your life?	(Reverse scored 0=4, 1=3, 2=2, ...)
8. How often have you felt that you were on top of things?	(Reverse scored 0=4, 1=3, 2=2, ...)
9. How often have you been angry because of things that happened that were outside of your control?	
10. How often have you felt that difficulties were piling up so high that you could not overcome them?	

only increase stress with time, and also can exacerbate anxiety and depression because the body develops resistance to these compounds so that higher doses are needed in the future. And once the antistress effect goes away the body responds by increasing significantly the amount of stress hormones that you can produce, which only increases your dependence on these drugs.

There are numerous stress questionnaires available on the internet that can be printed and answered by patients to be discussed with their health care professionals. For example, the Perceived Stress Scale (PSS) is retrospective over the previous month and has evolved over time. One modified example of PSS is found in Table 7.7 [385]. Answering these questions is empowering and therapeutic because it allows one to start taking control of your situation. Keeping a diary or notebook of stressors is also beneficial and encouraging patients to bring a companion the medical visit could help in remembering items at the visit and this can reduce stress and anxiety. A companion also further reduces stress because it is therapeutic to have someone that is able to discuss things when it comes to these important issues and how patients are feeling about them.

Additionally, creating a personal or modified PSS using additional questions that do not necessarily requiring scoring but personal commentary could be helpful [3]. These questions have tended to trigger some of the most informative answers from personal experience working with patients dealing with cancer and stress and/or anxiety. For example, some of the questions that appear important for cancer patients to answer that are not necessarily over the past month questions include the following:

How would you describe your energy level?

How have you been sleeping?

How has your mood been lately?

What kind of pressure have you been dealing with at work, home or in general?

What do you do to unwind at the end of the day and do you have difficulty unwinding?

Who do you turn to for support?

Are there any personal issues that need to be covered that you would like to share with your health care professional?

Have you felt sad, discouraged, or hopeless lately to the point where you wondered if anything was worthwhile?

B. Dietary supplements

Note: Any potential antistress supplement combined with medications to reduce stress, anxiety or depression could cause a drug interaction that can be dangerous, so the latest information on these products should be checked with the literature and for example a pharmacist to make sure there are no potential negative drug interactions that could occur. Also, sudden withdrawal of any supplement or drug that can reduce stress/anxiety and blood pressure may be dangerous by causing an increase in blood pressure or heart rate, so a gradual withdrawal over several weeks similar to a medication is encouraged. In other words, like every other supplement recommended in this book, please rereview the latest information.

Bacopa monnieri (also known as "Brahmi" or just "Bacopa," standardized to a minimum of 25 % bacopa a or 55 % total bacosides) at 200–450 mg/day for cognition/memory and/or anxiety. It has not been tested in breast cancer patients.

This is an alternative Ayurvedic medicine that in preliminary clinical trials has reduced stress and anxiety greater than a placebo [3]. This supplement also has come in a liquid or syrup form and may also have blood pressure lowering effects. Although this plant has been used in India and Pakistan for various ailments, the real focus lately has been on its potential for memory enhancement or to reduce anxiety.

This is a small herb with many branches, small leaves, and light purple flowers. It grows naturally in wet soil, marshes, and in shallow water [3]. It can be found to grow at higher altitudes (over 4000 ft) to sea level as long as there is some water around.

Many of the components of Bacopa were isolated years ago and include alkaloids, saponins, and sterols. For example, researchers have found beta-sitosterol as well as numerous compounds known as bacopasaponins and bacosides. The compounds being studied for their activity on cognitive and other brain effects are "Bacosides A and B."

Bacosides may be involved in nerve cell repair and production as well and improving nerve cell signaling. Bacosides also appear to have some antioxidant activity in different areas of the brain including hippocampus, frontal cortex, and striatum. Bacopa also has relaxing properties on the vascular system and perhaps even the lungs.

The dosages being studied for cognitive benefits have been for example 300 mg/day (55 % combined bacosides), and at the end of 12 weeks there appeared to be significant improvement in memory, learning, and speed of information processing, and these results were observed in the latter weeks of the study suggesting more long terms use is required to potentially receive a benefit [386]. A review of nine studies that included 518 participants and the overall quality of controls was a low risk of bias and significantly improved cognition ($p < 0.001$) and reduced choice reaction time ($p < 0.001$).

It is this level of cumulative research that is also sparking interest in Bacopa as an antianxiety herbal and laboratory studies of 25 % bacoside A has shown some favorable antianxiety ability similar to some prescriptions but without temporary issues with memory [387–389]. A clinical trial comparing 450 mg of Bacopa extract on healthy individuals against placebo over 12 weeks did not find any profound effects except for a trend for lower anxiety with Bacopa [390].

Bacopa monniera doses of 200–450 mg for a minimum of up to 12 weeks to determine the true benefit have been suggested, and dosage should be divided during the day [3]. Other areas of cognitive benefit have not been as consistently evaluated with Bacopa, but the potential for memory enhancement is its most notable potential feature. The most common side effect is mild gastrointestinal upset, which includes abdominal cramps, increased stool frequency, nausea, and minor blood pressure reductions. It is of interest that two proprietary brands have been used in numerous clinical trials including BacoMind® (Natural Remedies Pvt. Ltd, Karnataka, India) and KeenMind® (or CDRI 08, St Leonards, Australia) [391, 392].

GABA (also known as "gamma-amino butyric acid," an amino acid) at doses of 50–200 mg/day with or without food has been preliminarily tested. It has not been tested in breast cancer.
GABA is actually a known drug in some areas of the world for stress and anxiety, but in the USA it can be purchased as a dietary supplement [3]. GABA itself is a compound that is found in the brain normally that acts as an amino acid neurotransmitter to reduce stress and anxiety, and it is also found outside of the brain and in other body sites. There is research to suggest that it does other things apart from improving relaxation from modulating cardiovascular and kidney functions to keeping cell growth in check. Yet again its sole most-well known function is as a reducer of stress and anxiety. Doses of only 50–200 mg/day of this supplement have been effective in preliminary studies, and it has been taken with or without food. GABA has actually been used as a functional food ingredient in some foods in countries like Japan.

GABA actually also exists naturally in some foods at low levels but can be found in higher levels in some fermented foods [3]. It is for this reason some of the GABA supplements sold around the world actually are produced from a natural fermentation of strain-specific lactic acid bacteria (for example PharmaGABA®, one of the best studied from *Lactobacillus hilgardii*—used in the production of kimchi) [393–397]. It is interesting that in stressful situations the GABA content of the body can be reduced significantly. GABA dietary supplements also increase alpha wave activity of an EEG, and a reduction in beta waves, which shows that it works to promote relaxation but maintain concentration, and it may reduce levels of the stress hormone cortisol. Additionally, preliminary increases in salivary IgA are not with relaxation and GABA.

Side effects of this dietary supplement have not been well determined because most studies have not followed individuals long-term. Regardless, any antistress product always has drug interaction and dependency concerns in my opinion. Remember this is an effective preliminary supplement, but it also could promote sleep or reduce the time to fall asleep in some individuals, and temporary minor blood pressure reductions could.

Interestingly, some companies such as one from Japan are attempting to incorporate GABA into some foods such as chocolate, and one clinical study of using 28 mg of GABA and based on salivary testing of stress compounds it appeared to work quickly to reduce stress. It has been reported in some of these studies to work as quickly as 30 min [398].

l-*theanine (an amino acid found in green and black tea, how cool is that) at 100–250 mg/day in divided doses if needed. It has not been tested in breast cancer patients.*

l-theanine (gamma-glutamylethylamide or N-ethyl-l-glutamine) is a fascinating amino acid that comes from green and black tea, and it is believed that nature's placement of l-theanine in this product helped to counteract the stimulatory effects of caffeine in tea [3, 397, 399]. For example, when caffeine is given followed by theanine in the laboratory it can reduce the stimulant effects seen on an EEG. A cup of black tea has about 20 mg of theanine. Regardless, l-theanine has a fabulous record and has been used as an additive in candy, foods, and beverages in Japan for decades. How many times have individuals told me that their child was given a special drink to calm them down when traveling and it worked, and I told them that it had l-theanine in it. This is how common it is in certain parts of the world. l-THEANINE was first isolated in 1949 in tea and then in some mushrooms in the early 1950s. It has worked in studies in providing a "relaxing" effect by actually increasing GABA (the neurotransmitter and supplement mentioned earlier), blocking the uptake of glutamate in the nervous system, which can also promote relaxation, increasing other brain neurotransmitters such as dopamine and serotonin, encouraging the release of glycine that is an inhibitory neurotransmitter (relaxing effect), and even providing some protection for nerve cells of the brain. This relaxing or calming effect is why it is being used in clinical studies of stressful situations that can also cause anxiety.

l-theanine is a preliminary short-term antistress supplement when utilized at a dose of 100–250 mg/day (200–250 has shown more consistent impact) because it has demonstrated good safety short-term [397, 400–403]. L-theanine has also been found to promote or increase alpha waves in the brain (not as well as GABA), but it has a mild and consistent effect but its ability to profoundly reduce stress and anxiety is limited. This is not a disadvantage but another reason why it is safe and often used before GABA is used for example to determine the impact. A form of theanine known as "Suntheanine®" (Taiyo International, Mie, Japan) has been recognized as a Generally Recognized As Safe (GRAS) product since 2007, and this form has been patented has done arguably the best job of generating the most research [403]. Its biggest impact is in promoting "relaxation" in a variety of clinical studies. The 200 mg dose has the most research and not just for reducing subjective stress such as the person taking it feels less stress, but also objective measures of stress such as slightly reducing heart rate or increases alpha waves or increasing immune response (GABA does this also of course). However, some supplement companies are combining L-theanine with numerous other ingredients in order to have a unique blend, but this disregards the fact that L-theanine by itself was used in the most effective clinical trials. Doses even as low as 50 mg of L-theanine in some beverages have also provided antistress relief. The dietary supplement has been taken with or without food in studies and either as one daily dose or divided in half.

Rhodiola rosea (ideally find the extract known as "SHR-5") at 100–300 mg/day average given in divided doses (half in morning and afternoon). It has not been tested in breast cancer.

Rhodiola rosea (average dose in clinical trials of 100 mg) to is also known as "Roseroot" or "Rosenroot" and has received preliminary research with anxiety and stress induced fatigue [3, 397, 404–406]. Most of the positive research with this supplement was from a standardized proprietary extract from the root known as "SHR-5," and many trials had some methodological issues. Yet it still has enough clinical evidence that it should not be ignored either. It is also receiving attention as an antidepressant. It is not always easy to locate extract "SHR-5," but local health food stores or reputable online sources will reveal several companies that use the extract (for example Swedish Herbal Institute and Original Arctic Root Rhodiola Rosea and others and it is costly). Rhodiola listed in a supplement bottle does not equate to SHR-5, which is of course is also an issue. There are several active ingredients from this plant being studied including "rhodioloside, salidroside, triandrin, tyrosol, and rosavin." And the extract SHR-5 has at least the following active ingredients per tablet including "rhodioloside," "rosavin," "tyrosol," and "triandrin" from one clinical trial. The extracts used in some studies have also been standardized to what is believed to be the two more active ingredients 3 % rosavins and 0.8 % salidroside (naturally occurring ratio of these compounds in the root is 3:1), but with stress and anxiety the SHR-5 extract has dominated the majority of the studies so again I would put the technical jargon in the trash for a minute and look for that SHR-5 extract. There has been no consistent mention in studies or whether to take it with or without food. The total dose is usually divided during the day so that half is taken early in the day and the other half in the late afternoon or evening.

Rhodiola appears to favorably impact neurotransmitters in the brain and counteract the impact of adrenaline in the body [3, 397, 404–406]. Laboratory research suggests it has neuroendocrine modulating properties, which means it can also block cortisol release, and may favorably increase brain neurotransmitters. A dosage of 170 mg/day twice daily for 10 weeks demonstrated in a small study to reduce generalized anxiety disorder (GAD) using a well-known rating scale called the "Hamilton Anxiety Rating Scale" (HARS) [407]. Yet again the more impressive clinical trials overall were with the standardized extract SHR-5 reduced stress related fatigue and improved mental performance. For example, a typical dosage is 50 mg twice daily that was used in study of physicians on night shifts, but some studies have used SHR-5 extract to dosages as high as 680 mg/day, but again almost all of these studies were done with the extract "SHR-5." Rhodiola also appears to have an antistress effect and is being studied to reduce fatigue from stress, and potentially lethargic or asthenic depression [118]. It is for this reason that clinical trials using this herb to increase endurance exercise performance is a new area of interest [3].

The problem this herbal in the stress and anxiety trials is that there has not been enough safety information published on it and most clinical trials have reported no side effects beyond a placebo, but reducing heart rate in stressed or anxious individuals or in other situations can be a perceived benefit but is also a side effect [3, 397, 404–407]. Mild and uncommon side effects such as dizziness, dry mouth, irritability, allergy, fatigue, insomnia, and unpleasant feelings have been reported in rare cases especially as the dose increases.

Kava (a cautionary tale of an effective dietary supplement with an unknown future)
Kava has the most positive clinical research to reduce anxiety [3, 388], but it should not be utilized currently because of rare but concerning safety issues. If the safety issues are resolved then it could be one of the better supplements to test for anxiety. Kava or Kava Kava is an effective antianxiety supplement that is extract from the roots of a Polynesian plant (*Piper methysticum*) and is cultivated and used in the South Pacific (Polynesia, Melanesia, and Micronesia) for calming, relaxation, well-being, and even aphrodisiac effects [3, 388, 408, 409]. The active ingredient that is most interesting is the kava pyrones really known better as "kavalactones" and as many as 15 of them exist. It is used by many individuals as a substitute for Xanax or Valium prescription drugs. The recommended antianxiety dose is 50–70 mg kavalactones 2–4 times a day. And it has been suggested as a sleep aid before bed at a single dose of 150–210 mg. Side effects overall have been low in the range of 1–5 % in most studies. The problem is that the product has been tagged as hepatotoxic [410]. A past report of several individuals requiring liver transplantation along with a number of other liver issues and potentially death has led to withdrawal in the UK [3, 408–410]. The FDA issued a warning, and it is possible that the toxicity of Kava is due to some contaminant or a gene metabolism deficiency (CYP2D6) seen in a small percentage of the different populations around the world, which can also cause obscure drug interactions. The National Toxicology Program is a well known short- and long-term animal study that test things like supplements especially if one becomes popular [411]. They usually conduct 2-week, 3-month, and 2-year toxicity and carcinogenic studies in rats and mice and usually have no conflict of interest but just use funding to receive more answers. When they tested Kava there was some

hint of again liver issues, and it does appear to interact negatively with some prescription drugs, and some reviews now advocate routine monitoring of liver enzymes
[409], thus the risk exceeds the benefit at this moment. Yet this author is a little
biased because I worked on the state of Florida L-tryptophan dietary supplement
contaminant investigation that was responsible for thousands of injuries and even
deaths from Eosinophilia Myalgia Syndrome (EMS) in the USA [412].

Miscellaneous (dietary supplements with not evidence research or benefit), but
Music, Acupuncture and Aromatherapy have some preliminary research and benefit
generally outweighs risk for these options
Fish oil has not resulted in a consistent reduction in stress or anxiety. Valerian is not
a good antistress or antianxiety supplement in my opinion because it is a better sleep
aid and has drug interactions. Taking a sleeping pill to reduce stress makes me and
should make you nervous. Other herbal stress and anxiety supplements are not worthy of extensive discussion because there are a number of adequate prescription
stress and antianxiety aids with a know benefit-to-risk profile. For example,
Passionflower, Hops, Wild Lettuce, Jamaica Dogwood, California Poppy,
Chamomile, Lemon balm, Scullcap, Patrinia root, and others might sound interesting but save your money and the number of good studies that have looked at these
ingredients individually on stress and anxiety can be counted on one hand. Lemon
Balm (Melissa officinalis) for example is commonly combined with other active
herbals for different conditions (for example Valerian and Lemon Balm for sleep)
and although this looks good, it does not follow the effective research going on in
stress and anxiety.

Music has some preliminary research to reduce anxiety in adults while waiting
for medical procedures [413]. And acupuncture and aromatherapy despite having
mixed research with some questions of methodology are an option for cancer-
related stress and/or anxiety situations [414, 415].

• **Weight gain/excess belly fat/overweight/obesity**
Note: Please see Chap. 3 on lifestyle changes, Chap. 6 (and alpha-lipoic acid, berberine, …), and bone loss/sarcopenia section of this chapter for the preferred options to
prevent and treat weight/waist gain. In addition, the Chap. 3 on fiber intake for
example [416] is also pertinent to this section, as well as the discussion of a variety
of unconventional dietary plans that have enormous interest and will be generating
data in cancer in the next several years in terms of applicability [417].

Conclusion

Arguably, 20+ common and not so common side effects from breast cancer (and
overall cancer) treatment were reviewed in this chapter. Please see Table 7.8 for a
short but comprehensive list from A to Z of some of the integrative options that were
mentioned and recommended and also discouraged.

Table 7.8 A comprehensive rapid review of integrative medicines, especially dietary supplements that can reduced, have no impact or exacerbate a common or not so common side effect of breast cancer treatment

Side effects/supplements associated with breast cancer treatment from A to Z	Commentary on the role of integrative medicine and other options
1. Anemia from Hormone Manipulation Therapy/Chemotherapy and/or Neutropenia (Vitamin B12, Folate, Iron, Copper, Wheat grass juice)?	– Hormone suppression in prostate cancer generates a normochromic normocytic anemia that occurs in 90 % of patients acutely and is usually asymptomatic and requires no supplementation (not B6 or B12 or Folate or iron). This could occur in other cancer requiring hormone suppression
	– Hormone suppression or especially metabolism changes with aromatase inhibitors have very rarely been associated with erythrocytosis that does not need supplementation
	– Rarely, other forms of anemia can occur from overexposure to a supplement, or chronic use of a drug for example excessive zinc intake (80 mg or more) found in many eye health supplements could cause a copper deficiency and a sideroblastic anemia. Proton pump inhibitors or acid reflux drugs or metformin can cause a B12 deficiency. Iron absorption reduction can occur with excessive weight gain or obesity
	– Wheat grass (Triticum aestivum) juice daily versus a control group in breast cancer patients displayed some minimal promise to reduce hematologic toxicity after chemotherapy. However, wheat grass could just be acting as a proxy for nutritional support for some patients and has a multivitamin-like profile. Allergies to wheat grass and especially nausea was experienced these clinical studies when trying to drink several ounces (grassy taste) of this juice. Some experts credit benefit (if it really occurs) to the chlorophyll having a structural similarity to heme
2. Aromatase Inhibitor Arthralgia (AIA) and/or Aromatase Inhibitor Associated Musculoskeletal Symptoms (AIMSS)	– Exercise (aerobic and resistance) can provide substantial benefits over time from a well-done phase-3-like randomized trial
	– Weight loss appears to also improve and/or lower the risk of this condition from observational studies
	– Large trial is being conducted by SWOG to determine the impact of acupuncture on this side effect
	– The LEGS and MOVES Trials utilized glucosamine and chondroitin and potential structural and symptomatic benefit were observed with osteoarthritis patients
	– Glucosamine sulfate (1500 mg/day from a shellfish source) and chondroitin sulfate (1200 mg/day from a bovine source; both supplements from Thorne Research, Sandpoint, ID) utilized for 24 weeks in postmenopausal women experiencing pain from AI participated in a single-arm, open-label phase 2 study. This group demonstrated a significant ($p < 0.05$) improvement in pain and function, and 50 % of the patients experienced 20 % or more improvement in pain, stiffness, and function

(continued)

Table 7.8 (continued)

Side effects/supplements associated with breast cancer treatment from A to Z	Commentary on the role of integrative medicine and other options
	– A well-done 24-week randomized multicenter placebo-controlled trial (known as "SWOG S0927") of 240 patients found a 50 % reduction in pain/stiffness in both the 3360 mg/day omega-3 fatty acid group as well as the placebo group (soybean/corn oil). Triglyceride levels were significantly reduced (−22.1 mg/dl) in the omega-3 group versus no change in the placebo arm ($p=0.01$). Patients utilized six capsules per day and each omega-3 capsule contained 560 mg of EPA plus DHA in a 40-to-20 ratio (Ocean Nutrition, Dartmouth, Nova Scotia, Canada). However, why no difference could be found may also have to do with the choice of a potential anti-inflammatory placebo or simply lack of efficacy of omega-3. Should omega-3 be utilized?
	– Low-cost fish oil has overall good quality control and competes with prescription and other alternative marine sources for efficacy including lowering triglycerides
	– Preliminary research suggests higher blood levels of vitamin D with or without supplementation are associated with a lower risk of joint pain from Ais. Still yet to be published (since the publication of this text) randomized VITAL trial (Vitamin D for Arthralgias from Letrozole), One hundred and sixty postmenopausal women with a blood vitamin D level less than 40 ng/ml received 30,000 IU oral vitamin D3 weekly for 24 weeks or placebo. Approximately 38 % of the women on vitamin D reported an increase in pain compared to 61 % of the controls ($p=0.008$). However, a total of 113 postmenopausal women ingesting 600 IU D3 ($n=56$) or 4000 IU D3 ($n=57$) for 6 months was conducted (and presented at ASCO) and after this time the 25-OH vitamin D test was 33.8 ng/ml for the low-dose versus 46 ng/ml for the high-dose group. And no difference was found for AIMSS or other measures such as pain or stiffness between groups
	– Complicating matters are several issues including the potential for 25-OH vitamin D to potentially function as a negative acute phase reactant. A recent systematic review of eight relevant studies found that six demonstrated a drop in blood levels of vitamin D with an initial inflammatory insult and in another study there was a suggestion of hemodilution with no impact on inflammation. Does vitamin D really ameliorate AIA or do individuals with greater health parameters and a higher probability of having a sufficient vitamin D level (with or without supplementation) give the perception that vitamin D is effective when in reality it is the health status of the patient that really determines outcome (not vitamin D supplementation)?
	– Topical capsaicin needs to be studied for this condition because it has been utilized for controlled arthritis pains for joints near the surface of the skin. SAM-e(S-adenosyl-methionine) also needs research because it has been so effective and safe as an arthritis pain supplement. Other arthritis supplements abound that could be tested for AIA for example curcumin, ginger, and MSM

3. Bone Loss and Sarcopenia (Muscle Loss)	–	Obesity now appears to compromise bone quality despite a potential increase in bone quantity. Weight loss and exercise also improves vitamin D levels "naturally" and resistance exercises discourage bone loss, and taking an AI with increasing levels of testosterone could discourage sarcopenia when combined with exercise
	–	The Women's Health Initiative (WHI) was a double-blind, placebo-controlled clinical trial and the largest to address the issue of calcium and vitamin D supplementation (not in breast cancer). This trial included 36,282 postmenopausal US women to 1000 mg elemental calcium carbonate plus 400 IU of vitamin D3 (OsCal®, GSK) or placebo for 7 years. The mean BMI was 29 and there were a greater number of obese versus overweight women in the trial, which interestingly appears to reflect the current US population. No impact of supplementation was observed. However, among women compliant with the supplements (80 % or more utilization) there was a 29 % reduction in hip fracture risk, but this relationship cannot be accepted as solid evidence compared to an intention-to-treat analysis
	–	Vitamin D supplementation may simply help patients by reducing the risk of falls. The Institute of Medicine recommends 600–800 IU of vitamin D daily, but some may need more (1000 IU+). Excessive dosages of vitamin D should be discouraged due to the potential for toxicity and the lack of evidence of bone and muscle health improvement with mega-doses. The vitamin D blood test could have some application for a minority of patients deficient in vitamin D, but otherwise it is a costly test and should not be a screening test for the asymptomatic general population right now
	–	Calcium supplements have several forms but all (carbonate, citrate, phosphate) increase the risk of constipation (why magnesium is now in many supplements) and kidney stones except for calcium citrate. Regardless, many calcium supplements are not needed today because of the excessive amounts of calcium in the food supply (some almond milks contain 455 mg per 8-ounces for example)
	–	Vitamin D2 is derived from a plant source and vitamin D3 is generally derived from sheep lanolin, but D3 is produced by the body from UV-B light exposure, and D3 has been used in the most clinical trials. Both vitamin D2 and D3 have clinical efficacy and should be an individual choice (vegans for example usually need D2). D3 derived plant sources are making their way to the marketplace
	–	Whole body vibration in otherwise healthy women getting adequate exercise and calcium and vitamin D has not been shown to be a benefit
	–	Other supplements get a lot of hype for bone loss but should not be utilized due to the lack of long-term safety studies and some now with questionable cardiovascular risk like strontium (the drug has issues then so should the supplement for now). K1 and K2 need more consistent evidence—especially K2 in terms of fracture prevention
	–	Whey protein isolate (look for a no lactose, no sugar, no fat, approximately 25 g of protein per 100 calorie product with good taste—no protein bar can match it) and other animal and plant-based protein powders have evidence to suggest an improvement in muscle protein synthesis (MPS) that is synergistic with regular exercise. Chocolate milk is also beneficial but for endurance athletes and not others because of a high sugar and caloric content. Creatine powder has a good safety record but arguably does not offer any major advantage above protein powder unless do high-power quick burst exercises on a regular basis

(continued)

Table 7.8 (continued)

Side effects/supplements associated with breast cancer treatment from A to Z	Commentary on the role of integrative medicine and other options
4. Cardiovascular issues (dyslipidemia, glucose, blood pressure, …)	*Note:* Please see Chaps. 3, 4, 5, and 6 (statins, aspirin, and metformin) for detailed information on the preferred options Multiple other options exist for the S.A.M. chapters (Chaps. 4, 5, and 6) including: – Omega-3 supplements over triglycerides in breast cancer patients (FDA approved to lower high triglycerides in general—currently three drug omega-3 options in the USA for hypertriglyceridemia) – Red yeast rice or plant sterols for LDL lowering. Discouraging the use of niacin supplements at this time based on recent data. Berberine has some preliminary glucose controlling data – Metformin (from the French Lilac and a generic low cost drug) continues to garner impressive data in breast cancer patients to assist in reducing weight and improving metabolic parameters. B12 reductions are not uncommon with this drug (and associated magnesium deficiency)
5. Constipation (and Diarrhea)	– *Note:* Please see Chap. 3 on lifestyle changes and the different forms of fiber and please see the hot flash section of this chapter and the results with magnesium dietary supplements (stool softening) – Probiotics and antibiotic associated diarrhea (AAD) are garnering preliminary positive results especially in the area of Helicobacter pylori eradication. However, the actual risk or incidence in general is low and utilizing them in cancer patients for the prevention and treatment of diarrhea potentially increases the risk of a rare sepsis. Thus, until more research is conducted in cancer including long-term safety their use (but not food sources such as yogurt or kimchi which are healthy overall) as dietary supplements should be discouraged
6. Depression/Other Cognitive/Mental Health Issues (see also Stress and/or Anxiety section)	– Exercise should be first-line evidence to prevent or treat depression in addition to conventional medications – SAM-e appears to augment the response to SSRI medications (up to 1600 mg/day maximum) from a Harvard clinical trial and team experienced with these supplements. However, SAM-e supplements are costly. – St. John's wort also has good clinical evidence at 500–1200 mg/day (0.3 % hypericin) but should be used as a stand-alone or less often because of quality control issues and more importantly potential drug interactions – Watch the dietary supplement data for more options for difficult-to-treat depression such as L-methylfolate (15 mg/day), omega-3, 5-HTP; these are preliminary and need more data but interesting when other options are not effective. See the chapter for more specifics (as always)

7. Dry Eye/Dry Mouth/Dry Skin	– Aromatase inhibitors or just reduced levels of estrogen could increase the risk of dry eye or is at least associated with a higher prevalence of dry eye
	– Omega-3 and/or Omega-6 supplementation has good preliminary evidence to prevent and potentially treat dry eye from numerous etiologies
	– Vitamin A (retinyl palmitate 0.05 %—Viva Drops®) drops (Viva Drops®) have one large clinical trial to suggest they may be as effective as prescription cyclosporine options but more comparative research should be conducted
	– Yohimbine HCL (4–6 mg maximum three times a day) is the only supplements (it is really a drug) that has any data to combat dry mouth from other causes. However, there are quality control supplement issues and a host of side effects make it a last choice when nothing else is effective
	– The use of broad-spectrum moisturizers for the body are under appreciated as a method of combating and protecting dry skin from hormone suppression or alteration in cancer patients
8. Fatigue (Cancer-Related Fatigue or CRF)	– Aerobic and/or Resistance Exercise should be standard of care—Level 1 evidence to reduce CRF
	– American Ginseng (Panax quinquefolius 1000–2000 mg/day (3–5 % ginsenosides from Ginseng Board of Wisconsin) should be standard of care—Level 1 evidence to reduce CRF). This is from a Mayo Clinic directed phase-3-like trial. A small study from MD Anderson Cancer Center found that Panax ginseng (7 % or more ginsenosides) could also reduce CRF at a dosage of 800 mg/day within 1-month but it was not placebo-controlled (still fascinating)
	– Moderate caffeine intake (even Guarana supplements have preliminary data) intake should not be discouraged
	– B-vitamins for energy is tantamount to deceptive or false advertising. It does not help and B-12 shots overall do not work better than low cost pills to improve B-12 vitamin levels (unless there is a disease-based absorption issue in the GI tract)
	– CoQ10 at 300 mg/day recently failed a phase-3-like trial for CRF, and so did L-carnitine in an ECOG study of 2000 mg/day. D-ribose supplementation also has weak data. Mushrooms supplements are hyped but need higher methodology trials to prove they have any impact in CRF
9. Hot Flashes/Flushes/ Vasomotor Symptoms (hot flashes, night and/or cold sweats)	– Weight gain increases the frequency and/or severity of hot flashes and preliminary research suggest weight loss reduces hot flashes
	– Exercise, paced respiration and a variety of other lifestyle changes have modest data to suggest they may provide a benefit, but the overall benefit exceeds the risk, especially for exercise
	– Acupuncture has not worked significantly better than sham acupuncture
	– Almost all popular dietary supplements have failed to beat a placebo in phase-3 trials conducted in breast cancer patients (including black cohosh, flaxseed, magnesium, soy, and vitamin E). Red clover and omega-3 have also not worked better than placebo in menopausal women in larger more rigorous trials
	– However, of all these options flaxseed powder (and perhaps soy protein powder in some cases) has arguably the best benefit to risk ratio of all these dietary or supplemental interventions based on low caloric and nutritional value and as part of a weight loss regimen

(continued)

Table 7.8 (continued)

Side effects/supplements associated with breast cancer treatment from A to Z	Commentary on the role of integrative medicine and other options
	– Magnesium supplements could be a rare option for those with regular constipation and hot flashes (large placebo effect but does not work better than a placebo for phase-3-like trial) because it softens the stool (magnesium oxide was utilized in a clinical trial at 800 and 1200 mg/day) – Other options such as sage have no well-done trials
10. Insomnia/Difficulty Sleeping *Note:* Multiple sedative-like or drowsiness causing supplements with minimal to no data in breast cancer survivors include L-tryptophan and 5-HTP and countless others (Passionflower, Kava, …) should not be promoted for insomnia because of their lack of data in cancer and their potential ability to create dependence. Some of these should only be evaluated as an option when all other options have not been successful (very rare)	– Regular exercise should be utilized to promote sleep in breast cancer survivors as well as a review of sleep hygiene or potential behavioral changes to initiate sleep and maintain sleep – 1–3 mg of immediate release melatonin or 2 mg of Prolonged Release (PR) melatonin has shown some efficacy. A 2 mg PR melatonin is approved in Europe for insomnia (Circadin®—similar to a drug). And a melatonin receptor-binding drug is approved as a prescription in the USA (Ramelteon) – Recently, a 3 mg immediate release melatonin study from the Dana Farber Cancer Institute (Boston, MA) in breast cancer patients showed good efficacy. This trial consisted of 95 postmenopausal women with a previous history of stage 0–III breast cancers with a mean age of 59 years who completed conventional treatment were assigned to 3 mg of oral melatonin or placebo for 4 months. Melatonin was purchased from a single supplier who also guaranteed the composition and purity of these supplements (Rugby Laboratories, a subsidiary of Watson Laboratories—Duluth, GA, USA). Melatonin was ingested at 9 PM each evening because of the potential sedating effects of this supplement – Subjects utilizing melatonin had significantly greater improvements in sleep quality (PSQI, Pittsburgh Sleep Quality Index) including domains on sleep quality, daytime dysfunction and total score. Melatonin had no impact on depression or hot flashes. And melatonin is being studied in some breast cancer clinical trials as an adjunct to conventional treatment at high dosages (10–20 mg), which should not be encouraged now because of sedative effects and potential fugue (wait for the data) and keep in mind that 1–3 mg of melatonin (safer dosages) in many cases already exceeds physiologic dosages produced daily from the pineal gland – The Mayo Clinic along with numerous medical centers conducted a phase-3 like trial of 450 mg of Valerian (0.8 % valerenic acids) utilized 1-h before bedtime for 8-weeks in primarily breast cancer patients (64 % of the patients) receiving conventional treatment and although the primary endpoint (included 119 patients were evaluable out of 227 randomized) showed no difference with placebo, some secondary endpoints of improved sleep and reduced fatigue (Brief Fatigue Inventory and Profile of Mood States) demonstrated a significant benefit with valerian and the side effects were similar to a placebo. Patients reported less trouble with sleep and less drowsiness with valerian. The valerian utilized in this trial was "pure ground, raw root, from one lot and standardized to contain 0.8 % valerenic acid," which were supplied by Hi-Health (Scottsdale, Arizona) – Many of the counter sleep aids can be habit forming and impact memory such as the Benadryl-based pills (diphenhydramine) or supplements such as 5-HTP

11. Lymphedema and Improvement in Range of Motion/Mobility	– In stable lymphedema aerobic and/or resistance exercise should be encouraged for overall health benefits and they have not been found to exacerbate lymphedema based on previous theories. Decongestive therapy is a primary treatment and includes a comprehensive regimen and is not low cost and it is time consuming
	– Diosmin (and Daflon) has preliminary evidence to help prevent edema and venous issues in small weak methodology studies with some breast cancer patients.
	– Similarly horse chestnut seed extract has been studied in a small US trial and it appeared to provide no benefit for breast cancer patients. Rutin or rutosides are also being studied for this condition
	– Any supplement with a history of helping with chronic venous insufficiency (CVI) as the ones mentioned above also appear to assist with vein integrity and reducing edema (also used in hemorrhoids) and this is why they are being tested to prevent or treat lymphedema. However, keep in mind the evidence weak and they have some anticoagulant effects
12. Nausea and Vomiting (Chemotherapy-induced nausea and vomiting or CINV)	– Acupuncture and/or especially P6 acupressure point pressure has preliminary data in cancer patients to prevent nausea. There are many commercial products or bands that can be utilized today
	– A National Cancer Institute (NCI) sponsored Phase-3 like multicenter (23 private practice oncology groups participated) study with cancer patients (total of 744 participants randomized and 576 included in the final analysis) taking 500–1500 mg a day of ginger dietary supplements along with conventional medicines for nausea and vomiting showed that 500 or 1000 mg (used 3 days before and after chemotherapy was received) worked better than placebo. The ginger capsules were also standardized as a purified liquid extract of ginger root "with concentrated 8.5 mg of combined gingerols, zingerone, and shogaol content, equivalent to 250 mg of ginger root, in extra virgin olive oil …" Interestingly, the ginger was manufactured by Aphios Corporation in Woburn, MA, which is now testing their product (called Zindol®) in another phase III clinical trial and should be lauded for this wonderful dedication to research. Again, the difference between an effective drug and supplement is perception and not reality. The ginger product itself can be purchased right now as a dietary supplement (Zindol® DS). In addition, it is critical to mention that the majority of the patients in this clinical trial, approximately 74 %, were breast cancer patients. The greatest or most significant reduction in nausea intensity occurred with 500 mg ($p=0.017$) and 1000 mg ginger ($p=0.036$) supplements
	– In fact, currently in diverse clinical settings, not just chemotherapy-induced nausea and vomiting (CINV) ginger has now accumulated positive data from morning sickness, postoperative nausea and vomiting, and even antiretroviral-induced nausea and vomiting [258]. Additionally, 5-HT3 receptor antagonistic properties continued to be supported as one potential mechanism of action from these past trials
	– Vitamin B6 (Pyridoxine)—(Data is for pregnancy and even endorsed by the American College of Obstetrics and Gynecology (ACOG), but not tested for CINV). The doses used in pregnancy have been divided doses at a total of 25–75 mg of vitamin B6 or 10–25 mg three or four times a day. One study of 142 ovarian cancer patients utilized an injectable form of vitamin B6 (for 21 days), and when combined with P6 acupuncture was significantly more effective than either intervention alone. Dietary supplement studies of B6 and CINV are needed now

(continued)

Table 7.8 (continued)

Side effects/supplements associated with breast cancer treatment from A to Z	Commentary on the role of integrative medicine and other options
	– One small preliminary study of a higher whey protein intake in 28 cancer patients (19 with breast cancer) found that higher supplemental protein intake appeared to produce significant reductions in nausea and need for antiemetic medications versus normal protein intake or control. Protein powder supplementation needs more research (at 25–50 g/day) to determine the impact on CINV. Benefit exceeds the risk except when ingesting higher dosages of B6 (200–300 mg or more) over time could cause a sensory peripheral neuropathy
13. Peripheral Neuropathy or PN (Chemotherapy-Induced Peripheral Neuropathy or CIPN)	– Need to learn more form diabetic peripheral neuropathy supplement options to determine what could be effective for CIPN – For example, 0.075 % (or other OTC strengths) Topical Capsaicin (standard of care in diabetes and why not CIPN or neuropathic cancer pain/discomfort? Needs Research) and Rx 8 % Capsaicin Patch for post-herpetic neuralgia should also be tested in cancer patients for neuropathic pain (it is getting some research now—ASCEND trial …) – Alpha-Lipoic Acid (Thioctic Acid—endorsed for diabetic PN but looking for consistency with CIPN) at 600 mg/day has preliminary good data in diabetics but the IV drug form used in Europe has better data for PN. 1800 mg/day major study by MD Anderson Cancer Center have large dropouts with placebo and the supplement demonstrating that 1800 mg/day is too large to test in this patient population and is not realistic – Omega-3 Fatty Acids and Paclitaxel-Induced Peripheral Neuropathy (Preliminary but interesting) has a preliminary study at 1244.1 mg of EPA and DHA supplementation that showed some preventive benefit *Acetyl-l-carnitine should be avoided or discouraged to prevent or treat CIPN because it can make it worse based on a phase-3 like trial and other data!* *Acetyl-l-carnitine (ALC) supplements actually made PN significantly worse in a major study of breast cancer patients (women undergoing adjuvant taxane-based-docetaxel or paclitaxel chemotherapy breast cancer treatment (stage I–III) to reduce the risk of CIPN)* – Preliminary research on vitamin E supplements appeared promising, but a phase-3-like, randomized, double-blind, placebo-controlled multicenter clinical trial of 270 patients (61 % were being treated for breast cancer) receiving taxanes, cisplatin, carboplatin, oxaliplatin, or combinations with vitamin E (DL-alpha-tocopherol 300 mg twice daily) versus placebo was disappointing. Although some beneficial evidence for vitamin E against cisplatin toxicity is being debated

14. Sexual Dysfunction (Female Sexual Dysfunction or FSD) Note: Male sexual dysfunction was adequately covered in a previous integrative text written by the author [302]	– Comprehensive lifestyle changes in women with FSD and comorbidities have demonstrated benefit. Whether or not they can benefit women with breast cancer and FSD has not been adequately studied but it should be encouraged anyway for overall health promoting and side effect reducing evidence
	– It is remarkable that more studies of lubricants to potentially improve other aspects of FSD or even ED have not been attempted or published
	– Zestra is a female massage oil with some minimal clinical data to suggest it can increase warmth and sensitivity, and increase the probability of arousal when applied to the clitoris, labia, and vaginal opening (not tested in breast cancer patents). However, organic olive oil was tested as a lubricant in women with breast cancer (ages 37–66 years old) along with other methods and found to be acceptable and beneficial for the majority of participants (a small but unique clinical study). L-Citrulline especially and perhaps L-arginine should be studied in lubricants to determine if they can increase blood flow (similar to male studies of ED)
	– Korean Red ginseng (Panax ginseng) has preliminary data at 3000 mg (8 % ginsenosides) to improve arousal in postmenopausal women but not beneficial in premenopausal women (not tested in breast cancer and could have rare estrogenic activity)
	– A recent 12-week, double-blind, placebo-controlled trial of maca root 3000 mg/day in 45 female outpatients (mean age 41 years, from similar US research group earlier that tested Maca in women) with SSRI/SNRI-induced sexual dysfunction with remission of their depression was published showed a potential benefit (not studied in breast cancer). And SAM-e supplements need to be studied in patients with depression to see if they can augment or have no impact on sexual health (preliminarily found in men) because antidepressant used in women with breast cancer (for hot flashes …) also adds to the increase risk of FSD
	– An L-citrulline based dietary supplement (Lady Prelox) appears to improve sexual function in postmenopausal women (not studied in breast cancer) and should be studied in breast cancer
	ArginMax (combination supplement of *Panax ginseng*, L-arginine, …) has had some preliminary benefit for FSD. And a recent study in cancer patients utilizing three capsules of ArginMax (from Daily Wellness Company, Honolulu, HI) or placebo twice daily (six pills per day) and assessments were completed at 4, 8 and 12 weeks. A total of 78 % of the patients had breast cancer out of the 186 participants enrolled in the trial (median age 49–51 years and age range 23–72 years). At 12-weeks there were no differences between ArginMax and placebo for sexual desire, arousal, lubrication, orgasm, satisfaction, or pain. However, FACT-G (Functional Assessment of Cancer Therapy-General) was significantly better with ArginMax ($p=0.009$) versus placebo suggesting an improvement in overall quality of life, and side effects were similar to placebo. One has to commend these researchers and ArginMax for being involved in some clinical studies. Whether or not this is not enough or enough information to consider utilizing this supplement is a matter of debate and personal preference

(continued)

Table 7.8 (continued)

Side effects/supplements associated with breast cancer treatment from A to Z	Commentary on the role of integrative medicine and other options
	– DHEA supplements could theoretically increase the risk of recurrence of some hormonal-based cancers and can significantly drop HDL cholesterol. Unpredictable and wide variations in individual results. Quality control is also a large problem. The one rare exception to a potential benefit is adrenal insufficiency patients may potentially benefit in terms of FSD. Androgen and especially adrenal insufficiency (low DHEA or testosterone patients) may slightly benefit. Increased facial hair, weight gain, acne, temporary breast tenderness, and rarely loss of head hair and skin rash on dosages as low as 50 mg/day. Vaginal DHEA may be the most promising future option for DHEA, but daily application will be a potential compliance issue
15. Stress and/or Anxiety (and cognitive function-memory)	– Some form of exercise should be considered a first-line prevention and treatment of stress and/or anxiety for breast cancer patients (along with conventional treatment if needed) during and after breast cancer treatment. Also completing some online scale such as the PSS (Perceived Stress Scale) should be encouraged in patients
	– Bacopa monniera (also known as "Brahmi" or just "Bacopa," standardized to a minimum of 25 % bacopa a or 55 % total bacosides) at 200–450 mg/day for cognition/memory and/or anxiety. It has not been tested in breast cancer patients (BacoMind® or KeenMind®-CRI 08 are two of the more tested brand names in general)
	– GABA (also known as "Gamma-Amino Butyric Acid," an amino acid) at doses of 50–200 mg/day with or without food has been preliminarily tested. It has not been tested in breast cancer (PharmaGABA® is one of the more tested brand names in general)
	– L-theanine (an amino acid found in green and black tea, how cool is that) at 100–250 mg/day in divided doses if needed. It has not been tested in breast cancer patients (Suntheanine® is one of the more tested brand names in general and has safety data—GRAS approved)
	– Rhodiola rosea (ideally find the extract known as "SHR-5") at 100–300 mg/day average given in divided doses (half in morning and afternoon). It has not been tested in breast cancer
	– Kava has the most positive clinical research to reduce anxiety, but it should not be utilized currently because of rare but concerning liver safety issues that need to be resolved over many years. If safety issues are completely and satisfactorily resolved then it could make a return and some experts think that liver function tests need to be monitored in any patient still taking this product
	– Music, Acupuncture and Aromatherapy have some preliminary research, and benefit generally outweighs risk for these options

16. Weight Gain/Excess Belly Fat/Overweight/ Obesity or weight loss (cachexia) (*Note:* some rare methods especially protein powder supplementation can also be utilized for cancer cachexia or extreme weight loss from cancer treatment or cancer itself)	– Chapter 3 in this text include an adequate review of weight loss regimens that involve caloric restriction and/or increased physical activity. All forms of dieting are encouraged for weight loss especially if they can result in heart healthy parameter changes such as: Lower or normalize cholesterol (LDL and/or triglycerides), lower or normalized blood sugar, lower or normalized blood pressure, lower weight/waist, maintain or lower inflammatory markers such as hs-CRP and maintain stable or adequate mood during the regimen (should not increase depression, stress, and/or anxiety)
	– Low-fat, semi-ketogenic, ketogenic, high-protein, moderate protein … are all beginning to garner heart healthy data in the right patients. The main theme from breast cancer clinical trials is that even moderate weight loss and heart healthy changes and moderate caloric reduction could have an impact on relapse rates (WINS versus WHEL study…see Chap. 3)
	– Metformin arguably has the best benefit-to-risk ratio (arguably the only heart healthy weight loss medication on the market—which is why it is also being tested in over 100 cancer clinical trials from prevention or as an adjunct to treatment or to prevent remission—all preliminary) of any drug or supplement on the market and it is low-cost, generic and derived from a natural source (French Lilac). See Chap. 6. Metformin partial mimics in the dietary supplement world such as berberine or alpha-lipoic acid has some good preliminary clinical trial data but arguably not as good as metformin. Since metformin has proven that it can prevent type 2 diabetes (from the Diabetes Prevention Program trial first published in N Engl J Med in 2002) then one could argue that it has already been proven to reduce the risk of heart disease and cancer
	– Protein powder supplementation (25–50 g) with an animal-based product (whey has the most evidence) and plant based options can facilitate some weight loss programs and also helps maintain or improve muscle mass (which is also why they have some evidence for cachexia). At higher dosages it can act as an appetite suppressant
	– Fiber supplementation primarily from dietary sources at 20–30 g a day or more continues to garner good evidence to add to some weight loss regimens and it arguably one of the best internal antiaging compounds (see Chap. 3). In a recent metabolic syndrome large randomized trial it worked as well as comprehensive and timely dietary instructions for weight loss
	– Most prescription and especially dietary supplements for weight loss should be discouraged because of the risk of toxicity, lack of long-term studies and some ultimately (including prescriptions—remember sibutramine) turn out to be costly and heart unhealthy
	– Ketogenic diet clinical trials (using an MCT or medium-chain triglyceride supplement for fat intake=coconut oil and palm kernel oil) is being studied in multiple cancer clinical trials currently and should be followed and is just one of countless methods to lose weight in the right patient. Most diets have some merit that can be utilized to fit the right regimen with the right patient
	– Fish oil supplements are currently being studied for cancer cachexia (usually along with an anabolic stimulus) and also to prevent muscle loss from cancer cachexia

It must be remembered that in conventional medical treatment today for side effects (or any other treatment) that clinicians and patients need to review three areas currently to be completely and fully objectively educated (not just the patient but also the clinician). The three questions that need to be answered are:

1. What are some lifestyle options that can reduce side effects or not from cancer treatment (including things that can even make side effects worse)?
2. What are some dietary supplements or integrative medicines that can reduce side effects (including things that can even make side effects worse)?
3. What are some prescription agents and/or conventional procedures that can reduce side effects or not from cancer treatment (including things that can even make side effects worse)?

This is the ultimate goal in reviewing the benefit-versus-risk ratio but in cancer today not being able to provide or review integrative medicine options is tantamount to an incomplete, dangerous, and non-objective-based consult and one that can lead patients into following advice from someone that gives plenty of time to patients but has no credibility in this area and worse can take financial advantage of patients and hinder their overall care. The time has arrived for the complete three-question consult with cancer patients and anything less than this I would find personally disappointing. No one wants to buy a box with only half or three quarters of the puzzle pieces missing. No one deserves incomplete objective educational information, especially cancer patients where today the list of options becomes more exciting but more daunting by the day. Patients need an objective educational advocate and when the above three questions are adequately covered along with some of the information in this text then this is the paradigm of a win-win situation when fighting cancer.

References

1. Moyad MA. Promoting wellness: beyond hormone therapy. Ann Arbor, MI: Spry Publishing; 2013.
2. Strum SB, McDermed JE, Scholz MC, Johnson H, Tisman G. Anaemia associated with androgen deprivation in patients with prostate cancer receiving combined hormonal blockade. Br J Urol. 1997;79:933–41.
3. Moyad MA. The supplement handbook. New York, NY: Rodale Publishing; 2015.
4. Iyengar A, Sheppard D. A case of erythrocytosis in a patient treated with an aromatase inhibitor for breast cancer. Case Rep Hematol. 2013;2013:615198.
5. Wit JM, Hero M, Nunez SB. Aromatase inhibitors in pediatrics. Nat Rev Endocrinol. 2011;8:135–47.
6. Heidelbaugh JJ. Proton pump inhibitors and risk of vitamin and mineral deficiency: evidence and clinical implications. Ther Adv Drug Saf. 2013;4:125–33.
7. Alger E, Feldman A, Datz C. Obesity as an emerging risk factor for iron deficiency. Nutrients. 2014;6:3587–600.
8. Willis MS, Monaghan SA, Miller ML, McKenna RW, Perkins WD, Levinson BS, et al. Zinc-induced copper deficiency: a report of three cases initially recognized on bone marrow examination. Am J Clin Pathol. 2005;123:125–31.

9. Bar-Sela G, Tsalic M, Fried G, Goldberg H. Wheat grass juice may improve hematological toxicity related to chemotherapy in breast cancer patients: a pilot study. Nutr Cancer. 2007;58:43–8.

10. Ben-Arye E, Goldin E, Wengrower D, Stampfer A, Kohn R, Berry E. Wheat grass juice in the treatment of active distal ulcerative colitis: a randomized double-blind placebo-controlled trial. Scand J Gastroenterol. 2002;37:444–9.

11. Marawaha RK, Bansal D, Kaur S, Trehan A. Wheat grass juice reduces transfusion requirement in patients with thalassemia major: a pilot study. Indian Pediatr. 2004;41:716–20.

12. Pole SN. Wheat grass juice in thalassemia. Indian Pediatr. 2006;43:79–80.

13. Choudhary DR, Naithani R, Panigrahi I, Kumar R, Mahapatra M, Pati HP, et al. Effect of wheat grass therapy on transfusion requirement in beta-thalassemia major. Indian J Pediatr. 2009;76:375–6.

14. Singh K, Pannu MS, Singh P, Singh J. Effect of wheat grass tablets on the frequency of blood transfusions in Thalassemia Major. Indian J Pediatr. 2010;77:90–1.

15. Murphy CC, Bartholomew LK, Carpentier MY, Bluethmann SM, Vernon SW. Adherence to adjuvant hormonal therapy among breast cancer survivors in clinical practice: a systematic review. Breast Cancer Res Treat. 2012;134:459–78.

16. Irwin ML, Cartmel B, Gross CP, Ercolano E, Li F, Yao X, et al. Randomized exercise trial of aromatase inhibitor-induced arthralgia in breast cancer survivors. J Clin Oncol. 2015;33:1104–11.

17. DeNysschen CA, Burton H, Ademuyiwa F, Levine E, Tetewsky S, O'Connor T. Exercise intervention in breast cancer patients with aromatase inhibitor-associated arthralgia: a pilot study. Eur J Cancer Care (Engl). 2014;23:493–501.

18. Nyrop KA, Muss HB, Hackney B, Cleveland R, Altpeter M, Callahan LF. Feasibility and promise of a 6-week program to encourage physical activity and reduce joint symptoms among elderly breast cancer survivors on aromatase inhibitor therapy. J Geriatr Oncol. 2014;5:148–55.

19. Galantino ML, Desai K, Greene L, Demichele A, Stricker CT, Mao JJ. Impact of yoga on functional outcomes in breast cancer survivors with aromatase inhibitor-associated arthralgias. Integr Cancer Ther. 2012;11:313–20.

20. Crew KD, Capodice J, Greenlee H, Brafman L, Fuentes D, Awad D, et al. Randomized, blinded, sham-controlled trial of acupuncture for the management of aromatase inhibitor-associated joint symptoms in women with early stage breast cancer. J Clin Oncol. 2010;28:1154–60.

21. Oh B, Kimble B, Costa DS, Davis E, McLean A, Orme K, et al. Acupuncture for treatment of arthralgia secondary to aromatase inhibitor therapy in women with early breast cancer: pilot study. Acupunct Med. 2013;31:264–71.

22. Fransen M, Agailotis M, Nairn L, Votrubec M, Bridgett L, Su S, et al., for the LEGS study collaborative group. Glucosamine and chondroitin for knee osteoarthritis: a double-blind randomized placebo-controlled clinical trial evaluating single and combination regimens. Ann Rheum Dis 2015;74:851–8.

23. Hochberg MC, Martel-Pelletier J, Monfort J, Moller I, Castillo JR, Arden N, et al., on behalf of the MOVES investigative group. Ann Rheum Dis 2015, Epub ahead of print.

24. Singh JA, Noorbaloochi S, MacDonald R, Maxwell LJ. Chondroitin for osteoarthritis. Cochrane Database Syst Rev. 2015;1:CD005614.

25. Clegg DO, Reda DJ, Harris CL, Klein MA, O'Dell JR, Hooper MM, et al. Glucosamine, chondroitin sulfate, and the two in combination for painful knee osteoarthritis. N Engl J Med. 2006;354:795–808.

26. Greenlee H, Crew KD, Shao T, Kranwinkel G, Kallinsky K, Mauer M, et al. Phase II study of glucosamine with chondroitin on aromatase inhibitor-associated joint symptoms in women with breast cancer. Support Care Cancer. 2013;21:1077–87.

27. Goldberg RJ, Katz J. A meta-analysis of the analgesic effects of omega-3 polyunsaturated fatty acid supplementation for inflammatory joint pain. Pain. 2007;129:210–23.

28. Hershman DL, Loprinzi C, Schneider BP. Symptoms: aromatase inhibitor induced arthralgias. Adv Exp Med Biol. 2015;862:89–100.
29. Hershman DL, Unger JM, Crew KD, Awad D, Dakhill SR, Gralow J, et al. Randomized multicenter placebo-controlled trial of omega-3 fatty acids for the control of aromatase inhibitor-induced musculoskeletal pain: SWOG S0927. J Clin Oncol. 2015;33:1910–7.
30. Niravath P. Aromatase inhibitor-induced arthralgia: a review. Ann Oncol. 2013;24:1443–9.
31. Khan QJ, Reddy PS, Kimier BF, Sharma P, Baxa SE, O'Dea AP, et al. Effect of vitamin D supplementation on serum 25-hydroxy vitamin D levels, joint pain, and fatigue in women starting adjuvant letrozole treatment for breast cancer. Breast Cancer Res Treat. 2010;119: 111–8.
32. Khan Q, Kimler B, Reddy P, et al. Randomized trial of vitamin D3 to prevent worsening of musculoskeletal symptoms and fatigue in women with breast cancer starting adjuvant letrozole: the VITAL trial. J Clin Oncol 2012;30(Suppl; abstr 9000).
33. Shapiro AC, Adilis SA, Liang S, Robien K, Kirstein MN, Anderson E, et al. A randomized trial of vitamin D3 in aromatase inhibitor-associated musculoskeletal symptoms. J Clin Oncol 2015;33:(Suppl; abstract 9608).
34. Waldron JL, Ashby HL, Comes MP, Bechervaise J, Razavi C, Thomas OL, et al. Vitamin D: a negative acute phase reactant. J Clin Pathol. 2013;66:620–2.
35. Silva MC, Furlanetto TW. Does serum 25-hydroxyvitamin D decrease during acute-phase response? A systematic review. Nutr Res. 2015;35:91–6.
36. McAlindon T, LaValley M, Schneider E, Nuite M, Lee JY, Price LL, et al. Effect of vitamin D supplementation on progression of knee pain and cartilage volume loss in patients with symptomatic osteoarthritis: a randomized controlled trial. JAMA. 2013;309:155–62.
37. Laslett LL, Jones G. Capsaicin for osteoarthritis pain. Prog Drug Res. 2014;68:277–91.
38. Snedecor SJ, Sudharshan L, Cappelleri JC, Sadosky A, Mehta S, Botteman M. Systemic review and meta-analysis of pharmacological therapies for painful diabetic peripheral neuropathy. Pain Pract. 2014;14:167–84.
39. Derry S, Sven-Rice A, Cole P, Tan T, Moore RA. Topical capsaicin (high concentration) for chronic neuropathic pain in adults. Cochrane Database Syst Rev. 2013;2:CD007393.
40. Watson CP, Evans RJ. The postmastectomy pain syndrome and topical capsaicin: a randomized trial. Pain. 1992;51:375–9.
41. Watson CP, Evans RJ, Watt VR. The post-mastectomy pain syndrome and the effect of topical capsaicin. Pain. 1989;38:177–86.
42. Diaz-Laviada I, Rodriguez-Henche N. The potential antitumor effects of capsaicin. Prog Drug Res. 2014;68:181–208.
43. Lugman S, Meena A, Marler LE, Kondratyuk TP, Pezzuto JM. Suppression of tumor necrosis factor-alpha-induced nuclear factor kB activation and aromatase activity by capsaicin and its analog capsazepine. J Med Food. 2011;14:1344–51.
44. Mao JJ, Stricker C, Bruner D, Xie S, Bowman MA, Farrar JT, et al. Patterns and risk factors associated with aromatase inhibitor-related arthralgia among breast cancer survivors. Cancer. 2009;115:3631–9.
45. Madhu K, Chanda K, Saji MJ. Safety and efficacy of Curcuma longa extract in the treatment of painful knee osteoarthritis: a randomized placebo-controlled trial. Inflammopharmacology. 2013;21:129–36.
46. Pinsomsak P, Niempoog S. The efficacy of Curcuma Longa L. extract as an adjuvant therapy in primary knee osteoarthritis: a randomized controlled trial. J Med Assoc Thai. 2012;95 Suppl 1:S51–8.
47. Bayet-Robert M, Kwiatkowski F, Leheurteur M, Gachon F, Pianchat E, Abrial C, et al. Phase I dose escalation trial of docetaxel plus curcumin in patients with advanced metastatic breast cancer. Cancer Biol Ther. 2010;9:8–14.
48. Kumar P, Kadakol A, Shasthrula PK, Mundhe NA, Jamdade VS, Barua CC, et al. Curcumin as an adjuvant to breast cancer treatment. Anticancer Agents Med Chem. 2015;15:647–56.
49. Kanai M, Yoshimura K, Asada M, Imaizumi A, Suzuki C, Matsumoto S, et al. A phase I/II study of gemcitabine-based chemotherapy plus curcumin for patients with gemcitabine-resistant pancreatic cancer. Cancer Chemother Pharmacol. 2011;68:157–64.

50. Epelbaum R, Schaffer M, Vizel B, Badmaev V, Bar-Sela G. Curcumin and gemcitabine in patients with advanced pancreatic cancer. Nutr Cancer. 2010;62:1137–41.
51. Soeken KL, Lee W-L, Bausell B, Agelli M, Berman BM. Safety and efficacy of S-adenosylmethionine (SAMe) for osteoarthritis: a meta-analysis. J Fam Pract. 2002;51: 425–30.
52. Ringdahl E, Pandit S. Treatment of knee osteoarthritis. Am Fam Physician. 2011;83: 1287–92.
53. Sarkis KS, Pinheiro Mde M, Szejnfeld VL, Martini LA. High bone density and bone health. Endocrinol Nutr. 2012;59:207–14.
54. Zhang P, Peterson M, Su GL, Wang SC. Visceral adiposity is negatively associated with bone density and muscle attenuation. Am J Clin Nutr. 2015;101:337–43.
55. Mason C, Xiao L, Imayama I, Duggan CR, Bain C, Foster-Schubert KE, et al. Effects of weight loss on serum vitamin D in postmenopausal women. Am J Clin Nutr. 2011;94: 95–103.
56. Winters-Stone KM, Dobek J, Nail L, Bennett JA, Leo MC, Naik A, et al. Strength training stops bone loss and builds muscle in postmenopausal breast cancer survivors: a randomized, controlled trial. Breast Cancer Res Treat. 2011;127:447–56.
57. Irwin ML, Alvarez-Reeves M, Cadmus L, Mierzejewski E, Mayne ST, Yu H, et al. Exercise improves body fat, lean mass, and bone mass in breast cancer survivors. Obesity (Silver Spring). 2009;17:1534–41.
58. Jackson RD, LaCroix AZ, Gass M, Wallace RB, Robbins J, Lewis CE, et al. Calcium plus vitamin D supplementation and the risk of fractures. N Engl J Med. 2006;354:669–83.
59. Prentice RL, Pettinger MB, Jackson RD, Wactawski-Wende J, Lacroix AZ, Anderson GL, et al. Health risks and benefits from calcium and vitamin D supplementation: Women's Health Initiative clinical trial and cohort study. Osteoporos Int. 2013;24:567–80.
60. Martin-Herranz A, Salinas-Hernandez P. Vitamin D supplementation review and recommendations for women diagnosed with breast or ovary cancer in the context of bone health and cancer prognosis/risk. Crit Rev Oncol Hematol 2015, Epub ahead of print.
61. LeBlanc E, Chou R, Zakher B, Daeges M, Pappas M. Screening for vitamin D deficiency: systematic review for the U.S. Preventive Services Task Force Recommendation. Rockville, MD: Agency for Healthcare Research and Quality (US); Nov 2014. Report No.: 13-05183-EF-1.
62. LeBlanc ES, Zakher B, Daeges M, Pappas M, Chou R. Screening for vitamin D deficiency: a systematic review for the U.S. Preventive Services Task Force. Ann Intern Med. 2015;162: 109–22.
63. Ellis GK, Bone HG, Chlebowski R, Paul D, Spadafora S, Smith J, et al. Randomized trial of denosumab in patients receiving adjuvant aromatase inhibitors for nonmetastatic breast cancer. J Clin Oncol. 2008;26:4875–82.
64. Stopeck AT, Lipton A, Body JJ, Steger GG, Tonkin K, de Boer RH, et al. Denosumab compared with zoledronic acid for the treatment of bone metastases in patients with advanced breast cancer: a randomized, double-blind study. J Clin Oncol. 2010;28:5132–9.
65. Thacher TD, Obadofin MO, O'Brien KO, Abrams SA. The effect of vitamin D2 and vitamin D3 on intestinal calcium absorption in Nigerian children with rickets. J Clin Endocrinol Metab. 2009;94:1314–21.
66. Biancuzzo RM, Clarke N, Reitz RE, Travison TG, Holick MF. Serum concentrations of 1,25-dihydroxyvitamin D2 and 1,250dihydroxyvitamin D3 in response to vitamin D2 and vitamin D3 supplementation. J Clin Endocrinol Metab. 2013;98:973–9.
67. Holick MF, Biancuzzo RM, Chen TC, Klein EK, Young A, Bibuld D, et al. Vitamin D2 is effective as vitamin D3 in maintaining circulating concentrations of 25-hydroxyvitamin D. J Clin Endocrinol Metab. 2008;93:677–81.
68. Gordon CM, Williams AL, Feldman HA, May J, Sinclair L, Vasquez A, et al. Treatment of hypovitaminosis D in infants and toddlers. J Clin Endocrinol Metab. 2008;93:2716–21.
69. Gottschlich MM, Mayes T, Khoury J, Kagan RJ. Clinical trial of vitamin D2 vs D3 supplementation in critically ill pediatric burn patients. JPEN J Parenter Enteral Nutr 2015; Epub ahead of print.

70. Mangoo-Karim R, Da Silva Abreu J, Yanev GP, Perez NN, Stubbs JR, Wetmore JB. Ergocalciferol versus cholecalciferol for nutritional vitamin D replacement in CKD. Nephron 2015, Epub ahead of print.
71. Logan VF, Gray AR, Peddie MC, Harper MJ, Houghton LA. Long-term vitamin D3 supplementation is more effective than vitamin D2 in maintaining serum 25-hydroxyvitamin D status over the winter months. Br J Nutr. 2013;109:1082–8.
72. Osteoporosis-Part MA. Osteoporosis—Part II: Dietary and/or supplemental calcium and vitamin D. Urol Nurs. 2002;22:405–9.
73. Smith MR, Egerdie B, Harnandez Toriz N, Feldman R, Tammela TL, Saad F, et al., for the Denosumab HALT Prostate Cancer Study Group. Denosumab in men receiving androgen-deprivation therapy for prostate cancer. N Engl J Med 2009;361:745–55.
74. Kukuijan S, Nowson CA, Sanders KM, Nicholson GC, Seibel MJ, Salmon J, et al. Independent and combined effects of calcium-vitamin D3 and exercise on bone structure and strength in older men: an 18-month factorial design randomized controlled trial. J Clin Endocrinol Metab. 2011;96:955–63.
75. Kemmler W, von Stengel S, Engelke K, Haberle L, Kalender WA. Exercise effects on bone mineral density, falls, coronary risk factors, and health care costs in older women: the randomized controlled senior fitness and prevention (SEFIB) study. Arch Intern Med. 2010;170:179–85.
76. Uusi-Rasi K, Patil R, Karinkanta S, Kannus P, Tokola K, Lamberg-Allardt C, et al. Exercise and vitamin D in fall prevention among older women: a randomized clinical trial. JAMA Intern Med. 2015;175:703–11.
77. Lau EM, Woo J, Leung PC, Swaminathan R, Leung D. The effects of calcium supplementation and exercise on bone density in elderly Chinese women. Osteoporos Int. 1992;2: 168–73.
78. Slatkovska L, Alibhai S, Beyene J, et al. Effect of 12 months of whole-body vibration therapy on bone density and structure in postmenopausal women. Ann Intern Med. 2011;155: 668–79.
79. Lam TP, Ng BK, Cheung LW, Lee KM, Qin L, Cheng JC, et al. Effect of whole body vibration (WBV) therapy on bone density and bone quality in osteopenic girls with adolescent idiopathic scoliosis: a randomized, controlled trial. Osteoporos Int. 2013;24:1623–36.
80. Van Ruymbeke B, Boone J, Coorevitis P, Vanderstraeten G, Bourgois J. Whole-body vibration in breast cancer survivors: a pilot study exploring its effects on muscle activity and subjectively perceived exertion. Int J Rehabil Res. 2014;37:371–4.
81. Reid IR. Efficacy, effectiveness and side effects of medications used to prevent fractures. J Intern Med. 2015;277:690–706.
82. Medicines and Healthcare Products Regulatory Agency (MHRA). Strontium ranelate (Protelos): risk of serious cardiac disorders-restricted indications, new contraindications, and warnings. Drug Saf Update. 2013;6:S1.
83. Wohl GR, Chettle DR, Pejovic-Millic A, Druchok C, Webber CE, Adachi JD, et al. Accumulation of bone strontium measured by in vivo XRF in rats supplemented with strontium citrate and strontium ranelate. Bone. 2013;52:63–9.
84. Guralp O, Erel CT. Effects of vitamin K in postmenopausal women: mini review. Maturitas. 2014;77:294–9.
85. Theuwissen E, Teunissen KJ, Spronk HM, Hamulyak K, Ten Café H, Shearer MJ, et al. Effect of low-dose supplements of menaquinone-7 (vitamin K2) on the stability of oral anticoagulant treatment: dose-response relationship in healthy volunteers. J Thromb Haemost. 2013;11:1085–92.
86. Miller PE, Alexander DD, Perez V. Effects of whey protein and resistance exercise on body composition: a meta-analysis of randomized controlled trials. J Am Coll Nutr. 2014;33: 163–75.
87. Verreijen AM, Verlaan S, Engberink MF, Swinkels S, de Vogel-van den Bosch J, Weijs PJ, et al. A high whey protein-, leucine-, and vitamin D-enriched supplement preserves muscle mass during intentional weight loss in obese older adults: a double-blind randomized controlled trial. Am J Clin Nutr. 2015;101:279–86.

88. Pritchett K, Pritchett R. Chocolate milk: a post-exercise recovery beverage for endurance sports. Med Sports Sci. 2012;59:127–34.

89. Gualano B, Macedo AR, Alves CR, Roschel H, Benatti FB, Takayama L, et al. Creatine supplementation and resistance training in vulnerable older women: a randomized double-blind placebo-controlled clinical trial. Exp Gerontol. 2014;53:7–15.

90. Devries MC, Phillips SM. Creatine supplementation during resistance training in older adults—a meta-analysis. Med Sci Sports Exerc. 2014;46:1194–203.

91. Cooney GM, Dwan K, Greig CA, Lawlor DA, Rimer J, Waugh FR, et al. Exercise for depression. Cochrane Database Syst Rev. 2013;9:CD004366.

92. Bluementhal JA, Doraiswamy PM. Exercise to combat depression. JAMA. 2014;312: 2166–7.

93. Babyak M, Blumenthal JA, Herman S, Khatri P, Doraiswamy M, Moore K, et al. Exercise treatment for major depression: maintenance of therapeutic benefit at 10 months. Psychosom Med. 2000;62:633–8.

94. Blumenthal JA, Sherwood A, Babyak MA, Watkins LL, Smith PJ, Hoffman BM, et al. Exercise and pharmacological treatment of depressive symptoms in patients with coronary heart disease: results from the UPBEAT (Understanding the Prognostic Benefits of Exercise and Antidepressant Therapy) study. J Am Coll Cardiol. 2012;60(12):1053–63.

95. Bluementhal JA, Babyak MA, Doraiswamy PM, Watkins L, Hoffman BM, Barbour KA, et al. Exercise and pharmacotherapy in the treatment of major depressive disorder. Psychosom Med. 2007;69:587–96.

96. Travier N, Velthuis MJ, Steins-Bisschop CN, van den Buijs B, Monninkhof EM, et al. Effect of an 18-week exercise programme started early during breast cancer treatment: a randomized controlled trial. BMC Med. 2015;13:121.

97. Schmidt ME, Wiskemann J, Armbrust P, Schneeweiss A, Ulrich CM, Steindorf K. Effects of resistance exercise on fatigue and quality of life in breast cancer patients undergoing adjuvant chemotherapy: a randomized controlled trial. Int J Cancer. 2015;137:471–80.

98. Battaglini CL, Mills RC, Phillips BL, Lee JT, Story CE, Nascimento MG, et al. Twenty-five years of research on the effects of exercise training in breast cancer survivors: a systematic review of the literature. World J Clin Oncol. 2014;5:177–90.

99. Papakostas GI. Evidence for S-adenosyl-L-methionine (SAM-e) for treatment of major depressive disorder. J Clin Psychiatry. 2009;70 Suppl 5:18–22.

100. Nahas R, Sheikh O. Complementary and alternative medicine for the treatment of major depressive disorder. Can Fam Physician. 2011;57:659–63.

101. Papakostas GI, Mischoulon D, Shyu I, Alpert JE, Fava M. S-adenosyl methionine (SAMe) augmentation of serotonin reuptake inhibitors for antidepressant nonresponders with major depressive disorder: a double-blind, randomized clinical trial. Am J Psychiatry. 2010;167: 942–8.

102. Mischoulon D, Price LH, Carpenter LL, Tyrka AR, Papakostas GI, Baer L, et al. A double-blind, randomized, placebo-controlled clinical trial of S-adenosyl-L-methionine (SAMe) versus escitalopram in major depressive disorder. J Clin Psychiatry. 2014;75:370–6.

103. Sarris J, Papakostas GI, Vitolo O, Fava M, Mischoulon D. S-adenosyl methionine (SAMe) versus escitalopram and placebo in major depression RCT: efficacy and effects of histamine and carnitine as moderators of response. J Affect Disord. 2014;164:76–81.

104. Sarris J, Price LH, Carpenter LL, Tyrka AR, Ng CH, Papakostas GI, et al. Is S-adenosyl methionine (SAMe) for depression only effective in males? A re-analysis of data from a randomized clinical trial. Pharmacopsychiatry. 2015;48(4–5):141–4. Epub 26 May 2015.

105. Mischoulon D, Alpert JE, Aming E, Bottiglieri T, Fava M, Papakostas GI. Bioavailability of S-adenosyl methionine and impact on response in a randomized, double-blind, placebo-controlled trial in major depressive disorder. J Clin Psychiatry. 2012;73:843–8.

106. Dording CM, Mischoulon D, Shyu I, Alpert JE, Papakostas GI. SAMe and sexual functioning. Eur Psychiatry. 2012;27:451–4.

107. Rahimi R, Abdollahi M. An update on the ability of St. John's wort to affect the metabolism of other drugs. Expert Opin Drug Metab Toxicol. 2012;8:691–708.

108. Linde K, Berner MM, Kriston L. St John's wort for major depression. Cochrane Database Syst Rev. 2008;4:CD000448.
109. Luberto CM, White C, Sears RW, Cotton S. Integrative medicine for treating depression: an update on the latest evidence. Curr Psychiatry Rep. 2013;15:391.
110. Al-Akoum M, Maunsell E, Verreault R, Provencher L, Otis H, Dodin S. Effects of Hypericum perforatum (St. John's wort) on hot flashes and quality of life in perimenopausal women: a randomized pilot trial. Menopause. 2009;16:307–14.
111. He SM, Yang AK, Li XT, Du YM, Zhou SF. Effects of herbal products on the metabolism and transport of anticancer agents. Expert Opin Drug Metab Toxicol. 2010;6:1195–213.
112. Bloch MH, Hannestad J. Omega-3 fatty acids for the treatment of depression: systematic review and meta-analysis. Mol Psychiatry. 2012;17:1272–82.
113. Mischoulon D, Nierenberg AA, Schettler PJ, Kinkead BL, Fehling K, Martinson MA, et al. A double-blind, randomized controlled clinical trial comparing eicosapentaenoic acid versus docosahexaenoic acid for depression. J Clin Psychiatry. 2015;76:54–61.
114. Gertsik L, Poland RE, Bresee C, Rapaport MH. Omega-3 fatty acid augmentation of citalopram treatment for patients with major depressive disorder. J Clin Psychopharmacol. 2012;32:61–4.
115. Zimmer R, Riemer T, Rauch B, Schneider S, Schiele R, Gohlke H, et al., for the OMEGA-Study Group. Effects of 1-year treatment with highly purified omega-3 fatty acids on depression after myocardial infarction: results form the OMEGA trial. J Clin Psychiatry 2013;74:e1037–45.
116. Cockayne NL, Duffy SL, Bonomally R, English A, Amminger PG, Mackinnon A, et al. The Beyond Ageing Project Phase 2—a double-blind, selective prevention, randomized, placebo-controlled trial of omega-3 fatty acids and sertraline in an older age cohort at risk for depression: study protocol for a randomized controlled trial. Trials. 2015;16:247.
117. Papakostas GI, Shelton RC, Zajecka JM, Etemand B, Rickels K, Clain A, et al. L-Methylfolate as adjunctive therapy for SSRI-resistant major depression: results of two randomized, double-blind, parallel-sequential trials. Am J Psychiatry. 2012;169:1267–74.
118. Iovieno N, Dalton ED, Fava M, Mischoulon D. Second-tier natural antidepressants: review and critique. J Affect Disord. 2011;130:343–57.
119. Liu A, Ji J. Omega-3 essential fatty acids therapy for dry eye syndrome: a meta-analysis of randomized controlled studies. Med Sci Monit. 2014;20:1583–9.
120. Rosenberg ES, Asbell PA. Essential fatty acids in the treatment of dry eye. Ocul Surf. 2010;8:18–28.
121. Rashid S, Jin Y, Ecoiffier T, Barabino S, Schaumberg DA, Dana MR. Topical omega-3 and omega-6 fatty acids for treatment of dry eye. Arch Ophthalmol. 2008;126:219–25.
122. Al Mahmood AM, Al-Swailem SA. Essential fatty acids in the treatment of dry eye syndrome: a myth or reality? Saudi J Ophthalmol. 2014;28:195–7.
123. Jarvinen RL, Larmo PS, Setaia NL, Yang B, Engblom JR, Viltanen MH, Kallio HP. Effects of oral sea buckthorn oil on tear film fatty acids in individuals with dry eye. Cornea. 2011;30:1013–9.
124. Larmo PS, Jarvinen RL, Setaia NL, Tang B, Vitanen MH, Engblom JR, et al. Oral sea buckthorn oil attenuates tear film osmolarity and symptoms in individuals with dry eye. J Nutr. 2010;140:1462–8.
125. Kim EC, Choic JS, Joo CK. A comparison of vitamin a and cyclosporine a 0.05% drops for treatment of dry eye syndrome. Am J Ophthalmol. 2009;147:206–13.
126. Fraunfelder FW, Fraunfelder FT, Illingworth DR. Adverse ocular effects associated with niacin therapy. Br J Ophthalmol. 1995;79:54–6.
127. Turaka K, Nottage JM, Hammersmith KM, Nagra PK, Rapuano CJ. Dry eye syndrome in aromatase inhibitor users. Clin Experiment Ophthalmol. 2013;41:239–43.
128. Hutchinson CV, Walker JA, Davidson C. Oestrogen, ocular function and low-level vision: a review. J Endocrinol. 2014;223:R9–18.
129. Delli K, Spijkervet FK, Kroese FG, Bootsma H, Vissink A. Xerostomia. Monogr Oral Sci. 2014;24:109–25.

130. Hanchanale S, Adkinson L, Daniel S, Fleming M, Oxberry SG. Systematic literature review: xerostomia in advanced cancer patients. Support Care Cancer. 2015;23:861–8.
131. Bagheri H, Schmitt L, Berian M, Montasstruct JL. A comparative study of the effects of yohimbine and anetholtrithione on salivary secretion in depressed patients treated with psychotropic drugs. Eur J Clin Pharmacol. 1997;52:339–42.
132. Bagheri H, Schmitt L, Berian M, Montastruc JL. Effect of 3 weeks with yohimbine on salivary secretion in healthy volunteers and in depressed patients treated with tricyclic antidepressants. Br J Clin Pharmacol. 1992;34:555–8.
133. Cramp F, Byron-Daniel J. Exercise for the management of cancer-related fatigue in adults. Cochrane Database Syst Rev. 2012;11:CD006145.
134. Ruddy KJ, Barton D, Loprinzi CL. Laying to rest psychostimulants for cancer-related fatigue? J Clin Oncol. 2014;32:1865–7.
135. Barton DL, Liu H, Dakhil SR, Linquist B, Sloan JA, Nichols CR, et al. Wisconsin ginseng (Panax quinquefolius) to improve cancer-related fatigue: a randomized, double-blind trial, N07C2. J Natl Cancer Inst. 2013;105:1230–8.
136. Barton DL, Soori GS, Bauer BA, Sloan JA, Johnson PA, Figueras C, et al. Pilot study of Panax quinquefolius (American ginseng) to improve cancer-related fatigue: a randomized, double-blind, dose-finding evaluation: NCCTG trial N03CA. Support Care Cancer. 2010;18:179–87.
137. Yennurajalingam S, Reddy A, Tannir NM, Chisholm GB, Lee RT, Lopez G, et al. High-dose Asian ginseng (Panax ginseng) for cancer-related fatigue: a preliminary report. Integr Cancer Ther 2015, Epub ahead of print.
138. Kennedy DO, Haskell CF, Robertson B, Reay J, Brewster-Maund C, Luedemann J, et al. Improved cognitive performance and mental fatigue following a multi-vitamin and mineral supplement with added guarana (Paullinia cupana). Appetite. 2008;50:506–13.
139. de Oliveira Campos MP, Riechelmann R, Martins LC, Hassan BJ, Casa FB, Del Giglio A. Guarana (Paullinia cupana) improves fatigue in breast cancer patients undergoing systemic chemotherapy. J Altern Complement Med. 2011;17:505–12.
140. da Costa Miranda V, Trufelli DC, Santos J, Campos MP, Nobuo M, da Costa Mirand M, et al. Effectiveness of guarana (Paullinia cupana) for postradiation fatigue and depression: results of a pilot double-blind randomized study. J Altern Complement Med. 2009;15:431–3.
141. Vidal-Alaball J, Butler CC, Cannings-John R, Goringe A, Hood K, McCaddon A, et al. Oral vitamin B12 versus intramuscular vitamin B12 for vitamin B12 deficiency. Cochrane Database Syst Rev. 2005;3:CD004655.
142. Masucci L, Goeree R. Vitamin B12 intramuscular injections versus oral supplements: a budget impact analysis. Ont Health Technol Assess Ser. 2013;13:1–24.
143. Zhang SM, Cook NR, Albert CM, Gaziano JM, Buring JE, Manson JE. Effect of combined folic acid, vitamin B6, and vitamin B12 on cancer risk in women: a randomized trial. JAMA. 2008;300:2012–21.
144. Christen WG, Glynn RJ, Chew EY, Albert CM, Manson JE. Folic acid, pyridoxine, and cyanocobalamin combination treatment and age-related macular degeneration in women: the Women's Antioxidant and Folic Acid Cardiovascular Study. Arch Intern Med. 2009;169: 335–41.
145. Lesser GJ, Case D, Stark N, Williford S, Giguere J, Garino LA, et al. A randomized, double-blind, placebo-controlled study of oral coenzyme Q10 to relieve self-reported treatment-related fatigue in newly diagnosed patients with breast cancer. J Support Oncol. 2013;11:31–42.
146. Parkinson Study Group QE3 Investigators. A randomized clinical trial of high-dosage coenzyme Q10 in early Parkinson disease: no evidence of benefit. JAMA Neurol. 2014;71:543–52.
147. Teitelbaum JE, Johnson C, St Cyr J. The use of D-ribose in chronic fatigue syndrome and fibromyalgia: a pilot study. J Altern Complement Med. 2006;12:857–62.
148. Kerksick C, Rasmussen C, Bowden R, Leutholtz B, Harvey T, Earnest C, et al. Effects of ribose supplementation prior to and during intense exercise on anaerobic capacity and metabolic markers. Int J Sport Nutr Exerc Metab. 2005;15:653–64.

149. Cruciani RA, Zhang JJ, Manola J, Cella D, Ansari B, Fisch MJ. L-Carnitine supplementation for the management of fatigue in patients with cancer: an eastern cooperative oncology group phase III, randomized, double-blind, placebo-controlled trial. J Clin Oncol. 2012;30: 3864–9.

150. Cruciani RA, Revuelta M, Dvorkin E, Hormel P, Lesage P, Esteban-Cruciani N. L-Carnitine supplementation in patients with HIV/AIDS and fatigue: a double-blind, placebo-controlled pilot study. HIV AIDS (Auckl). 2015;7:65–73.

151. Mantovani G, Maccio A, Madeddu C, Serpe R, Massa E, Dessi M, et al. Randomized phase III clinical trial of five different arms of treatment in 332 patients with cancer cachexia. Oncologist. 2010;15:200–11.

152. Maccio A, Madeddu C, Gramignano G, Mulas C, Floris C, Sanna E, et al. A randomized phase III clinical trial of a combined treatment for cachexia in patients with gynecological cancers: evaluating the impact on metabolic and inflammatory profiles and quality of life. Gynecol Oncol. 2012;124:417–25.

153. Zhao H, Zhang Q, Zhao L, Huang X, Wang J, Kang X. Spore powder of Ganoderma lucidum improves cancer-related fatigue in breast cancer patients undergoing endocrine therapy: a pilot clinical trial. Evid Based Complement Alternat Med. 2012;2012:809614.

154. Mucke M, Mochamat S, Cuhls H, Peuckmann-Post V, Minton O, Stone P, et al. Pharmacological treatments for fatigue associated with palliative care. Cochrane Database Syst Rev. 2015;5:CD006788.

155. Walcott FL, Land SR, Constantino JP, Midthune D, Dunn BK. Vasomotor symptoms, BMI, and adherence to tamoxifen in the National Surgical Adjuvant Breast and Bowel Project (NSABP) Breast Cancer Prevention Trial (P-1). J Clin Oncol 2015;33(Suppl; abstr 1501).

156. Da Fonesca AM, Bagnoli VR, Suza MA, Azevedo RS, Couto Ede Jr B, Soares Jr JM, et al. Impact of age and body mass on the intensity of menopausal symptoms in 5968 Brazilian women. Gynecol Endocrinol. 2013;29:116–8.

157. Herber-Gast GC, Mishra GD, van der Schouw YT, Brown WJ, Dobson AJ. Risk factors for night sweats and hot flushes in midlife: results from a prospective cohort study. Menopause. 2013;20:953–9.

158. Huang AJ, Subak LL, Wing R, West DS, Hernandez AL, Macer J, et al. An intensive behavioral weight loss intervention and hot flushes in women. Arch Intern Med. 2010;170: 1161–7.

159. Ryu KJ, Park HT, Kwon DH, Yang KS, Kim YJ, Yi KW, et al. Vasomotor symptoms and metabolic syndrome in Korean postmenopausal women. Menopause 2015, Epub head of print.

160. Blumel JE, Chedraui P, Aedo S, Fica J, Mezones-Holquin E, Baron G, et al. Obesity and its relation to depressive symptoms and sedentary lifestyle in middle-aged women. Maturitas. 2015;80:100–5.

161. Imayama I, Alfano CM, Neuhouser ML, George SM, Wilder Smith A, Baumgartner RN, et al. Weight, inflammation, cancer-related symptoms and health related quality of life among breast cancer survivors. Breast Cancer Res Treat. 2013;140:159–76.

162. Daley A, Stokes-Lampard H, Thomas A, MacArthur C. Exercise for vasomotor menopausal symptoms. Cochrane Database Syst Rev. 2014;11:CD006108.

163. Newton KM, Reed SD, Guthrie KA, Sherman KJ, Booth-LaForce C, Caan B, et al. Efficacy of yoga for vasomotor symptoms: a randomized controlled trial. Menopause. 2014;21: 339–46.

164. Sternfeld B, Guthrie KA, Ensrud KE, LaCroix AZ, Larson JC, Dunn AL, et al. Efficacy of exercise for menopausal symptoms: a randomized controlled trial. Menopause. 2014;21: 330–8.

165. Duijts SF, van Beurden M, Oldenburg HS, Hunter MS, Kieffer JM, Stuvier MM, et al. Efficacy of cognitive behavioral therapy and physical exercise in alleviating treatment-induced menopausal symptoms in patients with breast cancer: results of a randomized, controlled, multicenter trial. J Clin Oncol. 2012;30:4124–33.

166. Carpenter JS, Burns DS, Wu J, Otte JL, Schneider B, Ryker K, et al. Paced respiration for vasomotor and other menopausal symptoms: a randomized, controlled trial. J Gen Intern Med. 2013;28:193–200.
167. Sood R, Sood A, Wolf SL, Linquist BM, Liu H, Sloan JA, et al. Paced breathing compared to usual breathing for hot flashes. Menopause. 2013;20:179–84.
168. Chandwani KD, Heckler CE, Mohile SG, Mustian KM, Janeisins M, Peppone LJ, et al. Hot flashes severity, complementary and alternative medicine use, and self-rated health in women with breast cancer. Explore (NY). 2014;10:241–7.
169. Chiu HY, Shyu YK, Chang PC, Tsai PS. Effects of acupuncture on menopause-related symptoms in breast cancer survivors: a meta-analysis of randomized controlled trials. Cancer Nurs 2015, Epub ahead of print.
170. Garcia MK, McQuade J, Haddad R, Patel S, Lee R, Yang P, et al. Systematic review of acupuncture in cancer care: a synthesis of the evidence. J Clin Oncol. 2013;31:952–60.
171. Dodin S, Blanchet C, Marc I, Ernst E, Wu T, Valliancourt C, et al. Acupuncture for menopausal symptoms. Cochrane Database Syst Rev. 2013;7:CD007410.
172. Pockaj BA, Gallagher JG, Loprinzi CL, Stella PJ, Barton DL, Sloan JA, et al. Phase III double-blind, randomized, placebo-controlled crossover trial of black cohosh in the management of hot flashes: NCCTG Trial N01CC1. J Clin Oncol. 2006;24:2836–41.
173. Pruthi S, Qin R, Terstreip SA, Liu H, Loprinzi CL, Shah TR, et al. A phase III, randomized, placebo-controlled, double-blind trial of flaxseed for the treatment of hot flashes: North Central Cancer Treatment Group N08C7. Menopause. 2012;19:48–53.
174. Pan A, Yu D, Demark-Wahnefried W, Franco OH, Lin X. Meta-analysis of the effects of flaxseed interventions on blood lipids. Am J Clin Nutr. 2009;90:288–97.
175. Anderson JW, Bush HM. Soy protein effects on serum lipoproteins: a quality assessment and meta-analysis of randomized, controlled studies. J Am Coll Nutr. 2011;30:79–91.
176. Park H, Qin R, Smith TJ, Atherton PJ, Barton DL, Sturtz K, et al. North Central Cancer Treatment Group N10C2 (Alliance): a double-blind placebo-controlled study of magnesium supplements to reduce menopausal hot flashes. Menopause. 2015;22:627–32.
177. Park H, Parker GL, Boardman CH, Morris MM, Smith TJ. A pilot phase II trial of magnesium supplements to reduce menopausal hot flashes in breast cancer patients. Support Care Cancer. 2011;19:859–63.
178. Herrada J, Gupta A, Campos-Gines AF, et al. Oral magnesium oxide for treatment of hot flashes in women undergoing treatment for breast cancer: a pilot study [Abstract]. In: 2010 ASCO annual meeting, Chicago, IL, 2010.
179. Cohen LS, Joffe H, Guthrie KA, Ensrud KE, Freeman M, Carpenter JS, et al. Efficacy of omega-3 for vasomotor symptoms treatment: a randomized controlled trial. Menopause. 2014;21:347–54.
180. Lethaby A, Marjoribanks J, Kronenberg F, Roberts H, Eden J, Brown J. Phytoestrogens for menopausal vasomotor symptoms. Cochrane Database Syst Rev. 2013;12:CD001395.
181. Fritz H, Seely D, Flower G, Skidmore B, Fernandes R, Vadeboncoeur S, et al. Soy, red clover, and isoflavones and breast cancer: a systematic review. PLoS One. 2013;28:e81968.
182. del Giorno C, Fonesca AM, Bagnoli VR, Assis JS, Soares Jr JM, Baracat EC. Effects of Trifolium pratense on the climacteric and sexual symptoms in postmenopausal women. Rev Assoc Med Bras. 2010;56:558–62.
183. Geller SE, Shulman LP, van Breeman RB, Banuvar S, Zhou Y, Epstein G, et al. Safety and efficacy of black cohosh and red clover for the management of vasomotor symptoms: a randomized controlled trial. Menopause. 2009;16:1156–66.
184. Bommer S, Klein P, Suter A. First time proof of sage's tolerability and efficacy in menopausal women with hot flashes. Adv Ther. 2011;28:490–500.
185. Quella SK, Loprinzi CL, Barton DL, Knost JA, Sloan JA, LaVasseur BI, et al. Evaluation of soy phytoestrogens for the treatment of hot flashes in breast cancer survivors: a North Central Cancer Treatment Group trial. J Clin Oncol. 2000;18:1068–74.
186. Barton DL, Loprinzi CL, Quella SK, Sloan JA, Veeder MH, Egner JR, et al. Prospective evaluation of vitamin E for hot flashes in breast cancer survivors. J Clin Oncol. 1998;16:495–500.

187. Scheffers CS, Armsrong S, Cantineau AE, Farquhar C, Jordan V, et al. Dehydroepiandrosterone for women in the peri- or postmenopausal phase. Cochrane Database Syst Rev. 2015;1: CD011066.
188. Wu WH, Kang YP, Wang NH, Jou HJ, Wang TA. Sesame ingestion affects sex hormones, antioxidant status, and blood lipids in postmenopausal women. J Nutr. 2006;136:1270–5.
189. Coulman KD, Liu Z, Hum WQ, Michaelides J, Thompson LU. Whole sesame seed is as rich a source of mammalian lignin precursors as whole flaxseed. Nutr Cancer. 2005;52:156–65.
190. Alipoor B, Haghighian MK, Sadat BE, Asghari M. Effect of sesame seed on lipid profile and redox status in hyperlipidemic patients. Int J Food Sci Nutr. 2012;63:674–8.
191. Florentino L, Ancoli-Israel S. Insomnia and its treatment in women with breast cancer. Sleep Med Rev. 2006;10:419–29.
192. Lis CG, Gupta D, Grutsch JF. The relationship between insomnia and patient satisfaction with quality of life in cancer. Support Care Cancer. 2008;16:261–6.
193. Courneya KS, Segal RJ, Mackey JR, Gelmon K, Friedenreich CM, Yasui Y, et al. Effects of exercise dose and type on sleep quality in breast cancer patients receiving chemotherapy: a multicenter randomized trial. Breast Cancer Res Treat. 2014;144:361–9.
194. Sprod LK, Palesh OG, Janelsins MC, Peppone LJ, Heckler CE, Adams MJ, et al. Exercise, sleep quality, and mediators of sleep in breast and prostate cancer patients receiving radiation therapy. Community Oncol. 2010;7:463–71.
195. Mustian KM, Sprod LK, Janelsins M, Peppone LJ, Chandwani K, Heckler C, et al. Multicenter, randomized controlled trial of yoga for sleep quality among cancer survivors. J Clin Oncol. 2013;31:3233–41.
196. FDA Drug Safety Communication: FDA warns of next-day impairment with sleep aid Lunesta (eszopiclone) and lowers recommended dose. www.fda.gov/Drugs/DrugSafety/ucm397260.htm. Accessed 15 June 2015.
197. Paulozzi LJ. Prescription drug overdoses: a review. J Safety Res. 2012;43:283–9.
198. Cardinali DP, Srinivasan V, Brzezinski A, Brown GM. Melatonin and its analogs in insomnia and depression. J Pineal Res. 2012;52:365–75.
199. Olde Rikkert MG, Rigaud AS. Melatonin in elderly patients with insomnia. A systematic review. Z Gerontol Geriatr. 2001;34:491–7.
200. Davis MP, Goforth HW. Long-term and short-term effects of insomnia in cancer and effective interventions. Cancer J. 2014;20:330–44.
201. Vural EM, van Munster BC, de Rooij SE. Optimal dosages for melatonin supplementation therapy in older adults: a systematic review of current literature. Drugs Aging. 2014;31: 441–51.
202. Wade AF, Farmer M, Harari G, Fund N, Laudon M, Nir T, et al. Add-on prolonged-release melatonin for cognitive function and sleep in mild to moderate Alzheimer's disease: a 6-month, randomized, placebo-controlled, multicenter trial. Clin Interv Aging. 2014;9: 947–61.
203. Rossignol DA, Frye RE. Melatonin in autism spectrum disorders: a systematic review and meta-analysis. Dev Med Child Neurol. 2011;53:783–92.
204. Schernhammer ES, Giobbie-Hurder A, Gantman K, Savoie J, Scheib R, Parker LM, et al. A randomized, controlled trial of oral melatonin supplementation and breast cancer biomarkers. Cancer Causes Control. 2012;23:609–16.
205. Chen WY, Giobbie-Hurder A, Gantman K, Savoie J, Scheib R, Parker LM, et al. A randomized, placebo-controlled trial of melatonin on breast cancer survivors: impact on sleep, mood, and hot flashes. Breast Cancer Res Treat. 2014;145(2):381–8.
206. Seely D, Wu P, Fritz H, Kennedy DA, Tsui T, Seely AJ, et al. Melatonin as adjuvant cancer care with and without chemotherapy: a systematic review and meta-analysis of randomized trials. Integr Cancer Ther. 2012;11:293–303.
207. Grossman E, Laudon M, Ylacin R, Zengil H, Peleg E, Sharabi Y, et al. Melatonin reduces night blood pressure in patients with nocturnal hypertension. Am J Med. 2006;119: 898–902.

208. Cagnacci A, Cannoletta M, Renzi A, Baldassari F, Arangino S, Volpe A. Prolonged melatonin administration decreases nocturnal blood pressure in women. Am J Hpertens. 2005; 18(12 Pt 1):1614–8.

209. Lusardi P, Piazza E, Fogari R. Cardiovascular effects of melatonin in hypertensive patients well controlled by nifedipine: a 24-hour study. Br J Clin Pharmacol. 2000;49:423–7.

210. Grossman E, Laudon M, Zisapel N. Effect of melatonin on nocturnal blood pressure: meta-analysis of randomized controlled trials. Vasc Health Risk Manag. 2011;7:577–84.

211. Khezri MB, Merate H. The effects of melatonin on anxiety and pain scores of patients, intra-ocular pressure, and operating conditions during cataract surgery under topical anesthesia. Indian J Ophthalmol. 2013;61:319–24.

212. Cook JS, Saunder CL, Ray CA. Melatonin differently affects vascular blood flow in humans. Am J Physiol Heart Circ Physiol. 2011;300:H670–4.

213. Kelber O, Nieber K, Kraft K. Valerian: no evidence for clinically relevant interactions. Evid Based Complement Alternat Med. 2014;2014:879396.

214. Fernandez-San-Martin MI, Masa-Font R, Palacios-Soler L, Sancho-Gomez P, Calbo-Caldentey C, Flores-Mateo G. Effectiveness of Valerian on insomnia: a meta-analysis of randomized placebo-controlled trials. Sleep Med. 2010;11:505–11.

215. Barton DL, Atherton PJ, Bauer BA, Moore DF, Mattar BI, LaVasseur BI, et al. The use of Valeriana officinalis (Valerian) in improving sleep in patients who are undergoing treatment for cancer: a phase III randomized, placebo-controlled, double-blind study (NCCTG Trial, N01C5). J Support Oncol. 2011;9(1):24–31.

216. Taavoni S, Ekbatani N, Kashaniyan M. Effect of valerian on sleep quality in postmenopausal women: a randomized placebo-controlled clinical trial. Menopause. 2011;18:951–5.

217. Kashani F, Kashani P. The effect of massage therapy on quality of sleep in breast cancer patients. Iran J Nurs Midwifery Res. 2014;19:113–8.

218. Wyatt RJ, Engelman K, Kupfer DJ, Fram DH, Sjoerdsma A, Snyder F. Effects of L-tryptophan (a natural sedative) on human sleep. Lancet. 1970;2(7678):842–6.

219. Wyatt RJ, Zarcone V, Engelman K, Dement WC, Snyder F, Sjoerdsma A. Effects of 5-hydroxytryptophan on the sleep of normal human subjects. Electroencephalogr Clin Neurophysiol. 1971;30:505–9.

220. Das YT, Bagchi M, Bagchi D, Preuss HG. Safety of 5-hydroxy-L-tryptophan. Toxicol Lett. 2004;150:111–22.

221. Fernstrom JD. Effects and side effects associated with the non-nutritional use of tryptophan by humans. J Nutr. 2012;142:2236S–44.

222. Loh SY, Musa AN. Methods to improve rehabilitation of patients following breast cancer surgery: a review of systematic reviews. Breast Cancer (Dov Med Press). 2015;7:81–98.

223. Shaitelman SF, Cromwell KD, Rasmussen JC, Stout NL, Armer JM, Lasinski BB, et al. Recent progress in the treatment and prevention cancer-related lymphedema. CA Cancer J Clin. 2015;65:55–81.

224. Fu MR. Breast cancer-related lymphedema: symptoms, diagnosis, risk reduction, and management. World J Clin Oncol. 2014;5:241–7.

225. Perera N, Liolitsa D, Iype S, Croxford A, Yassin M, Lang P, et al. Phlepotonic for haemorrhoids. Cochrane Database Syst Rev. 2012;8:CD004322.

226. Katsenis K. Micronized purified flavonoid fraction (MPFF): a review of its pharmacological effects, therapeutic efficacy and benefits in the management of chronic venous insufficiency. Curr Vasc Pharmacol. 2005;3:1–9.

227. Allaert FA. Meta-analysis of the impact of the principal venoactive drugs agents on malleolar venous edema. Int Angiol. 2012;31:310–5.

228. Bogucka-Kocka A, Wozniak M, Feldo M, Kockic J, Szewczyk K. Diosmin-isolation techniques, determination in plant material and pharmaceutical formulations, and clinical use. Nat Prod Commun. 2013;8:545–50.

229. Badger C, Preston N, Seers K, Mortimer P. Benzo-pyrones for reducing and controlling lypmhoedema of the limbs. Cochrane Database Syst Rev. 2004;2:CD003140.

230. Olszewski W. Clinical efficacy of micronized purified flavonoid fraction (MPFF) in edema. Angiology. 2000;51:25–9.
231. Pecking AP, Fevrier B, Wargon C, Pillion G. Efficacy of Daflon 500 mg in the treatment of lymphedema (secondary to conventional therapy of breast cancer). Angiology. 1997;48: 93–8.
232. Pecking AP. Evaluation by lymphoscintigraphy of the effect of a micronized flavonoid fraction (Daflon 500 mg) in the treatment of upper limb lymphedema. Int Angiol. 1995; 14(3 Suppl 1):39–43.
233. Pittler MH, Ernst E. Horse chestnut seed extract for chronic venous insufficiency. Cochrane Database Syst Rev. 2012;11:CD003230.
234. Horse Chestnut Seed Extract for Lymphedema. www.clinicaltrials.gov/ct2/show/ NCT00213928. Accessed 20 June 2015.
235. Hutson PR, Love RR, Cleary JF, Anderson SA, Vanummersen L, Morgan-Meadows SL, et al. Horse chestnut seed extract for the treatment of arm lymphedema. J Clin Oncol. 2004;22(14S(July 15 Suppl)):8095.
236. Wadsworth AN, Faulds D. Hydroxyethylrutosides. A review of their pharmacology and therapeutic efficacy in venous insufficiency and related disorders. Drugs. 1992;44:1013–32.
237. Kiesewetter H, Koscieiny J, Kalus U, Vix JM, Peil H, Petrini O, et al. Efficacy of orally administered extract of red vine leaf AS 195 (folia vitis viniferae) in chronic venous insufficiency (stages I–II). A randomized, double-blind, placebo-controlled trial. Arzneimittelforschung. 2000;50:109–17.
238. Rabe E, Stucker M, Esperester A, Schafer E, Otillinger B. Efficacy and tolerability of a red-vine-leaf extract in patients suffering from chronic venous insufficiency-results of a double-blind placebo-controlled study. Eur J Vasc Endovasc Surg. 2011;41:540–7.
239. Piller NB, Morgan RG, Casley Smith JR. A double-blind, cross-over trial of O-(beta-hydroxyethyl)-rutosides (Benzo-pyrones) in the treatment of lymphedema of the arms and legs. Br J Plast Surg. 1988;41:20–7.
240. Taylor HM, Rose KE, Twycross RG. A double-blind clinical trial of hydroxyethylrutosides in obstructive arm lymphedema. Phlebology. 1993;8 Suppl 1:22–8.
241. Pronk LC, van Putten WL, van Beurden V, de Boer-Dennert M, Stoter G, Verweii J. The venotonic drug hydroxyethylrutosiden does not prevent or reduce docetaxel-induced fluid retention: results of a comparative study. Cancer Chemother Pharmacol. 1999;43:173–7.
242. Schoonees A, Visser J, Musekiwa A, Volmink J. Pycnogenol (extract of French maritime pine bark) for the treatment of chronic disorders. Cochrane Database Syst Rev. 2012;4:CD008294.
243. Dennert G, Homeber M. Selenium for alleviating the side effects of chemotherapy, radiotherapy and surgery in cancer patients. Cochrane Database Syst Rev. 2006;3:CD005037.
244. Duffield-Lillico AJ, Slate EH, Reid ME, Turnbull BW, Wilkins PA, Combs Jr GF, et al., for the Nutritional Prevention of Cancer Study Group. Selenium supplementation and secondary prevention of nonmelanoma skin cancer in a randomized trial. J Natl Cancer Inst 2003;95:1477–81.
245. Stranges S, Marshall JR, Natarajan R, Donahue RP, Trevisan M, Combs GF, et al. Effects of long-term selenium supplementation on the incidence of type 2 diabetes: a randomized trial. Ann Intern Med. 2007;147:217–23.
246. Gontero P, Marra G, Soria F, Oderda M, Zitella A, Baratta F, et al. A randomized double-blind placebo controlled phase I–II study on clinical and molecular effects of dietary supplements in men with precancerous prostatic lesions. Chemopreventon or "chemopromotion"? Prostate. 2015;75:1177–86.
247. Kenfield SA, Van Blarigan EL, DuPre N, Stampfer MJ, Giovannucci E, Chan JM. Selenium supplementation and prostate cancer mortality. J Natl Cancer Inst. 2014;107:360.
248. Kristal AR, Darke AK, Morris JS, Tangen CM, Goodman PJ, Thompson IM, et al. Baseline selenium status and effects of selenium and vitamin e supplementation on prostate cancer risk. J Natl Cancer Inst. 2014;106:djt456.
249. Suh EE. The effects of P6 acupressure and nurse-provided counseling on chemotherapy-induced nausea and vomiting in patients with breast cancer. Oncol Nurs Forum. 2012; 39:E1–9.

250. Lee J, Dodd M, Dibbie S, Abrams D. Review of acupressure studies for chemotherapy-induced nausea and vomiting. J Pain Symptom Manage. 2008;36:529–44.
251. Chao LF, Zhang AL, Liu HE, Cheng MH, Lam HB, Lo SK. The efficacy of acupoint stimulation for the management of therapy-related adverse events in patients with breast cancer: a systematic review. Breast Cancer Res Treat. 2009;118:255–67.
252. Ryan JL, Heckler CE, Roscoe JA, Dakhil SR, Kirshner J, Flynn PJ, et al. Ginger (Zingiber officinale) reduces acute chemotherapy-induced nausea: a URCC CCOP study of 576 patients. Support Care Cancer. 2012;20:1479–89.
253. Zindol® for chemotherapy induced nausea and vomiting. http://www.aphios.com/products/therapeutic-product-pipeline/oncology/zindol.html. Accessed 1 June 2015.
254. Zindol® DS. http://www.aphioshwc.com/products/zindol-ds.html. Accessed 1 June 2015.
255. Zick SM, Ruffin MT, Lee J, Normolle DP, Siden R, Alrawi S, et al. Phase II trial of encapsulated ginger as treatment for chemotherapy-induced nausea and vomiting. Support Care Cancer. 2009;17:563–72.
256. Lua PL, Sailhah N, Mazlan N. Effects of inhaled ginger aromatherapy on chemotherapy-induced nausea and vomiting and health-related quality of life in women with breast cancer. Complement Ther Med. 2015;23:396–404.
257. Pillai AK, Sharma KK, Gupta YK, Bakhshi S. Anti-emetic effect of ginger powder versus placebo as an add-on therapy in children and young adults receiving high emetogenic chemotherapy. Pediatr Blood Cancer. 2011;56:234–8.
258. Marx W, Kiss N, Isenring L. Is ginger beneficial for nausea and vomiting? An update of the literature. Curr Opin Support Palliat Care. 2015;9:189–95.
259. Tan PC, Omar SZ. Contemporary approaches to hyperemesis during pregnancy. Curr Opin Obstet Gynecol. 2011;23:87–93.
260. ACOG Practice Bulletin. Clinical management guidelines for obstetrician-gynecologists. Number 52 (April), 2004;103:803–15.
261. Ensiyeh J, Sakineh MA. Comparing ginger and vitamin B6 for the treatment of nausea and vomiting in pregnancy: a randomized controlled trial. Midwifery. 2009;25:649–53.
262. Herrell HE. Nausea and vomiting in pregnancy. Am Fam Physician. 2014;89:965–70.
263. Persaud N, Chin J, Walker M. Should doxylamine-pyridoxine be used for nausea and vomiting of pregnancy? J Obstet Gynecol Can. 2014;36:343–8.
264. Matthews A, Haas DM, O'Mathuna DP, Dowswell T, Doyle M. Interventions for nausea and vomiting in early pregnancy. Cochrane Database Syst Rev. 2014;3:CD007575.
265. You Q, Yu H, Wu D, Zhang Y, Zheng J, Peng C. Vitamin B6 points PC6 injection during acupuncture can relieve nausea and vomiting in patients with ovarian cancer. Int J Gynecol Cancer. 2009;19:567–71.
266. Ghavanini AA, Kimpinski K. Revisiting the evidence for neuropathy caused by pyridoxine deficiency and excess. J Clin Neuromuscul Dis. 2014;16:25–31.
267. Levine ME, Gillis MG, Koch SY, Voss AC, Stern RM, et al. Protein and ginger for the treatment of chemotherapy-induced delayed nausea. J Altern Complement Med. 2008;14:545–51.
268. Jednak MA, Shadigian EM, Kim MS, Woods ML, Hooper FG, Owyang C, et al. Protein meals reduce nausea and gastric slow wave dysrhythmic activity in first trimester pregnancy. Am J Physiol. 1999;277(4 Pt 1):G855–61.
269. Paddon-Jones D, Short KR, Campbell WW, Volpi E, Wolfe RR. Role of dietary protein in the sarcopenia of aging. Am J Clin Nutr. 2008;87:1562S–6.
270. Fallon MT. Neuropathic pain in cancer. Br J Anaesth. 2013;111:105–11.
271. Bril V, England J, Franklin GM, Backonja M, Cohen J, Toro D, et al. Evidence-based guideline: Treatment of painful diabetic neuropathy: report of the American Academy of Neurology, the American Association of Neuromuscular and Electrodiagnostic Medicine, and the American Academy of Physical Medicine and Rehabilitation. PM R. 2011;3: 345–52.
272. Qutenza (capsaicin) 8% patch. www.qutenza.com. Accessed 15 June 2015.

273. Wagner T, Roth-Daniek A, Sell A, England J, Kern KU. Capsaicin 8% patch for peripheral neuropathic pain: review of treatment best practice from real-world clinical experience. Pain Manag. 2012;2:239–50.
274. Observation of the use of Qutenza in standard clinical practice (ASCEND). www.clinicaltrials.gov/ct2/show/NCT01737294. Accessed 15 June 2015.
275. Ziegler D, Low PA, Litchy WJ, Boulton AJ, Vinik AI, Freeman R, et al. Efficacy and safety of antioxidant treatment with alpha-lipoic acid over 4 years in diabetic polyneuropathy: the NATHAN 1 trial. Diabetes Care. 2011;34:2054–60.
276. Minhout GS, Kollen BJ, Alkhalaf A, Kleefstra N, Bilo HJ. Alpha lipoic acid for symptomatic peripheral neuropathy in patients with diabetes: a meta-analysis of randomized controlled trials. Int J Endocrinol. 2012;2012:456279.
277. Papanas N, Ziegler D. Efficacy of alpha-lipoic acid in diabetic neuropathy. Expert Opin Pharmacother. 2014;15:2721–31.
278. Gullo D, Evans JL, Sortino G, Goldfine ID, Vigneri R. Insulin autoimmune syndrome (Hirata Disease) in European Caucasians taking alpha-lipoic acid. Clin Endocrinol (Oxf). 2014;81:204–9.
279. Gedlicka C, Scheithauer W, Schull B, Kornek GV. Effective treatment of oxaliplatin-induced cumulative polyneuropathy with alpha-lipoic acid. J Clin Oncol. 2002;20:3359–61.
280. Guo Y, Jones D, Palmer JL, Forman A, Dakhil SR, Velasco MR, et al. Oral alpha-lipoic acid to prevent chemotherapy-induced peripheral neuropathy: a randomized, double-blind, placebo-controlled trial. Support Care Cancer. 2014;22:1223–31.
281. Koufaki M. Therapeutic applications of lipoic acid: a patent review (2011–2014). Expert Opin Ther Pat. 2014;24:993–1005.
282. de Aquiar Pastore Silva J, Emilia de Souza Fabre M, Waitzberg DL. Omega-3 supplements for patients in chemotherapy and/or radiotherapy: a systematic review. Clin Nutr. 2015;34:359–66.
283. Ghoreishi Z, Esfahani A, Djazayeri A, Djalali M, Golestan B, Ayromlou H, et al. Omega-3 fatty acids are protective against paclitaxel-induced peripheral neuropathy: a randomized double-blind placebo controlled trial. BMC Cancer. 2012;12:355.
284. Okuda Y, Mizutani M, Ogawa M, Sone H, Asano M, Asakura Y, et al. Long-term effects of eicosapentaenoic acid on diabetic peripheral neuropathy and serum lipids in patients with type II diabetes mellitus. J Diabetes Complications. 1996;10:280–7.
285. Fracasso PM, Picus J, Wildi JD, Goodner SA, Creekmore AN, Gao F, et al. Phase 1 and pharmacokinetic study of weekly docosahexaenoic acid-paclitaxel, Taxoprexin, in resistant solid tumor malignancies. Cancer Chemother Pharmacol. 2009;63:451–8.
286. Omega Swirl: Smoothie Taste & Texture. www.barleans.com/omega-swirl.asp. Accessed 15 June 2015.
287. Hershman DL, Unger JM, Crew KD, Minasian LM, Awad D, Moinpour CM, et al. Randomized double-blind placebo-controlled trial of acetyl-L-carnitine for the prevention of taxane-induced neuropathy in women undergoing adjuvant breast cancer therapy. J Clin Oncol. 2013;31:2627–33.
288. Campone M, Berton-Rigaud D, Joly-Lobbedez F, Baurain JF, Rolland F, Stenzi A, et al. A double-blind, randomized phase II study to evaluate the safety and efficacy of acetyl-L-carnitine in the prevention of sagopilone-induced peripheral neuropathy. Oncologist. 2013;18:1190–1.
289. Callander N, Markovina S, Eickhoff J, Hutson P, Campbell T, Hematti P, et al. Acetyl-L-carnitine (ALCAR) for the prevention of chemotherapy-induced peripheral neuropathy in patients with relapsed or refractory multiple myeloma treated with bortezomib, doxorubicin and low-dose dexamethasone: a study from the Wisconsin Oncology Network. Cancer Chemother Pharmacol. 2014;74:875–82.
290. Berger JR, Singhai D. The neurologic complications of bariatric surgery. Handb Clin Neurol. 2014;120:587–94.
291. Chopra K, Tiwari V. Alcoholic neuropathy: possible mechanisms and future treatment possibilities. Br J Clin Pharmacol. 2012;73:348–62.

292. Pacal L, Kuricova K, Kankova K. Evidence for altered thiamine metabolism in diabetes: is there a potential to oppose gluco- and lipotoxicity by rational supplementation. World J Diabetes. 2014;15:288–95.

293. Javed S, Petropoulos IN, Alam U, Malik RA. Treatment of painful diabetic neuropathy. Ther Adv Chronic Dis. 2015;6:15–28.

294. Ko SH, Ko SH, Ahn YB, Song KH, Han KD, Park YM, et al. Association of vitamin B12 deficiency and metformin use in patients with type 2 diabetes. J Korean Med Sci. 2014;29:965–72.

295. Gdynia HJ, Muller T, Sperfeld AD, Kuhnlein P, Otto M, Kassubek J, et al. Severe sensorimotor neuropathy after intake of highest dosages of vitamin B6. Neuromuscul Disord. 2008;18: 156–8.

296. Loven D, Levavi H, Sabach G, Zart R, Andras M, Fishman A, et al. Long-term glutamate supplementation failed to protect against peripheral neurotoxicity of paclitaxel. Eur J Cancer Care (Engl). 2009;18(1):78–83.

297. Kottschade LA, Sloan JA, Mazurczak MA, Johnson DB, Murphy BP, Rowland KM, et al. The use of vitamin E for the prevention of chemotherapy-induced peripheral neuropathy: results of a randomized phase III clinical trial. Support Care Cancer. 2011;19:1769–77.

298. Franconi G, Manni L, Schroder S, Marchetti P, Robinson N. A systematic review of experimental and clinical acupuncture in chemotherapy-induced peripheral neuropathy. Evid Based Complement Alternat Med. 2013;2013:516918.

299. Rostock M, Jaroslawski K, Guethlin C, Ludtke R, Schroder S, Bartsch HH. Chemotherapy-induced peripheral neuropathy in cancer patients: a four-arm randomized trial on the effectiveness of electroacupuncture. Evid Based Complement Alternat Med. 2013;2013:349653.

300. Schloss JM, Colosimo M, Airey C, Masci PP, Linnane AW, Vitetta L. Nutraceuticals and chemotherapy induced peripheral neuropathy (CIPN): a systematic review. Clin Nutr. 2013;32:888–93.

301. Eum S, Choi HD, Chang MJ, Choi HC, Ko YJ, Ahn JS, et al. Protective effects of vitamin E on chemotherapy-induced peripheral neuropathy: a meta-analysis of randomized controlled trials. Int J Vitam Nutr Res. 2013;83:101–11.

302. Moyad MA. Complementary and alternative medicine for prostate and urologic health. New York, NY: Springer Publishing; 2014.

303. Boquiren VM, Esplen MJ, Wong J, Toner B, Warner E, Malik N. Sexual functioning in breast cancer survivors experiencing body image disturbance. Psychooncology 2015, Epub ahead of print.

304. Lee M, Kim YH, Jeon MJ. Risk factors for negative impacts on sexual activity and function in younger breast cancer survivors. Psychooncology 2015, Epub ahead of print.

305. Schover LR, Baum GP, Fuson LA, Brewster A, Melhem-Bertrandt A. Sexual problems during the first 2 years of adjuvant treatment with aromatase inhibitors. J Sex Med. 2014;11:3102–11.

306. Bartula I, Sherman KA. The female sexual functioning index (FSFI): evaluation of acceptability, reliability, and validity in women with breast cancer. Support Care Cancer. 2015;23(9):2633–41. Epub 12 Feb 2015.

307. Taylor S, Harley C, Ziegler L, Brown J, Velikova G. Interventions for sexual problems following treatment for breast cancer: a systematic review. Breast Cancer Res Treat. 2011;130:711–24.

308. Esposito K, Ciotola M, Giugliano F, Schisano B, Autorino R, Iuliano S, et al. Mediterranean diet improves sexual function in women with the metabolic syndrome. Int J Impot Res. 2007;19:486–91.

309. Giugliano F, Maiorino MI, Di Palo C, Autorino R, De Sio M, Giugliano D, et al. Adherence to Mediterranean diet and sexual function in women with type 2 diabetes. J Sex Med. 2010;7:1883–90.

310. Esposito K, Giugliano F, Maiorino MI, Giugliano D. Dietary factors, Mediterranean diet and erectile dysfunction. J Sex Med. 2010;7:2338–45.

311. Esposito K, Giugliano F, Ciotola M, De Sio M, Armiento MD, Giugliano D. Obesity and sexual dysfunction, male and female. Int J Impot Res. 2008;20:358–65.

312. Aversa A, Bruzziches R, Francomano D, Greco EA, Violl F, Lenzi A, et al. Weight loss by multidisciplinary intervention improves endothelial and sexual function. J Sex Med. 2013;10(4):1024–33. Epub 24 Jan 2013.
313. Esposito K, Ciotola M, Malorino MI, Giugliano F, Autorino R, De Sio M, et al. Hyperlipidemia and sexual function in premenopausal women. J Sex Med. 2009;6:1696–703.
314. Veronelli A, Mauri C, Zecchini B, Peca MG, Turri O, Valitutti MT, et al. Sexual dysfunction is frequent in premenopausal women with diabetes, obesity, and hypothyroidism, and correlates with markers of increased cardiovascular risk. A preliminary report. J Sex Med. 2009;6:1561–8.
315. Alexander J, Crosby M, Ferguson D, Singh G, Steidle C, Weimiller M. Randomized, placebo-controlled, double-blind, crossover design trial of the efficacy and safety of Zestra for women in women with and without female sexual arousal disorder. J Sex Marital Ther. 2003;29 Suppl 1:33–44.
316. Pitel S, Raccah D, Gerbi A, Pieroni G, Vague P, Coste TC. At low doses, a gamma-linolenic acid-lipoic acid conjugate is more effective than docosahexaenoic acid-enriched phispholipids in preventing neuropathy in diabetic rats. J Nutr. 2007;137:368–72.
317. Hornych A, Oravec S, Girault F, Forette B, Horrobin DF. The effect of gamma-linolenic acid on plasma and membrane lipids and renal prostaglandin synthesis in older subjects. Bratisl Lek Listy. 2002;103:101–7.
318. Belch JJ, Shaw B, O'Dowd A, Saniabadi A, Leiberman P, Sturrock RD, et al. Evening primrose oil (Efamol) in the treatment of Raynaud's phenomenon: a double blind study. Thromb Haemost. 1985;54:490–4.
319. Herbenick D, Reece M, Hensel D, Sanders S, Jozkowski K, Fortenberry JD. Association of lubricant use with women's sexual pleasure, sexual satisfaction, and genital symptoms: a prospective daily diary study. J Sex Med. 2011;8:202–12.
320. Sutton KS, Boyer SC, Goldfinger C, Ezer P, Pukall CF. To lube or not to lube: experiences and perceptions of lubricant use in women with and without dyspareunia. J Sex Med. 2012;9:240–50.
321. Herbenick D, Reece M, Sanders SA, Dodge B, Ghassemi A, Fortenberry JD. Women's vibrator use in sexual partnerships: results from a nationally representative survey in the United States. J Sex Marital Ther. 2010;36:49–65.
322. Juraskova I, Jarvis S, Mok K, Peate M, Meiser B, Cheah BC, et al. The acceptability, feasibility, and efficacy (phase I/II study) of the OVERcome (Olive Oil, Vaginal Exercise, and MoisturizeR) intervention to improve dyspareunia and alleviate sexual problems in women with breast cancer. J Sex Med. 2013;10:2549–58.
323. Kim S-O, Kim MK, Lee H-S, Park JK, Park K. The effect of Korean red ginseng extract on the relaxation response in isolated rabbit vaginal tissue and its mechanism. J Sex Med. 2008;5:2079–84.
324. Lee H-S, Lee MN, Hwang IS, Kim SO, Ahn K, Park K. Effect of Korean red ginseng on vaginal blood flow and structure in hypercholesterolemic female rats. Kor J Androl. 2005;23:159–64.
325. Kim S-O, Kim MK, Chae MJ, Kim HY, Park JK, Park K. Effect of Korean red ginseng on the relaxation of clitoral corpus cavernosum in rabbit. Kor J Androl. 2006;24:29–34.
326. Oh K-J, Chae M-J, Lee H-S, Hong H-D, Park K. Effects of Korean red ginseng on sexual arousal in menopausal women: placebo-controlled, double-blind crossover clinical study. J Sex Med. 2010;7:1469–77.
327. Bottari A, Belcaro G, Ledda A, Luzzi R, Cesarone MR, Dugall M. Lady Prelox® improves sexual function in generally healthy women of reproductive age. Minerva Ginecol. 2013;65:435–44.
328. Bottari A, Belcaro G, Ledda A, Cesarone MR, Vinciguerra G, Di Renzo A, et al. Lady Prelox® improves sexual function in post-menopausal women. Panminerva Med. 2012;54(1 Suppl 4):3–9.
329. Cormio L, De Slati M, Lorusso F, Selvaggio O, Mirabella L, Sanquedolce F, et al. Oral L-citrulline supplementation improves erection hardness in men with mild erectile dysfunction. Urology. 2011;77:119–22.

330. Meston CM, Worcel M. The effects of yohimbine plus L-arginine glutamate on sexual arousal in postmenopausal women with sexual arousal disorder. Arch Sex Behav. 2002;31:323–32.

331. Lentz AC, Carson III CC, Marson L. Does the new herbal supplement "Maca" enhance erectile function or female sexual function. Sem Prev Alt Med. 2006;2:85–90.

332. Gonzales GF, Gonzales C, Gonzales-Castaneda C. Lepidium meyenii (Maca): a plant from the highlands of Peru—from tradition to science. Forsch Komplementmed. 2009;16: 373–80.

333. Gonzales GF, Cordova A, Vega K, Chung A, Villena A, Gonez C, et al. Effect of Lepidium meyenii (Maca) on sexual desire and its absent relationship with serum testosterone levels in adult healthy men. Andrologia. 2002;34:367–72.

334. Zenico T, Cicero AF, Valmorri L, Mercuriali M, Bercovich E. Subjective effects of Lepidium meyenii (Maca) extract on well-being and sexual performances in patients with mild erectile dysfunction: a randomized, double-blind clinical trial. Andrologia. 2009;41:95–9.

335. Dording CM, Fisher L, Papakostas G, Farabaugh A, Sonawalla S, Fava M, et al. A double-blind, randomized, pilot dose-finding study of maca root (L. meyenii) for the management of SSRI-induced sexual dysfunction. CNS Neurosci Ther. 2008;14:182–91.

336. Shin BC, Lee MS, Yang EJ, Lim HS, Ernst E. Maca (L. meyenii) for improving sexual function: a systematic review. BMC Complement Altern Med. 2010;10:44.

337. Dording CM, Schetter PJ, Dalton ED, Parkin SR, Walker RS, Fehling KB, et al. A double-blind placebo-controlled trial of maca root as treatment for antidepressant-induced sexual dysfunction. Evid Based Complement Alternat Med. 2015;2015:949036.

338. Zheng BL, He K, Kim CH, Rogers L, Shao Y, Huang ZY, et al. Effect of a lipidic extract from Lepidium meyenii on sexual behavior in mice and rats. Urology. 2000;55:598–602.

339. McCollom MM, Villinski JR, McPhail KL, Craker LE, Gafner S. Analysis of macamides in samples of Maca (Lepidium meyenii) by HPLC-UV-MS/MS. Phytochem Anal. 2005;16: 463–9.

340. Ganzera M, Zhao J, Muhammad I, Khan IA. Chemical profiling and standardization of Lepidium meyenii (Maca) by reversed phase high performance liquid chromatography. Chem Pharm Bull (Tokyo). 2002;50:988–91.

341. Gonzales GF. Ethnobiology and ethnopharmacology of Lepidium meyenii (Maca), a plant from the Peruvian Highlands. Evid Based Complement Alternat Med. 2012;2012:193496.

342. Ito TY, Trant AS, Polan ML. A double-blind placebo-controlled study of ArginMax, a nutritional supplement for enhancement of female sexual function. J Sex Marital Ther. 2001;27:541–9.

343. Ito TY, Polan ML, Whipple B, Trant AS. The enhancement of female sexual function with ArginMax, a nutritional supplement, among women differing in menopausal status. J Sex Marital Ther. 2006;32:369–78.

344. Greven KM, Case LD, Nycum LR, Zekan PJ, Hurd DD, Balcueva EP, et al. Effect of ArginMax on sexual functioning and quality of life among female cancer survivors: results of the WFU CCOP Research Base Protocol 97106. J Community Support Oncol. 2015;13(3): 87–94.

345. Kornblut Anne E, Wilson D. How one pill escaped place on steroid list. The New York Times, Sunday, 17 Apr 2005, p. 1, 20.

346. Brown GA, Vukovich M, King DS. Testosterone prohormone supplements. Med Sci Sports Exerc. 2006;38:1451–61.

347. Leder BZ, Longcope C, Catlin DH, Ahrens B, Schoenfeld DA, Finkelstein JS. Oral androstenedione administration and serum testosterone concentrations in young men. JAMA. 2000;283:779–82.

348. King DS, Sharp RL, Vukovich MD, Brown GA, Reifenrath TA, Uhl NL, et al. Effect of oral androstenedione on serum testosterone and adaptations to resistance training in young men: a randomized controlled trial. JAMA. 1999;281:2020–8.

349. Ritter RH, Cryar AK, Hermans MR. Oral androstenedione-induced impotence and severe oligospermia. Fertil Steril. 2005;84:217.

350. Broeder CE, Quindry J, Brittingham K, Panton L, Thomson J, Appakondu S, et al. The Andro Project: physiological and hormonal influences of androstenedione in men 35 to 65 years old

participating in a high-intensity resistance training program. Arch Intern Med. 2000;160: 3093–104.

351. Leder BZ, Leblanc KM, Longcope C, Lee H, Catlin DH, Finkelstein JS. Effects of oral androstenedione administration on serum testosterone and estradiol levels in postmenopausal women. J Clin Endocrinol Metab. 2002;87:5449–54.

352. Moyad MA. Dr. Moyad's guide to male sexual health: what works and what's worthless? Ann Arbor, MI: Spry Publishing; 2012.

353. Feldman HA, Goldstein I, Hatzichristou DG, Krane RJ, McKinlay JB. Impotence and its medical and psychological correlates results of the Massachusetts Male Aging Study. J Urol. 1994;151:54–61.

354. Reiter WJ, Pycha A, Schatzi G, Klingler HC, Mark I, Auterith A, et al. Serum dehydroepian-drosterone sulfate concentrations in men with erectile dysfunction. Urology. 2000;55: 755–8.

355. Traish AM, Kang P, Saad F, Guay AT. Dehydroepiandrosterone (DHEA)—a precursor steroid or an active hormone in human physiology. J Sex Med. 2011;8:2960–82.

356. Reiter WJ, Schatzi G, Mark I, Zeiner A, Pycha A, Marberger M. Dehydroepiandrosterone in the treatment of erectile dysfunction in patients with different organic etiologies. Urol Res. 2001;29:278–81.

357. Reiter WJ, Pycha A, Schatzi G, Pokorny A, Gruber DM, Huber JC, et al. DHEA in the treatment of erectile dysfunction: a prospective, double-blind, randomized, placebo-controlled study. Urology. 1999;53:590–4.

358. Hellbronn LK, de Jonge L, Frisard MI, DeLany JP, Larson-Meyer DE, Rood J, et al., for the Pennington CALERIE Team. Effect of 6-month calorie restriction on biomarkers of longevity, metabolic adaptation, and oxidative stress in overweight individuals: a randomized controlled trial. JAMA 2006;295:1539–48.

359. Niskanen L, Laaksonen DE, Punnonen K, Mustajoki P, Kaukua J, Rissanen A. Changes in sex hormone-binding globulin and testosterone during weight loss and weight maintenance in abdominally obese men with the metabolic syndrome. Diabetes Obes Metab. 2004;6: 208–15.

360. Ernst B, Wilms B, Thurnheer M, Schultes B. Reduced circulating androgen levels after gastric bypass surgery in severely obese women. Obes Surg. 2013;23:602–7.

361. Voznesensky M, Walsh S, Dauser D, Brindisi J, Kenny AM. The association between dehydroepiandosterone and frailty in older men and women. Age Ageing. 2009;38:401–6.

362. Panjari M, Bell RJ, Jane F, Wolfe R, Adams J, Morrow C, et al. A randomized trial of oral DHEA treatment for sexual function, well-being, and menopausal symptoms in postmenopausal women with low libido. J Sex Med. 2009;6:2579–90.

363. Panjari M, Davis SR. DHEA for postmenopausal women: a review of the evidence. Maturitas. 2010;66:172–9.

364. Panjari M, Bell RJ, Jane F, Adams J, Morrow C, Davis SR. The safety of 52 weeks of oral DHEA therapy for postmenopausal women. Maturitas. 2009;63:240–5.

365. Hackbert L, Helman JR. Acute dehydroepiandrosterone (DHEA) effects on sexual arousal in postmenopausal women. J Womens Health Gend Based Med. 2002;11:155–62.

366. Mortola JF, Yen SS. The effects of oral dehydroepiandrosterone on endocrine-metabolic parameters in postmenopausal women. J Clin Endocrinol Metab. 1990;71:696–704.

367. Panjari M, Davis SR. DHEA therapy for women: effect on sexual function and wellbeing. Hum Reprod Update. 2007;13:239–48.

368. Munarriz R, Talakoub L, Flaherty E, Giola M, Hoag L, Kim NN, et al. Androgen replacement therapy with dehydroepiandrosterone for androgen insufficiency and female sexual dysfunction: androgen and questionnaire results. J Sex Marital Ther. 2002;28 Suppl 1:165–73.

369. Davis SR, Panjari M, Stanczyk FZ. Clinical review: DHEA replacement for postmenopausal women. J Clin Endocrinol Metab. 2011;96:1642–53.

370. Arlt W, Callies F, van Villjmen JC, Koehler I, Reincke M, Bidlingmaier M, et al. Dehydroepiandrosterone replacement in women with adrenal insufficiency. N Engl J Med. 1999;341:1013–20.

371. Allollo B, Arlt W, Hahner S. DHEA: why, when, and how much—DHEA replacement in adrenal insufficiency. Ann Endocrinol (Paris). 2007;68:268–73.

372. Alkatib AA, Cosma M, Elamin MB, Erickson D, Swigio BA, Erwin PJ, et al. A systematic and meta-analysis of randomized placebo-controlled trials of DHEA treatment effects of quality of life in women with adrenal insufficiency. J Clin Endocrinol Metab. 2009;94:3676–81.

373. Nair KS, Rizza RA, O'Brien P, Dhatariya K, Short KR, Nehra A, et al. DHEA in elderly women and DHEA or testosterone in elderly men. N Engl J Med. 2006;355:1647–59.

374. Parasrampuria J, Schwartz K, Petesch R. Quality control of dehydroepiandrosterone dietary supplement products. JAMA. 1998;280:1565.

375. Baker WL, Karan S, Kenny AM. Effect of dehydroepiandrosterone on muscle strength and physical function in older adults: a systematic review. J Am Geriatr Soc. 2011;59: 997–1002.

376. Weiss EP, Shah K, Fontana L, Lambert CP, Holloszy JO, Villareal DT. Dehydroepiandrosterone replacement in older adults: 1- and 2-y effects on bone. Am J Clin Nutr. 2009;89:1459–67.

377. Labrie F, Archer D, Bouchard C, Fortier M, Cusan L, Gomez JL, et al. Effect of intravaginal dehydroepiandrosterone (Prasterone) on libido and sexual dysfunction in postmenopausal women. Menopause. 2009;16:923–31.

378. Panjari M, Davis SR. Vaginal DHEA to treat menopause related atrophy: a review of the evidence. Maturitas. 2011;70:22–5.

379. Labrie F, Martel C, Berube R, Cote I, Labrie C, Cusan L, et al. Intravaginal prasterone (DHEA) provides local action without clinically significant changes in serum concentrations of estrogens or androgens. J Steroid Biochem Mol Biol. 2013;138:359–67.

380. Mishra SI, Scherer RW, Geige PM, Berlanstein DR, Topalogiu O, Gotay CC, et al. Exercise interventions on health-related quality of life for caner survivors. Cochrane Database Syst Rev. 2012;8:CD007566.

381. Cramer H, Lange S, Klose P, Paul A, Dobos G. Yoga for breast cancer patients and survivors: a systematic review and meta-analysis. BMC Cancer. 2012;12:412.

382. Galantino ML, Callens ML, Cardena GJ, Piela NL, Mao JJ. Tai chi for well-being of breast cancer survivors with aromatase inhibitor-associated arthralgias: a feasibility study. Altern Ther Health Med. 2013;19:38–44.

383. Kim YH, Kim HJ, Ahn SD, Seo YJ, Kim SH. Effects of meditation on anxiety, depression, fatigue, and quality of life of women undergoing radiation therapy for breast cancer. Complement Ther Med. 2013;21:379–87.

384. Drackley NL, Degnim AC, Jakub JW, Cutshall SM, Thomley BS, Brodt JK, et al. Effect of massage therapy for postsurgical mastectomy recipients. Clin J Oncol Nurs. 2012;16:121–4.

385. Cohen S, Kamarck T, Mermelstein R. A global measure of perceived stress. J Health Soc Behav. 1983;24:385–96.

386. Kongkeaw C, Dilokthornsakul P, Thanarangsarit P, Limpeanchob N, Norman Scholfield C. Meta-analysis of randomized controlled trials on cognitive effects of Bacopa monnieri extract. J Ethnopharmacol. 2014;151:528–35.

387. Sarris J, McIntyre E, Camfield DA. Plant-based medicines for anxiety disorders: Part 2—A review of clinical studies with supporting preclinical evidence. CNS Drugs. 2013;27:301–19.

388. Ernst E. Herbal remedies for anxiety—a systematic review of controlled clinical trials. Phytomedicine. 2006;13:205–8.

389. Calabrese C, Gregory WL, Leo M, Kraemer D, Bone K, Oken B. Effect of a standardized Bacopa monnieri extract on cognitive performance, anxiety, and depression in the elderly: a randomized, double-blind, placebo-controlled trial. J Altern Complement Med. 2008;14: 707–13.

390. Sathyanarayanan V, Thomas T, Einother SJ, Dobriyal R, Joshi MK, Krishnamachari S. Brahmi for the better? New findings challenging cognition and anti-anxiety effects of Brahmi (Bacopa monniera) in healthy adults. Psychopharmacology (Berl). 2013;227:299–306.

391. BacoMind. www.bacomind.com. Accessed 15 June 2015.

392. KeenMind. www.keenmind.info. Accessed 15 June 2015.

393. PhamaGABA. www.natural-pharmagaba.com. Accessed 15 June 2015.

394. Weeks BS. Formulations of dietary supplement and herbal extracts for relaxation and anxiolytic action: Relarian. Med Sci Monit. 2009;15:RA256–62.
395. Abdou AM, Higashiguchi S, Horie K, Kim M, Hatta H, Yokogoshi H. Relaxation and immunity enhancement effects of gamma-aminobutyric acid (GABA). Biofactors. 2006;36:201–8.
396. Yoto A, Murao S, Motoki M, Yokoyama Y, Horie N, Takeshima K, et al. Oral intake of gamma-aminobutyric acid affects mood and activities of central nervous system during stressed condition induced by mental tasks. Amino Acids. 2012;43:1331–7.
397. Head KA, Kelly GS. Nutrients and botanicals for treatment of stress: adrenal fatigue, neurotransmitter imbalance, anxiety, and restless sleep. Altern Med Rev. 2009;14:114–40.
398. Nakamura H, Takishima T, Kometani T, Yokogoshi H. Psychological stress-reducing effect of chocolate enriched with gamma-aminobutyric acid (GABA) in human: assessment of stress using heart rate variability and salivary chromogranin A. Int J Food Sci Nutr. 2009;60 Suppl 5:106–13.
399. Mu W, Zhang T, Jiang B. An overview of biological production of L-theanine. Biotechnol Adv. 2015;33:335–42.
400. Rao TP, Ozeki M, Juneja LR. In search of a safe natural sleep aid. J Am Coll Nutr. 2015;11:1–12.
401. Camfield DA, Stough C, Farrimond J, Scholey AB. Acute effects of tea constituents L-theanine, caffeine, and epigallocatechin gallate on cognitive function and mood: a systematic review and meta-analysis. Nutr Rev. 2014;72:507–22.
402. Vuong QV, Bowyer MC, Roach PD. L-Theanine: properties, synthesis and isolation from tea. J Sci Food Agric. 2011;91:1931–9.
403. Suntheanine. www.suntheanine.com. Accessed 15 June 2015.
404. Panossian A, Wikman G, Sarris J. Rosenroot (Rhodiola rosea): traditional use, chemical composition, pharmacology and clinical efficacy. Phytomedicine. 2010;17:481–93.
405. Ishaque S, Shamseer L, Bukutu C, Vohra S. Rhodiola rosea for physical and mental fatigue: a systematic review. BMC Complement Altern Med. 2012;12:70.
406. Hung SK, Perry R, Ernst E. The effectiveness and efficacy of Rhodiola rosea L.: a systematic review of randomized clinical trials. Phytomedicine. 2011;18:235–44.
407. Bystritsky A, Kerwin L, Feusner JD. A pilot study of Rhodiola rosea (Rhodax) for generalized anxiety disorder (GAD). J Altern Complement Med. 2008;14:175–80.
408. Buchorntavakul C, Reddy KR. Review article: herbal and dietary supplement hepatotoxicity. Aliment Pharmacol Ther. 2013;37:3–17.
409. Sarris J, LaPorte E, Schweitzer I. Kava: a comprehensive review of efficacy, safety, and psychopharmacology. Aust N Z J Psychiatry. 2011;45:27–35.
410. Teschke R. Kava hepatotoxicity—a clinical review. Ann Heaptol. 2010;9:251–65.
411. Behl M, Nyska A, Chhabra RS, Travlos GS, Fomby LM, Sparrow BR, et al. Liver toxicity and carcinogenicity in F344/N rats and B6C3F1 mice exposed to Kava Kava. Food Chem Toxicol. 2011;49:2820–9.
412. Milburn DS, Myers CW. Tryptophan toxicity: a pharmacoepidemiologic review of eosinophilia-myalgia syndrome. DICP. 1991;25:1259–62.
413. Biddiss E, Knibbe TJ, McPherson A. The effectiveness aimed at reducing anxiety in health care waiting spaces: a systematic review of randomized and nonrandomized trials. Anesth Analg. 2014;119:433–48.
414. Errington-Evans N. Acupuncture for anxiety. CNS Neurosci Ther. 2012;18:277–84.
415. Boehm K, Bussing A, Ostermann T. Aromatherapy as an adjuvant treatment in cancer care—a descriptive systematic review. Afr J Tradit Complement Altern Med. 2012;9:503–18.
416. Ma Y, Olendzki BC, Wang J, Persuitte GM, Li W, Fang H, et al. Single-component versus multicomponent dietary goals for the metabolic syndrome: a randomized trial. Ann Intern Med. 2015;162:248–57.
417. Schwartz K, Chang HT, Nikolai M, Pernicone J, Rhee S, Olson K, et al. Treatment of glioma patients with ketogenic diets: report of two cases treated with an IRB-approved energy-restricted ketogenic diet protocol and review of the literature. Cancer Metab. 2015;3:3.

Chapter 8
Supplements/Diet/Other Integrative Method Vernacular and Controversies from A to Z: What is the Latest or Greatest, or Not So Great?!

Introduction

The impact of a variety of integrative medicines on breast cancer prevention, ancillary treatment, and the treatment of side effects has arguably more research accumulated compared to any other cancer. The field moves quickly and the ability to learn about the latest options that work and are worthless need to be reviewed whether they impact the consult with a patient directly or indirectly. Numerous integrative medicine terms or vernacular, along with lifestyle, diet, dietary supplement, environmental and other alternative medicine need a quick review and these can be found in this chapter and other sources [1–4].

Note: Many myths and misconceptions and integrative vernacular are already covered in the other chapters (especially Chap. 2), but included here are others that could not be addressed elsewhere in the book or simply needed more attention. There was also no need to include a table summary in this chapter versus the others because most subjects are brief overviews similar to a table format.

Acid reflux drugs and B12/magnesium and perhaps calcium and iron deficiency
Acid reflux drugs (not just proton pump inhibitors or PPI but also histamine 2 receptor antagonist or H2 blockers) could increase the risk or been associated with B12 and/or magnesium deficiency (via absorption issues) [5, 6]. And reductions in iron and calcium absorption (higher risk of bone loss and fractures) have also been reported. Chronic use of these medications in cancer patients should be generally discouraged unless there is a clear indication of need.

Adaptogens?
This is an often utilized term to describe the impact of an herbal supplement that provides a multitude of homeostatic or overall balancing effects to the body, which is apparently not due to a specific compound in the dietary supplement but all the

© Springer International Publishing Switzerland 2016   343
M.A. Moyad, *Integrative Medicine for Breast Cancer*,
DOI 10.1007/978-3-319-23422-9_8

products working synergistically together to improve the health of the body. I have found this term to be utilized in some clinical discussions with integrative medicine practitioners that cannot generally refer to positive consistent clinical research but instead redirect the discussion to inform their specific audience that the product has "adaptogenic" potential. *In reality, most of the herbal products I have researched are eventually found to have a standardized ingredient with efficacy if it works (or not)—just like a drug. For example, American and Panax ginseng were often referred to as adaptogens (almost the paradigm of the word adaptogen), but with increasing research it appears that "ginsensosides" are the active ingredients especially in the area of reducing cancer-related fatigue (CRF)* [7, 8]. For example, two phase-3-like clinical trials have found a potential benefit of ginsenoside contents of 3–5 %. Salicin appeared to be the active (standardized to 120 mg or 240 mg salicin) low-back pain relieving ingredient in willow bark extract [9], "gingerols" and other compounds in ginger for nausea [10], ….

Adult and childhood vaccines and side benefits (cardiovascular protection, cancer treatment and chronic disease prevention, herd immunity, …)
No integrative medicine appears to replace a vaccination despite some in the integrative world believing that they are "unnatural." However, it appears health care professionals could also do a better service by explaining the side benefits of some vaccines. For example, the reason that nothing replaces the flu shot is because it is designed based on the most current strains of virus that are infecting individuals around the world. It evolves and is up-to-date and no dietary supplement for the flu can do this. Second, the flu shot provides ancillary or side benefits just beginning to be appreciated, for example it appears to be reducing the risk of cardiovascular events such as heart attack and strokes [11]. And since cardiovascular disease is still the number 1 cause of death in women and men then any vaccine with that form of side benefit should receive more positive attention.

Flu and many other vaccinations do not just prevent disease but prevent the severity of disease even when infected [1]. And when receiving a vaccination such as the flu, one is conducting a selfless act via protecting more vulnerable elderly and children from being infected by life-threatening transmissible diseases. This is the concept called "Herd Immunity," which allows those that get vaccinated lower and lower disease prevalence and this also occurs for those individuals that are not vaccinated or those that were vaccinated but still highly susceptible to being infected (immune suppressed) [12, 13].

Multiple vaccines, via the pathway of preventing extreme systemic inflammatory reactions, appear to be cardioprotective. Interestingly, research on the shingles suggests it could increase the risk of a stroke, transient ischemic attack (TIA) and myocardial infarction even in younger individuals [14]. Thus, the shingles vaccine could potentially provide for cardiovascular protection. Hospitalization for pneumonia also appears to increase the risk of a cardiovascular short- and long-term cardiovascular disease (CVD) [15], and now two pneumonia vaccines are available to adults that qualify for them. Vaccines may also provide better immune regulation and surveillance and augment other treatment such as the recent tetanus toxoid injection that appeared to provide an enhanced neo-adjuvant preliminary treatment benefit in glioblastoma patients receiving immunotherapy treatment [16]. And the tetanus vaccination could be providing some protection against the risk of some autoimmune diseases (such as multiple sclerosis) [17, 18].

Andorra and dietary supplements or pills—only when really needed
What region of the world has the world's longest life expectancy right now [1, 19]?

A. Singapore
B. Okinawa
C. Australia
D. Canada

Answer: Andorra (a trick question)?!

Andorra, more officially known as "The Principality of Andorra," occupies a small area on the border between France and Spain. It is a popular destination for skiing and shopping (over 2000 shops and tax-free), but it is more. It is roughly the size of New Orleans, LA, and was established in 1278, but became a democracy in 1993 (jointly ruled by France and Spain prior to this). The only major town is the capital city known as "Andorra la Vella." Interestingly, Andorra was a poor country until after World War II when it became more of a skiing tourist spot. There are seven urbanized valleys that form separate political districts in this country, which are also known as "parishes." Andorra is not a member of the European Union, but still has an adequate relationship with it and uses the Euro. It has a population of only 82,000 and the official language is Catalan, but Spanish, French, and Portuguese are also commonly spoken here. There are many public and pristine swimming pools and gyms that are free or of low cost and used often by the young and old because regular exercise appears to be one of the secrets to longevity in this country. Andorra is located in the Pyrenees Mountains (Tour De France region) where the air is clean. A mountainous country also translates into an area replete with hiking and biking trials. The diet consists of a classic Mediterranean type fare with lean meat, red wine (even served in the hospitals), fish (trout is local and popular), vegetables, and olive oil. One of the most common winter dishes is "escudella," which is a soup of veal, chicken, potatoes, and vegetables. Socialization is another key component in this country and in the Mediterranean diet. There are leisure centers that are free in every parish of Andorra and tight family and friend connections are the rule not the exception.

Andorra also enjoys a fabulous health care service for its population, and it is not unusual for folks to have a surgery even in their 80s and even 90s. Andorra also enjoys a safe water supply, and sanitation is available to 100 % of the population in the rural and more urbanized areas. Andorra also enjoys 100 % employment and literacy, and minimal to no crime (one prison with approximately 50 inmates) which are also factors in health and longevity. Thus, stress appears to be very low in this country. Some government officials also credit the lack of long-term stress to the fact that there has been 700 years of peace in this country. Seven centuries without major conflict is unique. Yet there is also little concern about natural disasters since avalanches are the only real natural threat to life. Tourism accounts for about 80 % of the income and the banking sector is also formidable in this wealthy country. So, it is a smart, small, wealthy, and healthy country.

So, how long is the average life expectancy? It is 83.5 years, but for the women in this country it is about 85 years and for men about 81 years. Now, there is something really interesting that is often not reported in stories about this country perhaps because it puts a slight stigma of the perception of health in Andorra. *The fact is that there are still many Andorrans that smoke. Tobacco is still one of the only agricultural resources in this country. It appears to be the sum of what one does for their health compared to anything else.* The reason this is fascinating is that in many countries such as Canada and the USA smoking is associated with many bad behaviors (unhealthy diet, lack of exercise, excessive drinking, …), but not necessarily in Andorra. It is the opposite for many folks that live here. Still, this is no endorsement for smoking, just the opposite. It is argued that the male life expectancy in this country would approach that of females if more men quit smoking because less women compared to men in this country are smokers. Regardless, Andorra is number 1 so to speak in the race for more quantity and probably quality of life. Still, any country that is envied for its health can run into trouble because tourism, fast food, and other stressful and unhealthy behaviors can suddenly emerge, which is what has happened recently to Okinawa, Japan and what is also potentially threatening Andorra. So, whether or not 10 years from now this country will be number 1 in terms of longevity will be interesting. *And the last point to grasp from visiting this country and speaking with health care professionals—the use of dietary supplements (even prescription medications) does not appear to be prevalent among them, which is also apparently the case for most of the longest-lived populations. The mantra of only utilizing a pill when truly needed seems to be the rule and not the exception. Again, the foundation of longevity and quality of life revolves around simple or basic rules, which are not easy to follow and not easy to adhere to on a regular basis.*

Artificial Sweeteners (AS)—Friend or foe, or neither?

On December 10, 2013, the EFSA (European Food Safety Authority based in Parma, Italy) announced their investigation of aspartame (the artificial sweetener) and found that it was safe for human consumption [20]. "This opinion represents one of the most comprehensive risk assessments of aspartame ever undertaken" said the Chair of the EFSA's Panel Dr. Alicja Mortensen. A can of diet soda contains 180 mg of aspartame, which means an adult weighing 75 kg would need to drink more than 16 cans per day to exceed the EU acceptable daily intake level (EU level is 40 mg/kg of body weight and the US level is 50 mg/kg). Artificial sweeteners are easy targets but in reality they are not absorbed by the body and cause minimal blood sugar or insulin shifts and in the case of aspartame it consists of two amino acids (aspartic acid and phenylalanine). On the other hand, if someone believes they can consume seven diet sodas a day this type of overall lifestyle that encourages this kind of soda consumption will not be healthy. Someone that drinks too much soda also tends to have other unhealthy behaviors and a lack of good nutrition.

Artificial sweeteners (AS) are used in individuals with the common goals of losing weight, maintaining a healthy weight or reducing sugar intake. More clinical research or studies are always needed to determine the impact of these compounds on human health. Yet on a regular basis there appears a publication that promotes fear in many and rarely objective education when paraphrased for the public. For example, a series of laboratory experiments and observational data was utilized by a group of researchers to determine the impact of saccharin, sucralose, or aspartame added to the drinking water of lean 10-week-old mice [21]. Testing with antibiotics and transference of the flora were also achieved in animals. A small interventional and larger observational study of human consumption of AS was also conducted. AS mouse groups developed glucose intolerance ($p < 0.001$) and this did not occur in the mice consuming water, glucose and sucrose. Fecal transplant of the flora changes into non-AS consuming mice replicated the glucose intolerance phenotype ($p < 0.004$). Levels of glycosylated hemoglobin were significantly increased ($p < 0.002$) when comparing a subgroup of high AS consumers (40 individuals) compared to non-AS consumers (236 individuals). Researchers also followed seven healthy volunteers for a separate study where they consumed the FDA maximum acceptable daily intake of saccharin, and four of these individuals developed significantly poor glycemic response on 5–7 days after AS consumption versus days 1–4 ($p < 0.001$). AS appeared to alter friendly flora that could deter morbidity. *An acceptable daily intake of saccharin is from the FDA is 45 packets per day* [22]. And remember that saccharin was associated with the development of bladder cancer in laboratory rats in the 1970s, and since that time 30 human studies found the rat studies were not of significance (mechanism of action did not exist and/or high exposure to numerous items cause bladder cancer including vitamin C in these animals) to humans and in the year 2000 saccharin was removed from the potential carcinogen list [22, 23]. Additionally, the authors of the past observational study found glucose issues in the 40 "high-dose" AS users [21]. How high was this amount precisely, and what other unhealthy behaviors did these 40 individuals harbor? This was not answered.

At the same time I do not like the fact that AS causes changes in intestinal flora but this should not be the surprising part. The surprising part is that if these primarily animal studies are correct that in some individuals these flora changes may be associated with unhealthy changes. Yet most troubling in all of this preliminary and mostly animal based research is the hysteria this kind of story is able to generate and the deviation or distraction from real immediate health issues this stories have on society and individuals. AS alone have never shown consistent or significant clinical weight loss (just statistically significant) in individuals that switch to them except in some randomized trials there has been extremely modest or weak weight reduction, but in reality they occupy a position as part of a comprehensive weight loss regimens that allows some select individuals to lose weight [24]. In fact, arguably, one of the most comprehensive meta-analysis of AS examined 15 randomized trials and nine prospective studies and found significant reductions in weight parameters in the randomized trials, which included −0.80 kg (1.5–2 pounds) of body weight, −0.24 in BMI, and −0.83 cm (one-third of an inch) for waist circumference. Among prospective studies there were no beneficial effects except for a slight increase in BMI (+0.03) with AS [25].

B12 shot, B-vitamins (folic acid and B12) and cancer

There has been no benefit in terms of intramuscular B12 injections versus low-cost supplementation (for hematologic and neurologic responses) and no improvement demonstrated in fatigue in cancer patients (unless of course symptomatic macrocytic anemia from overt B12 deficiency) and this could save substantial health care dollars if this was implemented [26, 27].

Additionally, there has been concern that excessive dosages of supplemental high-dose B vitamins could theoretically increase the growth of some tumors including breast cancer, but it appears the more convincing data is in the area of colorectal cancer. Folate is needed for DNA synthesis and methylation, which are also important to cancer initiation and proliferation. Yet some believe that dietary folic acid and perhaps B12 are important as a cancer preventive, but once cancer occurs it could encourage cancer growth. In breast cancer currently there is some evidence from meta-analysis to suggest that dietary (not supplemental) folic acid is a breast cancer preventive in women that consume alcohol [28]. And arguably the largest review of data on 50,000 individuals from 13 randomized trials demonstrated no risk of cancer for treatment for at least 5 years of folic acid supplementation [29]. And the one trial that is receiving the most attention that for most women high-dose B-vitamin supplementation is safe is the WAFACS (Women's Antioxidant and Folic Acid Cardiovascular) study, which was a randomized, double-blind, placebo-controlled trial including over 5400 female health care professionals 40 years or older with preexisting cardiovascular disease or three or more cardiovascular disease risk factors. Participants were randomly assigned to 2.5 mg of folic acid, 50 mg of vitamin B-6, and 1 mg/day of B12 (all mega-doses of these B-vitamins) and after an average of 7.3 years there was 34 % significantly lower risk of age-related macular degeneration ($p = 0.02$), and no increased risk of cancer including breast cancer, and no impact on cardiovascular risk or mortality [30, 31]. Longer observations may be needed but at least this provides some initial comfort. What was not mentioned or seemed far more alarming in this US trial of health care professionals is that the average BMI was over 30 (obese), which should be more concerning compared to high-dose B-vitamins for health. Still, there is some preliminary evidence to suggest that in high-risk breast cancer individuals the use of folic acid supplements could increase the risk of disease or recurrence, but if this risk even exists it may be small since overall folic acid supplementation has not been correlated with overall prognosis [32–34].

Most recently, the B-PROOF (B-vitamins for the Prevention of Osteoporotic Fractures) concluded and found no overall benefit (subgroup above 80 years old showed a 73 % lower osteoporotic fracture risk) when taking 500 µg of B12 and 400 µg of folic acid in individuals with elevated homocysteine (12–50 µmol/L) for 2 years [35]. However, 63 versus 42 participants in the B-vitamin group versus placebo reported cancer diagnosis (56 % increase). The three cancers with the largest numerical cancer case difference was colorectal cancer, other gastrointestinal cancers (14 versus 5, 7 versus 1, and breast cancer 7 versus 3). The curves for cancer incidence in this trial began to separate shortly after the B-vitamins were utilized and more noticeable in elderly (greater than 80 years).

Beetroot juice

There is no known impact of beet root juice on breast cancer but it is one of the largest dietary sources of inorganic nitrate that may be converted to nitric oxide (NO) by flora, and it could improve athletic performance and slightly lower blood pressure from some clinical trials [36]. My biggest concern with this fad is the caloric content of drinking more than a cup a day. Otherwise this is interesting.

Beta-carotene supplements and lessons from the past that supplements are not always equal to dietary sources

Individual beta-carotene supplements have been found to increase the risk of lung cancer in current smokers from two past notable trials (ATBC used 20 mg and CARET used 30 mg/day) and should not even be used in patients who are former smokers based on preliminary evidence from the AREDS2 trial [37–40]. The amount in a single dose standard multivitamin is not the issue and neither is the amount in food. Only these larger amounts were associated with lung cancer risk. There has been no impact of these supplements on breast cancer (no increased or decreased risk).

A quick review here is needed for clarity. It was one of the most surprising findings in a large dietary supplements study ever recorded when in the 1990s the Alpha-Tocopherol Beta-Carotene Cancer Prevention (ATBC) trial, a randomized study of 50 mg of alpha-tocopherol and/or 20 mg of beta-carotene on over 29,000 male chronic smokers was stopped [37]. Participants receiving beta-carotene had a significant increase in the risk of lung cancer and of dying from all causes compared to placebo. Yet soon after the ATBC stopped, the Carotene and Retinol Efficacy (CARET) Trial, a randomized study of 30 mg of beta-carotene and 25,000 IU retinol for individuals with a history of smoking or asbestos exposure was also stopped for precisely the same reasons as ATBC [38]. A significant increase in lung cancer diagnoses and overall mortality occurred in the supplement versus the placebo arm. The third large prevention trial of beta-carotene, the Physicians' Health Study (PHS), did not show anything positive or negative, but PHS was not just conducted in smokers and it appears the median blood levels of beta-carotene (50 mg every other day) from supplementation were far lower in the PHS compared to the two other trials (1.2 μg/ml versus 3.0 μg/ml in ATBC and 2.1 μg/ml in CARET) [40]. In other words, researchers received a real indication that an excess of certain dietary supplements or antioxidants in certain populations could potentially increase the risk of cancer and early death. This was again a substantial change in the paradigm of thinking that really impacted present and future thoughts and beliefs and also suggested that similar to drug trials, large phase-3-like supplement trials need to have some phase I and II evidence before moving to a phase-3 trial that could be costly in dollars and in terms of morbidity and mortality without adequate preliminary evidence.

More recently, the result of one of the largest eye health studies in the world (conducted in the USA) was released. Interestingly, there was 15 mg of beta-carotene in the multivitamin type supplement that they used in this clinical trial. It was found that former smokers that took the supplement daily with the 15 mg of beta-carotene had a significantly higher risk of lung cancer (23 cases versus 11 cases) compared to those that did not take the supplement with beta-carotene [39]. This is not proof that beta-carotene in dietary supplements can increase the risk of lung cancer in former smokers, but we already know that it can do this in current and perhaps former smokers. Thus, former and current smokers need to try and eliminate beta-carotene in their dietary supplements going forward. It is not worth the risk—first do no harm. Dietary sources of beta-carotene include: carrots, sweet potatoes, spinach, collards, kale, cabbage, ... Many multivitamins have reduced their beta-carotene or eliminated it from their product but there are still many with it, so ask patients that are former and current smokers to check the dosage.

"Boosts the immune system"? No thanks!
This is a common phrase utilized to market a supplement to patients. And when approaching it superficially it does appear to make sense. Why not boost my immune system to prevent disease or fight cancer? For example, colds and the Flu are really called "cytokine diseases"—which means cytokines are protein molecules that the immune system makes when you are infected by a cold virus, and the cytokines travel to the site of the infection where they make sure an immune response occurs to the virus, but these pro-inflammatory cytokines are the reason for the symptoms you experience (not the virus itself) [1]. In other words, the body's response to the virus is what causes the symptoms. It is an over reacting immune system in a body that has never dealt with a strong virus like the flu that was part of the reason there are so many deaths from the flu. And the impact of the flu allows for other infections to take hold and cause pneumonia. *So supplements that claim they can really "enhance your immune system" or "boosts the immune system" is something that appears to make sense but does not. Clinical efficacy is what matters.* Weak or strong immune systems are just as likely to get a cold, and what is needed is better immune surveillance or modulation. Autoimmune diseases from rheumatoid arthritis to Crohn's to Celiac to Lupus to Allergies (food and otherwise) are immune systems that are "boosted." In other words, the body is being attacked by the immune system and this is why some immune boosting drugs for advanced cancer have can result in serious autoimmune toxic events (diarrhea, hepatotoxicity, colitis, renal, neurologic, ocular issues, ...) [41], but in this case (metastatic melanoma) the benefit outweighs the risk. Otherwise the risk exceeds the benefit.

Brown adipose tissue (BAT) versus white adipose tissue (WAT)
There are two types of adipose tissue that exists in the human body (BAT and WAT) [42]. WAT is the primary energy storage fat and the one correlated with inflammation and obesity. BAT is believed to be protective against weight gain and functions as an energy emitting area, which could reduce weight gain and functions as a glucose sponge (so to speak) in reducing glucose utilization from cancerous and other tissue (this last portion is a theory). Regardless one of the largest US retrospective studies included 98 cases of breast cancer with BAT (from PET CT scans, median age was 46 years) found the potential for women with advanced stages of breast cancer to have a greater survival benefit in those with more BAT.

Canola oil is evil? Olive oil is best? Ever heard of the Lyon Diet Heart Study? PREDIMED Overexcitement? Why patients and health care professionals need to always read the editorials?

It is obviously not possible to be an authority on every subject, or to be informed full-time on most issues in a discipline unless working and operating full-time in that specialty. For example, I follow the dietary supplement research daily and know the research occurring in the next 2–3 years because of the unlimited access to this field and the experts and meetings in this category of medicine. Still, after my experience and research I always check in to see what some of the real experts in the field are pondering in order to ensure my opinion is fair and balanced. It is for this reason that when one reads a major study you should be careful not to react to quickly or not read it at all, because there is always a story behind the story and one way to get an objective glimpse is to *read any editorial in the same issue of the medical journal as the groundbreaking study*. Why? The guest editorial column is usually written by the objective expert not involved in the study but still working full-time in the subject area, and this can transfer general knowledge in the field and how the study is similar or different to past research and how it may impact medical practice. *If more consumers and health care professionals read the editorial in the journal instead of the study it would provide more objectivity*. For example, when the headlining results of the NPC (Nutritional Prevention of Cancer) were published on December 25, 1996 in the Journal of the American Medical Association there seemed to be a palpable excitement because the trial suggested that selenium supplements were preventing all forms of major cancers, especially prostate cancer [43]. This ultimately led to a clinical trial (SELECT) that cost taxpayers at approximately 125+ million dollars to test this theory (which failed). If most consumers and health care professionals would have read the Editorial in the same issue only a few pages away by Dr. Colditz from Harvard (and just two pages in length) they would have learned about all the positives of this selenium study and also the many limitations in the study and made strong arguments of why one should not rush to judgment to assume selenium was working and more studies were needed [44]. He ended the editorial in the following way "For now, it is premature to change individual behavior, to market specific selenium supplements, or to modify public health recommendations based on the results of this one randomized trial." Fast forward 10–15 years later and he was 100 % correct and these supplements not only did not prevent cancer, including prostate cancer, but may actually have increased the risk of skin cancer returning in those previously treated for skin cancer, increased the risk of type 2 diabetes at the same dosage (200 µg daily), and arguably increased the risk of mortality from prostate cancer from more recent clinical data, and increase the risk of aggressive prostate cancer in those patients in the phase 3 SELECT trial already replete from dietary selenium [45–49].

Finding a credible expert that writes an objective editorial can be found from numerous sources and at times in addition to a medical journal despite journals being some of the best overall sources. When one of the largest randomized studies was published in the New England Journal of Medicine that showed such a large difference in favor of the Mediterranean diet (PREDIMED Study) over a reduced or low-fat diet [50], of course there was palpable verve. Dr. Dean Ornish (right or wrong, agree or disagree he changed the world for the better arguably by research-ing and promoting lifestyle to prevent disease long before it was proper to do so) provided a critical and primarily objective analysis [51]. In the PREDIMED study, total fat ingestion in the reduced fat group was reduced insignificantly from 39 % to 37 % (only 2 %-low-fat?), so in reality the PREDIMED Mediterranean diet with free access to extra-virgin olive oil (1 L/week) and nuts (30 g of mixed nuts per day-15 g of walnuts, 7.5 g of hazelnuts, and 7.5 g of almonds) and other changes was compared to no major dietary fat change. For example, the American Heart Association definition of low fat is less than 30 % fat and the Dr. Ornish diet is less than 10 % fat. Yet some physician experts quickly heralded this trial as evidence for why the Mediterranean diet trumps low-fat diets. This was reactionary, not objective and not a personal extensive review of the study which also contained numerous appendix data information that was evaluated by those that wrote the editorial in the journal and otherwise [51, 52]. What also appeared to be missed was the potential conflict of interest some of the primary researchers appeared to have with some companies or nutrition boards because this study was only about diet—calories intakes were not to be reduced, nor was exercise promoted.

It could also be argued that in the past had more individuals read the editorial to the once notable *Lyon Diet Heart Study, one of the first randomized trials on the Mediterranean diet, they would have realized that the researchers used a canola oil based margarine in the diet plan (not just olive oil) and it appeared to work very well* [53, 54]. The Lyon Diet Heart Study (initially published in the journal Lancet in 1994) was a randomized single blind secondary prevention trial for patients that suffered from a first myocardial infarction. Patients were randomized to the intervention/Mediterranean diet high in alpha-linolenic acid or ALA (from canola oil margarine) ($n = 302$) or control group ($n = 303$) for what was supposed to be 5 years. The ALA diet consisted of significantly less saturated fat, cholesterol, and linoleic acid but greater intakes of oleic and ALA confirmed by plasma measure-ments. Serum lipids, blood pressure and BMI continued to be similar in the two groups. After a mean of just 27 months, the trial was terminated by the Scientific and Ethics committee due to a 70 % reduction in dying from any cause primarily due to a dramatic reduction in heart disease deaths in the Mediterranean diet group. There were three cardiac deaths and five nonfatal myocardial infarctions in the intervention (ALA) group versus 16 and 17 in the control group (73 % reduction in risk from these two main endpoints, $p = 0.001$). Overall mortality was 8 in the Mediterranean diet group and 20 in the control (70 % reduction, $p = 0.02$). The conclusion of this unique randomized trial at the time was the following: "*An alpha-linolenic acid-rich Mediterranean diet seems to be more efficient than presently used diets in the secondary prevention of coronary events and death.*" The final report, published in the journal Circulation was even more surprising when follow-ing some of the participants for longer periods (almost 4 years) of time and included a 65 % reduction in cardiac deaths, 66 % reduction in deaths from all causes and a potential reduction in cancer risk in the Mediterranean canola oil ALA diet group [55, 56]. Researchers attempted to examine blood fatty acid markers from the diet that could predict prognosis and "only alpha-linolenic acid was significantly associated with an improved prognosis" and not other fatty acids [55]. This is not to advocate or imply that canola oil was the only reason for success but it appeared to be one of the primary reasons. Still, this was one of the first studies to lead to the excitement over the Mediterranean diet and olive oil, but the reason the Mediterranean diet group had such large improvements in their plant omega-3 levels is due to the fact that they and their family were given a supply of canola-rich margarine to use for the whole study (like the PREDIMED study and free olive oil or nuts). The researchers were concerned that the participants would not adhere to the diet if the only oil they could utilize were olive oil. So, they included a commercialized canola oil margarine from France (Astra-Calve, Paris, France), which again could have been one of the biggest reasons for the success of the Mediterranean diet in one of the most famous diet studies or at least Mediterranean diet studies. Interestingly, mean BMI on the last recorded visit of the study was 26.3 with the Mediterranean diet versus 26.9 with control (in more recent PREDIMED BMI was 30 and waist circumference was 100 cm—both would classify as obese) and LDL was 4.17 mmol/L (161 mg/dl) versus 4.23 (163 mg/dl), and caloric intake was −141 calories significantly less for the Mediterranean diet. Other significant differences were the following: higher fiber intakes, lower cholesterol intake, higher alpha-linolenic, and higher oleic acid with the Mediterranean diet but again it appeared only alpha-linolenic acid levels correlated with an improved prognosis. So, while "experts" still tout olive oil (with conflicts of interest) few experts appear to realize that canola oil arguably helped spur the sales of olive oil for health benefits based on this groundbreaking study where some thought the only oil used must have been olive oil. Perhaps this is why the editorial provided in the updated Lyon Diet Heart Study commented that few cardiac health care professionals at the time appeared to know about this study [55], and arguably today this statement is still true but includes many in the public that advocate for only olive oil in a Mediterranean diet as a path to success. The issue is that evidence-based medicine is suggesting that canola oil should be or should have arguably continued to be a major part of Mediterranean diet randomized trials but somehow this did not continue to occur. Canola oil is a primary product of Canada so is this some form of a Mediterranean diet country specific conspiracy? Spain for example appears to produce almost half of the world's olive oil supply. The real issue actually is the lack of reference or even deference to the Lyon Diet Heart Study, especially for all the websites that try to convince consumers that canola oil is harmful from a laboratory study or processing stand point (not a randomized trial).

Casino/Las Vegas/Lottery effect (selling probability versus select personal testimonials)

This is a common term I utilize in lectures and with patients to explain that cancer treatment is based on probability with no guarantee. Patients generally choose the treatments with the higher probability of success and clinicians are generally supposed to proffer options with higher probability or success rates. Some forms of alternative (and at times conventional) treatments focus on lower probability or a rare treatment success but do not refer to the greater research. This is tantamount to casino or lottery advertising that suggests one person has to win so why not you, and the evidence-based answer to that question is because I almost have a probability of winning that is arguably similar to the probability of not playing the game. The primary reason most humans do what they do is based on probability of an event or something they hope to achieve in making a choice, for example putting on a seatbelt to reduce the risk of receiving a ticket, injury, or death. How about stepping on an airplane, bus or train because it is rare to be in a catastrophic event in these scenarios (otherwise few individuals would utilize them). Most activities are preformed based on a probability-based event whose outcome is assumed will be achieved (not a guarantee). This is why personal testimonials are so powerful in convincing someone to do something without overt research because it distracts a patient from the fact that there is no credible research. When consulting with patients it should be mentioned how many websites promoting chelation utilize primarily testimonials but rarely high methodology research (because it does not exist). *Patients should be warned about lottery effect advertising with certain pills and procedures that could cost desperate individuals and families a fortune by certainly offering a temporary dash of hope, but with a potential pound of permanent disappointment.*

Chelation Therapy (reducing toxins? personal testimonials?)
Chelation to reduce compounds in the body that have truly been demonstrated to be harmful is one part of conventional medicine and this should be mentioned to patients; however, chelation therapy to promote cancer treatment by reducing "toxins" is another entirely separate non-evidence-based program that can be costly to susceptible cancer patients and compromise the window of opportunity for more evidence-based treatments. For example, iron overload and chelation could be utilized in myelodysplastic syndromes (or even thalassemia) and is not uncommon [57, 58], but iron overload or mercury overload chelation to treat breast cancer has no credible evidence but has a considerably personal detrimental cost. Again, chelation therapy is utilized in certain areas of cancer to reduce toxicity but it is currently not utilized to profoundly impact prognosis, especially in breast cancer. This does not imply that in the future there will be no role, but that currently it is advertised to many patients using the tactics of casino or lottery based advertising (plenty or personal testimonials and no evidence-based research).

Clinically significant versus statistically significant
Patients need to be informed about the difference between clinical significance and statistical significance. If cholesterol is statistically lowered or favorably changed with an agent but the clinical endpoints or outcomes do not change for the better then what is the point of using the treatment? For example, this is currently what niacin is suffering from in medicine [59]. Almost all clinically significant medicines (including some integrative) demonstrate statistical significance but the reverse is not always the case.

Coconut oil and water (what they have in common with chocolate and eggs)

Coconut water could be higher in potassium compared to a banana in some cases, and it is generally low in calories with some sugar, but coconut oil is different [1]. It is primarily saturated fat, which can increase your good cholesterol (HDL) but it can also increase your bad cholesterol (LDL). Coconut oil contains large amounts of the saturated fat known as "lauric acid" and this is what could also increase good cholesterol. Coconut oil could be utilized in diet after a baseline cholesterol examination to determine the eventual impact of the oil. Eggs do not cause significant increases in cholesterol as once thought. Eggs are low in calories (70–80 calories each), one of the best sources of high-quality protein (muscle support and to suppress appetite), one of the only natural sources of vitamin D, a natural source of choline that may improve brain health or memory, and is a large source of two compounds (lutein and zeaxanthin) that are being used as pills in clinical trials to potentially preserve eyesight from macular degeneration, which is one of the leading causes of vision loss in the world. And the cholesterol content of eggs continues to decrease over time thanks to more efficient farming methods. Both the egg white (main protein source, 15–20 calories) and the yellow part of the egg (choline, vitamin D, mineral, and eye health compound source) have value.

However, there are some rare situations where a few eggs a week can increase bad cholesterol or LDL. There have been only a few preliminary studies of coconut oil, for example at 30 ml a day to reduce body fat for 3 months in abdominally obese women and there was a *statistically significant waist reduction but not clinically significant (0.5 in.)* [60]. Still, coconut oil has been utilized regularly with a ketogenic diet (along with palm kernel oil) and this is the point. It appears the greatest flexibility with diet occurs in women and men that were able to achieve the goals set in Chap. 3 after normalization of LDL, glucose, blood pressure, and weight via exercise and caloric control whether or not it involves the rest of these selective items (chocolate or eggs) become less of a concern. These items should be consumed on a regular basis if desired (which is the point of this paragraph and could be utilized in patient consults) if one is able to achieve clinically significant results when dieting with them as part of a comprehensive effective program or after achieving weight loss results and then deciding to incorporate them in the diet.

Coenzyme Q10

CoQ10 arguably receives most of its attention for the potential to reduce statin-induced myalgia (SIM) or blood pressure reduction, but the data on the benefit has been mixed—not consistent [1]. Additionally, there is some indirect evidence to suggest CoQ10 could increase bleeding risk in patients on antiplatelet medicines such as aspirin and clopidogrel, but it could also harbor vitamin K like effects and could reduce the efficacy of warfarin [61]. Overall, and in large randomized trials thus far the side effects overall have been similar to placebo, but the results have been disappointing. For example, a phase 3 randomized, placebo-controlled, double-blind clinical trial known as "QE3" (Coenzyme Q10 in Early Parkinson Disease) was conducted at 67 North American sites [62]. This trial compared placebo to 1200 mg/day, or 2400 mg/day CoQ10 (all participants also received 1200 IU/day vitamin E).

The withdrawal rate was only 2.0–2.5 % among the groups and no clinical benefit was demonstrated over placebo. There were also no significant differences among groups in any laboratory parameter, vital signs or in EKG measures. Hypertension (2.6–3.5 % versus 0 %) and insomnia (3.1–6.5 % versus 3.0 %) were documented more often in the CoQ10 groups but the overall incidence was low.

CoQ10 currently holds no role in breast cancer but the data is limited. A randomized trial of 236 women with newly diagnosed breast cancer and planned adjuvant chemotherapy were randomized to 300 mg of Co10 or placebo and each group received 300 IU of vitamin E (all pills divided into three daily doses) [63]. Treatment was continued for 24 weeks and there was no difference in fatigue (the primary endpoint) or in the secondary endpoints of depression or quality of life scores. The goal of the trial was to prevent or reduce fatigue in patients and it was not able to accomplish this task. Regardless, side effects were similar to placebo. This is a costly supplement overall and unless there is future research with statins and CoQ10 (see Chap. 4) for side effect reduction there appears to be otherwise no role for CoQ10 supplementation currently in breast cancer.

Colon cleansing orally or rectally? Dietary fiber and perhaps adjunct fiber supplementation—Yes, as a prebiotic for the microbiome, but not pill dependence

Colon cleansing (high colonics or colon hydrotherapy) enema or cleansers where fluids are introduced through a tube inserted into the rectum could alter beneficial flora, perforate or injury the colon, cause hyponatremia, sepsis and become a medical emergency [64–68]. It is interesting that perforating the colon during a colonoscopy is rare but a real concern for some individuals but perforating the colon with an unregulated alternative treatment involves far more risk and has not prevented cancer or saved lives like a colonoscopy [69]. The ideal colon cleanse should be the incorporation of regular fiber intakes for overall health benefits and to establish and healthy microbiome or gut flora [1]. Fiber is arguably one of the best prebiotic sources available in medicine today, which have the ability to reduce the need for more pills such as probiotics (see Chap. 3). Dietary fiber should be the first source but supplemental options can also be helpful and now have an abundance of clinical research [70].

Cranberry dietary supplements versus cranberry juice

Increasing antibiotic resistance to multiple disease causing bugs are concerning. Other non-antibiotic options are needed as potential alternatives. Cranberry drink and supplements have garnered some interest as a potential viable option for recurrent UTIs, but longer duration trials are needed to provide more objective evaluations of supplements versus certain drugs. A double-blind trial of 221 premenopausal women that were randomized to a 12-month utilization of TMP-SMX 480 mg once daily, or 500 mg twice daily of cranberry capsules was published [71]. After 12 months the average number of participants with at least one symptomatic UTI was significantly reduced in the TMP-SMX group (1.8 versus 4.0) and the percentage of women with at least one symptomatic UTI was higher in the cranberry group (78 % versus 71 %). Median time to first UTI was 8 months on the antibiotic compared to 4 months with cranberry. Approximately 91 % of the asymptomatic specimens tested were TMP-SMX resistant after 1 month compared to 28 % with cranberry. Antibiotic resistance did not increase in the cranberry group. Thus, TMP-SMX at 480 mg/day was more effective than 500 mg twice a day of cranberry capsules to prevent recurrent UTIs in premenopausal women, but at the limitation of causing antibiotic resistance. It is concerning that the antibiotic resistance was so high in such a short period of time (1 month), and a "simultaneous increase" in resistance to other commonly used antibiotics (fluoroquinolones and amoxicillin) also occurred in this study. Antibiotics such as this one are more effective than a supplement and less costly in many cases [72], but when examining the overall risk-versus-benefit ratio some doctors will be more eager to recommend cranberry dietary supplements for some patients, especially since cranberry juice have questionable efficacy [73], and are replete with sugar and calories and arguably can increase weight gain that can also increase recurrent UTIs [3]. Additionally, cranberry supplements (a few calories per pill) have preliminarily been as effective as consuming large volumes of the juice [73]. And cranberry supplements are being studied to prevent urinary infections in patients undergoing cancer treatment [74].

Curcumin
Curcumin appears to be often embellished as a potential adjuvant treatment of cancer, and it lacks adequate clinical trial data to objectively access its potential for efficacy. Still, its potential for treating some side effects of cancer treatment is interesting and appears to have greater promise compared to the treatment of cancer itself. For example, the reduction in radiation dermatitis is preliminary but interesting [75], as is the potential for reducing arthralgia or even cognitive issues [76–79]. Arguably, more positive research in the future would provide more credibility for curcumin to be presented as a potential option for breast cancer patients with joint pain or major depressive disorder (not covered in Chap. 7), but more focused research in this area is still needed.

DIM (3,3′-diindolylmethane) or I3C or even sulforaphane? Food or cruciferous veggies—Yes. Supplements (Are you willing to contemplate and/or accept the risk of not knowing the risk long-term)? Remember beta-carotene, selenium, vitamin E, …
Indole derivatives or dietary indoles found "naturally" in foods are often touted as supplements that can prevent breast cancer. Indole-3-carbinol (I3C) is also often touted as a breast cancer supplement or in food, which is also converted to DIM, and sulforaphane (indole derived from the hydrolysis of glucosinolates) [1, 80]. *So, why not just consume more cabbage, broccoli and Brussels sprouts or just overall more cruciferous vegetables to ideally get all of these compounds from their "natural" source* and this is also where most of the positive research is derived from publications that also appear to espouse potential supplementation [80]. Other reasons cruciferous vegetables should be promoted more than the DIM supplementation (and other cruciferous supplements) is not just a cost issue, but lack of clinical research to support short- and long-term issues of supplementation. One small clinical study of 108 mg/day of DIM for just 30 days but with only 19 women (history of early stage

breast cancer) completing the trial (ten with DIM and nine with placebo) demonstrated a nonsignificant increase in the 2-OHE1/16alpha-OH1 ratio from 1.46 to 2.14 ($p = 0.059$) [81], which is tantamount to an interesting effect (since increasing this ratio could lower estrogenic stimulation of breast tissue), but it is a pilot study at best with no phase 1 or 2 or 3 data to support the clinical significance of this finding, and what happens long-term when ingesting this supplement in larger number of participants? Can it increase the risk of breast cancer, have no impact, or reduce the risk? Remember the beta-carotene or selenium information presented earlier in this chapter. All of these trials in cancer were really initiated because of early potentially positive pilot studies from food sources that turned out to be completely incorrect. A recent small study of 20 women with a BRCA1 mutation showed no impact on the 2:16 ratio mentioned earlier over 4–6 weeks with 300 mg DIM versus placebo [82]. And what about the observation that exercise can favorably impact this ratio and exercise is a more definitive risk reducing strategy for breast cancer [83]. Regardless, this ratio change is interesting but it is not a definitive marker of breast cancer risk or recurrence [84], and thus these supplements with such preliminary data such as DIM have to allow patients to address or contemplate the other potential consequence when ingesting them, which is the theoretical potential currently for it to increase, decrease or have no effect on personal risk of breast cancer when ingested long-term and is a person willing to accept that risk?

Essential oils, aromatherapy, RESPeRATE, and lipoid pneumonia
Aromatherapy essential oils could reduce stress, improve relaxation and sleep, which is why they could also assist with tension headaches for example [85, 86]. In reality it is a form of meditation or stress reducer that can have profound effects. People might not realize that one of the best selling devices for blood pressure reduction (called "RESPeRATE") is simply a device that teaches you how to breathe more slowly and deeply and relax and it helps temporarily lower blood pressure, but so do placebo comparative relaxation techniques such as soft music from some of their same clinical trials [87]. Essential oils are an interesting integrative medicine for some specific cancer treatment side effect reduction such as stress/anxiety but also there are greater risks when ingesting any of these oils orally such as the potential for lipoid pneumonia [88]. Thus, aromatherapy and topical treatments appear interesting and safer versus actual oral ingestion.

Farmed versus wild salmon (GMO is always bad?)—Why such hostility when there is enough room in the pool and other sources are desperately needed?
Ocean Farmed Salmon is not good for you? Ocean-farmed salmon has is now on a prestigious eco-friendly fish list. The Monterey Bay Aquarium Seafood Watch Program is the one many experts and food purchasing companies utilize to decide what types of fish are safe to order and consume for customers [89–91]. Verlasso® (based in Miami—sold in about 30+ states) farmed salmon from Chile has made the yellow list or a good alternative list. Up until now there were no ocean-based fish farms included on these lists.

It requires 4 pounds of wild fish to produce one pound of farmed salmon! This is because farmed fish are given feed high in omega-3 to thrive such as anchovies and ground-up herring. Now, it takes 2.5–3.5 pounds to produce a pound of salmon, so things are improving. Approximately 20 % of the world's fish catch (actually 17 %) is now used for fish oil or fishmeal. *Verlasso is a company that has now made this prestigious fish list by making some changes including using a genetically modified yeast (GMO-based) omega-3 feed instead of wild caught fish.* Verlasso is actually a ®company involved in a joint venture between AquaChile (raises the salmon) and Dupont (provides the feed). And their ratio is 1.34 (pounds of wild fish) to 1 (pound of farmed salmon), which is one of the best in the industry right now. Some fish are still needed in the feed because salmon are very selective eaters but this is good news for salmon farming because I believe Verlasso will make a lot of money from this and it will force other farmed raised salmons to keep up in order to maintain or increase profitability (similar to what is happening with fast food ingredients and improving quality or what happened to trans-fat). Salmon is now the third most consumed fish in the USA right now behind shrimp and tuna and I still prefer the taste of wild Alaskan salmon but at least some reputable farmed salmon companies. This is critical because the world supply or Alaskan supply of salmon is not large enough to handle global demand so there needs to be other sources of salmon. Perhaps this is the first of many companies that will have another option. And the nutritional profile of some of these farmed salmon do compete well with wild salmon, as do other farmed fish (such as trout), but there is always room for additional improvement from some specific farmed fish sources [92–94].

Fecal transplants and probiotics (perhaps the best example of probiotic power utilized with evidence-based medicine)

Probiotics pills sound healthy from all the advertising. What if you could transplant healthy bacteria with feces for some individuals and it would work far better than any other pill at treating or curing the issue? This is already being accomplished. Clostridium difficile (C difficile) is a bacterium infects the intestines and can cause significant recurring morbidity, and it can also be fatal. This infectious agent is also becoming more aggressive over time and even more resistant to most antibiotics. Yet currently fecal transplants (FT, also officially known as FMT or Fecal Microbiota Therapy) have a current 80–100 % cure rate, which surpasses any other therapy at the moment [95, 96]. The excitement of FT is it is low cost and addresses the reason for the issue (no antibiotic does this) and no serious side effects have been observed. Does it work like a perfect probiotic to colonize or take over an area of the intestine so the bacteria cannot reside, nor does it provide better immune surveillance or both? Researchers do not know, but they do know it is working.

Here is how FT work or are done in general [95, 96]. Donated feces from a healthy donor (feces is screened for infectious organisms) is used and homogenized and placed in the colon. There are three ways it can be given to the patient:

1. Upper gastrointestinal tract via nasogastric (NG) or nasoduodenal (ND) catheter
2. Colorectal route via colonoscopy or enema (called "retention enema")
3. Novel oral capsules or options are being created currently

Preliminary research suggests the colorectal route may be even more effective compared to the NG or ND approach. Still, all this research is preliminary and FT can take a week to set up because donors have to be screened. All donors are not only carefully reviewed but again stool tests and blood tests need to be done to make sure the donor has not been exposed to any infectious agents. This is why spouses or life partners are the ideal donors in many cases.

For example, an attention gathering randomized trial of FT was published in the New England Journal of Medicine and was completed at the University of Amsterdam and the study was stopped after interim analysis because of efficacy [96]. Patients received antibiotics (vancomycin) or basically this same regimen and then received fecal donation with a nasoduodenal tube. In the FT group 81 % had resolution of diarrhea after first treatment compared to 20–31 % in the antibiotic alone groups. There were no significant side effect differences between the groups except for mild diarrhea and abdominal cramping on the FT day. This was a small randomized study with only 16 patients in the FT group but the results were quick and noteworthy and patients were found to have "increased bacterial diversity" similar to the healthy donors and the FT.

Interestingly, the biggest barriers to more people being treated with FT (especially if they have a long history of C. difficile) were some physicians not completely understanding the research, data, or methods of this approach [95, 96]. *In many situations and surveys it was patient research and commentary that the led the doctor to begin to recommend or offer FT (a lesson for all of medicine when a patient is empowered with objective information).* This study and others demonstrate the power of healthy bacteria to occupy the intestinal tract and other research with this same concept for autoimmune disease treatment is just being initiated. This is why I am fixated with healthy diets, weight loss, fiber and other means to improve the immune health of the gut, and why probiotic supplements are interesting but need more research in many areas. My first choice is to change flora with heart healthy lifestyle changes outlined in Chap. 3, but when needed other approaches are looking interesting.

Garcinia cambogia—Here today, but where tomorrow?
One of the best and more recent studies to address this issue was a clinical trial of 2000 mg/day of garcinia cambogia extract compared to another supplement or placebo in 86 overweight subjects over 10 weeks [97]. The garcinia extract not only caused no significant weight loss or change in percent body fat but there were no effects on cholesterol compared to a placebo. So, despite a few studies suggesting profound weight loss with this supplement and some television channels and companies promoting this supplement the evidence is modest and there are some safety concerns [98, 99]. *In the meantime, there is the low-cost type 2 diabetes "natural" (from the French Lilac) generic drug known as "metformin" (see Chap. 6 for discussion and citations) that has already benefited some breast cancer patients in terms of changing metabolic parameters and it is a known heart healthy drug (first do no harm), and it is arguably of a considerably lower cost compared to any weight loss supplement including garcinia.*

So, garcinia needs more high methodology research, but whether or not this will really occur is the question.

High-dose supplements to prevent cancer recurrence (bladder cancer in this case and what can be learned for breast and other cancers)
There are few real well-done mega-dose cancer treatment studies in patients that do not have advanced cancer. In a small and randomized study from the 1990s, there was a suggestion that mega-doses of a supplement compared to a recommended daily allowance (RDA) supplement may reduce the risk of non-muscle invasive bladder cancer recurrence after BCG treatment [100]. However, a larger follow-up study was needed to confirm these preliminary findings, which to the researchers credit, occurred [101]. Patients were BCG naïve with carcinoma in situ, Ta or T1 bladder cancer were randomized to receive intravesical BCG or BCG + interferon alpha-2b, and then further randomized to receive an RDA (minimal intake) or mega-dose supplement. Each RDA tablet of vitamins contained 25 % of the recommended daily dose and patients took two tablets twice daily of either the RDA, or the mega-dose supplement. Each mega-dose tablet (again patient four tablets a day throughout the trial) contained:

- 9000 IU of vitamin A,
- 25 mg of B6,
- 500 mg of vitamin C,
- 400 IU of vitamin D3,
- 400 μg of folate,
- 100 IU of vitamin E, and
- 7.6 mg of zinc.

Induction BCG was given weekly for 6 weeks, and then at 4, 7, 13, 19, 25, and 37 months [101]. The primary endpoint was biopsy confirmed recurrence or cytology that was positive. A total of 670 patients were randomized and at 24-month median follow-up there were no significant differences between the RDA and mega-dose supplements groups. The following recurrence-free survival numbers were: BCG + RDA 63 %, BCG + mega-dose supplement 59 %, BCG + Interferon + RDA 55 %, and BCG + Interferon + mega-dose supplement 61 %. Mega-dose supplements, and/or interferon alpha-2b added to BCG did not impact time to recurrence in patients with non-muscle invasive bladder cancer. And there was a slight nonsignificant increased risk of recurrence with BCG and the mega-dose supplement.

When the first study small mega-dose study published in the 1990s in the Journal of Urology [101] it was visionary and impressive and served as an inspiration to continue to pursue integrative medicine using larger mega-doses. Mega-dose vitamins probably did reduce the risk of recurrence in my opinion from the earlier study because researchers were arguably dealing with a population of individuals with some minor and perhaps overt deficiencies in a variety of vitamins and minerals. Decades later in the USA for example patients are not generally deficient, but they appear to be over-supplemented or sufficient in most cases with antioxidants from foods, beverages, and supplements [1–3]. As I have argued throughout this book it will be difficult to truly conduct a large clinical trial of a truly deficient healthy population over a long period now and in the future. This is due to the consistent finding that clinical trials designed to supplement for nutritional deficiencies will no longer being dealing with a deficiency when the trial commences, which contaminates the ability of the trial to test the original hypothesis. And it should create some nervousness in treating any cancer, including breast cancer, with megadoses of supplements that the cancer itself could utilize for an advantage. It is for this reason I believe the greatest impact of integrative medicine in the future will be for treating side effects of treatment and not treatment itself. Currently, it is also easy to forget that apart from lung cancer, bladder cancer is second in terms of risk association with smoking-half the cases, and most major cancers have an increased risk of recurrence and mortality in those that continue to use tobacco [102–106].

Hygiene hypothesis and/or the "inflammation" buzzword
There is a well-known theory in medicine known as the "hygiene hypothesis" that was addressed in other chapters in this book, and essentially suggests that the diversity of exposure to germs (such as bacteria and fungi) when you are younger is inversely related to the risk of allergies and asthma for example [106–110]. In other words, excessive cleanliness and minimal exposure to germs as a child increases the risk of allergies because your immune system (while it is developing) is not allowed the time to be able to recognize outside friendly versus non-friendly invaders, and thus over-responds to many things that are not dangerous at a later point in life. Conversely, an individual exposed to some germs has a lower risk of allergies and asthma. Now, there is growing evidence that this theory may have at least some merit. For example, in some third world countries, individuals that live to an older age tend to have much lower rates of immune problems compared to Americans. And children growing up in farms (diverse germ exposure such as bacteria and fungi) in the USA and Europe tend to have lower risk of allergies and asthma compared to those that grew up in the same area, but were not raised on farms. A greater exposure to multiple types of germs that is measured from the house dust in the children's homes, the lower the risk of asthma from these studies. Another recent report showed that a greater attention to cleanliness for some individuals compared to others could partially explain why some adults have an increased risk or greater rates of some of these immune abnormalities. Research also suggests that certain bacteria and fungi may be more friendly and protective to the body, and when exposed to them at an early age, may actually protect a person from other germs that could increase the risk of immune problems. However, identifying which forms of germs are more protective or not is currently receiving a lot of research not just in the area of immunology but also in cancer research. The reason for this is that chronic inflammation of some tissues of the human body can increase the risk for certain cancers when that area is infected. Inflammation and immune enhancement is used to eradicate some cancers, for example, BCG against bladder cancer and the drug Yervoy® for melanoma treatment. However, there is also little doubt that something that can cause chronic inflammation in certain parts of the body can increase the risk of some cancers, for example:

- Hepatitis B or C and liver cancer
- *H. pylori* and stomach cancer
- Schistosomiasis and bladder cancer
- Acid reflux that is severe and esophageal cancer
- HPV and cervical cancer
- Inflammatory bowel disease and colon cancer

Researchers want to find ways to reduce chronic inflammation caused by some germs and find other germs that reduce it in the hope that they can solve some of the mysteries of why some individuals get certain cancers. Again, this is a lot of theory with some science but it is interesting. Another area of interest are the commercially available antibacterial soaps, for example, there is a common antimicrobial and preservative known as "triclosan" found in them that has become a concern. It was first introduced in the 1960s so that it could be used in personal care products, but now it has been added to some soaps, laundry detergents, toothpastes, deodorants, facial tissues, plastic kitchen utensils, medical devices, wound disinfection solutions, and even toys. Some researchers are recommending that triclosan be removed from the market. And recent research has found that antimicrobial soaps with triclosan provide no greater benefit beyond plain old soap and may promote antibiotic resistance. Now, there is emerging research that triclosan may have some association with allergies and asthma. For example, a recent US study examined triclosan levels in the urine and found that in some individuals younger than age 18 that they were more likely to be diagnosed with allergies and asthma with higher levels of triclosan. These results at least suggested that when the immune system is developing triclosan is not beneficial and may be harmful. Some animal studies suggest that triclosan may alter some hormone levels, so the FDA is currently working with other federal agencies to study the impact of triclosan on humans and the environment. What does this all imply for cancer? Again, rather than stocking up on immune supplements with promises allowing your body to receive a little immune workout once in a while is not such a bad thing (this can occur also with vaccine compliance). And chronic inflammation is not healthy but acute inflammation from exercise and other healthy lifestyle changes (reducing weight gain for example—a chronic inflammatory systemic state) helps to teach the body to become more fit and turns on immune protective mechanisms long-term. Thus, being exposed to germs just like accepting some temporary inflammation in life is one way to potentially reduce the risk of long-term immune and inflammatory issues. *It is for some of these same reasons new research in athletes is suggesting less body adaptability and negative health changes from exercise in those that consume large quantities of supplements because this suppresses oxidative stress, which is a trigger to help the body adapt to the health benefits of exercise itself (creating more efficient mitochondria for example)* [111].

Ketogenic diet (soft and hard versions) and low-fat … all fine to me after looking at your CT scan?
I do not believe there is only one type of anticancer diet and in fact I believe there are many different types of diet plans that if they are able to achieve heart healthy

numbers and mood improvement or preservation (as mentioned in Chap. 3) then I assume they will also be as effective as any other diet against cancer. Low carbohydrate dieting is not only still popular but really has become the basis of multiple diet plans. One extreme version of low-carbohydrate diets (LCD) is the classic "ketogenic diet," which contains a fixed ratio by weight of fat to combined protein and carbohydrate, which means most individuals simply exclude high-carbohydrate foods and increase their consumption of primarily fats and some protein [112]. This plan usually allows for 10–20 g of sugar daily and then it can be increased. In reality there are more extreme forms such as ketogenic low-carbohydrate (KLC) dieting and nonketogenic low-carbohydrate diets (NLC). For example, if allowed 1500 calories per day a KLC diet versus NLC will look like this:

- 30 g of carbohydrate daily versus 150 g
- 10 g of sugar versus 85 g
- 125 g of protein versus 115 g
- 100 g of fat versus 50 g
- 15 g of fiber versus 30 g

Basically in an average KLC about 10 % of calories comes from carbs, 30 % from protein, and 60 % from fat (some can go as high as 70–80 % fat intake). When these diets have been studied against other diets such as low fat dieting or just high protein dieting the weight loss and cardiovascular changes and loss of body fat appear to be similar, and appetite appears to be suppressed more on a KLC in some cases [113]. However, critics of low-carbohydrate dieting argue that if a study was done longer than 2 years (say 10–20 years) it would show that low-carb dieting is more detrimental to the human body and accelerate the risk of heart disease and cancer. I do agree but no one knows, but there are hints out there. The biggest problem is simply carrying too much weight or waist and there is no simple solution for every individual on how to get rid of the excess so people need to individually decide what works and what does not work for them. One of the best clinical trials conducted to test low-carbohydrate versus other types of dieting was the "POUNDS LOST" trial where participants were assigned one of four diets over 2-years [114]:

- Low-fat, average protein
- Low-fat, high protein
- High-fat, average protein
- High-fat, high protein

A subset of the patients in this study were given an imaging study after 6 months and 2 years to determine how the diets were effecting the inside of the body. *Interestingly, participants lost more fat than lean mass after consumption of all diets, and there were no differences in changes between diets when comparing abdominal or liver fat.* What does this all really mean? *It means that reduction in total calories, rather than a specific macronutrient (carb, protein, or fat) of the diet was the "most important determinant of fat loss."* In reality, there are many different diets or methods to lose weight. Coincidentally, at the time of this chapter submission the news reported for the first time in US history the number of obese are outnumbering overweight individuals in the USA [115], so multiple methods to achieve the same goal should be embraced.

Negative acute phase reactant and B6 and C, and selenium, vitamin A and D, and zinc inverse plasma correlations with CRP (but not intracellular nutrients or plasma copper or vitamin D). Iron also?

It is now known that several nutrients are reduced in the blood because of a systemic inflammatory response-known as "acute phase reactants." Therefore, lower levels of these nutrients do not always reflect a real "deficiency." One study over a decade reviewed 2217 blood samples from 1303 patients and conducted micronutrient blood screening for plasma zinc, copper, selenium, and vitamins A, B6, C, E and also vitamin D [116]. These results were then correlated with C-reactive protein concentrations (a positive acute phase reactant). Interestingly, except for only copper and vitamin E, all of the plasma nutrients levels were reduced with increasing severities of the acute inflammatory response. For example, selenium, vitamin B-6 and C decrease occurred with only minor increased CRP levels of 5–10 mg/L and then other tests also revealed interesting correlations. Thus, the real clinical understanding of plasma levels of nutrients can only be determined with adequate information on the severity of the inflammatory response. And remarkably, this research found that a dependable clinical understanding of zinc cold only occur if CRP is less than 20 mg/L, and for selenium and vitamins A and D less than 10 mg/L and for vitamin B6 and C less than 5 mg/L. Other reviews and studies are also suggesting for example that low levels of vitamin D could be consistently and strongly related to a systemic inflammatory response based on results of a meta-analysis [117]. And low levels of vitamin A and C could be inversely related to CRP levels in cancer patients (including potentially breast cancer) [118]. Yet even more fascinating is that other preliminary studies have suggested that despite the drop in plasma nutrient levels there is little to no impact on intracellular concentrations [119–121].

Iron may be the newest member of the group that is inversely associated with an inflammatory response and/or obesity in children and adults [122]. Obesity itself increases the risk of body inflammation that could independently drive down nutrient values not because intakes of these nutrients are inadequate but again because of the systemic inflammatory reaction.

"Scientifically formulated" dietary supplement? Equals no research itself?

In my experience of over 30 years I have found the words "scientifically formulated" supplement to be tantamount in some cases (not all) to a supplement that has not been researched in and of itself, but instead has added a diversity of compounds to a pill and utilized past research on each and every one of those compounds done by others (and many times for other conditions) to tout the benefits of their product that has no research. In other words, this is vernacular that always raises a red flag and should be discussed with patients. Consumers need to ask the specific question "How many studies have been done on your specific product and not the ingredient(s) in your product, but your specific product you are trying to sell me."

Snus (snuff) to quit smoking? Risk modification or "harm reduction" is better than doing nothing, but it is a controversial and flammable subject. Why?

A unique concept appears to have worked in Sweden with a product called "snus" (Swedish-type moist snuff) [123]. It has been shown that snuff and even chewing tobacco is dangerous to your health but it is less dangerous overall compared to smoking. This concept is called "*Harm reduction*" because if someone cannot quit smoking but can pick up a less risky alternative it is better than to continue smoking and I absolutely agree with this concept. However, it should be used as a last resort when everything else has been tried, and it frustrates some health "experts." Yet health care professionals and patients apply this concept daily in practice on some level by taking a cholesterol pill at a higher dosage instead of aggressively changing lifestyle to reduce the exposure to a higher dose of a drug such as cholesterol or for blood pressure or blood sugar in type-2 diabetes, and the subsequent serious risks of being on the higher dosage (for example type 2 diabetes and statins—see Chap. 4). It is better to produce or make an incremental change compared to none at all and this same philosophy should be applied to diet and lifestyle.

Soy (the healthy traditional products—edamame, protein powder, tofu, milk … not soy sauce or soy pills) is bad for breast cancer?

In one of the largest population studies of breast cancer survivors in the history of medicine, increasing soy food (not from dietary supplements) consumption up to 11 g of soy protein per day (and an increased isolflavone intake) reduced the risk of breast cancer recurrence and reduced the risk of dying from breast cancer [124]. A US California-based prospective (Life After Cancer Epidemiology Study) study concluded with somewhat similar positive soy observations [125]. Still, soy gets a lot of positive and negative news. Some think that it can prevent different diseases such as breast cancer and others think that it can abnormally change thyroid hormone levels, but the truth is a review of some traditional soy products (like soybeans, soy milk, soy protein powder, tempeh, tofu) demonstrates they contain the following healthy profile [1]:

- Low calories
- High quality protein
- Omega-3 fatty acids
- Natural vitamin E
- Low in saturated fat
- No cholesterol
- Enzymes (proteases)
- B-vitamins
- Calcium
- Fiber

However, soy also contains compounds known "plant estrogens," which are also known as "isoflavones" that look similar to estrogen, but they are so weak in potency that they rarely result in the ability to increase estrogen levels in women or men, unless you are willing to mega-dose on pills for example [1]. Still, there has always been a concern for breast cancer patients and many health care professionals that consuming soy products may increase the risk of breast cancer returning or reducing the ability of conventional medicine to treat breast cancer. This had never been adequately studied, but the idea was to be safe rather than sorry and that is completely understandable. However, then things began to change recently as some of these well-done studies were completed. For example, a study mentioned earlier of more than 5000 surgically treated breast cancer survivors in China was conducted (Shanghai Breast Cancer Survival Study) [124]. Surveys were conducted 18, 36, and 60 months after diagnosis. Women were divided into four groups based on how much soy they consumed. The low dose soy group consumed about a half of cup of soymilk a day while the high-dose group ingested about three cups a day. After 4 years, 7.4 % of those that ate the most soy died compared to 10.3 % of those that ate the least soy, and there were also somewhat similar reductions in the risk of cancer returning. In other words, there was approximately a 30–40 % reduction in risk of dying earlier or of cancer coming back. *What these results suggest is that it is probably safe for women with breast cancer to consume natural or whole food sources of soy, but this does NOT mean that soy dietary soy supplements are safe so I would not use these right now.* Some researchers believe that soy may partially work by acting somewhat like a breast cancer drug by not allowing estrogen to stimulate breast cancer cells. *The more interesting finding of the study is the reduction in risk was not just found in women with estrogen-receptor-positive breast cancer patients and tamoxifen users, but also those with estrogen-receptor-negative or more aggressive breast cancers, and in premenopausal and postmenopausal women.* Perhaps the reason dietary soy is beneficial is for the reasons I mentioned earlier that it contains so many other compounds and benefits. *However, it is also important to keep in mind that women consuming the most soy exercised more, consumed more cruciferous vegetables (broccoli, Brussels sprouts, kale, …), more fish, drank tea, used vitamin supplements, but also consumed more meat, so soy food was generally associated with a healthier lifestyle.* Meat consumption itself was not related to breast cancer survival. Additionally, in many Asian countries soy consumption starts very early in life and continuous into older age, so that the benefits may be greater from lifelong consumption and not only recent consumption of these foods [126]. And most of the positive studies have been in Asian populations where the caloric intake, obesity rates and cardiovascular rates are far lower than the USA [127, 128]. And arguably this is the real reason for the benefits, so increased soy could be a marker of healthy behavior. This is the main message I believe, that soy does not really have any magical powers, but soy tends to be associated with a diet that is low in calories and that can help some patients lose weight and keep heart healthy. In case there is curiosity—the majority Shanghai Breast Cancer Survival Study over 3270 of the 5042 participants (65 %) had a BMI of 24 or less and 5.5 % of the participants were obese [124]! Where in the USA or world can one find women or men with those numbers? Again, this reiterates the baseline characteristics of the average soy utilizer in some studies compared to others.

"Superfood" = Super embellished advertisement?
This is vernacular for a food that appears to offer a health advantage over other foods including healthy foods, but this is not supported in the literature. In the Chap. 3 on lifestyle changes is a review of varieties of fruits and vegetables and how they were no greater at reducing heart disease compared to another—only quantity to a point was relevant [1, 129]. In other words, plain vegetables and fruits without a higher antioxidant content have as much to offer as the brightly colored products in terms of health benefits (see Chap. 3). Additionally, many "superfoods" are then touted as supplements, which in many cases have no clinical evidence of serious value (story of some acai berry products and weight loss for example with the FDA and FTC) [130, 131].

Vitamin C (IV or oral)—Does not appear to treat advanced cancer but could it treat some of the side effects of advanced cancer treatment? Let's find out now!
After a review of five randomized trials ($n=322$), 12 phase I/II trials ($n=287$), six observational studies ($n=7599$), and 11 case reports ($n=267$) authors from Canada reported the following "There is no high-quality evidence to suggest that ascorbate supplementation in cancer patients either enhances the antitumor effects of chemotherapy or reduces its toxicity. Given the high financial and time costs to patients of this treatment, high quality placebo-controlled trials are needed" [132]. I have personally observed patients handled by other health care professionals and receiving IV vitamin C for decades and this previous review appears accurate but it is not my contention that it will become a form of cancer treatment soon because there is no adequate evidence that suggests it has anticancer effects, but rather it could have some potential application for treating side effects of conventional treatment for some highly selective advanced cancer patients. It is simply not known because no high methodology trial has been completed. It has not appeared to significantly harm (except it can be costly which is arguably the biggest concern) despite all the previous concerns of immediate kidney stone production from high levels of oxalate ..., which is arguably why it must move forward to a larger study for side effect reduction (fatigue, pain, ...) [133]. In the meantime, a review of benefits (questionable) and side effects (primarily cost) should be conducted with patients interested in this alternative medicine. *It should not be dismissed because for some cancer patients it is a very relevant topic today especially since some advanced cancer patients that have serious challenges with conventional cancer treatment side effects.*

Vitamin D
Although low levels (19 ng/ml or less) are associated with a more aggressive type of breast cancer (hormone negative, later stage, ...) in some studies [134], it could be that vitamin D is more a marker of health and disease activity than panacea ....Vitamin D is a misnomer because it is really a hormone since it is produced by the body and released in the blood and is involved in so many diverse body functions [1]. It keeps cells from proliferating out of control, promotes bone health, and even prevents infections by helping to produce antimicrobial products in the human body. This is part of the reason vitamin D gets so much attention in so many areas

of health. Still, I think today most patients realize that when you get as little as 15–30 min of sunlight it can activate the body's ability to make its own vitamin D. However, why would I want you to get more sunlight when the sun and ultraviolet light is a carcinogen?! Skin cancer rates continue to increase in most age groups in the USA and especially in the younger age groups. The other option is to take large doses of vitamin D to increase your blood level and although it is a quick fix it never makes sense or cents to me to solve something initially with a pill if it is not needed. So, what is left to do? Arguably the best and safest initial option is the one that receives the least attention—how about increasing your vitamin D level naturally without the sun and/or pills?

Have you ever heard the following: "If diet and exercise does not work then there is _____(insert name of a popular and well advertised cholesterol lowering drug)" [1]. These words have become so common (as they should—I agree with this approach) that most patients would never even react if the doctor used those words. Yet what is missed in this cholesterol lowering cliché is that if the world of healthcare were perfect then these words would feel just as jaded in almost every aspect of preventive medicine. What I am trying to say is whether someone is worried not just about cholesterol but about high blood pressure, blood sugar, weight loss, kidney stones, bone loss, low testosterone, erectile dysfunction (ED), female sexual dysfunction (FSD) … you name it, a doctor should say when diet and exercise does not work then there is _____(insert the drug or supplement here). So, would it seem that in countless cases you could change your health numbers "naturally" (I do not like that word as much today because I think a lot of folks today use the word natural to simply charge folks more money) with diet, exercise or other lifestyle changes and if successful you do not need a pill for that condition or side effect of treatment. And if not successful at least you know that you actually need a pill or even need a lower dose of a pill—the ultimate truth serum.

So, how do you raise vitamin D levels "naturally" before taking an individual vitamin D pill or injection? And how can you raise it without increasing sun or tanning bed exposure (the most well known way to raise vitamin D without pills), which increases skin cancer risk [1, 117, 135–138]?

1. Lose weight/waist
2. Exercise
3. Lower LDL cholesterol
4. Reduce chronic inflammation and other heart disease risk factors
5. Mental health = Vitamin D health?
6. Eat more "natural" foods with natural vitamin D
7. Eat more fortified foods with vitamin D
8. Read the new amount of vitamin D in your low-dose one pill a day maximum multivitamin
9. Be patient and it pays off (half-life of 25-OH vitamin D is formidable at least 2–3 weeks)

Weight gain is associated with lower vitamin D levels. Recent research now shows that vitamin D and its production is suppressed or reduced when body inflammation and weight increases [1, 117, 135–138]. It is for this reason that patients with more disease burden and systemic inflammation have lower levels of vitamin D compared to healthy individuals. Thus, if you can reduce chronic inflammation then you increase vitamin D blood levels. Some statin studies demonstrate in certain patients that lowering LDL cholesterol improves the ability of the body to produce its own vitamin D. So, lower your cholesterol by diet and exercise and increase your vitamin D level. If one can reduce blood pressure (if high) and stress one could increase vitamin D blood levels. Depression and decreased mental health appears to also reduce vitamin D levels from preliminary research. Fatty fish high in omega-3 are also higher in vitamin D. Additionally, mushrooms and egg yolks are also good natural sources. Just a cup of almond milk can provide 25–50 % of your daily intake of vitamin D, and flax milk contains 25 %. Many foods (not just cow's milk anymore) are being fortified with vitamin D and look for it and add it to your total intake. Most multivitamins have dramatically increased vitamin D levels so if one consumes a daily multivitamin. Remember when diet and exercise does not work there are always individual vitamin D pills!

I find it interesting that when some doctors discover a low vitamin D level they want to immediately fixit by recommending super high doses of vitamin D, which is concerning for three reasons. First, it ignores the ability of a person to raise them naturally through lifestyle changes mentioned earlier and sends the message to first solve a problem with a pill. Second, it increases the risk of toxicity such as hypercalcemia and kidney stones, although rare, by trying to rapidly increase the number using mega-doses of vitamin D. And third and most importantly it does not recognize the fact that 25-OH remains in the blood for some time before the levels can change (half life of at least 2–3 weeks but could be longer based on patient characteristics). In other words, it can take 3–6 months or more to experience lifestyle alterations vitamin D blood level.

Water (alkaline versus tap)—profit and no adequate evidence and in fact cancer can do well in an acid or alkaline environment and tap water is not only safe but has more anticancer studies than other types of water

Alkaline water or the purchase of an alkaline water system can be very costly (hundreds to thousands of dollars over the short- and long-term) and it is generally safe and arguably as healthy as tap water, and if any type of water has any ounce of anticancer activity it is tap water more than any other. However, the problem is that one of alkaline waters primary selling points (in my experience) to patients concerned about cancer (diagnosed or not) is the claim, without clinical evidence, that cancer apparently cannot survive in an alkaline environment and thrives in an acidic environment and I will explain why this cannot make sense, but believing this inaccuracy could cost a patient many cents.

Parts of the body that are more acidic—do they have a higher risk for cancer? No, and in fact the most acidic part of the body is the normal functioning stomach at an average pH of 2–3 (highly acidic) [139, 140]. And the pH of the small and large intestines are primarily alkaline or become more alkaline along the length of each separate intestinal tract (small and large). *If cancer thrives in an acidic environment, then the stomach would be the most common site where cancers would survive and thrive, and arguably the largest source of cancer deaths. However, one of the most common cancers in women and men and one of the top causes of cancer deaths in the past and present is colorectal cancer (alkaline or almost neutral pH area), while stomach cancer is a rare cause of overall cancer deaths and in fact is currently at an almost 100-year low in the USA in terms of age-adjusted cancer deaths in women and men* [141]. And with or without cancer the pH of the colon is approximately the same [139, 140], which is why testing the pH of the colon or any other part of the body directly cannot detect cancer or even establish the stage or prognosis of cancer. How about the esophagus? If acid from the stomach escapes upward and chronically touches the esophagus over time it causes long-term inflammation and changes the cells of the esophagus (metaplasia), which can increase the risk of esophageal cancer [142], but there are approximately four times as many deaths yearly from colorectal cancer compared to esophageal cancer. However, if I wanted to push the pro-alkaline anticancer agenda I would just focus on the small intestine (not the large intestine) where it is alkaline and an uncommon site of cancer and then mention acid striking the esophagus as a cancer risk factor (despite obesity and smoking also being major risk factors as with many other cancers) [141], and not mention the rest of the body, but again this would provide a skewed picture if one was not told about the entire gastrointestinal tract and overall cancer rates and deaths. *So, in reality, just using the entire gastrointestinal tract (esophagus thru colon) as an objective example—cancer can actually start, thrive and can be quite common or not common in an alkaline, neutral, or acidic environment and the gastrointestinal tract is a classic example of this observation (as is the rest of the body). And whatever the pH of any part of the mouth to the rectum (basic, neutral or acidic) it is so tightly regulated (like the rest of the internal body) and does not like to change dramatically (more on this later) or else there are serious health consequences. So, why would I want to try and change the pH of any part of the body when it functions optimally at its current pH and cancer grows in acidic or alkaline environments?*

What would happen if humans could actually change the pH of a specific area of the body with some kind of supplement or drug? Would this prevent, cause or treat cancer or other diseases? As was mentioned earlier the esophagus does not like to be exposed to a highly acidic environment, but what about medication altering pH medications? There are only a small number of pills that patients utilize regularly that can cause a dramatic alkaline pH change in a specific part of the body. For example, if someone ingests acid reflux medications (proton pump inhibitors or PPIs) chronically then it removes the ability of the stomach to produce acid and then what happens when it becomes more alkaline or even less acidic? *Long-term use of these drugs increases the risk of nutrient deficiencies, serious and in some cases life-threatening intestinal infections, pneumonia, bone loss and fractures, and there is some preliminary new evidence that suggests they could increase the risk of car-diovascular disease* [143, 144]. Thus, the human body does not like to have any of its normal functioning parts change their inherent pH dramatically unless a medical condition requires an immediate need for this to occur. For example, for a serious case of acid reflux or ulcer risk due to a bacterium (*H. pylori*) is to administer a combination drug regimen to eliminate the bacterium to reduce the risk of ulcer or gastric cancer [145]. Some "experts" tout drinking alkaline water to reduce body acidity in the gastrointestinal tract and even in the blood but obviously trying to dramatically change the pH of the gastrointestinal tract (to a more alkaline state) or any part of the body can increase the risk of numerous problems or other unintended problems. So, even if you can temporarily change the stomach pH to more basic with a highly alkaline drinking water source, pH 8.8 for example, the potential to denature critical enzymes for health could occur similar to what is observed with high potency acid reflux drugs [146]. Why would one want to do this?

What would happen if humans could change the pH of the blood or cells of the body? The blood is slightly basic between 7.35 and 7.45, and the area right outside of human cells is also slightly basic while the pH inside the cells is almost neutral to slightly acidic (pH of 6.8–7.0). And in all of these areas of the body (head-to-toe) the pH is so tightly regulated that any small shift toward more basic or more acidic milieu could result in a life-threatening emergency [147]. If the blood or cells in the body were to increase their pH (more alkaline) or reduce their pH (more acidic) significantly it would be a medical emergency. Severe body acidosis (too much acid) can cause shock and even death, but so can severe alkalosis (too alkaline), and this is why the body again does not like a shift in pH that is too high or low—it likes to be exactly where it was intended in terms of its tight pH range to maintain life and normal body functions. *It is like the thermostat of the body or a house maintaining a temperature balance or narrow range for comfort and if the barometer is not working well and allows the temperature to go too high (fever) or too low (hypothermia) then again it is a life-threatening emergency. So, why would someone want to do anything that risked changing the body pH dramatically—I would not want to do this.*

What happens when a person ingests food or beverages that vary in pH? Can that dramatically change the pH of the body?

This is virtually impossible as mentioned before because the body does not like to leave its pH or temperature comfort zone because this can be a medical emergency [147]. In fact, almost anything that one eats or drinks enters the stomach and becomes normally bathed in an acidic environment, then it is transferred to the small intestine, where it becomes slightly basic in pH, and eventually is absorbed into the blood [148, 149]. Although water is absorbed in the small and large intestine, the end result is the pH of that ingested water also becomes slightly neutral to basic because it becomes part of the fluid of the cells or the blood. So, why would I drink a fluid that is slightly basic or acidic when it just ends up changing the pH of the internal body little to nothing and it was reviewed earlier what can happen when trying to change the pH dramatically of any body part (such as the stomach with acid reflux drugs). Coffee and caffeine are slightly acidic and is being studied for its anticancer and anti-disease effects [150–152]. Most fruits and especially vegetables including the type that receive arguably the most research for cancer prevention, the cruciferous vegetables (broccoli, Brussels sprouts, cabbage, cauliflower, garden cress, ...) are basically all acidic. And this is true of many healthy foods (salmon …) so why aren't these foods associated with an increase rather than a decrease in cancer?

What about pills to prevent and treat cancer or other diseases?

Aspirin (acetylsalicylic acid) is acidic and appears to have the ability to prevent numerous cancers including colorectal cancer [153, 154]. Metformin hydrochloride (HCL) is being studied to prevent breast, prostate and many others cancers and it prevents type 2 diabetes, and diabetes itself increases the risk of cancer, but metformin HCL the drug is also slightly acidic (note also see Chap. 6 of this book) [155]. Many of the most effective drugs are neutral or slightly acidic or basic (nothing dramatic). And what about vitamin C supplements, which are arguably one of the most acidic dietary supplements ever invented—hence its other name "ascorbic acid." In fact, when health care professionals have difficulty with a less acidic stomach and need to create a temporary acidic environment to increase the digestion and absorption of another supplement or drug then vitamin C is added to that pill regimen. For example, vitamin C is recommended with iron supplements or present in most prenatal vitamins to increase the absorption of iron [156]. And what about vitamin C and cancer? Obviously it has not been linked to an increased risk of cancer, but to no change in cancer risk or a potential reduction in cancer risk [157]. So, some of the most popular supplements and/or effective drugs are slightly acidic and they do not cause or encourage cancer growth but could prevent it and may even slow its progression (in the case of aspirin and metformin for example).

Now what about the one compartment of the body that has not been discussed, which alkaline diet enthusiasts utilize as evidence—the urinary tract? Some that advocate alkaline water usage contend that this is where their water really exerts its health effects. One of the only places in the human body that has a slightly larger pH range than the rest is the urinary tract or urine itself, because it is one of the primary disposal areas of the body that needs a little more pH latitude in order to keep the whole body itself tightly pH regulated (remember the thermostat of the house example). This is a somewhat similar reason as to why humans sweat because it allows the internal body to stay tightly temperature regulated to function normally, while the urinary tract allows the internal body to stay tightly pH regulated. So, humans need some latitude (not a lot) in the urinary tract, but this also receives a lot of embellishment by some alkaline water enthusiasts. *A large pH shift in the urine is a marker for something already wrong with the human body and usually not a cause of some disease process, but a consequence of the disease process somewhere else.* Think of dirty ashtrays as the place where people dump their cigarettes pieces—the ashtrays are not the cause of the problem or cancer, but a consequence of the real carcinogen (tobacco) being used by humans. And, for example, some individuals with metabolic syndrome (higher-risk for diabetes, cardiovascular disease, cancer, …) could have a lower urinary pH as a consequence of this medical situation [158–164]. Excessive weight gain can also dramatically shift the urinary pH as can serious urinary tract infections. Otherwise, the pH of the urine is actually tightly regulated but just not as tightly regulated as the rest of the human body. A more alkaline pH favors calcium phosphate or struvite containing kidney stones for example, and more acidic urine increases the risk of uric acid or cystine stones. A normal urine pH is from approximately 5.0–8.0 and if too high (kidney failure) or too low (diabetic ketoacidosis) it can indicate a disease process or medical emergency. One of the only consistent solutions to help prevent kidney stones recurrence with almost every type of stone is to consume adequate fluids or increase fluid intake daily especially water (for urine output of 2–2.5 L/day). And most of the studies showing the ability to reduce kidney stones, including the longest randomized trial of diet to prevent recurrent kidney stones encouraged greater fluid intake or regular water (not alkaline) consumption or one with reduced calcium and sodium similar to most US tap waters [165–167]. And if greater fluid intake could result in a lower risk of any cancer, and the data is mixed, it is bladder cancer where water in one of the largest US prospective studies (Health Professionals Follow-up Study, 47,909 participants over 10 years) demonstrated a reduced risk of bladder cancer, which appeared to be primarily from municipal sources or tap water [168]. Although, the risk reduction was attenuated when participants were followed an additional 12 more years (total of 22 years), but it is still an interesting observation [169]. This is yet another one of the countless reasons I recommend plain water or tap water. If patients have a private well water source they should have it tested regularly for arsenic amounts because high levels of arsenic from these sources have been associated with an increased risk of bladder cancer [170], which is another reason to consume tap water (virtually zero or almost undetectable levels) [171].

Has there been any other interesting research on the subject? After a 1-year (equivalent to 30-years in humans) exposure to alkaline water old rats (6 or 12 weeks old) had significantly lower body weights than the control, and the authors wrote "dull and patchy fur seen in some of the test animals suggests a systemic toxic or metabolic response to alkaline drinking water" [172]. The rats with the lowest body weights from the alkaline water were the age of 6 weeks. Interestingly, in human studies severe pH alterations in children can lead to growth stunting or reduction [173]. This is not to imply that alkaline drinking water is unsafe at all, but again suggests that the human body pH is tightly regulated for a reason and anything (disease, environmental hazard, …) that chronically changes that pH could cause a health problem. Yet that was just a laboratory study. It is also interesting that a recent report of severe alkaline drinking water contamination of a town near Bonn, Germany in North Rhine-Westphalia might provide more insight [174]. The town was exposed to a concentrated sodium hydroxide solution that washed into the drinking water at a pumping station, which increased the pH of the water to 12 (highly basic). The residents that were in contact briefly with this water had an immediate toxicity (contact dermatitis over the entire body exposed to the water, gastrointestinal side effects—inflammation of mouth …), and this was immediately and fortunately recognized and resolved because otherwise it could have been a large public health problem.

It is interesting that tap water in the USA generally falls between 6.5 and 8.5, which is slightly acidic, neutral, or slightly alkaline [175], which is just like the different areas of the human body (nothing extreme). *Again, the human body needs to remain in a tight pH range to survive and function and any slight increase in acidity or alkalinity in the body signals the activation of three major lines of defense by the human body to save it from disaster, starting immediately with the blood buffers, followed soon by the respiratory system's control of carbon dioxide, and finally the kidney excretion of the excess acid or base.* Thus, whatever one eats, drinks, or ingests in terms of pills or potions, or even when a disease occurs (including cancer) it will fight to remain in a narrow pH zone to survive and thrive (not too basic and not too acidic). And it is not the acidity or alkalinity of products that prevents cancer, nor does the acidity or alkalinity of the body, but extreme pH is a consequence (along for the ride) of the disease process and not the cause of it. *Thus, spending time and money on reducing the known major cancer risk factors or those that can reduce the risk of cancer recurrence such as eliminating tobacco, reducing obesity, exercising more, improving diet, or even decreasing ultraviolet light exposure makes more sense than spending more cents and large sums of money on other methods that might sound logical at first, but when one peels back the layers of this argument there is no real proof and no real convincing argument, but only a distraction from what really matters in the fight against cancer.*

References

1. Moyad MA. The supplement handbook. New York, NY: Rodale Publishing; 2014.
2. Moyad MA. Complementary and alternative medicine for prostate and urologic diseases. New York, NY: Springer Publishing; 2013.
3. Moyad MA. Beyond hormone therapy. Updated 2nd ed. Ann Arbor, MI: Spry Publishing; 2014.
4. Moyad MA. Promoting wellness for prostate cancer patients. 4th ed. Ann Arbor, MI: Spry Publishing; 2013.
5. Lam JR, Schneider JL, Zhao W, Corley DA. Proton pump inhibitor and histamine 2 receptor antagonist use and vitamin B12 deficiency. JAMA. 2013;310:2435–42.
6. Wilhelm SM, Rjater RG, Kale-Pradhan PB. Perils and pitfalls of long-term effects of proton pump inhibitors. Expert Rev Clin Pharmacol. 2013;6:443–51.
7. Barton DL, Liu H, Dakhil SR, Linquist B, Sloan JA, Nichols CR, et al. Wisconsin ginseng (Panax quinquefolius) to improve cancer-related fatigue: a randomized, double-blind trial, N07C2. J Natl Cancer Inst. 2013;105:1230–8.
8. Barton DL, Soori GS, Bauer BA, Sloan JA, Johnson PA, Figueras C, et al. Pilot study of Panax quinquefolius (American ginseng) to improve cancer-related fatigue: a randomized, double-blind, dose-finding evaluation: NCCTG trial N03CA. Support Care Cancer. 2010;18:179–87.
9. Oltean H, Robbins C, van Tulder MW, Berman BM, Bombardier C, Gagnier JJ. Herbal medicine for low-back pain. Cochrane Database Syst Rev. 2014;12:CD004504.
10. Ryan JL, Heckler CE, Roscoe JA, Dakhil SR, Kirshner J, Flynn PJ, et al. Ginger (Zingiber officinale) reduces acute chemotherapy-induced nausea: a URCC CCOP study of 576 patients. Support Care Cancer. 2012;20:1479–89.
11. Udell JA, Zawi R, Bhatt DL, Keshtkar-Jahromi M, Gaughran F, Phrommintikul A, et al. Association between influenza vaccination and cardiovascular outcomes in high-risk patients: a meta-analysis. JAMA. 2013;310:1711–20.
12. Pollard SL, Malpica-Lianos T, Friberg IK, Fischer-Walker C, Ashraf S, Walker N. Estimating the herd immunity effect of rotavirus vaccine. Vaccine. 2015;33(32):3795–800. Epub 23 Jun 2015.
13. Rashid H, Khandaker G, Booy R. Vaccination and herd immunity: what more do we know? Curr Opin Infect Dis. 2012;25:243–9.

14. Breuer J, Pacou M, Gautier A, Brown MM. Herpes zoster as a risk factor for stroke and TIA: a retrospective cohort study in the UK. Neurology. 2014;83:e27–233.
15. Corrales-Medina VF, Alvarez KN, Weissfeld LA, Angus DC, Chirinos JA, Chang CC, Newman A, et al. Association between hospitalization for pneumonia and subsequent risk of cardiovascular disease. JAMA. 2015;313:264–74.
16. Mitchell DA, Batich KA, Gunn MD, Huang MN, Sanchez-Perez L, Nair SK, et al. Tetanus toxoid and CCL3 improve dendritic cell vaccines in mice and glioblastoma patients. Nature. 2015;519:366–9.
17. Hernan MA, Alonso A, Hernandez-Diaz S. Tetanus vaccination and risk of multiple sclerosis: a systematic review. Neurology. 2006;67:212–5.
18. Farez MF, Correale J. Immunizations and risk of multiple sclerosis: systematic review and meta-analysis. J Neurol. 2011;258:1197–206.
19. Thompson P. Why Andorrans live longer than everyone else. www.cnn.com/2009/HEALTH/04/23/andorra.life.expectancy/index.html?_s=PM:HEALTH. Accessed 15 June 2015.
20. EFSA completes full risk assessment on aspartame and concludes it is safe at current levels of exposure. www.efsa.europa.eu/en/press/news/131210.htm. Accessed 15 June 2015.
21. Suez J, Korem T, Zeevi D, Zilberman-Schapira G, Thaiss CA, Maza O, et al. Artificial sweeteners induce glucose intolerance by altering gut microbiota. Nature. 2014;514:181–6.
22. US Food and Drug Administration. Additional information about High-Intensity Sweeteners Permitted for use in Food in the United States. www.fda.gov/Food/IngredientsPackagingLabeling/FoodAdditivesIngredients/ucm397725.htm#Saccharin. Accessed 15 June 2015.
23. Weihrauch MR, Diehl V. Artificial sweeteners—do they bear a carcinogenic risk? Ann Oncol. 2004;15:1460–5.
24. Roberts JR. The paradox of artificial sweeteners in managing obesity. Curr Gastroenterol Rep. 2015,17.423.
25. Miller PE, Perez V. Low-calorie sweeteners and body weight and composition: a meta-analysis of randomized controlled trials and prospective cohort studies. Am J Clin Nutr. 2014;100:765–77.
26. Butler CC, Vidal-Alaball J, Cannings-John R, McCaddon A, Hood K, Papaioannou A, et al. Oral vitamin B12 versus intramuscular vitamin B12 for vitamin B12 deficiency: a systematic review of randomized controlled trials. Fam Pract. 2006;23:279–85.
27. Masucci L, Goeree R. Vitamin B12 intramuscular injections versus oral supplements: a budget impact analysis. Ont Health Technol Asses Ser. 2013;13:1–24.
28. Chen P, Li C, Li X, Li J, Chu R, Wang H. Higher dietary folate intake reduces the breast cancer risk: a systematic review and meta-analysis. Br J Cancer. 2014;110:2327–38.
29. Vollset SE, Clarke R, Lewington S, Ebbing M, Halsey J, Lonn E, et al., for the B-vitamin Treatment Trialists' Collaboration. Effects of folic acid supplementation on overall and site-specific cancer incidence during the randomized trials: meta-analyses of data on 50,000 individuals. Lancet 2013;381:1029–36.
30. Christen WG, Glynn RJ, Chew EY, Albert CM, Manson JE. Folic acid, pyridoxine, and cyanocobalamin combination treatment and age-related macular degeneration in women: the Women's Antioxidant and Folic Acid Cardiovascular Study. Arch Intern Med. 2009;169:335–41.
31. Zhang SM, Cook NR, Albert CM, Gaziano JM, Buring JE, Manson JE. Effect of combined folic acid, vitamin B6, and vitamin B12 on cancer risk in women: a randomized trial. JAMA. 2008;300:2012–21.
32. Kotsopoulos J, Kim YI, Narod SA. Folate and breast cancer: what about high-risk women? Cancer Causes Control. 2012;23:1405–20.
33. Deghan Manshadi S, Ishiguro L, Sohn KJ, Medline A, Renlund R, Croxford R, et al. Folic acid supplementation promotes mammary tumor progression in a rat model. PLoS One. 2014;9, e84635.
34. McEligot AJ, Ziogas A, Pfeiffer CM, Fazili Z, Anton-Culver H. The association between circulating total folate and folate vitamers with overall survival after postmenopausal breast cancer diagnosis. Nutr Cancer. 2015;67(3):442–8.

35. van Wijngaarden JP, Swart KM, Enneman AW, Dhonukshe-Rutten RA, van Dijk SC, Ham AC, et al. Effect of daily vitamin B12 and folic acid supplementation on fracture incidence in elderly individuals with an elevated plasma homocysteine concentration: B-PROOF, a randomized controlled trial. Bone Abstr. 2014;3:OC2.2.

36. Siervo M, Lara J, Ogbonmwan I, Mathers JC. Inorganic nitrate and beetroot juice supplementation reduces blood pressure in adults: a systematic review and meta-analysis. J Nutr. 2013;143:818–26.

37. Albanes D, Heinonen OP, Taylor PR, Virtamo J, Edwards BK, Rautalahti M, et al. Alpha-tocopherol and beta carotene supplements and lung cancer incidence in the alpha-tocopherol, beta-carotene cancer prevention study: effects of base-line characteristics and study compliance. J Natl Cancer Inst. 1996;88:1560–70.

38. Omenn GS, Goodman GE, Thornquist MD, Balmes J, Cullen MR, Glass A, et al. Risk factors for lung cancer and for intervention effects in CARET, the beta-carotene and retinol efficacy trial. J Natl Cancer Inst. 1996;88:1550–9.

39. Age-Related Eye Disease Study 2 Research Group. Lutein + zeaxanthin and omega-3 fatty acids for age-related macular degeneration: the Age-Related Eye Disease Study 2 (AREDS2) randomized clinical trial. JAMA. 2013;309:2005–15.

40. Duffield-Lillico AJ, Begg CB. Reflections on the landmark studies of beta-carotene supplementation. J Natl Cancer Inst. 2004;96:1729–31.

41. Quirk SK, Shure AK, Agrawal DK. Immune-mediated adverse effects of anticytotoxic T lymphocyte-associated antigen 4 antibody therapy in metastatic melanoma. Transl Res 2015, Epub ahead of print.

42. Silva OE, Warsch SM, Torres AE, Arteaga AG, Westin G, Dawar R, et al. "Fight fat with fat": the impact of brown adipose tissue (BAT) on breast cancer prognosis—a retrospective analysis. J Clin Oncol 2015;33(Suppl; abstr 1585).

43. Clark LC, Combs Jr GF, Turnbull BW, Slate EH, Chalker DK, Chow J. Effects of selenium supplementation for cancer prevention in patients with carcinoma of the skin. A randomized controlled trial. Nutritional Prevention of Cancer Study Group. JAMA. 1996;276:1957–63.

44. Colditz GA. Selenium and cancer prevention. Promising results indicate further trials required. JAMA. 1996;276:1984–5.

45. Duffield-Lillico AJ, Slate EH, Reid ME, Turnbull BW, Wilkins PA, Combs Jr GF, et al., for the Nutritional Prevention of Cancer Study Group. Selenium supplementation and secondary prevention of nonmelanoma skin cancer in a randomized trial. J Natl Cancer Inst 2003;95:1477–81.

46. Stranges S, Marshall JR, Natarajan R, Donahue RP, Trevisan M, Combs GF, et al. Effects of long-term selenium supplementation on the incidence of type 2 diabetes: a randomized trial. Ann Intern Med. 2007;147:217–23.

47. Gontero P, Marra G, Soria F, Oderda M, Zitella A, Baratta F, et al. A randomized double-blind placebo controlled phase I–II study on clinical and molecular effects of dietary supplements in men with precancerous prostatic lesions. Chemoprevention or "chemopromotion"? Prostate. 2015;75:1177–86.

48. Kenfield SA, Van Blarigan EL, DuPre N, Stampfer MJ, Giovannucci E, Chan JM. Selenium supplementation and prostate cancer mortality. J Natl Cancer Inst. 2014;107:360.

49. Kristal AR, Darke AK, Morris JS, Tangen CM, Goodman PJ, Thompson IM, et al. Baseline selenium status and effects of selenium and vitamin e supplementation on prostate cancer risk. J Natl Cancer Inst. 2014;106:djt456.

50. Estruch R, Ros E, Salas-Salvado J, Covas MI, Corella D, Aros F, et al., for the PREDIMED Study Investigators. Primary prevention of cardiovascular disease with a Mediterranean diet. N Engl J Med 2013;368:1279–90.

51. Ornish D. Does a Mediterranean diet really beat low-fat for heart health? http://www.huffingtonpost.com/dr-dean-ornish/mediterranean-diet_b_2755940.html. Accessed 15 June 2015.

52. Appel LJ, Van Horn L. Did the PREDIMED trial test a Mediterranean diet? N Engl J Med. 2013;368:1353–4.

53. de Lorgeril M, Renaud S, Mamelle N, Salen P, Martin JL, Monjaud I, et al. Mediterranean alpha-linolenic acid-rich diet in secondary prevention of coronary heart disease. Lancet. 1994;343:1454–9.
54. McKeigue P. Diets for the secondary prevention of coronary heart disease: can linolenic acid substitute for oily fish? Lancet. 1994;343:1445.
55. de Lorgeril M, Salen P, Martin JL, Monjaud I, Delaye J, Mamelle N. Mediterranean diet, traditional risk factors, and the rate of cardiovascular complications after myocardial infarction: final report of the Lyon Diet Heart Study. Circulation. 1999;99:779–85.
56. Leaf A. Dietary prevention of coronary heart disease: the Lyon Diet Heart Study. Circulation. 1999;99:733–5.
57. Temraz S, Santini V, Musallam K, Taher A. Iron overload and chelation therapy in myelodysplastic syndromes. Crit Rev Oncol Hematol. 2014;91:64–73.
58. Fisher SA, Brunskill SJ, Doree C, Chowdhury O, Gooding S, Roberts DJ. Oral deferiprone for iron chelation in people with thalassaemia. Cochrane Database Syst Rev. 2013; 21:CD004839.
59. Mani P, Rohatgi A. Niacin therapy, HDL cholesterol, and cardiovascular disease: is the HDL hypothesis defunct? Curr Atheroscler Rep. 2015;17:521.
60. Assuncao ML, Ferreira HS, dos Santos AF, Cabral Jr CR, Florencio TM. Effect of dietary coconut oil on the biochemical and anthropometric profiles of women presenting abdominal obesity. Lipids. 2009;44:593–601.
61. Wyman M, Leonard M, Morledge T. Coenzyme Q10: a therapy for hypertension and statin-induced myalgia? Clev Clin J Med. 2010;77:435–42.
62. The Parkinson Study Group QE3 Investigators. A randomized clinical trial of high-dosage coenzyme Q10 in early Parkinson Disease. JAMA Neurol. 2014;71:543–52.
63. Lesser GJ, Case D, Stark N, Williford S, Giguere J, Garino LA, et al. A randomized, double-blind, placebo-controlled study of oral coenzyme Q10 to relieve self-reported treatment-related fatigue in newly diagnosed patients with breast cancer. J Support Oncol. 2013;11:31–42.
64. No authors listed. Colon cleansing. Med Lett Drugs Ther 2009;51:39–40.
65. Ratnaraja N, Raymond N. Extensive abscesses following colonic hydrotherapy. Lancet Infect Dis. 2005;5:527.
66. Handley DV, Rieger NA, Rodda DJ. Rectal perforation from colonic administered by alternative practitioners. Med J Aust. 2004;181:575–6.
67. Tan MP, Cheong DM. Life-threatening perineal gangrene from rectal perforation following colonic hydrotherapy: a case report. Ann Acad Med Singapore. 1999;28:583–5.
68. Norlela S, Izham C, Khalid BA. Colonic irrigation-induced hyponatremia. Malays J Pathol. 2004;26:117–8.
69. Schreuders EH, Ruco A, Rabeneck L, Schoen RE, Sung JJ, Young GP, et al. Colorectal cancer screening: a global overview of existing programmes. Gut 2015, Epub ahead of print.
70. Singh B. Psyllium as therapeutic and drug delivery agent. Int J Pharm. 2007;334:1–14.
71. Beerepoot MJ, Riet GT, Nys S, van der Wall WM, de Borgie CA, et al. Cranberries vs antibiotics to prevent urinary tract infections: a randomized double-blind noninferiority trial in premenopausal women. Arch Intern Med. 2011;171:1270–8.
72. Bosmans JE, Beerepoot MA, Prins JM, ter Riet G, Geerlings SE. Cost-effectiveness of cranberries vs. antibiotics to prevent urinary tract infections in premenopausal women: a randomized clinical trial. PLoS One. 2014;9:e91939.
73. Jepson RG, Williams G, Craig JC. Cranberries for preventing urinary tract infections. Cochrane Database Syst Rev. 2012;10:CD001321.
74. Hamilton K, Bennett NC, Purdie G, Herst PM. Standardized cranberry capsules for radiation cystitis in prostate cancer patients in New Zealand: a randomized double blinded, placebo controlled pilot study. Support Care Cancer. 2015;23:95–102.
75. Ryan JL, Heckler CE, Ling M, Katz A, Williams JP, Pentland AP, et al. Curcumin for radiation dermatitis: a randomized, double-blind, placebo-controlled clinical trial of thirty breast cancer patients. Radiat Res. 2013;180:34–43.

76. Yu JJ, Pei LB, Zhang Y, Wen ZY, Yang JL. Chronic supplementation of curcumin enhances the efficacy of antidepressants in major depressive disorder: a randomized, double-blind, placebo-controlled pilot study. J Clin Psychopharmacol. 2015;35:406–10.

77. Lopresti AL, Maes M, Maker GL, Hood SD, Drummond PD. Curcumin for the treatment of major depression: a randomized, double-blind, placebo controlled study. J Affect Disord. 2014;167:368–75.

78. Madhu K, Chanda K, Saji MJ. Safety and efficacy of Curcuma longa extract in the treatment of painful knee osteoarthritis: a randomized placebo-controlled trial. Inflammopharmacology. 2013;21:129–36.

79. Pinsomsak P, Niempoog S. The efficacy of Curcuma longa L. extract as an adjuvant therapy in primary knee osteoarthritis: a randomized controlled trial. J Med Assoc Thai. 2012;95 Suppl 1:S51–8.

80. Higdon JV, Delage B, Williams DE, Dashwood RH. Cruciferous vegetables and human cancer risk: epidemiologic evidence and mechanistic basis. Pharmacol Res. 2007;55:224–36.

81. Dalessandri KM, Firestone GL, Fitch MD, Bradlow HL, Bjeldanes LF. Pilot study: effect of 3,3-diindolylmethane supplements on urinary hormone metabolites in postmenopausal women with a history of early-stage breast caner. Nutr Cancer. 2004;50:161–8.

82. Nikitina D, Llacuachaqui M, Sepkovic D, Bradlow HL, Narod SA, Kotsopoulos J. The effect of oral 3,3′-diindolylmethane supplementation on the 2:16alpha-OHE ratio in BRCA1 mutation carriers. Fam Cancer. 2015;14:281–6.

83. Bentz AT, Schneider CM, Westerlind KC. The relationship between physical activity and 2-hydroxyestrone, 16alpha-hydroxyestrone, and the 2/16 ratio in premenopausal women (United States). Cancer Causes Control. 2005;16:455–61.

84. Ursin G, London S, Yang D, Tseng CC, Pike MC, Bernstein L, et al. Urinary 2-hydroxyestrone/16alpha-hydroxyestrone ratio and family history of breast cancer in premenopausal women. Breast Cancer Res Treat. 2002;72:139–43.

85. Lillehei AS, Halcon LL. A systematic review of the effect of inhaled essential oils on sleep. J Altern Complement Med. 2014;20:441–51.

86. Kligler B, Chaudhary S. Peppermint oil. Am Fam Physician. 2007;75:1027–30.

87. Cernes R, Zimlichman R. RESPeRATE: the role of paced breathing in hypertension treatment. J Am Soc Hypertens. 2015;9:38–47.

88. Prather AD, Smith TR, Poletto DM, Tavora F, Chung JH, Nallamshetty L, et al. Aspiration-related lung diseases. J Thoracic Imaging. 2014;29:304–9.

89. Monterey Bay Aquarium Seafood Watch. http://www.seafoodwatch.org/. Accessed 15 June 2015.

90. Weise E. First ocean-farmed salmon makes eco-friendly list. http://www.usatoday.com/story/news/nation/2013/08/26/verlasso-farmed-salmon-seafood-watch/2693365/. Accessed 15 June 2015.

91. Verlasso. www.verlasso.com/. Accessed 15 June 2015.

92. Harris WS. Fish oil supplementation: evidence for health benefits. Cleve Clin J Med. 2004;71:208–10. 212, 215–8.

93. Nichols PD, Glencross B, Petrie JR, Singh SP. Readily available sources of long-chain omega-3 oils: is farmed Australian seafood a better source of the good oil than wild-caught seafood? Nutrients. 2014;6:1063–79.

94. Cladis DP, Kleiner AC, Freiser HH, Santerre CR. Fatty acid profiles of commercially available finfish fillets in the United States. Lipids. 2014;49:1005–18.

95. Senior K. Faecal transplantation for recurrent C difficile diarrhea. Lancet. 2013;13:200–1.

96. van Nood E, Vrieze A, Nieuwdorp M, Fuentes S, Zoetendal EG, de Vos WM, et al. Duodenal infusion of donor feces for recurrent Clostridium difficile. N Engl J Med. 2013;368:407–15.

97. Kim JE, Jeon SM, Park KH, Lee WS, Jeong TS, McGregor RA, et al. Does Glycine max leaves or Garcinia Cambogia promote weight-loss or lower plasma cholesterol in overweight individuals: a randomized control trial. Nutr J. 2011;10:94.

98. Kim YJ, Choi MS, Park YB, Kim SR, Lee MK, Jung UJ. Garcinia Cambogia attenuates diet-induced adiposity but exacerbates hepatic collagen accumulation and inflammation. World J Gastroenterol. 2013;19:4689–701.

99. Lopez AM, Kornegay J, Hendrickson RG. Serotonin toxicity associated with Garcinia cambogia over-the-counter supplement. J Med Toxicol. 2014;10:399–401.

100. Lamm DL, Riggs DR, Shriver JS, vanGilder PF, Rach JF, DeHaven JI. Megadose vitamins in bladder cancer: a double-blind clinical trial. J Urol. 1994;151:21–6.

101. Nepple KG, Lightfoot AJ, Rosevear HM, O'Donnell MA, Lamm DL, for the Bladder Cancer Genitourinary Oncology Study Group. Bacillus Calmette-Guerin with or without interferon alpha-2b and megadose versus recommended daily allowance vitamins during induction and maintenance intravesical treatment of nonmuscle invasive bladder cancer. J Urol 2010;184:1915–9.

102. Grossman HB, Stenzl A, Moyad MA, Droller MJ. Bladder cancer: chemoprevention, complementary approaches and budgetary considerations. Scand J Urol Nephrol Suppl. 2008; 218:213–33.

103. Vilensky D, Lawrentschuk N, Hersey K, Fleshner NE. A smoking cessation program as a resource for bladder cancer patients. Can Urol Assoc J. 2012;6(5):E167–73. Epub 1 May 2011.

104. Freedman ND, Silverman DT, Hollenbeck AR, Schatzkin A, Abnet CC. Association between smoking and risk of bladder cancer among men and women. JAMA. 2011;306:737–45.

105. Rink M, Xylinas E, Babjuk M, Hansen J, Pycha A, Comploj E, et al. Impact of smoking on outcomes of patients with a history of recurrent nonmuscle invasive bladder cancer. J Urol. 2012;188:2120–7.

106. Letasiova S, Medveova A, Sovcikova A, Dusinska M, Volkovova K, Mosolu C, et al. Bladder cancer, a review of environmental risk factors. Environ Health. 2012;11 Suppl 1:S11.

107. Ege MJ, Mayer M, Normand AC, Genuneit J, Cookson WO, Braun-Fahrlander C, et al. Exposure to environmental microorganisms and childhood asthma. N Engl J Med. 2011;364:701–9.

108. Clough S. Gender and the hygiene hypothesis. Soc Sci Med. 2011;72:486–93.

109. Rook GA, Dalgleish A. Infection, immunoregulation, and cancer. Immunol Rev. 2011; 240:141–59.

110. Clayton EM, Todd M, Dowd JB, Aiello AE, et al. The impact of bisphenol A and triclosan on immune health parameters in the U.S. population, NHANES 2003–2006. Environ Health Perspect. 2011;119:390–6.

111. Gomes EC, Silva AN, de Oliveira MR. Oxidants, antioxidants, and the beneficial roles of exercise-induced production of reactive species. Oxid Med Cell Longev. 2012;2012:756132.

112. Johnston CS, Tjonn SL, Swan PD, White A, Hutchins H, Sears B. Ketogenic low-carbohydrate diets have no metabolic advantage over nonketogenic low-carbohydrate diets. Am J Clin Nutr. 2006;83:1055–61.

113. de Souza RJ, Bray GA, Carey VJ, Hall KD, LeBoff MS, Loria CM, et al. Effects of 4 weight-loss diets differing in fat, protein, and carbohydrate on fat mass, lean mass, visceral adipose tissue, and hepatic fat: results from the POUNDS LOST trial. Am J Clin Nutr. 2012;95:614–25.

114. Johnstone AM, Horgan GW, Murison SD, Bremmer DM, Lobley GE. Effects of a high-protein ketogenic diet on hunger, appetite, and weight loss in obese men feeding ad libitum. Am J Clin Nutr. 2008;87:44–55.

115. Yang L, Colditz GA. Prevalence of overweight and obese in the United States, 2007–2012. JAMA Intern Med 2015, Epub ahead of print.

116. Duncan A, Talwar D, McMillan DC, Stefanowicz F, O'Reilly D. Quantitative data on the magnitude of the systemic inflammatory response and its effect on micronutrient status based on plasma measurements. Am J Clin Nutr. 2012;95:64–71.

117. Silva MC, Furlanetto TW. Does serum 25-hydroxyvitamin D decrease during acute-phase response? A systematic review. Nutr Res. 2015;35:91–6.

118. Mayland C, Allen KR, Degg TJ, Bennet M. Micronutrient concentrations in patients with malignant disease: effect of the inflammatory response. Ann Clin Biochem. 2004;41(Pt 2):138–41.

119. Oakes EJC, Lyon TDB, Duncan A, Gray A, Talwar D, O'Reilly DS. Acute inflammatory response does not affect erythrocyte concentrations of copper, zinc and selenium. Clin Nutr. 2008;27:115–20.

120. Vasilaki AT, Leivaditi D, Talwar D, Kinsella J, Duncan A, O'Reilly DS, et al. Assessment of vitamin E status in patients with systemic inflammatory response syndrome: plasma, plasma corrected for lipids or red blood cell measurements? Clin Chim Acta. 2009;409:41–5.

121. Vasilaki AT, McMillan DC, Kinsella J, Duncan A, O'Reilly DS, Talwar D. Relation between riboflavin, flavin mononucleotide and flavin adenine dinucleotide concentrations in plasma and red cells in patients with critical illness. Clin Chim Acta. 2010;411(21–22):1750–5.

122. Cepeda-Lopez AC, Osendarp SJ, Meise-Boonstra A, Aeberli I, Gonzalez-Salazar F, Feskens E, et al. Sharply higher rates of iron deficiency in obese Mexican women and children are predicted by obesity-related inflammation rather than by differences in dietary iron intake. Am J Clin Nutr. 2011;93:975–83.

123. Gartner CE, Hall WD, Vos T, Bertram MY, Wallace AL, Lim SS. Assessment of Swedish snus for tobacco harm reduction. Lancet. 2007;369:2010–4.

124. Shu XO, Zheng Y, Cai H, Hu K, Chen Z, Zheng W, et al. Soy food intake and breast cancer survival. JAMA. 2009;302:2437–43.

125. Guha N, Kwan ML, Quesenberry Jr CP, Weitzen EK, Castillo AL, Caan BJ. Soy isoflavones and risk of cancer recurrence in a cohort of breast cancer survivors: the Life After Cancer Epidemiology Study. Breast Cancer Res Treat. 2009;118:395–405.

126. Hilakivi-Clarke L, Andrade JE, Helferich W. Is soy consumption good or bad for the breast? J Nutr. 2010;140:2326S–34.

127. Dong JY, Qin LQ. Soy isoflavones consumption and risk of breast cancer incidence or recurrence: a meta-analysis of prospective studies. Breast Cancer Res Treat. 2011;125:315–23.

128. Xie Q, Chen ML, Qin Y, Zhang QY, Xu HX, Zhou Y, et al. Isoflavone consumption and risk of breast cancer: a dose-response meta-analysis of observational studies. Asia Pac J Clin Nutr. 2013;22:118–27.

129. Bhupathiraju SN, Wedick NM, Pan A, Manson JE, Rexrode KM, Willett WC, et al. Quantity and variety in fruit and vegetable intake and risk of coronary heart disease. Am J Clin Nutr. 2013;98:1514–23.

130. Fake News Sites Promote Acai Supplements. www.consumer.ftc.gov/articles/0299-fake-news-sites-promote-acai-supplements. Accessed 30 June 2015.

131. Public Notification: "Acai Berry Soft Gel ABC" Contains Undeclared Drug Ingredient. www.fda.gov/Drugs/ResourcesForYou/Consumers/BuyingUsingMedicineSafely/MedicationHealthFraud/ucm276098.htm. Accessed 30 June 2015.

132. Jacobs C, Hutton B, Ng T, Shorr R, Clemons M. Is there a role for oral or intravenous ascorbate (vitamin C) in treating patients with cancer? A systematic review. Oncologist. 2015;20:210–23.

133. Carr AC, Vissers MC, Cook JS. The effect of intravenous vitamin C on cancer- and chemotherapy-related fatigue and quality of life. Front Oncol. 2014;4:283.

134. Peppone LJ, Tejani MA, Mustian KM, Janelsins MC, Kamen CS, Mohile SG, et al. Prognostic characteristics of 492 newly diagnosed breast cancer patients by serum vitamin D levels. J Clin Oncol 2015;33(Suppl; abstr e12619).

135. Moyad MA. Vitamin D: a rapid review. Dermatol Nurs. 2009;21:25–30.

136. Datta S, Pal M, De A. The dependency of vitamin d status on anthropometric data. Malays J Med Sci. 2014;21:54–61.

137. Jones KS, Assar S, Vanderschueren D, Bouillon R, Prentice A, Schoenmakers I. Predictors of 25(OH)D half-life and plasma 25(OH)D concentrations in the Gambia and the UK. Osteoporos Int. 2015;26:1137–46.

138. Sathyapaian T, Shepherd J, Arnett C, Coady AM, Kilpatrick ES, Atkin SL. Atorvastatin increases 25-hydroxy vitamin D concentrations in patients with polycystic ovary syndrome. Clin Chem. 2010;56:1696–700.
139. McDougall CJ, Wong R, Scudera P, Lesser M, DeCosse JJ. Colonic mucosal pH in humans. Dig Dis Sci. 1993;38:542–5.
140. Fallingborg J. Intraluminal pH of the human gastrointestinal tract. Dan Med Bull. 1999;46:183–96.
141. American Cancer Society. www.cancer.org/acs/groups/content/@editorial/documents/document/acspc-044552.pdf. Accessed 15 June 2015.
142. Runge TM, Abrams JA, Shaheen NJ. Epidemiology of Barrett's esophagus and esophageal adenocarcinoma. Gastroenterol Clin North Am. 2015;44:203–31.
143. Fashner J, Gitu AC. Common gastrointestinal symptoms: risks of long-term proton pump inhibitor therapy. FP Essent. 2013;413:29–39.
144. Shah NH, LePendu P, Bauer-Mehren A, Ghebremariam YT, Iyer SV, Marcus J, et al. Proton pump inhibitor usage and the risk of myocardial infarction. PLoS One. 2015;10:e0124653.
145. Yang JC, Lu CW, Lin CJ. Treatment of Helicobacter pylori infection: current status and future concepts. World J Gastroenterol. 2014;20:5283–93.
146. Koufman JA, Johnston N. Potential benefits of pH 8.8 alkaline drinking water as an adjunct in the treatment of reflux disease. Ann Otol Rhinol Laryngol. 2012;121:431–4.
147. Ayers P, Dixon C. Simple acid-base tutorial. JPEN J Parenter Enteral Nutr. 2012;36:18–23.
148. Barrett KE. Water and electrolyte absorption and secretion. In: Barrett KE, editor. Gastrointestinal physiology. New York: McGraw-Hill; 2006. Chapter 5. http://www.accessmedicine.com/content.aspx?aID=2307040. Accessed 1 Mar June 2015.
149. Fenton TR, Tough SC, Lyon AW, Eliasziw M, Hanley DA. Causal assessment of dietary acid load and bone disease: a systematic review and meta-analysis applying Hill's epidemiologic criteria for causality. Nutr J. 2011;10:41.
150. pH values of common foods and ingredients. https://foodsafety.wisc.edu/business_food/files/Approximate_pH.pdf. Accessed 15 June 2015.
151. Crippa A, Discacciati A, Larsson SC, Wolk A, Orsini N. Coffee consumption and mortality from all causes, cardiovascular disease, and cancer: a dose-response meta-analysis. Am J Epidemiol. 2014;180:763–5.
152. Tse G, Eslick GD. Cruciferous vegetables and risk of colorectal neoplasms: a systematic review and meta-analysis. Nutr Cancer. 2014;66:128–39.
153. Dotevall G, Ekenved G. The absorption of acetylsalicylic acid from the stomach in relation to intragastric pH. Scand J Gastroenterol. 1976;11:801–5.
154. Usman MW, Luo F, Cheng H, Zhao JJ, Liu P. Chemopreventive effects of aspirin at a glance. Biochim Biophys Acta. 1855;2015:254–63.
155. Graham GG, Punt J, Arora M, Day RO, Doogue MP, Duong JK, et al. Clinical pharmacokinetics of metformin. Clin Pharmacokinet. 2011;50:81–98.
156. Atanassova BD, Tzatchev KN. Ascorbic acid—important for iron metabolism. Folia Med (Plovdiv). 2008;50:11–6.
157. Wang L, Sesso HD, Glynn RJ, Christen WG, Bubes V, Manson JE, et al. Vitamin E and C supplementation and risk of cancer in men: posttrial follow-up in the Physicians' Health Study II randomized trial. Am J Clin Nutr. 2014;100:915–23.
158. Nakanishi N, Fukui M, Tanaka M, Toda H, Imai S, Yamazaki M, et al. Low urine pH is a predictor of chronic kidney disease. Kidney Blood Press Res. 2012;35(2):77–81.
159. Najeeb Q, Masood I, Bhaskar N, Kaur H, Singh J, Pandey R, et al. Effect of BMI and urinary pH on urolithiasis and it composition. Saudi J Kidney Transpl. 2012;24:60–6.
160. Hara S, Tsuji H, Ohmoto Y, Amakawa K, Hsieh SD, Arase Y, et al. High serum uric acid level and low urine pH as predictors of metabolic syndrome: a retrospective cohort study in a Japanese urban population. Metabolism. 2012;61:281–8.
161. Curhan GC, Willett WC, Rimm EB, Stampfer MJ. A prospective study of dietary calcium and other nutrients and the risk of symptomatic kidney stones. N Engl J Med. 1993;328:833–8.

162. Wagner CA, Mohebbi N. Urinary pH and stone formation. J Nephrol. 2010;23 Suppl 16:S165–9.
163. Frassetto L, Kohlstadt I. Treatment and prevention of kidney stones: an update. Am Fam Physician. 2011;84:1234–42.
164. Heilberg IP, Goldfarb DS. Optimum nutrition for kidney stone disease. Adv Chronic Kidney Dis. 2013;20:165–74.
165. Borghi L, Meschi T, Amato F, Briganti A, Novarini A, Giannini A. Urinary volume, water and recurrences of idiopathic calcium nephrolithiasis: a 5-year randomized prospective study. J Urol. 1996;155:839–43.
166. Azoulay A, Garzon P, Eisenberg MJ. Comparison of the mineral content of tap water and bottle waters. J Gen Intern Med. 2001;16:168–75.
167. Cheungpasitporn W, Rossetti S, Friend K, Erickson SB, Lieske JC. Treatment effect, adherence, and safety of high fluid intake for the prevention of incident and recurrent kidney stones: a systematic review and meta-analysis. J Nephrol 2015, Epub ahead of print.
168. Michaud DS, Spiegelman D, Clinton SK, Rimm EB, Curhan GC, Willett WC, et al. Fluid intake and the risk of bladder cancer in men. N Engl J Med. 1999;340:1390–7.
169. Zhou J, Smith S, Giovanucci E, Michaud DS. Reexamination of total fluid intake and bladder cancer in the Health Professionals Follow-up Study Cohort. Am J Epidemiol. 2012;175:696–705.
170. Malats N, Real FX. Epidemiology of bladder cancer. Hematol Oncol Clin North Am. 2015;29:177–89.
171. United States Environmental Protection Agency. Basic information about arsenic in drinking water. http://water.epa.gov/drink/contaminants/basicinformation/arsenic.cfm. Accessed 15 June 2015.
172. Merne ME, Syrjanen KJ, Syrjanen SM. Systemic and local effects of long-term exposure to alkaline drinking water in rats. Int J Exp Pathol. 2001;82:213–9.
173. Chan JC. Acid-base disorders and the kidney. Adv Pediatr. 1983;30:401–71.
174. Lendowski L, Farber H, Holy A, Darius A, Ehrich B, Wippermann C, et al. Accidental contamination of a German town's drinking water with sodium hydroxide. Int J Hyg Environ Health. 2015;218:366–9.
175. United States Environmental Protection Agency. http://safewater.supportportal.com/link/portal/23002/23015/Article/22806/What-is-the-federal-standard-for-pH-in-drinking-water. Accessed 15 June 2015.

Index

© Springer International Publishing Switzerland 2016
M.A. Moyad, *Integrative Medicine for Breast Cancer*,
DOI 10.1007/978-3-319-23422-9

Printed in the United States
By Bookmasters